PLASTIC SURGERY

Editor
JOSEPH G. McCARTHY, M.D.
Lawrence D. Bell Professor of Plastic Surgery and
Director of the Institute of Reconstructive Plastic Surgery
New York University Medical Center
New York, New York

Editors, Hand Surgery Volumes
JAMES W. MAY, JR., M.D.
Director of Plastic Surgery and Hand Surgery Service
Massachusetts General Hospital
Associate Clinical Professor of Surgery
Harvard Medical School
Boston, Massachusetts

J. WILLIAM LITTLER, M.D.
Past Professor of Clinical Surgery
College of Physicians and Surgeons
Columbia University, New York
Senior Attending Surgeon
The St. Luke's–Roosevelt Hospital Center
New York, New York

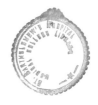

PLASTIC SURGERY

VOLUME 6
THE TRUNK
AND
LOWER EXTREMITY

1990
W.B. SAUNDERS COMPANY
Harcourt Brace Jovanovich, Inc.
Philadelphia ▪ London ▪ Toronto
Montreal ▪ Sydney ▪ Tokyo

W. B. SAUNDERS COMPANY
Harcourt Brace Jovanovich, Inc.

The Curtis Center
Independence Square West
Philadelphia, PA 19106

Library of Congress Cataloging-in-Publication Data

Plastic surgery.
    Contents: v. 1. General principles—v. 2–3.
The face—v. 4. Cleft lip & palate and craniofacial
anomalies—[etc.]
    1. Surgery, Plastic.   I. McCarthy, Joseph G., 1938–
[DNLM: 1. Surgery, Plastic. WO 600 P7122]

RD118.P536   1990   617′.95   87–9809

ISBN 0–7216–1514–7   (set)

25/7/94

Editor: W. B. Saunders Staff
Designer: W. B. Saunders Staff
Production Manager: Frank Polizzano
Manuscript Editor: David Harvey
Illustration Coordinator: Lisa Lambert
Indexer: Kathleen Garcia
Cover Designer: Ellen Bodner

Volume 1 0–7216–2542–8
Volume 2 0–7216–2543–6
Volume 3 0–7216–2544–4
Volume 4 0–7216–2545–2
Volume 5 0–7216–2546–0
Volume 6 0–7216–2547–9
Volume 7 0–7216–2548–7
Volume 8 0–7216–2549–5
8 Volume Set 0–7216–1514–7

Plastic Surgery

Printed in the United States of America.

Last digit is the print number: 9   8   7   6   5   4   3   2   1

Contributors

SHERRELL J. ASTON, M.D.
Associate Professor of Surgery (Plastic Surgery), New York University School of Medicine; Attending Surgeon, University Hospital and Manhattan Eye, Ear & Throat Hospital, New York, New York.

JOHN BOSTWICK III, M.D.
Professor of Surgery, Emory University School of Medicine; Chief of Plastic Surgery, Emory University Hospital, Atlanta, Georgia.

LEO CLODIUS, M.D.
Docent for Plastic Surgery, Zurich University Medical School; Visiting Surgeon, American Medical International Hospital, Zurich, Switzerland.

STEPHEN R. COLEN, M.D., D.D.S.
Assistant Professor of Surgery (Plastic Surgery), New York University School of Medicine; Attending Surgeon, University Hospital, Bellevue Hospital Center, Manhattan Eye, Ear & Throat Hospital, and New York Eye & Ear Infirmary, New York, New York.

CHARLES J. DEVINE, JR., M.D.
Professor of Urology, The Eastern Virginia Medical School of the Medical College of Hampton Roads, Norfolk, Virginia.

GREGORY S. GEORGIADE, M.D.
Associate Professor of Surgery, Division of Plastic, Maxillofacial and Reconstructive Surgery, Duke University School of Medicine, Durham, North Carolina.

NICHOLAS G. GEORGIADE, M.D.
Professor of Surgery, Division of Plastic, Maxillofacial and Reconstructive Surgery, Duke University School of Medicine, Durham, North Carolina.

FREDERICK M. GRAZER, M.D.
Associate Clinical Professor, Division of Plastic Surgery, University of California, Irvine, School of Medicine; Clinical Associate Professor in Plastic and Reconstructive Surgery, Pennsylvania State University School of Medicine; Chairman, Baromedical Committee, Hoag Memorial Hospital Presbyterian, Newport Beach, California.

JAMES C. GROTTING, M.D., F.A.C.S.
Associate Professor of Surgery, Division of Plastic Surgery, University of Alabama Medical School, Birmingham, Alabama.

CHARLES E. HORTON, M.D.
Professor of Plastic Surgery, The Eastern Virginia Medical School of the Medical College of Hampton Roads, Norfolk, Virginia.

CHARLES E. HORTON, JR., M.D.
Fellow in Urology, Harvard School of Medicine, Boston, Massachusetts.

GERALD H. JORDAN, M.D.
Assistant Professor of Urology, The Eastern Virginia Medical School of the Medical College of Hampton Roads, Norfolk, Virginia.

JOHN B. McCRAW, M.D.
Professor of Plastic Surgery, The Eastern Virginia Medical School of the Medical College of Hampton Roads, Norfolk, Virginia.

RONALD RIEFKOHL, M.D.
Associate Professor of Surgery, Division of Plastic, Maxillofacial and Reconstructive Surgery, Duke University School of Medicine, Durham, North Carolina.

RICHARD C. SADOVE, M.D.
Assistant Professor of Plastic Surgery, University of Kentucky Medical Center, Lexington, Kentucky.

PAUL F. SAUER, M.D.
Assistant Professor, Department of Plastic Surgery, Medical College of Virginia, Richmond, Virginia.

WILLIAM W. SHAW, M.D.
Associate Professor of Surgery (Plastic Surgery), New York University School of Medicine; Attending Surgeon, Institute of Reconstructive Plastic Surgery, New York University Medical Center; Chief, Plastic Surgery, Bellevue Hospital, New York, New York.

JOHN W. SIEBERT, M.D.
Assistant Professor of Surgery, New York University Medical Center; Chief of Plastic Surgery, Bellevue Hospital, New York; Director of Microsurgery, New York University Medical Center and Bellevue Hospital, New York, New York.

MICHAEL R. SPINDEL, M.D.
Fellow, Reconstructive Urology, The Eastern Virginia Medical School of the Medical College of Hampton Roads, Norfolk, Virginia.

JOHN F. STECKER, M.D.
Professor of Urology, The Eastern Virginia Medical School of the Medical College of Hampton Roads, Norfolk, Virginia.

CHARLES H. M. THORNE, M.D.
Assistant Professor of Surgery (Plastic Surgery), New York University School of Medicine; Attending Surgeon, Manhattan Eye, Ear & Throat Hospital, University Hospital, Bellevue Hospital, and Manhattan Veterans Administration Hospital, New York, New York.

LUIS O. VASCONEZ, M.D.
Professor and Chief, Division of Plastic Surgery, University of Alabama at Birmingham, Birmingham, Alabama.

BARRY M. ZIDE, D.M.D., M.D.
Assistant Professor of Surgery (Plastic Surgery), New York University Medical Center; Attending Surgeon, Bellevue Hospital Center, Manhattan Veterans Administration Hospital, and Manhattan Eye, Ear & Throat Hospital, New York, New York.

Contents

87

88

PLASTIC SURGERY

76

William W. Shaw
Sherrel J. Aston
Barry M. Zide

Reconstruction of the Trunk

CHEST WALL RECONSTRUCTION

The earliest surgical experiences with the chest wall were necessitated by penetrating chest injuries resulting from wars and accidents. While these injuries were considered generally hopeless, the surgical dilemma was whether or not to close them. Hewson and later Larrey, Napoleon's military surgeon, were credited with the practice of closing sucking chest wounds to prevent death from respiratory failure (Meade, 1961). Larrey astutely observed the importance of drainage in order to allow retained blood and other material to egress from the wound. During the American Civil War, Billings also adopted the practice of early closure and noted the improved survival rate. Many patients, however, suffered late chronic empyema cavities as a result of retained contaminated hematomas (Seyfer, Graeber and Wind, 1986). By World War I, the practice of early closure was adopted by all allied medical services. The not infrequent occurrence of empyema was treated by aggressive and repeated thoracentesis and, if needed, eventual conversion to an open empyema cavity.

Around the turn of the century, with the introduction of general anesthesia, more aggressive surgery became possible. Surgeons began to resect tumors of the chest wall. Initially, when such surgery was attempted, every effort was made to avoid entering the pleura to avoid the potentially fatal situation of an open pneumothorax. In fact, many ingenious methods were devised to avoid collapse of the lungs at the time of resection by preliminary procedures to create adhesions between the lung and rib cage (Seyfer, Graeber, and Wind, 1986).

Parham (1899) described two patients who underwent chest wall tumor resection. In the first patient he mobilized surrounding soft tissue to close a sucking surgical wound and saved the patient. In the second patient with inadvertent pleural rent and lung collapse, he employed a crude form of endotracheal tube to stabilize ventilation. This allowed him to close the wound in layers by soft tissue mobilization. He was thus credited for introducing positive pressure ventilation in surgery by using a respirator device originally described by Fell for physiologic experiments in dogs and the laryngeal endotracheal tube devised by Odwyer. In the ensuing decades, as the experience with pneumonectomy for the treatment of tuberculosis and lung cancer became more common, the basic principles of chest surgery using endotracheal ventilation, closed drainage and antibiotics became established. In World War II, with the increased firepower of the weapons resulting in more massive chest injuries, a manual for thoracic surgery was published in 1943 by the U.S. Government (Graham and associates, 1943; Ahnfeldt and Berry, 1963, 1965) and the concepts of surgical debridement and tension free soft tissue closure were emphasized. Numerous methods of closure were described, including the use of adjacent muscles such as the pectoralis major.

During the Korean and the Vietnam wars, with the improved survival from more rapid evacuation and resuscitation for shock, many more soldiers survived the initial injuries to become candidates for chest wall reconstruction. Radiation therapy to the chest wall became popular for various tumors, and not infrequently the resultant ulceration or necrosis became reasons for elaborate and multi-staged reconstructions. Recognizing the importance of maintaining semirigid support of the chest wall, surgeons introduced fascia and other synthetic materials for providing support. In addition, a number of local skin flaps, such as the deltopectoral flap, or distant transfers were introduced (Seyfer, Graeber, and Wind, 1986).

In the mid-1970's the use of muscle and musculocutaneous flaps was rediscovered and popularized. The availability of the latissimus dorsi, pectoralis major, and rectus abdominis muscle flaps greatly expanded the ability to provide coverage and to seal dead space. These major advances came fortuitously at a time associated with an increase

Table 76–1. Clinical Problems in Chest Wall Reconstruction

Coverage
Pressure sores, radiation necrosis, tumor resection, burns

Skeletal stabilization
Severe pectus deformities, sternal clefts, major resections

Obliteration of Dead Space
Chronic empyema cavity, bronchopleural fistula

Complex Chest Wall Reconstructions
Median sternotomy dehiscence, massive chest wall resection for tumor or radiation necrosis, massive injuries

Esthetic Contour Corrections
Pectus deformities, Poland's syndrome, scoliosis

in surgically related chest wounds such as dehiscence from median sternotomy following cardiac surgery and chest wall necrosis from radiation for breast cancer. The muscle flaps, along with customized implants, have also expanded the surgeon's ability to correct congenital or developmental contour deformities of the chest wall, such as pectus excavatum or Poland's syndrome. A major reassessment of the scope and methods of chest wall reconstruction has evolved (Dingman and Argenta, 1981; Scheflan, Bostwick, and Nahai, 1982; Arnold and Pairolero, 1984). Plastic surgeons have much to contribute to chest wall reconstruction (Table 76–1).

Anatomy and Physiology

The intimate correlation between anatomy and function throughout the body is uniquely illustrated in the design of the chest wall to provide simultaneously a hard shell for protection of the vital visceral organs (heart, liver, spleen, pancreas, and kidneys) while serving as a flexible frame for respiratory movements (Seyfer, Graeber, and Wind, 1986; Lambertsen, 1980). To accomplish this, the ribs are hinged posteriorly and superiorly against the spine and anteriorly and inferiorly at the sternal junction. With the sternum serving as a "bucket-handle" controlling the expansion of the rib cage, superior and anterior movement of the sternum results in an "unfolding" of the ribs and a greater thoracic volume. The costal cartilage provides additional flexibility between the ribs and sternum (Fig. 76–1).

Inspiratory Muscles. The sternocleidomastoid and the scalene muscles insert onto the clavicle and the first and second ribs, serving as elevators of the "superior aperture" of the rib cage and helping to expand the chest volume. Major resections of the upper sternum and ribs result in a partial "collapse" of the ribs inferiorly and a measurable functional loss in ventilation. Maximum inspiratory effort, for example, requires complete upward and lateral expansion of the ribs to achieve maximum chest circumference. This enlarges the frame for the diaphram to contract against, and it therefore further expands the chest cavity against the abdomen.

Expiratory Muscles. The muscles attached to the much larger "inferior aperture" of the rib cage (rectus abdominis, internal oblique, and external oblique muscles) serve to constrict the rib cage downward and to force the abdominal content upward against the diaphragm. In addition to postural control, they are important in the expiratory phase of respiration and during "cough" and "sneeze."

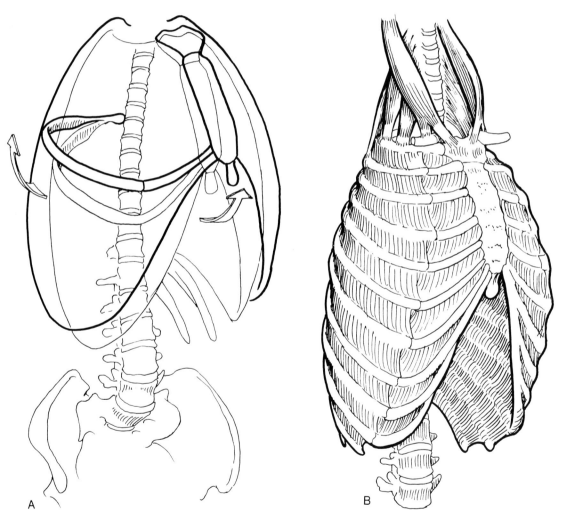

A

B

Figure 76–1. *A,* Forced inspiration depends on the "bucket-handle" motion of the ribs and the "pump-handle" motion of the sternum. This energy-consuming effort is mediated through the accessory muscles of respiration and occurs when metabolic demand outstrips ventilatory capabilities at rest. Excessive removal of the chest wall in the wrong patient can activate this response and lead to exhaustion. *B,* The accessory muscles of inspiration include the sternocleidomastoids, the scalene muscles, the external intercostals, and the parasternal intercartilaginous muscles. These activate the bucket-handle and pump-handle mechanisms. (From Seyfer, A., Graeber, G., and Wind, G. (Eds.): Atlas of Chest Wall Reconstruction. Rockville, MD, Aspen Publications, 1986, p. 28.)

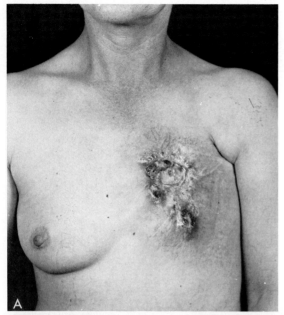

Figure 76–2. *A,* Large, recurrent carcinoma of the chest wall following radical mastectomy and irradiation therapy. The patient could not tolerate additional irradiation. The lesion was widely excised, together with the underlying ribs and sternum. Split-thickness skins grafts were applied directly to the pericardium and chest wall. *B,* Position of the graft-covered pericardium in forced expiration. *C,* The grafted pericardium is drawn inward at the beginning of inspiration. Photographs *B* and *C* were taken more than three years after operation.

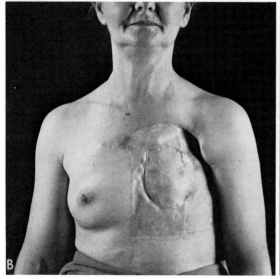

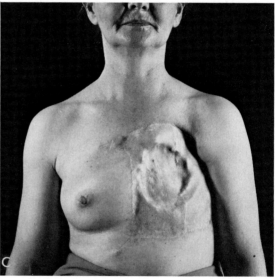

The muscles attached to the clavicle, scapula, and humerus (such as the pectoralis major, trapezius, and the latissimus dorsi and others) are designed primarily for movement of the shoulder and arm. Their contraction and relaxation, however, exert an important secondary influence on the rib cage, as evidenced by the arm motions and postures of the opera singer.

The overall expansion of the rib cage is critically important in creating the "negative pressure" necessary for lung expansion during inspiration. Loss of the rigid support over a large area of the rib cage may result in an inward motion of the chest walls, so-called paradoxical movement (Fig. 76–2), which compromises the efficiency of ventilatory excursions. Small paradoxical movements are well tolerated as a result of the considerable functional reserve of the lungs. Excessive paradoxical movements, on the other hand, severely reduce effective vital capacity and promote lung atelectasis caused by poor alveolar expansion. Similarly, interruption in the integrity of the chest wall would result in a "sucking wound" when outside air rushes into the chest during inspiration. This not only causes the collapse of the affected lung but also may produce a "tension pneumothorax" when the air is unable to escape. Such a patient may go into shock and respiratory failure as a result of pressure on the cardiovascular system and the opposite lung.

Principles of Chest Wall Reconstruction

FUNDAMENTAL GOALS

The need to restore absolute integrity of the chest wall demands that the surgeon understand clearly the anatomic requirements involved, whether treating an open chest injury or resecting ribs to improve appearance. Failure to accomplish the essential reconstructive goals endangers the patient's survival and usually necessitates additional surgical procedures as well. The common components of the reconstructive problems encountered are listed (Table 76–2), and the specific reconstructive goals are discussed individually.

Debridement and Resection

An adequate debridement or resection prior to closure is essential. In trauma cases it entails removal of contaminated tissues to minimize the likelihood of infection; in radiation injuries it allows uncomplicated primary wound healing; and in tumor cases it maximizes the chances of cure or palliation. The inelasticity of the rib cage makes primary closure after any significant debridement difficult and prone to dehiscence and potentially serious complications. Inadequate margins of resection, on the other hand, result in the approximation of infected or irradiated tissue,

Table 76–2. Principles of Chest Wall Reconstruction

Debridement and resection
Remove devitalized bone or cartilage; healthy margins

Requirements for Skeletal Reconstruction
Bone, fascia, synthetic mesh, acrylic

Coverage
Leak-free, tension-free, well vascularized

Obliteration of Potential Cavities (Dead Space)
Suction, mediastinal/diaphragm shifts, lung expansion, distant flaps

Esthetic Considerations

a situation likely to result in persistent infection and breakdown. Even muscle flaps with their vigorous blood supply cannot be expected to "clean up" an infected wound. Placing a valuable muscle flap in an inadequately debrided wound commits one of the most unforgivable sins in reconstructive surgery, i.e., the wasting of precious tissue and rendering it unavailable for future use. With the many flaps available today, one should no longer be restricted in the initial debridement of a chest wound.

When aggressive wide debridement is difficult, such as in wounds involving deep sinuses around the heart or granulation tissue over coronary bypass grafts, the wound should be left open and treated with topical dressing changes until the gross infection is cleared. Flap reconstruction can then be done with more limited debridement.

Flap Requirements

The "semirigid" skeletal frame of the chest renders the surrounding soft tissue less mobile for use in closure, as compared with the abdomen. A large soft tissue defect, therefore, requires addition of tissue from a distance. The rigidity makes the chances less likely of a chronic chest cavity closing spontaneously by gradual contraction; therefore, any residual "dead space" must be filled with a sufficiently bulky flap. The closure of the surface defect or the dead space must also be "leak-free" to avoid the development of a pneumothorax. A secure closure of the surface and the dead space, which can withstand the repetitive and forceful respiratory movement of the ribs, must also be "tension-free." Finally, the flap should be "well vascularized" to offer the best chance for uncomplicated primary wound healing. In chest wall reconstruction any "minor" wound healing problems are likely to evolve into a "major" complication associated with significant morbidity and possible mortality.

Skeletal Reconstruction

Some loss or disruption of the sternum-rib complex is usually seen whether in penetrating injury or following tumor resection. Optimal skeletal restoration should always be the goal. Failure to stabilize the "semirigid skeletal framework" may result in paradoxical movement with ventilatory compromise, which may not be noticeable at rest but may manifest itself as limitations in exercise tolerance. Malangoni and associates (1980) reported a 31 to 74 per cent reduction of the forced vital capacity in six children who had undergone tumor resection and Marlex reconstruction. The importance of minimizing further loss of vital capacity cannot be over-emphasized. Another reason for skeletal restoration is that the constant motion of the wound edges also interferes with healing.

Unless compromised by other associated factors, most patients can tolerate the loss of segments of up to four ribs without skeletal replacement. When the defect is covered by a thick flap, such as a latissimus dorsi musculocutaneous flap, the amount of flailing is also reduced compared with that of a thin skin flap. The loss of the lower portion of the sternum is less critical in the overall expansion of the rib cage, and skeletal reconstruction is often not needed. Finally, in many chronic conditions, there may be sufficient rigid scar formation to minimize the need for skeletal reconstruction.

In most massive chest wall resections, some form of skeletal stabilization should be considered. This goal may be accomplished with autogenous bone grafts, rigid synthetic materials, such as acrylic, or a semirigid replacement (fascia or synthetic mesh). Over the body of the ribs, this is effectively accomplished by any rigid membrane to minimize gross flailing of the defect and reconstruction with bone is needed only occasionally.

When the sternum is removed, however, the instability results in a more serious paradoxical movement of the entire chest. When the diaphragm contracts to expand the lungs, the rib cage is pulled toward the center, resulting in a counterproductive constriction of the chest and a reduction of the total lung capacity. Conversely, when the diaphragm relaxes during expiration, the ribs spring back to a larger frame, inhibiting a more complete expiration. Bisgard and Swenson (1948) used autogenous rib grafts to span the gap in the anterior ribs to prevent collapse of the ribs during inspiration. This maneuver converts the "median tie-beam" type of construction of the anterior chest to a continuous arch, or "Quonset hut" type of structure.

Obliteration of Potential Cavities (Dead Spaces)

In lobectomies or pneumonectomies, the potential void created is readily filled by lung expansion and shifting of the surrounding structures and elevation of the diaphragm aided by negative suction drainage. Following irradiation, chronic inflammation, or chronic cavitation, the lung and the surrounding structures are no longer pliable and a permanent cavity results. In cases such as chronic emphysema cavities, the cavity can be obliterated only by (1) exteriorizing the cavity, (2) surgically collapsing the rib cage, or (3) filling the cavity with soft tissue. The first two options may be functionally satisfactory, but the result is esthetically grotesque and functionally inconvenient. Omentum or muscle, therefore, is the preferred material for filling the dead space to achieve wound healing.

Esthetic Considerations

Although patients are always grateful for the restoration of function by successful chest wall reconstruction, the appearance remains important, especially in women. Massive wounds with depressed contours, hyperpigmented skin grafts, tight contractural bands, or distorted nipples and breasts are disturbing reminders to the patient. With the wide variety of flaps available today, every attempt should be made to achieve an esthetically acceptable reconstruction along with basic functional restoration (Arnold, 1981).

AVAILABLE FLAPS

The flaps used for chest wall reconstruction closely parallel the evolution of flap surgery in general. With the popularization of skin flap surgery following World War I and II, the previous simple type of closure was supplemented with a variety of local rotation flaps, often delayed in stages (Aston and Pickrell, 1977) (Fig. 76–3). For difficult wounds, flaps from the abdomen were carried via the wrist in stages as "jump flaps" and eventually transferred to the chest (Fig. 76–4). "Tube flaps" were also "waltzed" from the back or abdomen in many laborious stages (Fig. 76–5). The opposite breast was divided or mobilized to cover defects resulting from irradiation injuries. Such multistaged flaps were often limited in size, disfiguring, cumbersome, and often unsuccessful. They have been largely replaced by the newer generation of flaps that entail shorter periods of reconstruction and provide a more reliable blood supply. The principles previously learned regarding

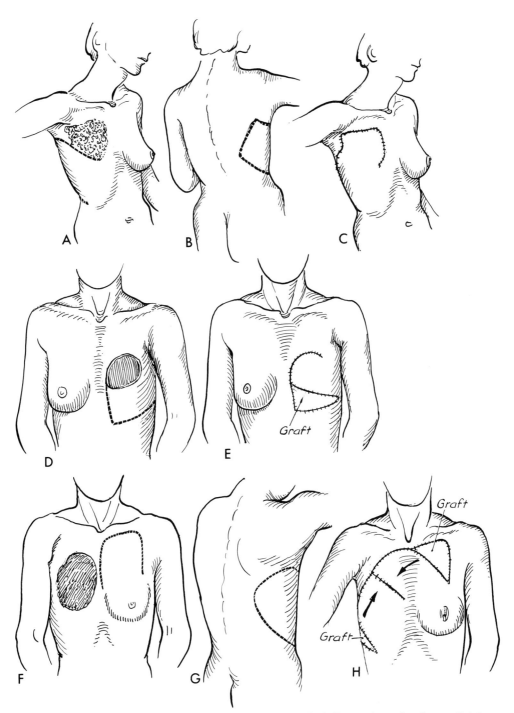

Figure 76–3. Various local flaps for chest wall reconstruction. *A to C,* Axillary and anterior chest wall defect covered by a dorsal flap. *D,* Anterior chest wall defect covered by a transposition flap. *E,* Note that split-thickness skin grafts were used to cover the defect remaining after flap transposition. *F to H,* Large anterior chest wall defect covered by a dorsal and anterior chest wall transposition flap.

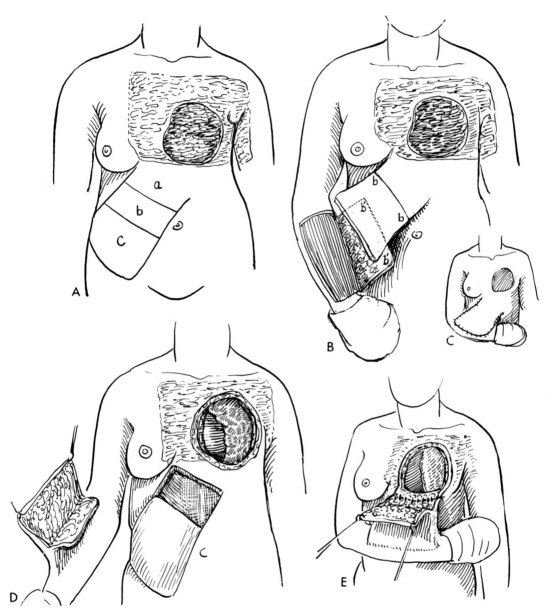

Figure 76–4. Closed carried flap for closure of a thoracic defect. *A,* Chest wall defect, pericardium exposed. The shaded area represents the scarred, previously irradiated skin. The flap is outlined. Portion *a* will remain attached to the abdomen; portion *b* is the intermediary part of the flap; portion *c* will be attached to the forearm. *B,* The abdominal and hinge forearm flaps are raised and are in position for suturing. *C,* The closed carried flap is established. A split-thickness skin graft is used to cover the secondary abdominal wall defect after elevation of the flap. *D,* Devitalized tissue is excised, exposing the pericardium and the lung. The proximal end of the flap is detached from the abdomen. *E,* The distal end of the forearm flap is sutured to the inferior end of the thoracic wall defect.

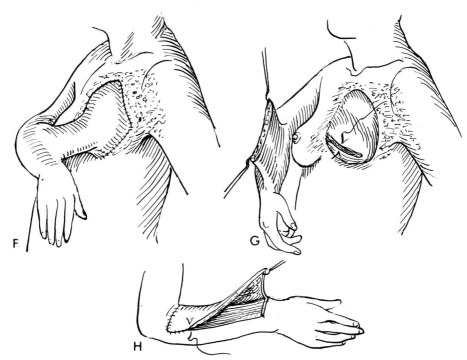

Figure 76–4 *Continued F,* Suture of the flap to the thoracic defect is completed. *G,* The flap is cut from its attachment to the chest. *H,* The forearm flap is returned to its original position. (From Converse, J., Campbell, R., and Watson, W.: Repair of ulcers situated over the heart and brain. Ann. Surg., *133*:95, 1951.)

chest wall reconstruction, however, remain valid.

The development of the epigastric (Shaw and Payne, 1946) and deltopectoral (DP) (Bakamjian, Culf, and Bales, 1967) flaps represented the beginning of trunk flaps based on specific arterial supply. Muscles, although used earlier by Campbell (1950), became popular and were more systematically studied in the 1970's and 1980's. Arnold and Pairolero (1984) utilized 142 muscle flaps in 92 of 100 consecutive patients for chest wall reconstruction. More experience was also gained with using omentum, initially for treatment of lymphedema and later as microvascular free flaps. The excitement generated over muscle and axial-pattern arterial skin flaps eventually matured into a more comprehensive view of the regional blood supply of the trunk and a more versatile concept of fasciocutaneous flaps. Finally, microvascular free flaps from the lower extremity or lower abdomen provided large flaps when regional flaps were not available. An understanding of the regional blood supply and the characteristics of the commonly used flaps is critical in the planning of any chest wall reconstruction (Table 76–3).

Skin Flaps

Vascular Architecture of the Trunk Skin. Palmer and Taylor (1986) studied the arterial blood supply of the chest. The skin blood supply of the upper torso more or less mirrors that of the lower torso (abdomen) (see Chapter 10). A series of "segmental" vessels branch off the intercostal vessels and supply the skin through anterior, lateral, and posterior perforators. They interconnect extensively in the subcutaneous layer across "choke zones" with a predominantly horizontal orientation (Fig. 76–6). Thus, in addition

Table 76–3. Common Flaps in Chest Wall Reconstruction

Skin Flaps
Simple rotation, deltopectoral, lateral thoracic, scapular, etc.

Muscle or Musculocutaneous Flaps
Pectoralis, serratus, latissimus, rectus abdominis

Other Regional Tissues
Omentum, double breast, total arm, diaphragm, etc.

Free Flaps
Rectus abdominis, latissimus, tensor, lateral thigh, etc.

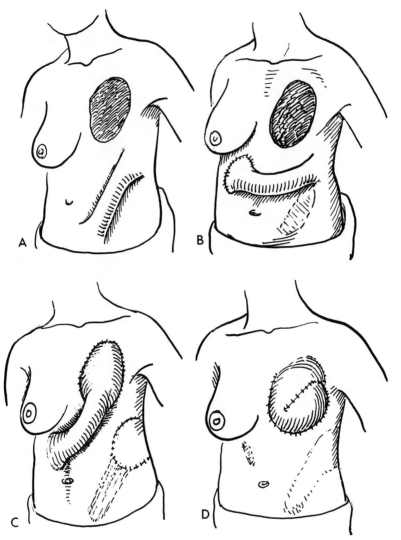

Figure 76–5. A full-thickness defect of the anterior chest wall with exposed pericardium. *A*, Construction of a thoracoabdominal tube. *B*, Inferior end of tube migrated to the epigastrium. *C*, Lateral tube attachment migrated to the defect. *D*, Inferior inset of tube transposed to the area of the defect. (After Rees, T. D.: Radiation necrosis of the chest wall, full-thickness reconstruction with pedicle flap and diced homologus cartilage over the pericardium complicated by cardiac arrest. Plast. Reconstr. Surg., 28:67, 1961.)

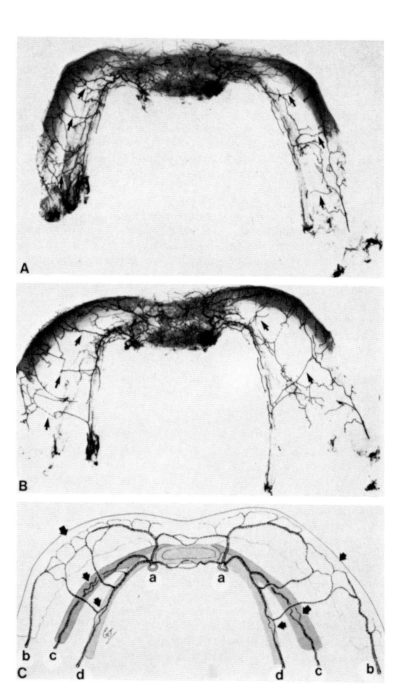

Figure 76–6. Cross section study of the anterior chest wall at the level of the inframammary crease in a female cadaver. *A,* Intact specimen. Note large cutaneous perforators arising from the anterior and posterior intercostal arcade (*arrows*). *B,* Specimen separated laterally into its three layers consisting of the integument, the pectoralis major muscle, and the rib cage. *C,* Schematic diagram of the internal thoracic artery (a) highlighting its choke arterial connections with branches of the lateral thoracic (b), pectoral (c), and posterior intercostal (d) arteries. Note: These interconnections occur at corresponding regions in each layer (*arrows*). (From Taylor, G. I.: Discussion of Carramenha e Costa, M. A., Carriquiry, C., Vasconez, L. O., Grotting, J. C., Herrera, R. H., and Windle, B. H.: An anatomic study of the venous drainage of the transverse rectus abdominis musculocutaneous flap. Plast. Reconstr. Surg., 79:214, 1987.)

to the well-known DP flap based on the large second or third internal mammary perforators, other medially based flaps can be designed throughout the trunk. From the axilla and the groin, a more distinct axial pattern vessel is seen, the lateral thoracic and the superficial inferior epigastric vessels, respectively. Utilization of these "axial" arteries running from the axilla and the groin allows for the design of long regional flaps. The internal mammary vessels send off a sizable direct cutaneous artery between the xiphoid and the costal margin to supply the upper abdominal skin (superior superficial epigastric). The circumflex scapular artery consistently has large cutaneous branches supplying the upper lateral back, which can be utilized for the construction of microvascular free flaps and regional flaps. A vertical row of medial posterior perforators on the two sides of the spine is similar to that of the internal mammary perforators of the anterior aspect. Between the anterior and posterior perforators, a row of lateral perforators is located approximately along the midaxillary line. Intramuscular and subcutaneous interconnections of the three systems occur in a network fashion that is oriented horizontally.

Planning of Skin Flaps. Whenever possible, flaps should be designed to contain the maximal blood supply and to take advantage of well-known principles of flap surgery. The length-to-width (base) ratio, although convenient for descriptive purposes, is not important in determining the blood supply of the flap. More important, the base of the flap should center over one of the sources of the regional blood supply and the direction of the flap should be aligned along the principal direction of the subcutaneous vessel network. Inclusion of the deep fascia also generally improves the reliability of the skin flap (Ponten, 1981). These recently clarified concepts have been, in retrospect, confirmed by the well-established reliability of the DP flap or the groin flap. Because of the greater elasticity of the skin along the vertical axis and because of the more limited circumference transversely, tension is better tolerated vertically than horizontally. Rotation or transposition flaps generally should be designed sufficiently large to ensure adequate movement and closure without tension.

Deltopectoral Flap. Deltopectoral flaps were first described by Bakamjiam (1965) for pharyngeal reconstruction. This report was historically important because it broke the existing rules for the length-to-width ratio and the dependence on time-consuming delays. Its reliability and versatility have been well tested for more than two decades, and it remains a useful flap for the head and neck region and for local chest reconstruction (Fig. 76–7) (Aston and Pickrell, 1977). McGregor and Jackson (1970) described the applications of the DP flap in an upper semicircle for head and neck reconstructions. Robinson (1976) advanced the concept of using the lower half of the semicircle of the DP flap reach for chest wall reconstruction, including defects of the opposite side. Leonard (1980) deepithelized the DP flap and turned it over to cover a defect of the opposite side. The dermis was used to provide fascia-like support, and the exposed subcutaneous undersurface was skin grafted.

Surgical Anatomy and Elevation. The principal blood supply of the DP flap is derived from one or two large perforating arteries from the second or the third interspace located lateral to the sternal border. The axial arteries pass just above the muscle fascia for a short distance and disappear into the subcutaneous fatty layer heading toward the shoulder. Laterally, they form collateral connections with the thoracoacromial perforators over the coracoid process, extending the potential vascular territory of the flap to the skin over the anterior shoulder. Extension of the flap in an inferior direction over the upper arm has also been described, the additional skin probably based on additional collateral connections with the muscular cutaneous perforators over the deltoid muscle (Fig. 76–7). The flap width can cover the entire chest, although excessive width would limit its ability to rotate and does not add to the useful length of the flap. The upper margin of the flap usually lies over the medial half of the clavicle and continues superolaterally toward the acromion. A parallel lower margin usually spares the nipple and heads toward the anterior axillary fold. Most flaps are raised without delay, whereas longer flaps are better delayed during the first stage by elevating the lateral part of the flap to ligate the thoracoacromial vessels. Flap elevation is commenced laterally to medially in the plane above the muscle. Some authors prefer to include the pectoralis major muscle fascia with the flap to minimize injury to the axial vessels. Near the lateral border of the ster-

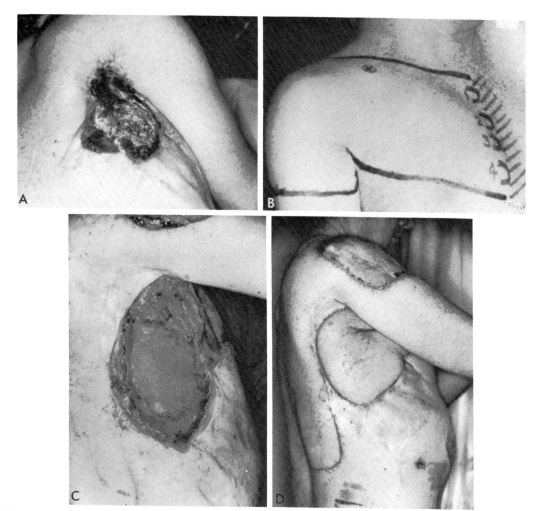

Figure 76–7. *A,* Recurrent squamous cell carcinoma in the posterolateral aspect of the thorax. Note the surrounding area of healed skin grafts, which necessitates the use of a distant flap. *B,* Outline of a deltopectoral flap with a paddle extension over the deltoid region. The latter was delayed as a preliminary procedure. *C,* Intraoperative view following full-thickness resection of the chest wall and insertion of a Marlex mesh. *D,* Appearance of the flap two weeks following surgery. A superiorly based dorsal flap that had been delayed was not used in the chest wall reconstruction. (Courtesy of Dr. Joseph G. McCarthy, Institute of Reconstructive Plastic Surgery, NYU Medical Center.)

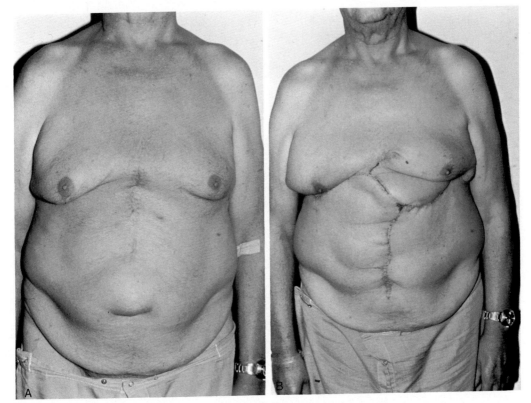

Figure 76–8. *A,* Recurrent gastric carcinoma involving the abdominal and chest wall requiring full-thickness resection. *B,* Reconstruction was accomplished with a local double rotation flap. (Courtesy of Dr. Norman Godfrey.)

num the dissection must be done carefully, preferably with magnifying loupes. When the second or the third perforators are observed exiting the muscle, the dissection has reached its absolute limit. Back cuts can be done on the skin at the base to improve rotation, only if the perforating vessels are not compromised.

Other Arterialized (Fasciocutaneous) Skin Flaps. Aside from the DP flap, other skin flaps can be designed in the chest and abdomen and they are based on the cutaneous perforators from the internal mammary, lateral intercostal, paraspinal, thoracoacromial, lateral thoracic, and circumflex scapula arteries (Fig. 76–8). In fact, the vascular architecture of the posterior chest skin is remarkably similar to that of its anterior counterpart. Similar flaps, based medially on the posterior perforators, can be designed. Most of the time, a simple rotation or transposition flap is designed similar to, but not as long as, the DP flap and the cutaneous perforators are usually not seen. In the case of the lateral thoracic or the parascapular

flap, these can be dissected as island flaps and the vessels may be skeletonized for better reach and versatility. The possible designs of various arterialized flaps are limited mainly by the knowledge and ingenuity of the surgeon. Maruyama, Ohnishi, and Chung (1985) used "vertical abdominal fasciocutaneous flaps" of length-to-width ratio of 3:1 or more based on the superficial vessels from the superior epigastric artery at the costal margin.

Muscle and Musculocutaneous Flaps

Tansini (1906) described the use of the latissimus dorsi muscle for chest wall reconstruction. Campbell (1950) used the muscle with a skin graft to cover a fascial graft that had been utilized to stabilize a large anterior chest defect. Olivari (1976), Muhlbauer and Olbrisch (1977), Mendelson and Masson (1977) and McCraw, Penix, and Baker (1978) improved the understanding of the latissimus dorsi flap and popularized its uses for breast and chest wall reconstructions. Chang and Mathes (1982) suggested that muscle flaps

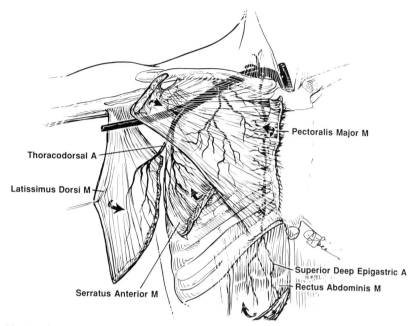

Figure 76–9. Muscles frequently used in chest wall reconstruction. Note the vascular pedicles in the axilla directly over the chest wall. Division of the humeral and scapular insertions of the muscles can produce remarkable reach of the muscles medially.

may be advantageous for reconstruction of contaminated wounds, as there is improved ability to reduce the bacterial count, compared with random-pattern skin flaps (see also Chapter 11).

The pectoralis major and the rectus abdominis muscle flaps came a bit later to provide three reliable techniques for chest wall reconstruction. The serratus anterior muscle is also useful but is limited in size. The trapezius muscle is of satisfactory size, but it reaches only the upper chest and its functional loss is not always well tolerated. The latissimus dorsi, pectoralis major, and rectus abdominis muscles are excellent donor muscles for chest wall reconstruction because of their large mass, length, and consistent vascular pedicle and functional expendability. A complete understanding of the muscle anatomy, arc of rotation, and reconstructive capabilities is essential (Mathes and Nahai, 1982; McCraw and Arnold, 1986; Tobin, 1986) (Fig. 76–9).

Lastissimus Dorsi Muscle. The anatomy and clinical applications of this muscle have been amply described (see also Chapter 79). The functional loss is minimal, except, perhaps, in mountain climbers, gymnasts, or paraplegics when forceful upward pull of the body weight by the arms is important. Several anatomic features deserve special consideration for chest wall reconstruction.

The anteriorly located vascular pedicle makes it highly efficient for transfer to the anterior chest wall. To gain maximum reach, the vascular pedicle can be skeletonized, the branches to the serratus anterior muscle divided, and the tendinous insertion of the muscle detached from the humerus. This maneuver allows it to reach easily across the midline (Fig. 76–10). Matsuo and associates (1988) tunneled the contralateral latissimus muscle between the pectoralis major and minor muscles to reach the contralateral anterior axilla and upper chest (Fig. 76–11). On the back, the latissimus dorsi flap can reach most of the upper back, shoulder, and neck (Fig. 76–11). When the main subscapular artery or the upper thoracodorsal artery is ligated during mastectomy, the muscle remains reliable (May, Toth, and Cohen, 1982), although the distal aspect of the skin flap can develop partial ischemia or necrosis. The serratus anterior branch must be preserved to provide retrograde flow, thus restricting the movement somewhat. In cases of previous thoracotomy, the muscle may have been transected and, therefore, the lower portion of the muscle (near the origins) may not be reliable.

For chest wall reconstruction, it is important to have comfortable obliteration of any potential dead space. One should therefore be aware of the dimensions of the fan-shaped

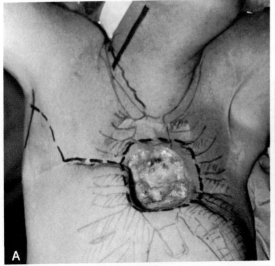

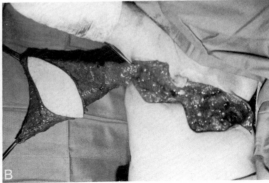

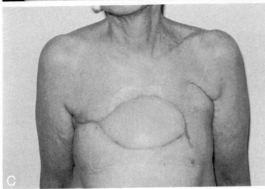

Figure 76–10. *A,* After bilateral mastectomy and mediastinal radiation for breast carcinoma, a 55 year old woman had a chronic draining fistula of the lower sternum that required debridement to unroof the cavity. Radical debridement ten days later removed all necrotic cartilage and sternum. The manubrium was well vascularized and was therefore preserved. *B,* After the humeral insertion was divided, the latissimus dorsi musculocutaneous flap was attached only by the vascular pedicle and could be mobilized anteriorly to reach beyond the midline. *C,* Appearance one year postoperatively.

distal aspect of the muscle, so as to ensure adequate direct contact between the muscle and the wound. If skin is carried with the muscle, it becomes particularly important to plan its location properly on the muscle. Although the major skin perforators follow the course of the two main branches of the thoracodorsal artery along the anterior and the superior border, any skin island over the muscle should be more than adequately supplied. When needed, the skin island may extend beyond the muscle as a fasciocutaneous component. Primary skin closure may be accomplished for up to 7 to 10 cm and is easier when the skin island is oriented transversely. A closure with excessive tension is prone to dehiscence or an extremely widened scar.

The subscapular artery supplies three reliable microvascular free flap donor sites: the latissimus dorsi muscle, the serratus anterior muscle, and the skin of the parascapular region. When needed, two or three of the components can be taken together on the same pedicle to cover a large defect or to fill a dead space at the same time.

The latissimus dorsi muscle has a dual blood supply (see Fig. 76–9). Along the posterior medial border, it is supplied by multiple posterior perforators (McCraw, Penix, and Baker, 1978). The humeral insertion and the thoracodorsal vessels can be divided and the muscle rotated, based on the posterior perforators. In addition, segments of the muscle can be utilized in the same way for smaller posterior defects.

Flap Elevation. When a skin island is taken with the flap, the incision is made completely and the skin flaps are elevated in both directions to reveal the superior and the anterior borders of the muscle. When skin is not included, similar skin flaps are elevated to reveal the entire extent of the muscle. At the midportion of the muscle, near the tip of the scapula, the muscle is dissected away from the underlying serratus muscle, thereby creating a tunnel under the muscle between the two borders. The broad expansion of the muscle's origin from the posterior ribs is detached by sharp and blunt dissection. The body of the muscle is lifted away from the chest, leaving it attached by its humeral insertion and the vascular pedicle. The pedicle runs through the axillary fat to become adherent to the undersurface of the muscle at approximately 10 cm from the humerus (see Fig. 76–9). The posterosuperior border of the muscle needs to be separated from the skin to allow comfortable anterior transposition of the muscle through a subcutaneous tunnel or a direct skin incision. If maximum anterior movement is needed, the space between the vascular pedicle and the humeral insertion is dissected free to allow detachment of the tendinous insertion. Without the protection of the normal insertion, one must be careful to avoid excessive tension or torsion of the vascular pedicle. If only a part of the muscle is needed, one can split the muscle between the major branches of the vessels as seen on the under surface of the muscle (Tobin and associates, 1981). The distal muscle (origin side) can also be divided along the direction of its fibers into many tails for obliteration of multiple dead spaces.

Pectoralis Major Muscle. Sisson, Straehley, and Johnson (1962) described a flap from the medial aspect of the pectoralis major muscle, based on the medial perforators from the internal mammary vessels; it was used to close a midline sternal defect. Hueston and McConchie (1968) reported a pectoralis major musculocutaneous flap to close a manubrial defect. Brown, Fleming, and Jurkiewicz (1977) used bilateral pectoralis major flaps with skin grafts for closure of an anterior chest wall defect. Arnold and Pairolero (1979) recommended a rotated island pectoralis major flap along with rib grafts to reconstruct a sternal defect and prevent flailing (Fig. 76–12).

Like the latissimus dorsi muscle, the pectoralis major is supplied by a dominant pedicle (thoracoacromial vessels) that extends from the axilla and emerges medial to the pectoralis minor muscle. The secondary supply is by a roll of perforators from the internal mammary vessels along its sternal origin. With the humeral insertion and the medial rib origins detached, the muscle can be easily moved medially and superiorly to fill defects in the superior mediastinum, laterally to re-

surface the shoulder and through a window in the anterior ribs to fill the upper chest cavity (de la Rocha and Robertson, 1984).

A skin island can be carried with the muscle, preferably including some element of medial muscle with large segmental perforators. The skin beyond the inferior edge of the muscle origin can be carried reliably if the deep muscle fascia of the serratus and rectus abdominis is included.

When the lateral humeral insertion is detached, the muscle can be turned on itself, based on the medial perforators, and used to fill mediastinal defects. Care must be taken not to damage the roll of perforators near the edge of the sternum. In cases of extensive mediastinal radiation, the internal mammary artery and its perforators may have been destroyed; thus, such a flap should not be considered. As part of the muscle is also wasted when turned on itself, the useful bulk is limited.

The pectoralis major flap is generally highly reliable and technically easy to raise. Few data are available regarding complications in chest wall reconstruction. In the head and neck region, a 10 to 20 per cent flap loss of some degree has been noted (Maisel, Liston, and Adams, 1983). Robbins and Woodson (1984) reported two cases of rapid spreading of squamous cell carcinoma of the larynx and base of tongue to the chest following immediate reconstruction with pectoralis major flaps. It was recommended that the wounds be irrigated thoroughly during surgery and that separate drains be used for the resection site and the flap donor site.

Flap Dissection. When a skin island is used, the incisions are made and extended in the appropriate directions. Skin flaps are elevated to reveal the margins of the muscle. The origin of the muscle from the ribs is detached, starting from the well-defined lateral border. Medially, the muscle is detached from its sternal origin. Superiorly, the muscle is separated at the deltopectoral groove and from its clavicular origin. Care is exercised in the region of the lateral half of the clavicle, medial to the coracoid process. The thoracoacromial vessels enter the undersurface of the muscle medial to the insertion of the pectoralis minor muscle on the coracoid process (see Fig. 76–9). When medial rotation is needed, the humeral insertion of the muscle is divided. When the flap is based on the medial perforators, the insertion and the

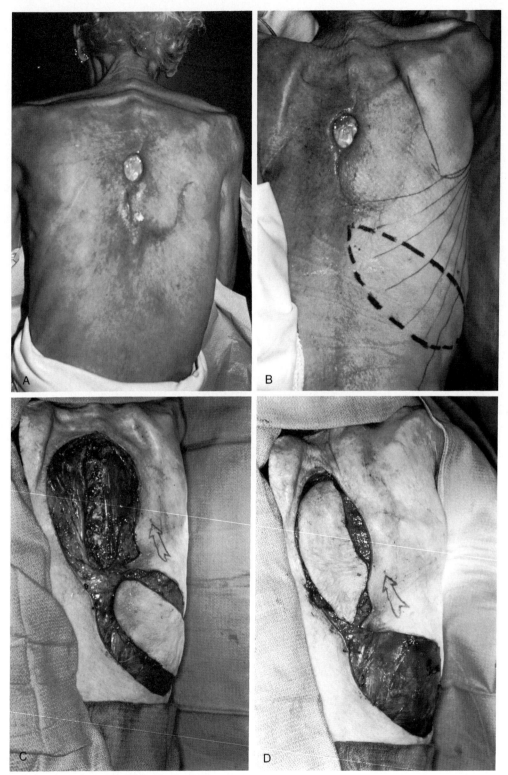

Figure 76–11. *A,* A 79 year old woman with previous mediastinal radiation and posterior spine pressure necrosis. *B,* Note the location of the skin island on the latissimus dorsi muscle to ensure adequate reach. After wide debridement *(C),* the flap is transposed into the defect *(D)* and the donor area is closed primarily *(E).*

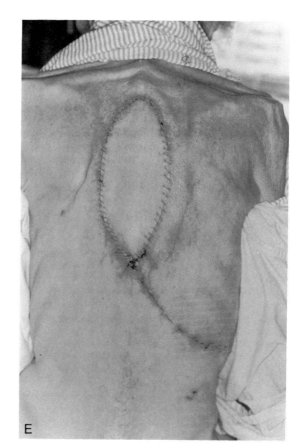

Figure 76–11 *Continued*

E

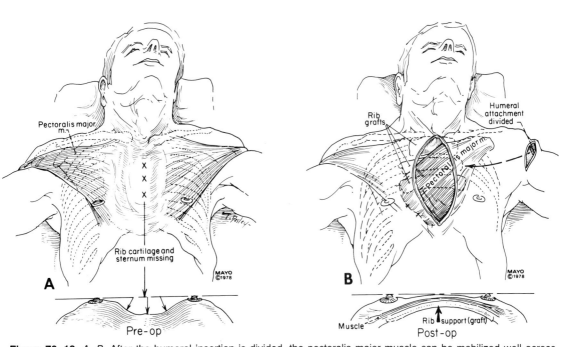

Figure 76–12. *A, B,* After the humeral insertion is divided, the pectoralis major muscle can be mobilized well across the midline and into the median sternotomy defect. (From Arnold, P. G., and Pairolero, P. C.: Use of pectoralis major muscle flaps to repair defects of anterior chest wall. Plast. Reconstr. Surg., *63:*205, 1979.)

thoracoacromial pedicles are divided and the undersurface of the muscle is easily separated from the pectoralis minor muscle, the serratus anterior muscle, and the ribs. The lower origins of the muscle from the ribs and the clavicular origins are sharply detached. Medial elevation of the flap can proceed quickly until a line 2 cm from the sternal border. Further dissection should proceed cautiously with loupe magnification to avoid injury to the perforators from the internal mammary vessels as they pass through the interspaces.

Rectus Abdominis Muscle. Since its description by Hartrampf, Scheflan, and Black (1982) for breast reconstruction, the rectus abdominis muscle has been used extensively for chest reconstruction as well (see also Chapter 79). As a lower transverse rectus abdominis musculocutaneous (TRAM) flap, it has been used to cover irradiated defects of the chest wall. Ishii and associates (1985) used double-pedicled flaps, as a single skin unit or two independent skin units for greater versatility and reliability. This technique was thought to improve the poor vascularity in the contralateral tip of the transverse skin island of the unilateral muscle flap. Dinner and Dowden (1983) described a vertical skin island over the muscle rather than the transverse skin island for greater reliability of the skin component. The superiorly based muscle may be turned on itself to fill the defect in the mediastinum. Finally, when based on the inferior epigastric artery and vein, it can be transferred as a free flap in different configurations, depending on the requirements of the chest defect (Pennington and Pelly, 1980; Shaw, 1983).

Taylor, Corlett, and Boyd (1984) and Boyd, Taylor, and Corlett (1984), through extensive anatomic studies of the abdominal wall blood supply (see also Chapter 10), provided an excellent description of the vascular anatomy of the rectus abdominis muscle and its overlying skin (Figs. 76–13 and 76–14). Miller and associates (1988) studied the variations of the arterial anatomy at the upper attachment of the rectus muscle and recommended preserving the costal marginal artery as an important collateral supply in cases of compromised internal mammary vessels. In view of the possibility of poor intramuscular connections between the superior and the inferior systems, it may also be worthwhile to preserve the entire width of the muscle pedicle. Carramenha e Costa and associates

(1987) studied the venous anatomy of the rectus muscle and recommended preservation of a sufficient skin island over the upper muscle to ensure more anatomic venous drainage (Fig. 76–15). The vertically oriented intramuscular arterial network is supplied inferiorly from the inferior epigastric artery, superiorly from the internal mammary artery, and laterally from the segmental intercostal arteries. The watershed area between the superior and inferior systems is located generally mid-distance between the costal margin and the umbilicus. The lower abdominal muscle and its overlying skin, therefore, are supplied principally from the inferior epigastic artery. When this is divided, as in the superiorly based flaps, the blood supply must come superiorly through intramuscular collaterals of variable caliber. Shaw and Feng (1988) studied intraoperative arterial pressures within the muscle based superiorly versus inferiorly and confirmed the hemodynamic dominance of the inferior system. Microvascular anastomoses of the inferior vessels or use of the muscle as inferiorly based microvascular free flaps can provide a more reliable flap with a larger skin territory. The technique also has the advantage of sacrificing only a small piece of muscle for less functional loss and easier abdominal closure (Fig. 76–15).

With careful attention to anatomic detail and preoperative preparation, however, the superiorly based TRAM flap remains useful and convenient for chest wall reconstruction. Many of the complications with the TRAM flaps are due to poor patient selection, i.e., extreme obesity, smoking, or abdominal wall weakness. The tips of the transverse skin island represent secondary or tertiary zones of blood supply and are therefore prone to fat necrosis. Skin taken directly over the muscle as an island or the entire muscle by itself, however, have been consistently reliable. The quality of perfusion of these somewhat tenuous flaps is also easily affected by systemic hemodynamic changes such as hypotension, vasospasm, or cold exposure. Hartrampf (1988) emphasized the importance of adequate blood volume and fluid replacement along with warm ambient temperature and pharmacologic supplementation with steroids and vasodilators.

Flap Dissections. The techniques of the TRAM flap for breast reconstruction are well described (see Chapter 79). Only the dissec-

Figure 76–13. Arterial supply of the rectus abdominis flap. Note that the connections between the anterior and posterior intercostals are either by true anastomoses or by choke arteries: the musculophrenic (MP) artery; the costomarginal (CMA) branch of the deep superior epigastric artery, which links with the eighth posterior intercostal artery; the involvement of the ascending branch (a) of the deep circumflex iliac artery and the lower posterior intercostals in the blood supply of the anterior abdominal wall; the anastomosis across the midline, which is rich in the chest but sparse in the abdomen. Note also that the anastomosis between the deep superior epigastric artery and the deep inferior epigastric artery is situated in the segment of rectus muscle above the umbilicus. The arcuate line and the direction of flow of the arteries are indicated by arrows. (From Taylor, G. I.: Discussion of Miller, L. B., Bostwick, J. III, Hartrampf, C. R., Jr., Hester, T. R., Jr., and Nahai, F.: The superiorly based rectus abdominis flap: predicting and enhancing its blood supply based on an anatomic and clinical study. Plast. Reconstr. Surg., *81*:721, 1988.

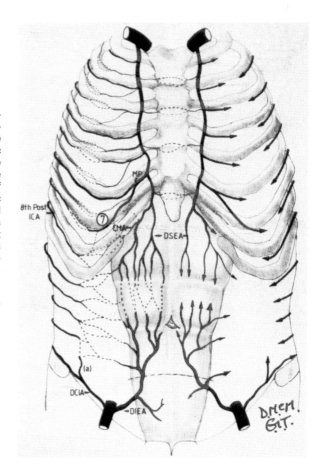

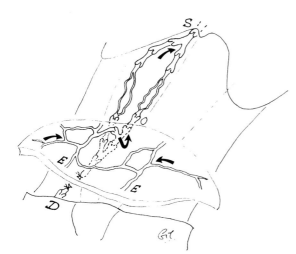

Figure 76–14. Venous drainage of the rectus abdominis flap. The superficial inferior epigastric system (E) communicates across the midline and by large channels in the periumbilical region with the deep inferior epigastric veins (D). The flow is then against the valves of this system and across the choke system of venules in the rectus muscle to reach the deep epigastric veins (S). (From Taylor, G. I.: Discussion of Carramenha e Costa, M. A., Carriquiry, C., Vasconez, L. O., Grotting, J. C., Herrera, R. H., and Windle, B. H.: An anatomic study of the venous drainage of the transverse rectus abdominis musculocutaneous flap. Plast. Reconstr. Surg., 79:214, 1987.

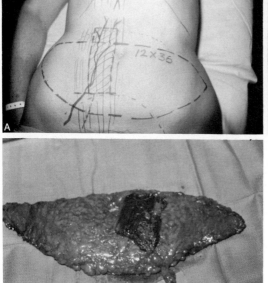

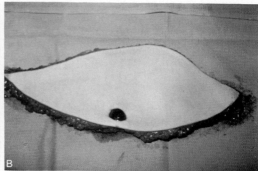

Figure 76–15. Transverse rectus abdominis musculocutaneous (TRAM) flap as a free flap based on the inferior epigastric vessels. *A,* Note the approximate location of the long vascular pedicle and the intended muscle cuff marked by the dashed rectangle. *B,* Flap after being harvested. *C,* Note the small amount of muscle taken.

tion of the superiorly based muscle, with the inclusion of a modest skin island on top of the muscle, are discussed. Although a transverse abdominal incision leaves a more esthetic scar, the much longer operating time and the more extensive dissection are rarely justified in patients in need of chest wall reconstruction. Usually a midline or paramidline incision is made, incorporating the skin island in the design. Minimal skin flaps are elevated on the two sides to allow more precise anterior sheath and skin closure later. The anterior rectus sheath is incised longitudinally throughout the length of the muscle needed and is then peeled from the muscle to expose the medial and lateral borders of the muscle and the inscriptions. If there is sufficient laxity of the anterior sheath, a 4 to 5 cm strip of it may be preserved with the muscle to facilitate dissection across the inscriptions. At each inscription the muscle segments condense into a tendinous insertion that is densely adherent to the anterior sheath. Care must be taken to stay close to the sheath to avoid dissecting through to the posterior aspect of the muscle. The medial and lateral dissections are connected underneath the muscle, and the muscle is divided

with a cautery at the intended level. If preservation of the inferior epigastric pedicle is desired for later anastomosis, this can first be identified and protected. At the lateral border of the muscle, the numerous intercostal vessels and nerves are identified and individually cauterized and divided. The posterior aspect of the muscle can be easily separated from the posterior sheath with blunt dissection to the region of the costal margin. If extra length is needed, the lateral margin of the muscle can be detached for some distance above the costal margin, as the main superior blood supply comes into the undersurface of the muscle between the xiphoid and the costal margin. It is helpful to leave as many of the intercostal contributions as possible, in case the upper internal mammary artery may have been compromised during previous chest surgery. The eighth intercostal artery, the so-called costal marginal artery, can support the entire rectus muscle. It is usually large and is a major collateral to the mammary system; thus, it should be preserved.

In contrast to the superiorly pedicled flap, the transverse skin island is more reliable as a microvascular free flap and the dissection of the abdomen is more limited, in that no upper abdomen tunnel is needed. The surgical dissection of the free flap is relatively easy (Shaw and Hidalgo, 1987). The skin flap is elevated to a point 1 cm lateral to the midline and 3 to 4 cm medial to the semilunar line. Since few major musculocutaneous perforators exist in the lower abdomen, the anterior rectus sheath is usually incised transversely at a level halfway between the umbilicus and the pubis, often superior to the lower border of the skin flap. After the medial and lateral borders of the muscle are ascertained, the medial and lateral sheaths are incised longitudinally, taking only 4 to 5 cm of anterior sheath transversely with the skin and muscle flap. Superiorly, a similar transverse incision is made in the sheath a few centimeters above the umbilicus at the level of the skin incision. If no skin is taken, the anterior sheath is simply incised and the entire muscle is exposed. The upper muscle is divided at the desired level. The inferior epigastric artery and vein can be identified coming toward the undersurface of the muscle along a line drawn from the midpoint of the inguinal ligament to the umbilicus. The vessels enter the muscle at approximately mid-distance between the pubis and umbilicus. The space between the lower part of the muscle and the pedicle is cleaned, and the lower muscle divided with a cautery. The large-caliber artery and veins (2 to 3 mm) can be easily followed to their origins from the iliac vessels and ligated and transected. To facilitate the final phases of pedicle dissection and fascial closure, the patient is given maximal muscle relaxation.

Serratus Anterior Muscle. The blood supply of this muscle is derived mainly from a branch of the thoracodorsal artery shortly before its entry into the latissimus-dorsi muscle (see Fig. 76–9). The conveniently long pedicle makes this moderate-sized flat muscle a useful second-line muscle for upper chest reconstruction. It is rarely indicated as the first choice muscle, in that its loss results in the well-known "winged scapula" deformity. In patients with difficult major upper chest wall reconstruction, when the latissimus dorsi and pectoralis major muscles are not sufficient, the use of the serratus anterior muscle is well justified. After the vascular supply is visualized on the surface of the muscle, a part or the entire muscle can be mobilized for local transfer.

Tensor Fasciae Lata Muscle. The deep fascia over the lateral muscles of the hip and thigh is thicker than usual and is known as the fascia lata. Its central condensation, the iliotibial band, stretches from the anterior portion of the iliac crest to the bony and tendinous attachments of the lateral knee. This fascia has excellent tensile strength and has long been a favorite source of fascial grafts for various suspension procedures, fascial patches, or as grafts for ligaments. The broad fascia has also been utilized for abdominal repairs. Hill, Nahai, and Vasconez (1978) described its neurovascular anatomy and suggested its use as island flaps and as free flaps.

Anatomy and Flap Dissection. The tensor muscle originates from the anterior 5 cm of the anterior iliac crest just behind the anterior iliac spine and the origin of the rectus femoris muscle (see Chapter 77). Its keel-shaped muscle belly is enveloped by the two layers of the fascia lata and is wedged between the rectus femoris muscle and gluteus medius muscles. Its contraction tightens the fascia lata and aids in lateral stability of the hip, but its loss is rarely noticed.

The tensor muscle has a dominant blood supply from the transverse branch of the lateral femoral circumflex artery passing off the profundus femoris artery. It enters the underside of the muscle at a point approximately 10 cm inferior from the anterior iliac spine (Fig. 76–16). The skin over the muscle receives musculocutaneous perforators, which travel longitudinally over the deep fascia and interconnect with fasciocutaneous networks in the lower thigh to allow the lower thigh skin to be carried on the same vascular pedicle. Up to 7 to 9 cm of skin width can be taken; yet, primary closure of the defect can be achieved for excellent esthetic results. Skin as wide as the entire lateral half of the thigh can be carried on the same pedicle; however, the donor defect would require a split-thickness skin graft for closure and the cosmetic appearance is not ideal. A sheet of fascia lata longer or wider than the skin can be taken for fascial repair of the abdomen or chest (Fig. 76–17).

The inferior skin incision is first made, and the fascia lata is exposed. The fascia lata is incised at the level determined by the size needed. Its undersurface is separated from the underlying vastus lateralis and rectus femoris muscles by blunt dissection. The longitudinal vessels on the surface of the vastus lateralis muscle can be used as a guide as to

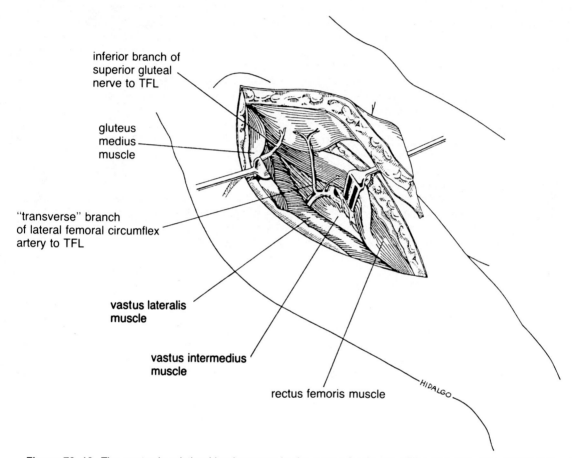

inferior branch of
superior gluteal
nerve to TFL

gluteus
medius
muscle

"transverse" branch
of lateral femoral circumflex
artery to TFL

vastus lateralis
muscle

vastus intermedius
muscle

rectus femoris muscle

HIDALGO

Figure 76–16. The anatomic relationships important in the tensor fascia lata (TFL) free flap. The lateral femoral cutaneous nerve enters the skin from just anterior to the anterior iliac spine and is not illustrated in the drawing. (From Hidalgo, D. A., and Shaw, W. W.: Tensor fascia lata free flaps. *In* Shaw, W. W., and Hidalgo, D. A. (Eds.): Microsurgery in Trauma. Mount Kisco, Futura Publishing Company, 1987, p 317.)

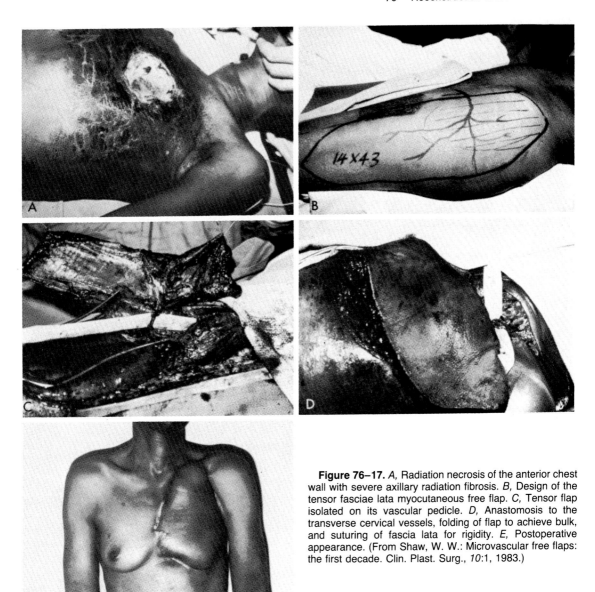

Figure 76–17. *A,* Radiation necrosis of the anterior chest wall with severe axillary radiation fibrosis. *B,* Design of the tensor fasciae lata myocutaneous free flap. *C,* Tensor flap isolated on its vascular pedicle. *D,* Anastomosis to the transverse cervical vessels, folding of flap to achieve bulk, and suturing of fascia lata for rigidity. *E,* Postoperative appearance. (From Shaw, W. W.: Microvascular free flaps: the first decade. Clin. Plast. Surg., *10*:1, 1983.)

the location where the lateral femoral circumflex vessels emerge under the rectus femoris muscle to enter the tensor muscle. After this has been identified, the upper skin incision is made and the separation between the tensor muscle and the rectus muscle anteriorly and the gluteus medius muscle pos-

teriorly is completed as far as the ilium as needed. For maximum mobility, the origin from the ilium is detached and the island flap can be easily moved to cover sizable defects of the lower abdomen. If needed, the continuation of the vessels posteriorly to the gluteus muscles can be divided to give more anterior mobility. The vessels can also be divided after the rectus femoris branch in order to use it as a microvascular free flap.

For chest wall reconstruction, the long vascular pedicle allows anastomoses to the axillary cervical vessels. The strong fascia lata can also be useful in reconstruction of the chest wall for stability with autologous tissue, avoiding the need for synthetic material (Shaw and associates, 1980). If a large skin surface is needed, the flap may include the entire lateral half of the thigh and the rectus femoris muscle may be included on the same vascular pedicle.

Omentum

Omentum has been used by surgeons to cover difficult abdominal wounds for decades. Alday and Goldsmith (1972) studied the omentum's blood supply to allow its mobilization into the extremities for treatment of lymphedema. Dupont and Menard (1972) described using the omentum based on either the right or left gastroepiploic vessels for extra-abdominal transfers for chest wall reconstruction (Fig. 76–18). The exposed omentum was covered with a skin graft in one stage. Marlex mesh was used under the omentum in one of their patients (Dupont and Menard, 1972). Others have since reported similar types of reconstruction, most commonly for recurrent breast carcinoma or for radiation necrosis (Jurkiewicz and Arnold, 1977; Jacobs and associates, 1978). Nakao and associates (1986) reported a series of nine patients who underwent omentum reconstruction following wide resection of the chest wall for recurrent, advanced breast carcinoma. They reported significant improvement in the quality of life of the patients. In two of the patients, an acryl-resin plate was placed under the omentum. The largest defect was 15 by 20 cm. Hakelius (1978), however, reported a case of fatal complication of intestinal strangulation from the use of a pedicled omentum for chest wall reconstruction. Although such complications are rare and potentially correctable, the need for a laparotomy to harvest the omentum makes it a less ideal technique compared to the use of regional muscles as a primary flap for chest wall reconstruction. It is, however, an important option when no other flaps are available or when laparotomy is performed for other reasons at the same time.

Flap Dissection. To utilize the omentum for pedicled transfer, there should be two major anatomic considerations: the dissection of the omentum from the transverse colon and the selective division of the omental vessels to gain flap length. Although they were separate structures originally, in the course of development, the posterior surface of the omentum generally becomes adherent to the transverse colon and its mesocolon from the hepatic to splenic flexure. Separation of the two structures along the potentially avascular plane requires care to avoid injury to the colon or the middle colic vessels within the mesocolon. The omentum is partially detached from the greater curvature of the stomach by dividing either the right or the left gastroepiploic vessels while preserving the vascular arcade with the omentum. Depending on the pattern of the vascular arcades within the omentum, it can usually be further subdivided and unfolded to increase its reach (Hidalgo, 1987) (Fig. 76–19). Care must be taken to avoid twists or compression of the pedicle. Potential holes or loops of the omentum within the abdomen should be obliterated to avoid possible internal bowel herniation.

Miscellaneous Flaps

Total Arm Flaps. In a patient with a large recurrent breast carcinoma involving the subclavian vessels and the brachial plexus, Fuentes (1986) described a total arm flap for reconstruction of the left shoulder and upper two thirds of the anterior chest. The upper arm skin and muscles, as inferior as the elbow, were harvested as a bulky flap based on the shoulder collaterals around the subscapular vessels. Although five ribs were resected, the rigidity of the flap was sufficient to prevent postoperative respiratory problems without the use of bone grafts or Marlex. The patient, unfortunately, succumbed several months later to massive systemic metastases.

The circumference of the arm or the forearm, indeed, is sufficiently large to cover an entire anterior or posterior hemichest. Its use as a flap is obviously justified only in extremely desperate cases or in situations when the arm would otherwise be amputated. In this case, with the tumor encased around the brachial plexus, the arm, if left, would have been totally flail and insensate after the resection of the clavicle, trapezius muscle and the brachial plexus.

The arm and the forearm can be "de-boned"

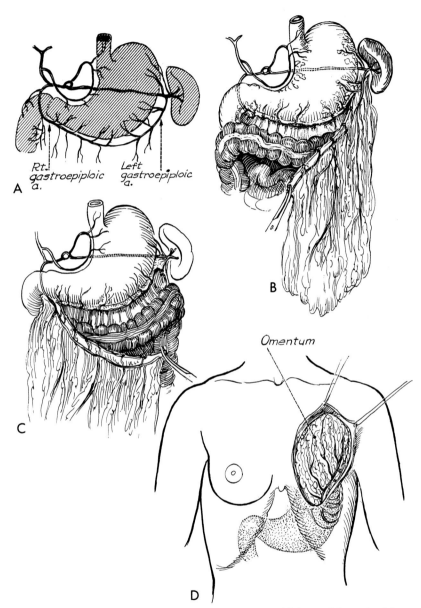

Figure 76–18. Closure of a chest wall defect with greater omentum. *A,* Main arterial supply of the greater omentum. *B, C,* The greater omentum can be pedicled on the right or left gastroepiploic artery, depending on the site of the defect to be closed. The omental flap is freed from the stomach at the muscularis layer in order to maintain the integrity of the vascular gastroepiploic arch. *D,* The greater omentum is transferred to the thoracic defect through the superior portion of the abdominal wall incision or through a separate stab wound. A subcutaneous tunnel may be utilized to pass the omentum to the defect. (After Dupont, C., and Menard Y.: Transposition of the greater omentum for reconstruction of the chest wall. Plast. Reconstr. Surg., *49:*263, 1972.)

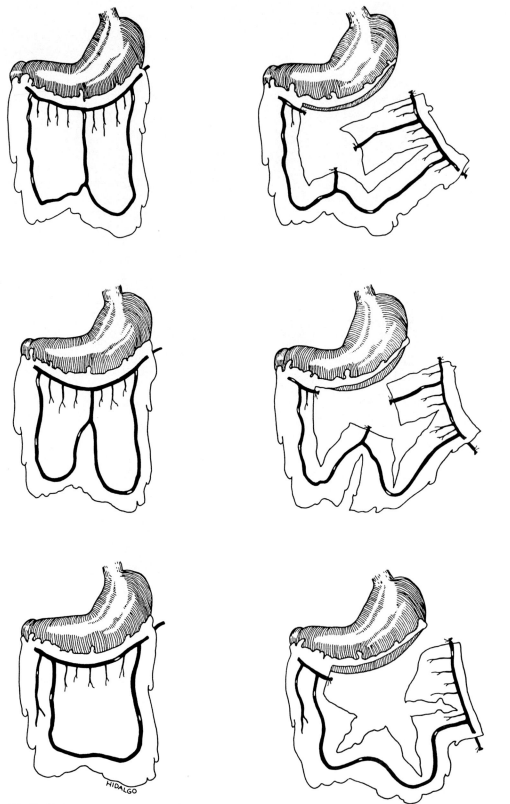

Figure 76–19. Variations in the omental vascular anatomy and the methods of flap lengthening. (From Hidalgo, D. A.: Omentum free flaps. *In* Shaw, W. W., and Hidalgo, D. A. (Eds.): Microsurgery in Trauma. Mount Kisco, Futura Publishing Company, 1987, p. 386.)

and utilized as a free flap for large coverage. In a patient with traumatic disarticulation at the shoulder with exposed chest, the deboned arm and forearm can be reattached to cover the large upper chest-shoulder defect (Fig. 76–20) (Colen and associates, 1983).

Unilateral or Bilateral Breast Flaps. The use of the opposite breast as a flap was first described in 1924 by Achepelman (Aston and Pickrell, 1977), who split the breast to gain additional width. Maier (1947), Pickrell, Kelley, and Marzoni (1948), Beardsley (1950), Urban (1951), Whalen (1953), Rees and Converse (1965), and Latham (1966) also reported similar procedures. In women with moderate or large breasts, this technique can provide a readily accessible source of adjacent skin flap for coverage and protection of the underlying synthetic graft material. The esthetic appearance of the distorted breast or a "cyclops"-like chest is rarely justified today, except in the most desperate cases (Fig. 76–21). In poor-risk patients less concerned with appearance, the opposite breast skin may be split and used as flaps while the excess breast tissue is removed. This technique provides large surface areas as well as a somewhat less grotesque appearance. (Fig. 76–22). Tsur, Shafir, and Lieberman (1982) mobilized both breasts to reconstruct a midline anterior chest wall defect and achieved a reasonably good esthetic result.

External Oblique Muscle. Hodgkinson and Arnold (1980) rotated a laterally based external oblique muscle from the lower abdomen to fill a defect in the lower anterior chest. The segmental blood supply to this muscle comes superolaterally from the lateral intercostal perforators, and the distal insertion of the muscle is along the lateral edge of the rectus abdominis muscle forming the semilunar line. For limited defects, this technique appears to be a reasonable option because of its convenience.

Diaphragm Mobilization. In patients with poor risk or cancer prognosis, Tsur, Lieberman, and Heim (1984) advocated a relatively simple procedure to reconstruct lower chest defects by detaching the anterior portion of the diaphragm and reinserting it superiorly at the edge of chest wall resection. This technique effectively restores the integrity of the chest cavity by reducing its volume. Local skin rotation flaps or skin grafts can complete the surface coverage required.

Free Flaps

Although the availability of musculocutaneous flaps and muscles has greatly expanded our ability to reconstruct many previously difficult defects, free flaps remain useful in certain special situations. The latissimus dorsi muscle may have been transected by prior thoracotomy, or its pedicle may have been severely compromised by irradiation. The pectoralis major muscle often has been removed by previous mastectomy or may have become scarred or destroyed by irradiation. Mediastinal irradiation or surgery can render both the ipsilateral and contralateral rectus abdominis muscles unreliable. The omentum may not be easily available in cases of previous upper abdominal surgery. Finally, the defect may be sufficiently large, so that it cannot be reconstructed with the available regional flaps. In most cases, a significant part of a muscle flap may be wasted in the transfer to the defect, so that the useful part of the flap is limited. Microvascular free flaps, on the other hand, can be harvested from any part of the body with relatively little wastage of their pedicles.

During the past decade, with improving results and a survival rate of 95 per cent, the indications for free flaps have broadened (Shaw, 1983). As in other parts of the body, the technique is no longer indicated only when no other choices are available. Free flaps are chosen over regional flaps because of convenience, less functional loss, versatility of reconstruction, and better esthetic results. The surgeon, however, must be aware of the special problems associated with microvascular free flaps in chest wall reconstruction so as to be able to achieve results more reliable than and superior to regional flaps.

Recipient Vessels. An ideal free flap recipient vessel should be of reasonable caliber (1.5 mm to 2.5 mm), outside of the zone of injury, easily accessible, anatomically consistent, potentially dispensable, and conveniently located near the defect. Because of the large area of the chest and the paucity of large trunk vessels in the anterior aspect, the selection of proper recipient vessels must come from the axilla, neck, or mediastinum. At times, long vein grafts are also required.

The axilla provides several significant arterial branches, in addition to the potential

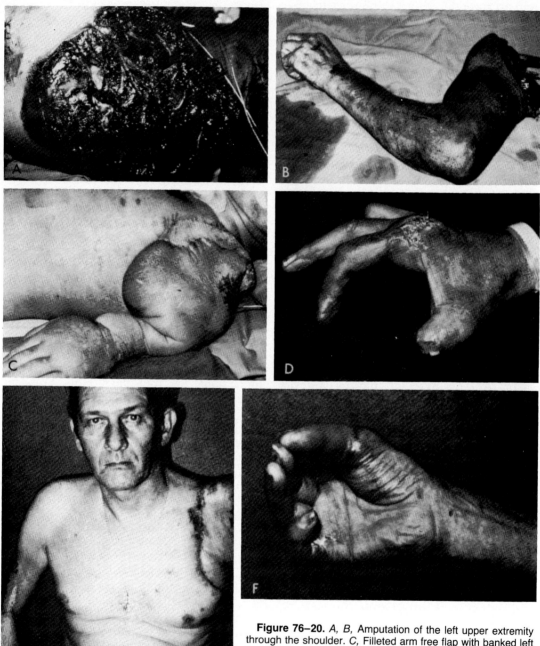

Figure 76–20. *A, B,* Amputation of the left upper extremity through the shoulder. *C,* Filleted arm free flap with banked left hand. *D,* Amputation of the right thumb. *E, F,* Appearance nine months after surgery. (From Colen, S. R., Romita, M. C., Godfrey, N. V., and Shaw, W. W.: Salvage replantation. Clin. Plast. Surg., *10:*125, 1983.)

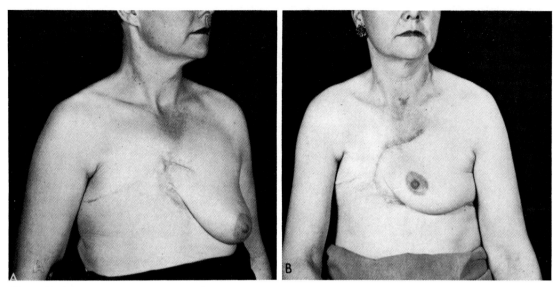

Figure 76–21. *A,* A recurrent carcinoma of the sternum and ribs in a 47 year old woman who had a radical mastectomy one year previously. The patient had received a full course of irradiation postoperatively. An en bloc excision of the sternum and third, fourth, fifth, sixth, and seventh ribs was performed. The operative defect was covered and closed by transposing the left breast on a superior pedicle. *B,* Four years after operation.

for vein grafts directly onto the axillary artery. It is therefore the most common source for recipient arteries. The *subscapular* and *thoracodorsal system* may be utilized at any convenient point. When taken above the serratus branch for end-to-end anastomosis, the distal flow to the latissimus dorsi muscle is preserved via the collaterals from the serratus anterior and its potential use as a flap is maintained. The *thoracoacromial artery,* or a stump of it, is nearly always available. The pectoralis major muscle may need to be split and retracted or temporarily divided at its insertion and then repaired. When the axilla is not convenient, the *transverse cervical artery* can be found through a collar incision that is esthetically well concealed. The *internal mammary artery* can be predictably exposed by resecting a single segment of costal cartilage and is always of satisfactory caliber (2 mm or larger). The *intercostal arteries,* on the other hand, are usually smaller (1 mm or under) and have many muscular branches that make dissection difficult. Finally, the omentum and the *gastroepiploic artery* have been used by Harii and Ohmori (1973) as recipient arteries when no other vessels are available.

Donor Sites. The most common requisite in chest wall reconstruction is usually the need for large surface coverage. Thickness to fill out or restore contour is also a require-

ment. Bone or fascia as a part of a microvascular free flap may be an additional feature when structural support is needed. The *contralateral latissimus dorsi,* lower *rectus abdominis* or *tensor fascia lata* musculocutaneous free flaps are the most commonly considered donor flaps for chest wall reconstruction. The tensor fasciae lata microvascular free flap has the advantage of being located at a distance away from the chest, therefore, allowing for simultaneous dissection while the chest is debrided. The flap also does not further compromise the postoperative respiratory care, as may be the case with abdominal or back flaps. When a very large flap is needed, one can also incorporate the rectus femoris or the vastus lateralis muscles in the flap.

Technical Considerations. Aside from basic principles applicable to all microvascular free flap surgery and chest wall reconstructions, certain problems deserve special attention. The *exposure* for microvascular anastomoses around the chest is generally much more awkward than in the extremities. Often the surgeon or the assistant may have difficulty sitting comfortably, and the anastomoses may even need to be done with the surgeon in the standing position. *Respiratory movement* of the chest may cause the structures under the microscope to go in and out of focus, making suturing technically diffi-

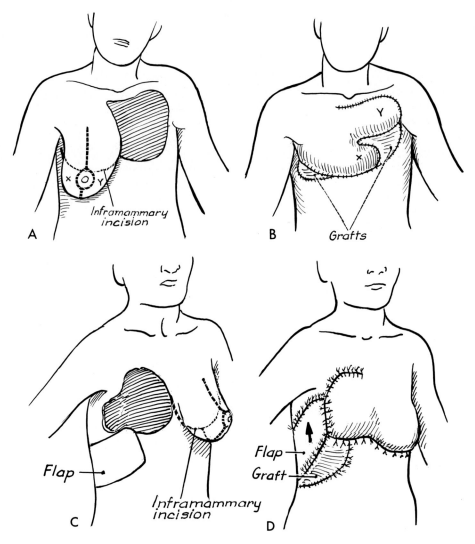

Figure 76–22. *A, B,* Complete split breast flap technique with cleavage of the breast extending from the inframammary crease to the superior limit of breast tissue. The nipple in this case has been discarded, but it can be retained if additional tissue is needed. This technique provides the largest amount of readily available tissue for defect closure. *C, D,* The complete split breast technique used in conjunction with a local transposition flap to close a defect of the anterior thoracic wall with extension into the axilla. (After Whalen, W. P.: Coverage of thoracic wall defects by a split breast flap. Plast. Reconstr. Surg., *12:*64, 1953.)

cult. During the critical period of the anastomoses, it may be necessary to reduce the tidal volume and to use more frequent but smaller chest excursions. The need for *rigid support* may be more important for free flaps than regional flaps. The vulnerable vascular pedicle must be protected from excessive movement associated with the positive lung ventilations from the respirator. The anastomoses must also be well protected from the possibility of compression or kinking. The excessive intrathoracic pressure generated postoperatively may be minimized by using "jet ventilators" instead of the usual volume respirators.

GRAFTS AND SYNTHETIC MATERIALS FOR STRUCTURAL SUPPORT

Indications for Skeletal Support

Not all skeletal components of chest wall defects need to be specifically replaced. The semirigid frame of ribs, sternum, cartilage, joints, and muscles cannot be fully substituted by either rigid materials or by fascia. Small defects in healthy patients with satisfactory functional reserves are extremely well tolerated. Radiation and other chronic inflammatory conditions generally result in sufficient adhesion formation and rigidity so that surgical stabilization is not needed (Boyd and associates, 1981). Finally, the inherent stiffness and bulk of musculocutaneous flaps,

such as the latissimus dorsi, would tend to minimize significant paradoxical movements.

Patients with compromised pulmonary functional reserve from emphysema or other causes are more vulnerable to any loss of skeletal support. This is usually manifested by diminished exercise capacity. The functional loss is proportional to the size of the defect. If the relative importance of any established paradoxical movement is in question, the need for skeletal stabilization can be determined by pulmonary function tests. Finally, surgical loss of the sternum may be poorly tolerated and skeletal reconstruction should be considered. Chronic sternotomy dehiscence, on the other hand, may be associated with sufficient scar and the need for prolonged intubation and positive ventilatory support is thus alleviated. The preoperative pulmonary function evaluation is important.

Methods of Skeletal Stabilization

A wide variety of methods have been used for chest wall stabilization. Autogenous sources include pedicled ribs, free rib grafts, iliac bone, or fascia lata. Synthetic materials include Marlex, polytef (Teflon)-felt patch, acrylic, and Marlex-acrylic sandwich (McCormack and associates, 1981) (Fig. 76–23). Comparisons of the different methods are difficult because the number of cases reported with each method is small, there is a lack of

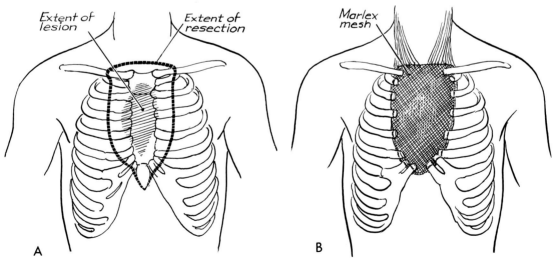

Figure 76–23. Reconstruction following total resection of the sternum. *A,* The extent of the total sternal resection. *B,* Reconstruction was accomplished with Marlex mesh sutured to the margins of the defect and covered with the pectoralis muscles approximated in the midline. (After Baue, A.: Total resection of the sternum. J. Thorac. Cardiovasc. Surg., *45:*559, 1963.)

objective physiologic data, and the indications are inconsistent. The selection of the different methods is generally based on presumptions about the properties of different material. Bone grafts are ideal, in that they become permanently incorporated and do not deteriorate with time. The sources and available sizes, however, are limited.

Pers and Medgyesi (1973) described using lower ribs pedicled on the serratus muscle to reconstruct an upper chest defect (Fig. 76–24). Mauer and Blades (1946) cut an adjacent rib obliquely to wire its free end to the next rib to provide more stabilization (Fig. 76–25).

Arnold (1981) emphasized the importance of tailoring the bone grafts to achieve satisfactory esthetic results (Fig. 76–26). Fascia or synthetic meshes have sufficient flexibility to conform to the required contour and can be easily sutured in place. There is, however, always some residual paradoxical movement. Acrylic can be easily molded in the operating room to fit the skeletal defect, but its edges tend to move against the rest of the chest wall with motion and respiration. The Marlex-methacrylate sandwich has the advantage of allowing suturing of the edges, yet providing rigidity in the center. In general,

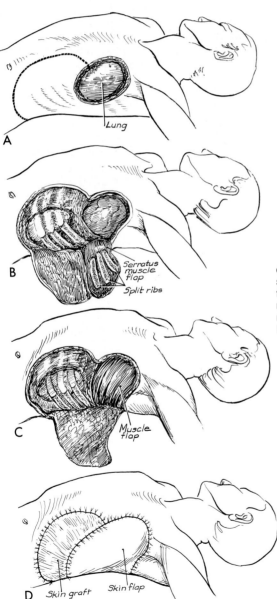

Figure 76–24. Muscle-rib flap closure of a lateral thoracic defect. *A,* Defect with exposed lung. *B,* Serratus muscle-split rib flap developed. *C,* Muscle-rib flap closing the thoracic defect. *D,* Large local skin flap used to cover the muscle-rib flap. (After Pers, M., and Medgyesi, S.: Pedicle muscle flaps and their applications in the surgery of repair. Br. J. Plast. Surg., 26:313, 1973.)

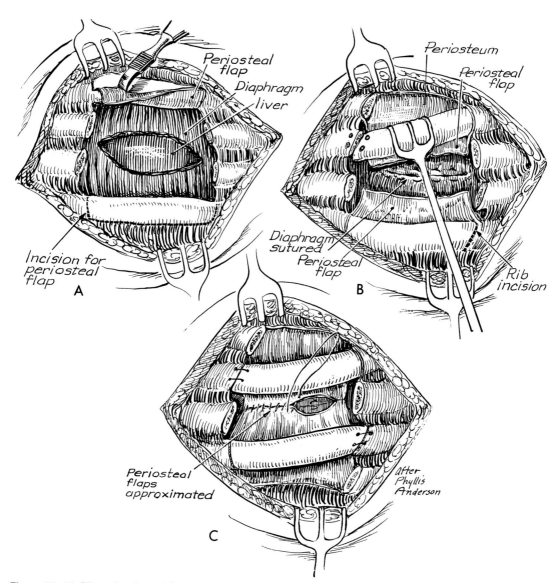

Figure 76–25. Rib and periosteal flap closure of thoracic defects. *A,* Full-thickness chest wall defect. Periosteum being elevated from the ribs for periosteal flaps. *B,* Rib cut tangentially and displaced to the cut end of the adjacent rib. Drill holes placed through the cut ends of the ribs for suture stabilization. *C,* Periosteal flaps approximated under tension over the chest wall defect. The displaced ribs are secured to the tangentially cut ends by chromic catgut sutures. (After Mauer, E., and Blades, B.: Hernia of the lung. J. Thorac. Surg., *15:*77, 1946.)

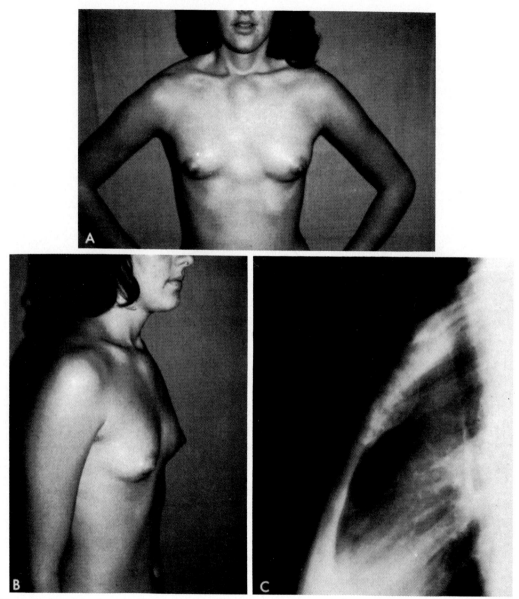

Figure 76–26. *A* to *D,* An 18 year old woman with a 12 month history of upper sternal mass diagnosed as chondrosarcoma. After wide resection of the upper one third of the sternum, the adjacent first three ribs, and the clavicles, the anterior bony thorax was reconstructed with three whole rib grafts (two horizontal and one vertical strut—secured with a rabbit joint laterally and wired to each other centrally). The superior horizontal strut is back-cut in multiple areas to allow the rig to be "bowed" out to prevent its direct contact with the aortic outflow tract. *E,* The left "nondominant" pectoralis major muscle is divided at its insertion and freed from the subcutaneous and chest wall attachments to be moved medially to cover the reconstructed bony anterior chest. *F,* The appearance of the wound at the time of closure. *G, H,* Appearance ten months following resection. (From Arnold, P. G.: Reconstruction of the sternum and anterior chest wall: aesthetic considerations. Clin. Plast. Surg., *8:*391, 1981.)

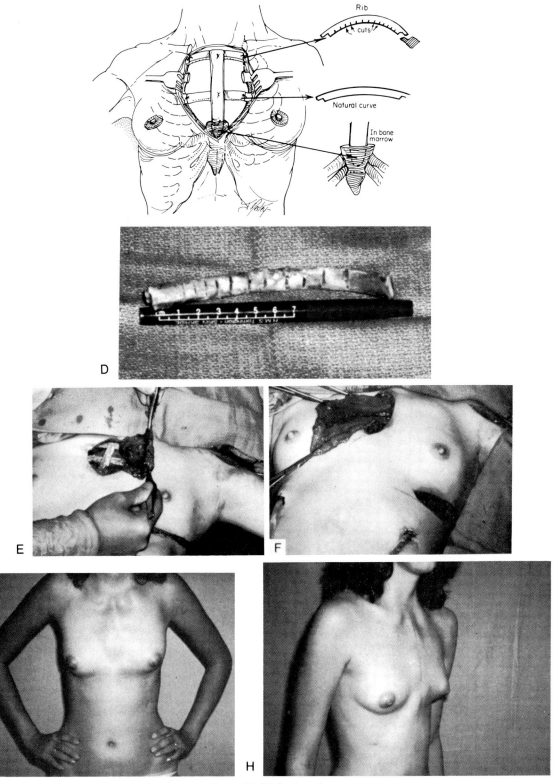

Figure 76–26 *Continued*

large defects with radiation injury or poor soft tissue coverage are better reconstructed with autogenous bone or fascial grafts to minimize the risks of infection or extrusion of the synthetic material. If necessary, a wide resection and replacement with a well-vascularized flap for coverage should be done first or simultaneously.

Reconstructive Problems

CHEST WALL INJURY

Emergency Care

Minor chest wall injuries with *fractures of a few ribs* are common. Although the physiologic derangements are minor, the pain from movements of the ribs with respiration or activities is often excruciating. The main therapeutic goal is to relieve pain by medication or to minimize rib motion by splinting or taping of the chest.

Major chest wall injuries from penetrating or blunt trauma are frequently associated with life-threatening emergencies of the cardiovascular or respiratory systems. The initial efforts are dominated by massive efforts to combat cardiorespiratory failure, hemorrhage, or shock. The use of positive pressure respirators has allowed a more elective management of chest wall problems. Plastic surgeons are generally called to reconstruct chest wall defects only after the patient has survived the initial stages of resuscitation. Some general understanding of the emergency management of chest wounds is, however, essential to the plastic surgeon involved with the chest surgeon in both acute and long-term reconstructions.

Aside from general resuscitative measures, few emergency surgical procedures are indicated. Open or "sucking" wounds should be simply covered with petroleum jelly (Vaseline) gauze and occlusive dressings to minimize gross leaks. "Stab wounds" with knives or sticks still in the chest are best brought to the hospital with the penetrating objects in place. Such objects may serve as temporary seals, and their removal results in sudden uncontrollable bleeding or pulmonary collapse. Romero and associates (1978) reported a case of a 29 year old man impaled in the right upper chest by a 6 foot long, 4 by 4 inch wooden post during an automobile accident. The patient was rapidly transported to the hospital with the wooden post protruding anteriorly and posteriorly. The wooden post was removed in the operating room under direct vision after a thoracotomy was first performed and the great vessels secured. After partial lung resection for contusion, skin grafts and later musculocutaneous flap coverage of the entry wound, the patient survived and was discharged. Attempts to remove the pole at the site of injury would have certainly resulted in prompt exsanguination and death. If, however, there is evidence of respiratory distress from "tension pneumothorax," a chest tube or temporary one-way trephine may be life saving. In rare instances, those with cardiac tamponade or restrictive hemothorax may benefit briefly from aspiration and decompression. Quick transfer of the patient to a properly equipped hospital emergency room and operating room is usually more important than wasting time performing risky procedures under suboptimal circumstances.

The mortality of the "multiple trauma" patients tends to fall into three peaks in relation to the time of injury (Trunkey, 1983). Approximately 50 per cent die at the scene of the accident and basically cannot be salvaged regardless of the type of medical care. A second phase of deaths occurs within the next few hours, resulting mostly from *hemorrhage* and *shock*. Rapid transportation and aggressive resuscitation may salvage some of these patients. Finally, 20 per cent of the trauma deaths occur days or weeks later, largely as a result of *sepsis* and the attendant *multiple organ failure.*The survivors typically require prolonged intensive care and at times multiple surgical procedures. These are grim reminders that in all of these patients one must be prepared to deal with multiple injuries as well as difficult systemic problems. Decisions regarding the type of flaps or reconstruction, therefore, must always be considered relative to the patient's overall situation.

Emergency Surgery

Incision and Soft Tissue Restoration. For patients with sizable soft tissue loss resulting from injuries such as blast wounds, the plastic surgeon should be involved in the planning of the incisions for the emergency thoracic surgical procedure. Depending on the injury, the surgery may involve simple debridement and wound closure or wide exposure of the chest for control of bleeding, removal of foreign bodies, repair of lacerations, lung resection, or repair of bronchial lacerations. Most standard thoracotomy incisions in the fourth to sixth interspaces result in transections across the valuable latissimus dorsi or pectoralis major muscles. With a few minutes of extra time, these muscles and their overlying skin can be preserved as invaluable large regional flaps. Instead of a tight closure after debridement, one can achieve a more generous debridement and a well-vascularized, tension-free closure. The regional muscles can also be utilized to wrap around bronchial stumps or repairs.

Skeletal Stabilization. Occasionally, *grossly displaced fractured ribs* may protrude into the pleural cavity requiring early surgical intervention. In isolated rib protrusions, simple resection may be sufficient. With multiple fractures, stabilization can be accomplished with Kirschner wires, looped wires, or screw plates (Hood, 1986). Most sternal fractures can be treated conservatively. *Subluxed sternal fractures* should be surgically reduced and maintained with heavy wire sutures or plates.

Late Reconstructions after Trauma

Complex surgical reconstructions involving *bone* or *synthetic grafts* or *distant flaps* are rarely indicated acutely. The patients are generally in poor condition for prolonged surgery and the wounds may be contused and partially contaminated. In most cases, a few days of systemic resuscitation, positive pressure respirator therapy and aseptic occlusive local wound care allow delayed, definitive reconstruction with a greater chance of success. After the patient is stabilized, the reconstructive methods are not substantially different from the elective reconstructions associated with tumor resections. *Costal cartilage fractures* that may persist as painful non-union are best treated by resection. *Infected cartilage* also requires wide debridement, although the perichondrium may be preserved to provide later stability. When the costal arch is involved, it may be difficult to resect the entire arch and wide resection is followed with well-vascularized muscle coverage.

BENIGN AND MALIGNANT NEOPLASMS

Tumors of the chest wall from primary, metastatic, or adjacent neoplasms are rela-tively infrequent. Except for patients with extremely poor prognoses, surgical resection along with immediate reconstruction is the primary treatment. The reconstructive possibilities are important in planning the management of these problems.

In a series of 100 consecutive patients, Pairolero and Arnold (1985) reported 50 primary malignant neoplasms, 32 metastatic lesions, and 18 benign tumors. Surgical resection included multiple ribs, sternum, and, in 47 per cent, an en bloc resection of the overlying soft tissue. There was one operative death. At a median follow-up of 32 months, all patients with benign tumors, 95 per cent of patients with primary tumors, and 59 per cent of patients with metastatic tumors were living. The authors concluded that aggressive resection for chest wall tumors with reliable reconstruction can be accomplished safely and that early, wide resection is potentially curative for most and at least palliative in the remainder. The more aggressive philosophy of wide resection and definitive reconstruction is also supported by others (Ramming and associates, 1982).

Primary Chest Wall Tumors

Primary tumors of the chest wall are uncommon, and therefore some questions remain regarding the incidence, prognosis, and treatment options. Pascuzzini, Dahlin, and Clagett (1957) in a survey of 2000 bone tumors from the Mayo Clinic found 6 per cent originating from the ribs and 1 per cent from the sternum. The presence of a mass or pain is the most common presentation, but neither is a reliable indicator of malignancy. Tumors in children or the elderly are more prone to be malignant as Ewing's sarcoma or myelomas, respectively. Anterior lesions of the costal cartilage or sternum and tumors larger than 4 cm in diameter are also likely to be malignant (Boyd, 1986). Except for fever, adenopathy, elevated erythrocyte sedimentation rates (ESR), and abnormal lelukocytes in the cases of systemic diseases like myeloma, systemic diagnostic evaluations are generally unrevealing. Radiologic studies with plain radiographs, computed tomographic (CT) scans, and magnetic resonance imaging (MRI) provide the most useful information regarding the extent and nature of the tumors. Frozen section diagnosis at the time of resectional surgery is notoriously unreliable. Because of the extensive resection and reconstruction often required, unequivocal preoperative tissue diagnosis should be established by permanent histologic studies. Needle biopsy or aspiration may be successful; in cases of metastases or systemic disease, it may obviate the need for open biopsy. Smaller lesions of likely benign nature can often be primarily excised at the time of biopsy followed by limited local reconstruction. For larger tumors (greater than 4 cm) of suspicious pathology, open biopsy with a well-planned small incision is usually indicated prior to definitive resection and reconstruction.

Benign Tumors (Table 76–4)

Wide local resection is generally indicated in the following conditions.

Chondroma. This tumor typically occurs at the costochondral junction in young adults and presents as a slow-growing, painless mass, frequently of enormous size. Radiographs show the tumors as medullary masses often with stipled calcifications but without penetration of the overlying cortex.

Fibrous Dysplasia. This tumor is usually seen prior to puberty as a painless, slow growing mass in the posterior rib area. On radiographic study, the tumors appear as

Table 76–4. Histologic Classification of Benign Chest Wall Neoplasms

Type of Tumor	No. of Patients	Per Cent of Total
Chondromatous	19	37.3
Fibrous dysplasia	8	15.7
Osteogenic	7	13.7
Lipoma	3	5.9
Giant cell	2	3.9
Miscellaneous	12	23.5
Eosinophilic granuloma	1	
Osteomyelitis	1	
Mesenchymoma	1	
Fibroxanthoma	1	
Bone cyst	1	
Hemangioendothelioma	1	
Benign hemangiopericytoma	1	
Granuloma (noncaseating)	1	
Lymphangioma	1	
Benign mass (not histologically classified)	2	
Tuberculoma	1	
Total	51	100%

*From Graeber, G. M., Snyder, R. J., Fleming, A. W., et al.: Initial and long-term results in the management of primary chest wall neoplasms. Ann. Thorac. Surg., *34:*665, 1982. Reprinted with permission from The Society of Thoracic Surgeons.

fusiform expanding osteolytic lesions with a thin, overlying cortex.

Osteochondroma. This rare, small, painless, hard tumor in young patients ceases growing with the closure of the nearest bony epiphysis. Later growth or pain suggests malignant degeneration, which occurs in about 20 per cent.

Neurogenic Tumor. This is usually a small tumor arising from the intercostal nerve with accompanying pain. The tumors may be multiple, and approximately 15 per cent are reported as malignant.

Desmoid Tumor. This rare benign, but locally aggressive, fibrous tumor, usually arises from the intercostal muscles. Despite clinically adequate resection, local recurrence is common and may necessitate secondary resection.

Eosinophilic Granuloma. This disease of the reticuloendothelial system may be associated with fever, malaise, leukocytosis, and eosinophilia. Approximately 10 to 20 per cent of patients have isolated lesions of the rib or sternum presenting as painful lytic lesions with cortical destruction. Local resection or irradiation is usually curative.

Lipoma. Isolated small lipomas are common and are excised generally for esthetic reasons. After the capsule is partially freed from the surrounding tissue, it can almost be "delivered" by squeezing and pulling it out through a relatively small incision placed in the direction of the skin lines. Multiple or large lipomas are less common. Excision is often indicated for discomfort and inconvenience (Fig. 76–27). Occasionally, sensory nerves may be closely involved with excessive fatty accumulation and resultant pain with pressure-adiposis dolorosa (Dercum's disease).

Neurofibromatosis (von Recklinghausen's disease). Multiple cutaneous tumors of nerve sheath origin are scattered all over the body (Fig. 76–28). Surgical excision is done mainly for esthetic reasons. There are sometimes deeper lesions in the major nerve sheaths, and there is an associated propensity for malignant degeneration of the large, initially benign, lesions. Larger and rapidly growing lesions should be excised or a biopsy specimen should be obtained.

Malignant Tumors (Table 76–5)

Chondrosarcoma. This large tumor is most common at the costochondral junctions

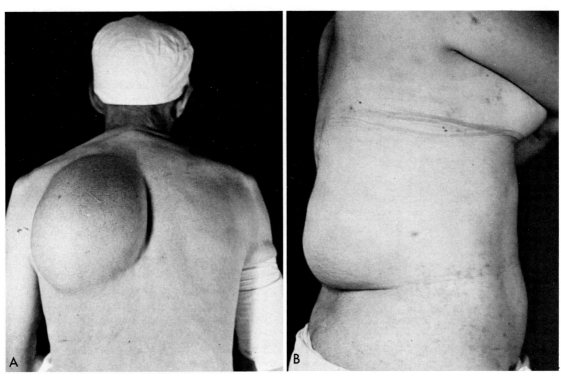

Figure 76–27. *A,* A football-sized lipoma of the back. *B,* A diffuse lipoma of the lower back. The specimen weighed more than 5 lb.

and over the sternum. They are usually slow-growing and may be painful and tender to touch. The skin over the tumor may be fixed and reddened. Radiographs show large lobulated destructive lesions with involvement of the surrounding soft tissue. Stipple calcifica-

Table 76–5. Histologic Classification of Primary Malignant Chest Wall Neoplasms

Type of Tumor	No. of Patients	Per Cent of Total
Fibrosarcoma	19	32.2
Chondrosarcoma	10	16.9
Multiple myeloma	8	13.6
Ewing's sarcoma	6	10.2
Osteogenic sarcoma	4	6.8
Miscellaneous	12	20.3
Hemangioendothelioma, malignant	3	
Rhabdomyosarcoma	3	
Liposarcoma	3	
Reticulum cell sarcoma	1	
Undifferentiated sarcoma	1	
Anaplastic carcinoma	1	
Total	59	100%

*From Graeber, G. M., Snyder, R. J., Fleming, A. W., et al.: Initial and long-term results in the management of primary chest wall neoplasms. Ann. Thorac. Surg., *34:*666, 1982. Reprinted with permission from The Society of Thoracic Surgeons.

tions may be present. Until Jaffe and Lichtenstein (1943) characterized the tumors histologically, such cartilaginous lesions were frequently considered as benign, only to recur later.

Surgery generally involves a full-thickness resection of the chest wall with a macroscopic margin of approximately 5 cm. The ribs above and below, along with a large segment of adjacent sternum, are excised as well. The large skeletal defect (usually three to five ribs) is prone to flailing and is usually reconstructed with a mesh of Marlex, polypropylene (Prolene), Gore-tex, bone, or other material (Arnold and Pairolero, 1978; Larsson and associates, 1984). The overlying soft tissue may be reconstructed with a number of regional musculocutaneous flaps, most commonly the latissimus dorsi or pectoralis major (Fig. 76–29).

These tumors respond poorly to radiation or chemotherapy. McAfee and associates (1985) reviewed the Mayo Clinic's experience and reported a 10 year recurrence rate after wide resection of 17 per cent with 96 per cent survival compared with 50 per cent recurrence and 65 per cent survival after local excision.

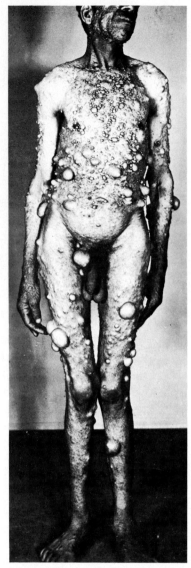

Figure 76–28. Diffuse nodular neurofibromatosis in a 50 year old man. Only the larger masses were excised.

Fibrosarcoma. These large painful tumors may occur anywhere on the chest with frequent skin involvement. Radiographs show large, ill-defined masses with adjacent involvement of the soft tissue and destruction of bone. Wide excision with postoperative chemotherapy is recommended.

Myeloma (Plasmacytoma). Even when this presents as a localized rib lesion, systemic disease invariably develops later. Fever, weakness, and abnormal serum proteins are frequently present. A search for other lesions, particularly multiple punched-out lytic lesions of the skull, should be performed.

A needle biopsy may be sufficient, and systemic chemotherapy is the treatment of choice.

Osteogenic Sarcoma. These painful and rapidly growing tumors occur primarily in adolescents and young adults. A characteristic "sunburst" appearance is seen on radiographic study. Pulmonary metastases occur frequently and early; resection may be done later if indicated. Wide resection with preoperative and postoperative chemotherapy is the treatment of choice.

Ewing's Sarcoma. The tumor generally occurs in adolescents and affects the ribs, and is often with associated fever, malaise, and increased ESR. Early metastases are common in approximately one third of cases at the time of diagnosis. Radiographs show typical "onionskin" calcifications from periosteal elevation. Radical local excision is followed by radiation and chemotherapy.

Miscellaneous Tumors. Angiosarcoma, neurosarcoma, liposarcomas, Hodgkin's disease, and reticulum cell sarcoma can also arise from the chest wall.

Metastatic Tumors

With bone metastases, solitary tumors of the chest wall are as likely to represent a metastasis as a primary tumor. Sternum metastases are most likely to be from lesions of the breast, thyroid, kidney, testicle, lung, stomach, and colon. Ribs may be the site for invasive as well as metastatic breast carcinoma. Lesions of the clavicle and scapula are most likely to be metastases from visceral organs.

Local resection of metastatic lesions is rarely indicated, especially in cases of multiple lesions.

Invasive Chest Wall Tumors

Carcinomas of the lung, breast, and skin not infrequently may involve the chest wall and may be amenable to local resection and reconstruction (Fig. 76–30). When carcinoma of the lung involves the lateral pleura, away from the anterior and posterior midline areas, resection can usually be done en bloc along with the primary tumor. With medial lesions, the spine or the anterior mediastinum is involved and en bloc resection is not feasible (LeRoux and Shama, 1983). The 5 year survival following such en bloc resection is ap-

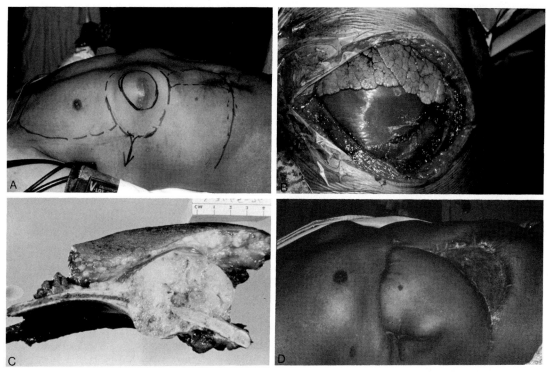

Figure 76–29. A 60 year old man with one year history of a painless enlarging mass of the lower ribs. *A,* Biopsy confirmed the diagnosis of chondrosarcoma. *B,* The wide resection of chest wall with the exposed lung and diaphragm. *C,* The resected specimen on cross section. *D,* Closure with a Marlex mesh to the ribs and a simple rotation skin flap and skin graft to the donor area.

proximately 35 per cent. In the Mayo Clinic experience, the tumor type was not important but the presence of lymph nodes reduced the survival to 7 per cent instead of 54 per cent. Tumors in the apical region invading the upper ribs and brachial plexus—the Pancoast tumor—are generally considered to be of grave prognosis and of questionable resecta-bility. Paulson (1979), however, showed a 31 per cent 5 year survival with preoperative radiation followed by radical resection.

Breast carcinomas may occasionally involve the chest wall as large and deep-seated primary lesions or, more frequently, as a recurrence after mastectomy. In the presence of multiple metastases, local resection must

Figure 76–30. Recurrent breast carcinoma of the chest wall after mastectomy and radiation. (Courtesy of Dr. Sumner Slavin.)

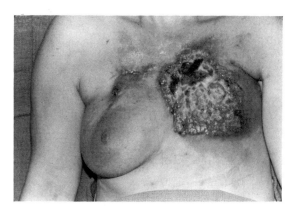

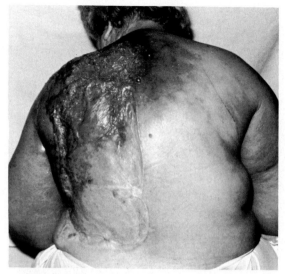

Figure 76–31. Postirradiation injury of the skin of the posterior trunk.

be tempered against the prognosis of the patient and should not interfere with the patient's appropriate program of chemotherapy. On occasions, such lesions may be relatively isolated and resection may be worthwhile. Particularly when it is associated with radiation necrosis, resection and reconstruction may represent the best palliation.

Squamous and basal cell carcinomas of the skin rarely necessitate full-thickness resection of the chest wall. Occasionally, large lesions or recurrent lesions after radiation may best be treated by wide local resection and reconstruction (Fig. 76–31).

THE IRRADIATED CHEST WALL

Therapeutic radiation may be given to the chest preoperatively as the primary treatment for certain diseases, such as Hodgkin's, to facilitate resection and postoperatively as a prevention of local recurrence or as part of the primary treatment of breast carcinoma along with a partial mastectomy. The biology of radiation injury becomes an important factor in surgical reconstruction in dealing with necrosis and ulceration from radiation, recurrence after regional radiation, and wound dehiscence in a previously irradiated area.

Biology of Radiation and Wound Healing

The biologic consequences of tissue irradiation are well known. However, several fundamental principles pertinent to chest wall

reconstruction need to be emphasized (Arnold and Pairolero, 1986).

Radiation results in permanent microvascular fibrosis and compromise of the circulation. The tissue fibrosis also impedes leukocyte migration and inflammatory response, which are essential to wound healing. The extent of radiation injury is invariably wider than the observable area of necrosis or severe skin changes. Wound edges involving irradiated tissue heal more slowly and are prone to dehiscence and breakdown. The effect of radiation is permanent and progressive; thus any ulceration is more likely to become worse with time rather than better. The affected soft tissue becomes progressively more scarred and rigid, making skin flaps less pliable and successful. Because the path of radiation is across all layers of tissue, the area of necrosis and damage is often full-thickness, requiring a through-and-through resection and reconstruction (Hines and Lee, 1983). Finally, radiation may result in necrosis of the soft tissue, cartilage, and bone, converting them into sequestra vulnerable to persistent infection. Pulmonary fibrosis may require lobectomy or partial resection. Patients with subclavian-axillary artery thrombosis or hemorrhage may require emergency surgery.

Surgical Plan

The fundamental principles for surgery involving irradiated tissues are as follows:

1. Excise as much of the irradiated tissue as possible to minimize the presence of compromised tissue vulnerable to chronic infection.

2. Reconstruct with healthy, well-vascularized tissue to maximize the chances of primary wound healing.

3. Avoid foreign material, poorly vascularized tissue, or closure under tension. In practice, this means wide excision of the necrotic center along with adjacent irradiated margins and reconstruction with a large regional musculocutaneous flap or microvascular free flap.

The above concepts are well borne out by clinical experience over the years. With occasional exceptions, simple excision with primary closure or skin grafting is notorious for poor wound healing with propensity for recurrent ulcerations (Robinson, 1975; Rees and Converse, 1965; Woods and associates, 1979). The usefulness of bringing to the irradiated area a new and permanent blood supply that does not have to be interrupted later was well known to earlier plastic surgeons involved in treating these problems (Brown, Fryer, and McDowell, 1951). The flaps available for reconstruction of such large defects have improved significantly. Laterally or medially based abdominal flaps provided the first of the more reliable flaps (Woods and associates, 1979). Omentum became popular because of its availability and familiarity to the general surgeon (Dupont and Menard, 1972; Jurkiewicz and Arnold, 1977; Jacobs and associates, 1978; Nakao and associates, 1986). The latissimus dorsi, pectoralis major, and rectus abdominis muscle and musculocutaneous flaps are currently most commonly used when available. Finally, microvascular free flaps can provide, consistently, the largest coverage and have the additional advantage of not borrowing from the adjacent area. The newer and larger flaps have reduced the complication rate of reconstruction probably because of the more adequate resection of the irradiated margin along with the more vigorous blood supply supplied by the flaps. Boyd and associates (1981) reported an incidence of 36 per cent flap necrosis with 11 random pattern skin flaps, a problem that did not occur with ten consecutive musculocutaneous or microvascular free flaps.

Radiation Ulcerations Associated with Breast Cancer

Following mastectomy, radiation therapy may be given to the internal mammary node region, axilla, or chest wall. Despite improvements in radiation therapy, occasional cases of radiation tissue necrosis and ulceration are still seen (Woods and associates, 1979). The lesions start as erythematous, hyperpigmented, and atrophic skin changes that progress to ulceration, necrosis of the underlying bone and cartilage, and chronic infection (Fig. 76–32).

Local wound care can minimize the level of gross infection but rarely results in spontaneous healing. Untreated wounds tend to progress with more ulceration, necrosis, infection, and scarring. This results in a foul-smelling, purulent infection, extension of the ulcer, and ultimately systemic evidence of sepsis. The patient may eventually succumb to pneumonia, sepsis, or massive arterial hemorrhage. After chest wall ulceration is present, this should be considered as a life-threatening problem. Inadequate resection and faulty flap reconstruction are almost certainly doomed to recurrent breakdown and infection (Fig. 76–33). Aggressive, wide resection of the affected chest wall and reconstruction with a large flap are needed. In the early stages, adequate excision followed by reconstruction with well-vascularized flaps can be accomplished relatively easily (Fig. 76–34). The addition of healthy tissue to the area frequently appears to improve the overall condition of the irradiated bed as well (Figs. 76–35 and 76–36).

Mediastinal Radiation and Sternal Dehiscence

The combination of mediastinal radiation and median sternotomy may be seen in patients with Hodgkin's disease or in patients with a history of radiation therapy who later underwent coronary bypass surgery. The internal mammary vessels may be destroyed, and the superiorly based rectus abdominis muscle flap or the pectoralis major turnover flaps, therefore, may not be reliable. The latissimus dorsi muscle, however, is generally spared and can reach across the midline if the tendinous insertion on the humerus is divided and the vascular pedicle skeletonized. With larger defects, free flaps are needed with anastomoses to the take-off of the internal mammary vessels or the transverse cervical vessels.

Axillary Radiation with Brachial Plexus Palsy, Arm Lymphedema, and Clavicular Osteoradionecrosis

Severe radiation to the axilla results in extensive fibrosis of the interstitium and a high incidence of lymphedema. Brachial plexus palsy and chronic pain may be due to the direct effect of radiation on the nerves or secondary compression of the nerves from the resulting scar tissue. Skin ulcerations are often associated with pathologic fractures of the clavicle. The shoulder is constricted with limited abduction of the arm because of dense scarring around the axillary vessels and brachial plexus.

Any surgery to excise the ulcer or release the brachial plexus invariably necessitates immediate, massive soft tissue replacement. Omentum is used both as a pedicled flap and

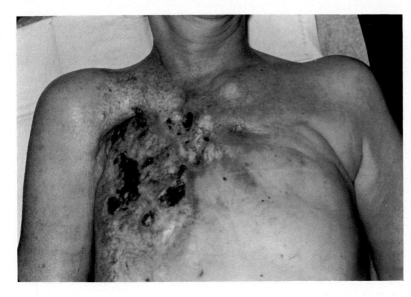

Figure 76–32. A patient 20 years after mastectomy and radiation with progressive necrosis, infection, and pain involving the right upper chest wall. Episodes of life-threatening massive arterial bleeding finally prompted a wide chest wall resection, right upper lobectomy, subclavian artery graft, and arm amputation. Attempted reconstruction with a "fillet of arm" flap failed as a result of thrombosed axillary artery; a wide microvascular tensor fascia lata flap was transferred with anastomoses via vein grafts to the subclavian artery and azygos vein. The patient could not be extubated, partially because of the unstable chest wall, and eventually died from multiple organ failure and venous thrombosis of the flap. Note the extensive destructions of the clavicle, ribs, scapula, and upper lobe of the lung.

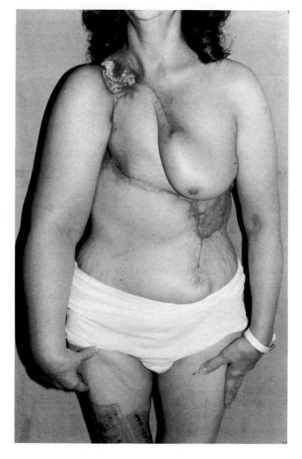

Figure 76–33. Recurrence of chest wall radiation necrosis caused by previous inadequate resection and suboptimal flap reconstruction.

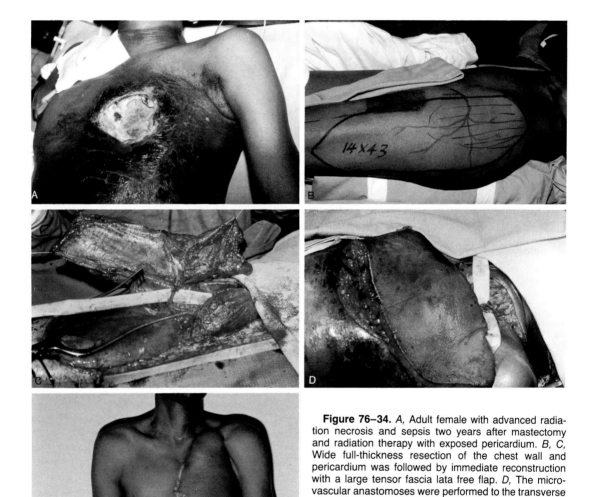

Figure 76–34. *A,* Adult female with advanced radiation necrosis and sepsis two years after mastectomy and radiation therapy with exposed pericardium. *B, C,* Wide full-thickness resection of the chest wall and pericardium was followed by immediate reconstruction with a large tensor fascia lata free flap. *D,* The microvascular anastomoses were performed to the transverse cervical vessels outside the zone of radiation injury. *E,* Fascia lata was used to stabilize the chest. Appearance one year later. (From Shaw, W. W.: Microvascular free flaps: the first decade. Clin. Plast. Surg., *10:*1, 1983.)

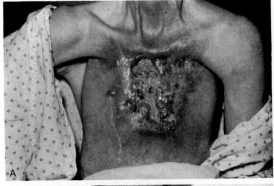
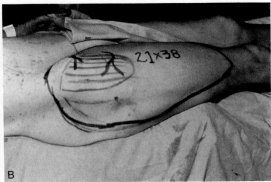
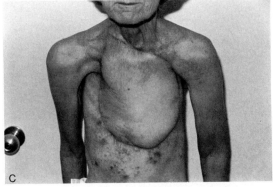

Figure 76–35. *A,* Adult female with recurrent chest wall carcinoma after bilateral mastectomy and mediastinal radiation. *B, C,* After wide resection the defect was reconstructed with a 21 cm wide tensor fascia lata free flap with anastomoses to the internal mammary artery and the external jugular vein. (Courtesy of Dr. Stephen Colen, Institute of Reconstructive Plastic Surgery, NYU Medical Center.)

as a microvascular free flap. Clodius, Uhlschmid, and Hess (1984), in a series of 31 patients with neurolysis and well-vascularized flap coverage, reported improvements in the pain symptoms and cessation of the functional deterioration but not functional improvement. Excision of the scar tissue and release of the plexus are extremely treacherous, and the surgeon must be prepared to handle any vascular emergencies that may arise. A preoperative angiogram is advised. Severe fibrosis of the axilla may make the ipsilateral latissimus dorsi muscle pedicle unreliable. Matsuo and associates (1988) used the contralateral latissimus dorsi and tunneled it between the pectoralis major and minor muscles to reach the opposite axilla. A microvascular free flap from the abdomen or the lower extremity is generally preferred. Anastomoses can be done to the transverse cervical vessels beyond the zone of radiation injury.

MEDIAN STERNOTOMY DEHISCENCE

Following its introduction in 1957 by Julian and associates, median sternotomy has become the standard approach used to ex-

pose the heart, great vessels, and mediastinum. The incidence of infection and dehiscence—"mediastinitis"—varies between 0.4 and 5 per cent and is generally accepted to be low at approximately 1 to 2 per cent (Culliford and colleagues, 1976; Ott and associates, 1980; Jurkiewicz and associates, 1980; Sarr, Gott, and Townsend, 1984). As a result of the large number of coronary bypass procedures being done since the 1970's, however, this dreaded complication occurs now with alarming regularity in most major medical centers. Infection of the suture line, the prosthetic grafts, the pledget material, or the adjacent cartilage may result in life-threatening complications, chronic sinuses, or even sepsis. Plastic surgeons are increasingly called upon to help manage these problems early. The improved understanding of wound biology and the availability of musculocutaneous flaps have greatly improved the results achieved.

Several factors may contribute to the occurrence of such infections: prolonged operating time, improper closure, previous surgery, postoperative hemorrhage, sternal disruption from closed cardiac massage, low-output cardiac state, tracheostomy, or con-

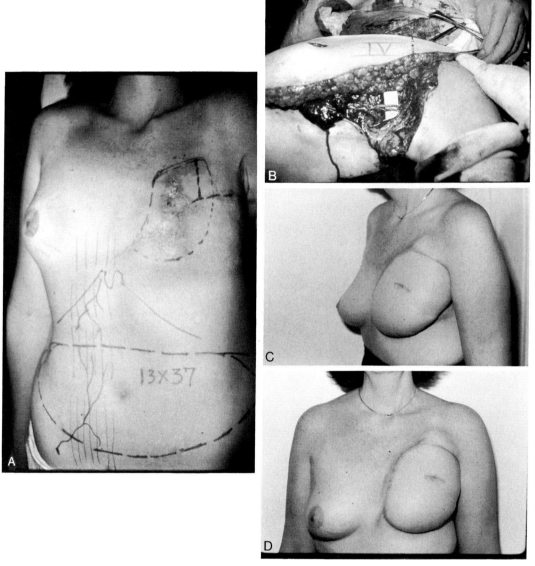

Figure 76–36. *A,* Adult female with radiation skin changes with early ulceration treated by local resection of all irradiated skin along with partial debridement of the involved ribs and (*B*) immediate superiorly pedicled transverse rectus abdominis musculocutaneous flap augmented by microvascular anastomosis of the inferior epigastric vessels. *C, D,* Appearance one year later.

comitant systemic infection (Cohen and associates, 1988). A variety of bacteria have been isolated from these wounds, frequently including *Staphylococcus aureus* and *albus* along with gram-negative rods (Firmin and Wood, 1987). It is generally felt that the infection plays a secondary role to other causes in the etiology of the dehiscence. The possible role of the disruption of the blood supply of the sternum, resulting from the increasing preference for using internal mammary arteries for coronary bypass, is unclear (Grmoljez and associates, 1975; Hutchingson and associates, 1975). The sternum receives multiple direct perforators from the two internal mammary arteries with a rich collateralization on its anterior and posterior surfaces (Arnold, 1972). The periosteum, however, is well connected through the adjacent soft tissue to the intercostal blood supply, and care should be taken to minimize trauma to that region.

The majority of mediastinal dehiscences present several days to a few weeks after cardiac surgery. It is often first noted as serous drainage from the wound along with a failure of the suture line to heal and excessive instability of the sternal closure. Fever, malaise, pleural effusion, or frank sepsis may ensue.

Management

In early cases, the patient should be returned to the operating room and the sternotomy reopened. The wound is debrided and the sternum closed over irrigation-suction catheters. In many cases, healing will be satisfactory if the extent of infection or necrosis is limited. If the wound cannot be closed with confidence, it should be left open for a period of approximately 7 to 10 days of dressing changes until the bacterial count is less than 10^5 (Pearl and Dibbell, 1984) or until a healthy layer of granulation tissue is seen (Johnson and associates, 1985). Patients presenting weeks or months later, however, generally have well-established scar tissue, and a direct closure is not recommended. A preliminary debridement is often needed to gain control of the wound prior to definitive flap reconstruction. Well-vascularized flaps are needed to obliterate the dead space and prevent recurrent infection. Systemic antibiotics should be used judiciously on the basis of wound culture.

A difficult decision at the time of reconstruction is the management of the split sternum. Closed wiring risks hiding underlying infection and makes elimination of the substernal dead space uncertain. Leaving the two halves of the sternum results in a narrow slit, which alternately opens and closes tightly with respiratory movements. The pounding together of the sternum may cause necrosis of the healthy muscle placed into the narrow bony defect. Ultimately, the decision to preserve and stabilize the sternum, as opposed to removing it, is based on the assessment of the viability of the sternum. When extensive sternal necrosis or costal cartilage infection is evident, radical resection of the sternum and the adjacent costal cartilage and ribs is essential. Muscle flaps can be placed into a widely open defect. If the sternal surfaces, particularly the upper part, bleed well, it is safe to wire it together after adequate debridement of any apparent infected portion. The lower part of the sternum should be widely debrided to allow comfortable passage of the muscle flap. The rectus abdominis muscle is well suited to enter the defect from below.

Another difficult decision is that regarding the need for bony stabilization. In acute cases with large defects, clean surgical margins, and borderline pulmonary function studies preoperatively, immediate stabilization with synthetic mesh, acrylic, or bone graft should be considered. In chronic cases, there may be sufficient rigidity, so that skeletal stabilization is usually not necessary. Others (Voegele and associates, 1985), however, recommended using Kirschner wires or immediate rib grafts to stabilize the rib cage underneath the muscle flaps. After the chest is healed, the recurrence of localized osteomyelitis may be treated with local debridement.

Flaps for Reconstruction

The pectoralis major, rectus abdominis, latissimus dorsi muscles, and omentum have been used in different combinations to cover the sternotomy defect. The *pectoralis major muscles* may be used singly or bilaterally (Arnold and Pairolero, 1979) (Fig. 76–37). Most commonly, the muscle origin is detached from the ribs and the insertion on the humerus is transected to allow medial movement of the muscle into the upper defect. The muscle can also be turned over, based

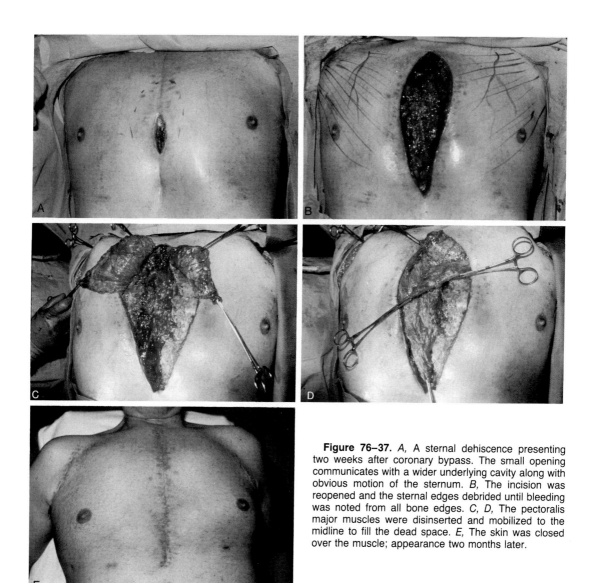

Figure 76–37. *A,* A sternal dehiscence presenting two weeks after coronary bypass. The small opening communicates with a wider underlying cavity along with obvious motion of the sternum. *B,* The incision was reopened and the sternal edges debrided until bleeding was noted from all bone edges. *C, D,* The pectoralis major muscles were disinserted and mobilized to the midline to fill the dead space. *E,* The skin was closed over the muscle; appearance two months later.

on its medial internal mammary perforators. This technique is particularly helpful in the lower chest, where the perforators are a little more laterally situated and less likely to be destroyed by previous surgery. The *rectus abdominis muscle* is usually based on its superior blood supply from the mammary and the marginal costal arteries (Milloy, Anson, and McAfee, 1960; Miller and associates, 1988). A midline abdominal incision is usually used, and the superiorly pedicled rectus muscle is turned on itself to obliterate the inferior defect. The *latissimus dorsi muscle* can also be mobilized to reach beyond the midline when its humeral insertion is divided and its vascular pedicle isolated. The *omentum* can be harvested through a limited upper abdominal extension and brought into the chest through a window in the diaphragm.

Since no skin is removed, in most cases the existing skin of the chest can be approximated over the muscle flaps. If there is doubt, the muscles can be simply covered with skin grafts. Multiple suction drains placed in the depth of the wound are well secured and left for several days until the wound is healed.

Infant Sternotomy Wounds

The increasing success with infant cardiac surgery has brought with it occasional reconstructive problems related to the median sternotomy (Stahl and Kopf, 1988). In neonates, life-threatening cardiorespiratory compromise may occasionally result from the tight spaces of the chest and postoperative edema. In desperation, silicone rubber (Silastic) sheets have been sutured to the skin to cover temporarily the open mediastinum. A few days or weeks later, closure may be achieved secondarily by muscle flaps, as in the adult. Bilateral pectoralis major muscles are generally sufficient. In infants the rectus abdominis muscle appears to be proportionately wider than in the adult but it is much more delicate to dissect. If there is established infection, resection of the sternum or ribs is done. The long-term effect of such resection on growth remains to be seen.

BRONCHOPLEURAL FISTULA AND CHRONIC EMPYEMA

Following partial lung resection, lobectomy, or pneumonectomy, the potential dead space is usually filled, eventually, by lung expansion, mediastinal shift, and elevation of the diaphragm. Incomplete obliteration of this dead space or early removal of chest tubes results in a cavity filled with blood or serum, an invitation for wound infection, known as *empyema*. Failure of the bronchial stump to heal in such an environment results in a *bronchopleural fistula*, which can be notoriously difficult to close secondarily.

In the acute phase, the patient may become septic and external drainage with chest tubes must be reestablished expediently. Subacute or chronic empyema may require surgical resection of the ribs to open a *pleurocutaneous fistula* for a vigorous regimen of chronic irrigation and packing to allow healing from within. With well-established cavities, however, spontaneous closure cannot be expected. One should wait until the cavity has contracted maximally and the wound is free of gross infection to undertake definitive reconstruction. The latter usually involves additional debridement of the cavity, obliterating the dead space with muscle or omentum and the reestablishment of negative suction drainage. For smaller defects, the pectoralis muscle is most commonly used, particularly to cover the bronchial stump (Figs. 76–38 and 76–39). For larger cavities, multiple muscles (Fig. 76–40) or even a microvascular free flap may be needed (see Fig. 76–40).

PRESSURE NECROSIS AND OTHER CHRONIC COVERAGE PROBLEMS

In quadriplegic patients and chronically debilitated patients with severe wasting or prolonged bed rest, pressure necrosis may develop over the bony prominences of the spine or costal margins. The management plan follows that for other chronic wounds: (1) debridement of the necrotic tissue, (2) control of the infection, (3) resection of obvious bony protrusions, and (4) coverage with a well-vascularized flap (see also Chapter 77). In the thorax, local rotation flaps based on the posterior cutaneous perforators, the latissimus dorsi muscle (McCraw, Penix, and Baker, 1978), and occasionally the trapezius muscle may be useful.

CONGENITAL DEFORMITIES

Congenital or developmental deformities of the chest do not usually result in severe functional problems as in major limb anom-

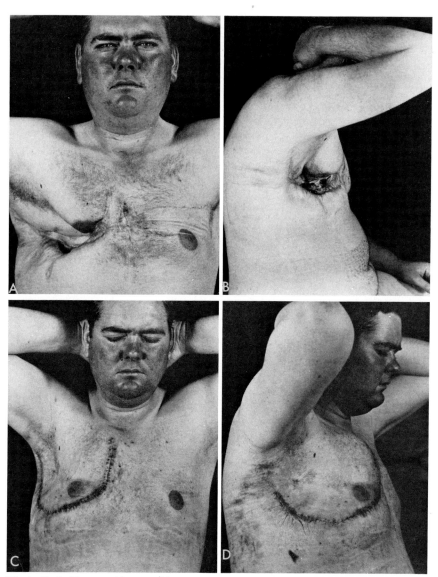

Figure 76–38. *A, B,* A 26 year old man with a severe deformity of the chest and a bronchial fistula following a penetrating wound of the right chest five years previously. It was impossible for the patient to go swimming and even dangerous to take a tub bath. Four attempts to close the defect had been unsuccessful. The bronchial fistula was closed, and a pectoralis muscle flap was transposed to fill the defect. *C, D,* Primary healing occurred, and the patient was discharged on the 11th postoperative day.

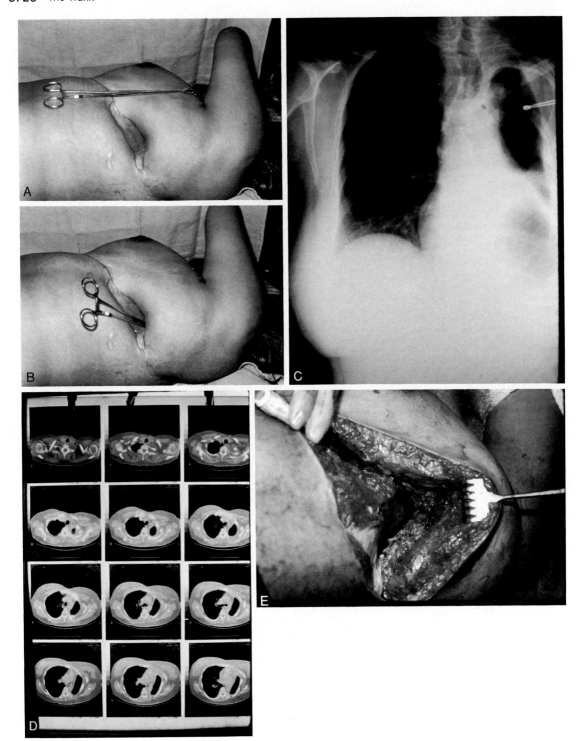

Figure 76–39. *A, B,* A 49 year old woman with chronic empyema cavity and pleural cutaneous fistula. *C, D,* Chest radiograph and CT scan showing the air-filled space. *E,* The cavity was decorticated and the opening of the cavity was enlarged by resecting adjacent ribs; the pectoralis major, the serratus, and the remnant of the latissimus dorsi muscles were also mobilized. Suction drains were placed to ensure collapse of the dead space as well as draining of any blood or fluid.

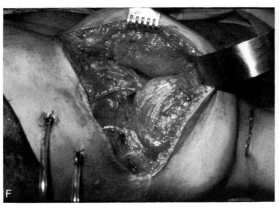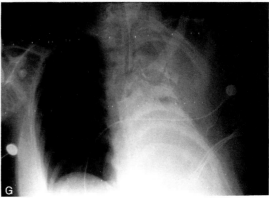

Figure 76–39 *Continued F,* The muscles were mobilized into the cavity and the skin was closed. *G,* Postoperative radiograph showing obliteration of the previous air-filled space.

alies. The appearance is also much better tolerated and more easily camouflaged compared with major facial clefts. Surgical correction, however, may be important in the prevention of progressive scoliosis, exertional cardiopulmonary restriction, and adverse psychologic developments. The most common problems encountered are pectus excavatum, pectus carinatum, sternal clefts, rib deformities, and Poland's syndrome. Ravitch (1977), in a comprehensive text, first organized the management of these deformities into rational therapeutic patterns.

Surgery during early infancy is indicated only rarely for functional reasons. Most of the deformities are mild, and no major surgical reconstruction is required. Lesser procedures, such as custom implants, may be done later in life or after stabilization of the deformity. If the deformity is severe, surgical correction should be completed by the time the child is 4 to 5 years of age, prior to starting school. In females with Poland's syndrome, there is usually associated breast hypoplasia and asymmetry and it is generally preferable to wait until full growth and development to correct both the chest and breast deformity at the same time.

Pectus Excavatum

Pectus excavatum (funnel chest, schusterbrust, thorax embudo) is the most common chest deformity. The depression of the anterior chest wall usually begins at the manubriogladiolar junction (angle of Louis) and reaches the deepest point at the xiphisternal junction (Fig. 76–41). The deformity is occasionally so severe that the sternum reaches

the vertebral bodies, or the sternum may actually pass to one side of the vertebral bodies into the paravertebral gutter (Ravitch, 1951). This finding is associated with a compensatory potbelly. With growth, a characteristic posture may develop with rounded and forward thrust shoulders and some evidence of dorsal kyphosis of the spine.

Pectus excavatum is usually noted soon after birth. The rate and degree of progression are inconstant. In some patients, the deformity is not noticed at birth and becomes obvious only months later. On the other hand, because of the great flexibility of the anterior chest wall of the newborn, paradoxical motion of the lower portion of the sternum from brief increases in negative intrathoracic pressure during crying or gasping is common. Such newborn sternal retractions are not pectus excavatum.

Occasionally, an older patient may report that the deformity became obvious only in early adolescence. When the deformity progresses beyond the adolescent years, it is characteristically associated with lumbodorsal scoliosis, slumped shoulders, and a protruding abdomen.

Etiology. The cause of pectus excavation is not known, although a familial tendency does exist. Four generations with the anomaly in one family and six involved members of another family were documented (Troisier and Monnerot, 1930). Males are affected four times more often than females. Many theories have been proposed for the development of this condition, e.g., arrested development of the sternum, failure of ossification of the lower sternum, congenitally short rectus muscles, pressure on the anterior chest wall

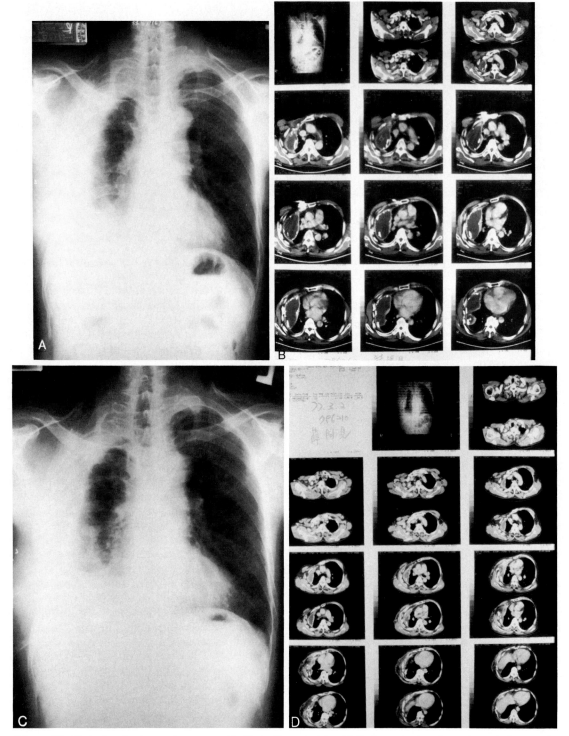

Figure 76–40. A chronic pleurocutaneous cavity filled with contralateral latissimus dorsi and serratus anterior muscles as free flaps because of the inadequate bulk of the previously transsected ipsilateral latissimus dorsi muscle. *A, B,* Preoperative. *C, D,* Postoperative. (Courtesy of Dr. H. Chang.)

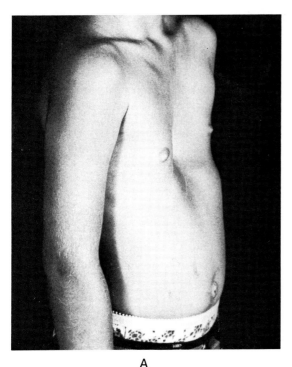
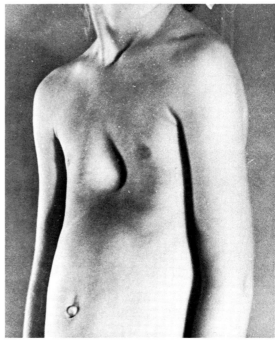

A   B

Figure 76–41. *A,* Pectus excavatum deformity beginning at the level of the manubriosternal junction. The narrowest vertebrosternal distance is at the level of the xiphisternal junction. *B,* Severe cavitary pectus excavatum beginning at the third costochondral junction. (Both photos, courtesy of Dr. Mark M. Ravitch, Pittsburgh, PA.)

in utero, birth injuries, hereditary syphilis, fibrous bands at the lower end of the sternum, or shortened central tendon of the diaphragm (Aston and Pickrell, 1977). Currently, the most accepted concept is that the deformity results primarily from an overgrowth of the costal cartilages, forcing the sternum posteriorly in the case of pectus excavatum and anteriorly in the case of pectus carinatum (Hausmann, 1955). This explanation may be supported by the occurrence of pectus excavatum and pectus carinatum in different members of the same family (Sweet, 1944; Becker and Schneider, 1962). Excision of the involved cartilages, therefore, is considered an important component of the surgical correction (Haller and associates, 1970).

Symptoms. The majority of patients with pectus excavatum are essentially asymptomatic, although adolescents and young adults may have slight dyspnea, palpitations, or mild limitation of activity. Patients with the most severe pectus excavatum deformities complain, more often, of limitation of their ability to perform strenuous exercises and may actually suffer respiratory and cardiac insufficiency.

Cardiopulmonary Function. Most studies of cardiopulmonary function in the majority of patients with pectus excavatum report normal heart rate, venous pressure, blood pressure, circulation time, oxygen saturation, arteriovenous difference, vital capacity, and maximal breathing capacity (Brewer, 1958; Becker and Schneider, 1962). Likewise, evaluation of patients with cardiac catheterization has yielded normal or nearly normal intracardiac pressures and cardiac output in most patients (Fabricius, Davidsen, and Slaughter, 1957; Reusch, 1961). Although some abnormal cardiac catheterizations have been reported (Ravitch, 1951; Lindskog and Felton, 1955; Lyons, Zuhdi, and Kelly, 1955), Brown and Cook (1951), in extensive studies of the respiratory status, found maximum breathing capacity reduced 50 per cent in nine of 11 patients with pectus excavatum. The electrocardiogram (ECG) is normal in most patients, but a few show mild axis changes or right bundle branch block findings thought to be secondary to cardiac displacement rather than intrinsic cardiac disease (Wachtel, Ravitch, and Grishman, 1956; Brewer, 1958, Haller and associates, 1970).

Many patients with mild symptoms, primarily limitation of strenuous activity, receive significant symptomatic benefit from surgical correction, but the physiologic basis for improvement has been questioned because of reported normal, or near-normal, cardiac catheterization studies.

It is clear that pectus excavatum, by displacement and compression of the heart, may cause cardiac symptoms to appear in adolescence or young adult life with lesser degrees of exercise tolerance. Occasionally, severe cardiac stress occurs, with arrhythmias and cardiac failure (Ravitch, 1951). Ravitch (1956) reviewed the recorded experience with pectus excavatum, and the reported cardiac disabilities included (1) a decreased return of blood to the right heart, (2) cardiac arrhythmias secondary to atrial compression, (3) restriction of diastolic filling, and (4) a decrease of respiratory reserve. These findings are limited to patients with severe pectus excavatum.

Beiser and associates (1972) obtained normal data on cardiac catheterization of the right side of the heart and found normal hemodynamic responses to supine exercise in patients with pectus excavatum deformity. However, the cardiac output and stroke volume response to mild upright exercise differed from the norm. The cardiac output and stroke volume during intense upright exercise was reduced in five of six patients. After operative repair in three patients, cardiac output during intense upright exercise increased an average of 38 per cent and hemodynamic response to mild upright exercise also changed toward normal. The investigators hypothesized that the sternal deformity is most severe at its caudal end and the upright position of the torso interferes with the pumping capacity as the heart descends into the portion of the thorax most compromised by the depression of the lower sternum. This finding is significant, since most exercise studies performed on patients with pectus excavatum during cardiac catheterization have been performed in the supine position. Bevegard (1962) had previously found anomalies in patients studied in the upright position. The stroke volume was considerably less during exercise in the supine position. The author suggested an alteration in the abdominothoracic pumping mechanism secondary to the anterior chest wall deformity. Thus, the discrepancy between the symptomatic status of the patients and the catheterization data

may be due to the position in which the patients were studied. Weg, Krumholz, and Harkleroad (1967) studied 25 U.S. Air Force basic trainees who complained of exercise intolerance associated with pectus excavatum. A decrease in maximum voluntary ventilation and forced expiratory flow was well documented. Additional cardiac catheterization, in symptomatic patients, has shown a right ventricular diastolic dip and pressure plateau similar to that observed in patients with constrictive pericarditis. This finding suggests that the restriction between the sternum and the vertebral bodies can cause functional compression of the ventricles, particularly during increased cardiac output.

Roentgenographic Studies. The most common finding on anteroposterior projection is an increase in the extension of the cardiac silhouette into the left chest, although patients with wide pectus excavatum deformities may show a "flattened" heart on the lateral view and extension to the right and left on the anteroposterior film.

The deformity observed on radiographic study obviously varies with the degree of the bony abnormality. The normal distance from the anterior surface of the vertebral column to the posterior surface of the sternum averages approximately 9 cm in adult women and 10.5 cm in men (Roesler, 1934; DeLeon, Perloff, and Twigg, 1965). Fabricius, Davidsen, and Hansen (1957) defined the pectus excavatum deformity as being "slight" when the distance was over 7 cm, "marked" when the distance was 5 to 7 cm, and "severe" when the distance was less than 5 cm. Ben-Menachem, O'Hara, and Kane (1973) reported radiographic paradoxical cardiac enlargement during inspiration in children with pectus excavatum and stressed the necessity of inspiratory and expiratory films to evaluate heart size adequately.

Indications for Surgical Correction. Surgical correction is required for cosmetic reasons and in more advanced cases for improvement of cardiorespiratory dysfunction. Although most patients are relatively asymptomatic, the psychologic implications resulting from an anterior thoracic wall deformity may be significant to the patient or the parents. This is an adequate indication for surgical correction (Becker and Schneider, 1962; Haller and associates, 1970; Jensen and coworkers, 1970; Johnson, 1972; Vidne and Levy, 1973).

Although in the past it was felt that the

affected individuals were suffering primarily from the psychologic standpoint, the now well-established cardiopulmonary restriction that may develop along with the drooped shoulders, protuberant abdomen, kyphosis, and scoliosis are clear indications for surgical correction. Likewise, the deformity is unpredictably progressive, and surgical correction is indicated in (1) infants with severe deformity, (2) infants with a documented progression of the deformity, (3) children and young adults with the deformity, and (4) adults who are symptomatic. It is generally believed that surgery should be performed in the younger group between 2 and 6 years of age before disturbance of the child's developing personality and before the development of orthopedic problems (Vidne and Levy, 1973; Holcomb, 1977; Humphrey and Jaretzki, 1980). It is felt that earlier surgery was also technically easier and better tolerated by the patients.

Operative Procedure. Surgical correction of pectus excavatum began with Meyer's (1911) and Sauerbruch's (1927) attempts to alleviate the cardiorespiratory symptoms. Lexer (as reported by Hoffmeister, 1927) performed the first bilateral resection of costal cartilages and transverse sternal osteotomy and reversed the anteroposterior surfaces of the sternum. Ochsner and DeBakey (1939) reviewed the techniques of surgical correction of pectus excavatum until the time of their report. Brown (1939) established the basis for most present-day techniques with bilateral resection of the costal cartilages, excision of the xiphoid, division of the attachments of the diaphragm and rectus muscles, transverse cuneiform osteotomy at the manubriosternal junction, stabilization by wiring the fifth costal cartilage to the sternum, and traction on the sternum by wires placed in the gladiolus. This method was modified by Ravitch (1956) to include posterior osteotomy of the sternum and wedge bone grafting. Other authors have recommended less radical resection of the cartilages, but supplemented the technique by internal support with metallic struts (Jensen and associates, 1970; Vidne and Levy, 1973; Holcomb, 1977) or Kirschner wires (Barnard and DeWet Lubbe, 1973). The use of rib grafts for support (Dormer, Keil, and Schissel, 1950; Adkins and Gwathmey, 1958) has now been largely abandoned as a result of resorption and softening. External devices to maintain correction of the sternum during the early postoperative period have also been advocated. This technique generally consisted of a wire placed through or around the sternum, brought through the skin, and tied over a fixation device of some sort (Lester, 1946; Fish, Baxter, and Moran, 1954; Lindskog and Felton, 1955). Because of the discomfort and the limited duration of usefulness, they are seldom used today. Wada and associates (1970) reintroduced the sternal turnover operation first described by Lexer and also described using multiple incisions and wedge resections of the ribs and cartilages, the so-called costoplasty, to correct asymmetric deformities. Finally, for smaller and purely cosmetic deformities, standard or custom-made silicone implants have been used (Masson, Payne, and Gonzalez, 1970; Stanford and associates, 1972; Lavey and associates, 1982; Marks, Argenta, and Lee, 1984).

Most methods involve a midline vertical skin incision or, frequently, a transverse submammary curvilinear incision severing the muscle attachments from the sternum and costal cartilages; resection of the deformed cartilages; transverse sternal osteotomy; and elevation of the sternum. The procedure described by Ravitch (1965) and Haller and coworkers (1970) remains the most commonly performed procedure. It is generally agreed that limited operations designed to free the diaphragm from the anterior chest wall are not adequate for functional correction and should be abandoned. Resection of the lower cartilages is essential. The sternum must also be returned to its normal anatomic position and stabilized. Finally, internal support to maintain correction for a prolonged period may be helpful to prevent recurrence.

Operative Techniques

Ravitch's Technique. With this technique (Aston and Pickrell, 1977), the chest is arched forward by placing a folded towel between the scapulas (Fig. 76–42). A vertical skin incision in the midline of the sternum provides maximum exposure. A transverse curvilinear submammary skin incision is frequently used and is particularly indicated in young females. Flaps of skin, subcutaneous tissue, and pectoralis muscles are elevated bilaterally and extended cephalad to expose the entire area of the deformity (Fig. 76–42*B*). Injury to the perichondrium must be avoided in elevating the flaps. Longitudinal incisions are made through the perichon-

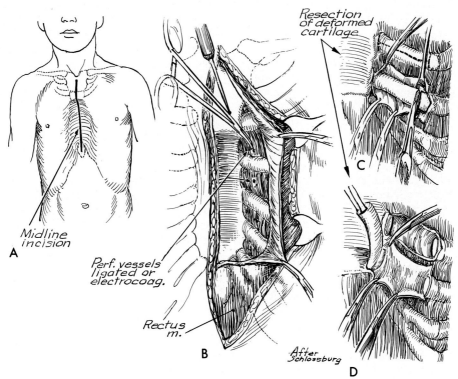

Figure 76–42. Correction of pectus excavatum (Ravitch technique). *A,* A midline incision gives better exposure with less dissection and smaller flaps. A transverse submammary incision does not provide adequate exposure in older patients or in those whose defect begins at the manubriosternal junction. *B,* Flaps of skin, subcutaneous fat, and pectoralis major muscle are dissected, exposing the deformed ribs and cartilage. *C,* Rectangular perichondrial flaps are developed to provide access to the deformed cartilage. *D,* The deformed cartilages are resected for the full extent of their deformity.

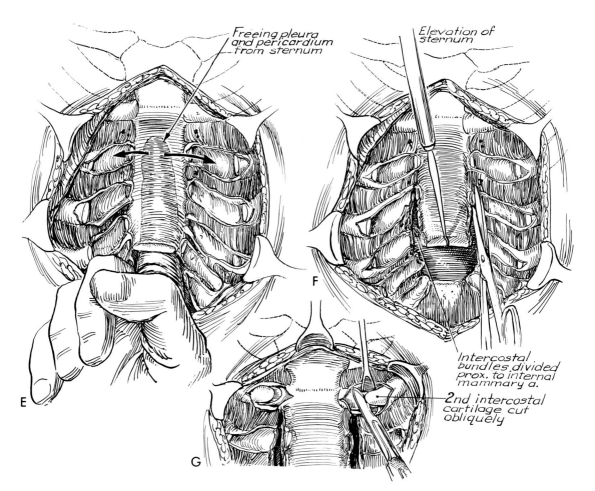

Figure 76–42 *Continued E,* The xiphoid is divided from the sternum, and blunt finger dissection separates the posterior surface of the sternum from the pleura and pericardium. *F,* The sternum is retracted upward, and the intercostal bundles are divided medial to the internal mammary vessels. *G,* The next higher cartilage above the level of the deformity is divided obliquely for later three-point fixation.

Illustration continued on following page

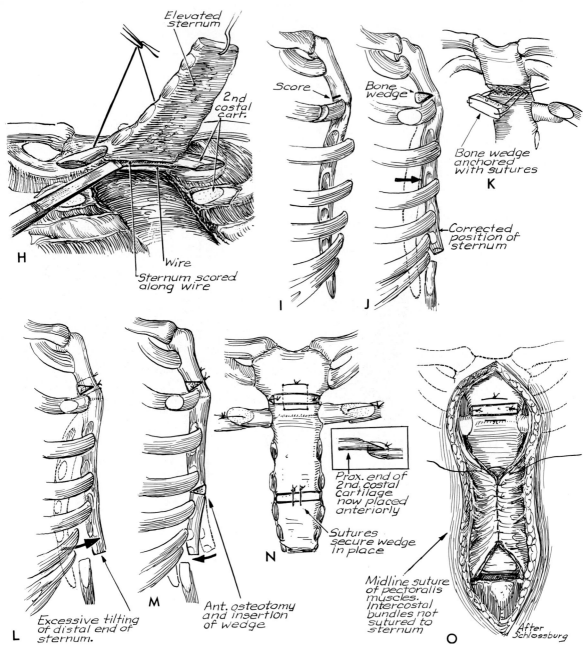

Figure 76–42 *Continued H, I,* A posterior transverse osteotomy is performed at the next higher interspace above the transected normal cartilage. The wire passed around the sternum gives a guideline to the exact site of the desired osteotomy. *J, K,* A bone block is placed in the osteotomy defect produced by anterior movement of the sternum. The bone block can be held in place with sutures placed either through it or around the sternum. *L, M,* When the distal sternum points excessively anteriorly following the superior transverse osteotomy, a distal anterior transverse osteotomy is performed and stabilized with a bone block. *N,* The superior osteotomy is secured by using silk sutures placed through and through the sternum across the osteotomy site. The beveled, transected, normal cartilages are secured as shown to provide "tripod fixation" of the sternum in its new position (two cartilages and anterior periosteum). *O,* The pectoralis muscles are sutured together and to the sternum in the midline. The intercostal bundles are not sutured back to the sternum because of a tendency to recreate the deformity. (After Ravitch, M. M.: General Thoracic Surgery. Philadelphia, Lea & Febiger, 1972.)

drium of the involved cartilages and are complemented by transverse incisions so that rectangular flaps of perichondrium can be reflected. An upper flap of perichondrium is first released by grasping the upper edge of the incised perichondrium and by dissecting with a Joseph nasal periosteal elevator or with a blunt staphylorrhaphy elevator. The lower edge of the perichondrium is elevated in a similar fashion. The perichondrium is thin over the upper and lower borders of the rib, and careful dissection in these areas is required to avoid disruption. It may be possible to pass a blunt instrument behind the cartilage, leaving the perichondrium intact, and to divide the cartilage at the two ends. In other instances it is difficult to strip the perichondrium behind the cartilage. A Kocher clamp is used to hold the cartilage while it is incised in its midportion until one half of the cartilage is lifted from the underlying perichondrium. The perichondrium is dissected from both halves of the cartilage, and the two ends of the cartilage are divided medially and laterally (Fig. 76–42C) to remove the specimen (Fig. 76–42D). The deformed cartilages are resected for the full length of their deformity. The costochondral junction is preserved when possible. In infants and small children, the resection includes 3 to 5 cm of the upper cartilages. In older children and young adults, the deformity usually extends laterally into the bony rib. As few as three cartilages may be removed, but usually four and frequently five on each side must be resected.

The postoperative result may be unsatisfactory if the cartilages are not resected sufficiently lateral or if a sufficient number of cartilages are not excised. When all deformed cartilages have been removed, the next higher cartilages, usually the second or third, are transected anteriorly and medially to behind and laterally to allow overlap of the medial fragment upon the lateral when the sternum is lifted to its corrected position. Suture fixation of the overlapped cartilages is established later in the procedure.

With the sternum elevated by a bone hook (Fig. 76–42F), the xiphoid process is divided from the sternum and allowed to retract. A finger is inserted into the mediastinum through the opening made by division of the sternum and xiphoid, and reflected pleura is displaced laterally on both sides. When the sternum is raised by upward traction on the bone hook, it is possible to cut the intercostal bundles away from the sternum on both sides, preferably medial to the internal mammary vessels, to isolate the sternum as a peninsula attached only above.

A posterior transverse osteotomy of the sternum is performed at the next higher interspace above the transected normal cartilage. A wire is passed around the sternum at the desired level of the osteotomy, the sternum is elevated, and a sharp osteotome scores the posterior surface of the sternum until the sternum is fractured forward (Fig. 76–42H). A block of rib bone may then be placed in the defect, resulting from the posterior osteotomy (Fig. 76–42J). If a bone block is used, it should be sutured in place or around the sternum to prevent it from being dislodged into the mediastinum postoperatively. The posterior sternal osteotomy came into practice because it was noted that in some patients undergoing an anterior cuneiform osteotomy and fracture of the posterior cortical lamella, the posterior periosteum stripped back, allowing the distal sternal fragment to assume a recessed position subsequently. After posterior osteotomy, any tendency for regression to the original deformity produces a desired anterior tilting of the distal segment of the sternum. In some patients, especially older children, the sternum may be rather sharply rotated toward the right, i.e., counterclockwise. This can usually be corrected by dividing the right half of the osteotomy completely and twisting the sternum back into position.

The sternum is held in a somewhat overcorrected position by two or three mattress sutures of heavy braided silk placed through the bone anteriorly across the level of the posterior osteotomy (Fig. 76–42N). A saddler's awl or a heavy-gauge Reverdin needle can be helpful in passing sutures through the sternum. The transected, overlapped, unaffected cartilages are sutured into their new position. This maneuver establishes a natural fixation, referred to as "tripod fixation," because the sternum is supported by its anterior periosteum as well as by the two cartilages. The pectoral muscles are sutured and the sternal periosteum is sutured in the midline (Fig. 76–42O). The intercostal bundles are not sutured back to the sternum because this has the tendency to reproduce the deformity. Likewise, the xiphoid process is not sutured back to the sternum. A large suction catheter

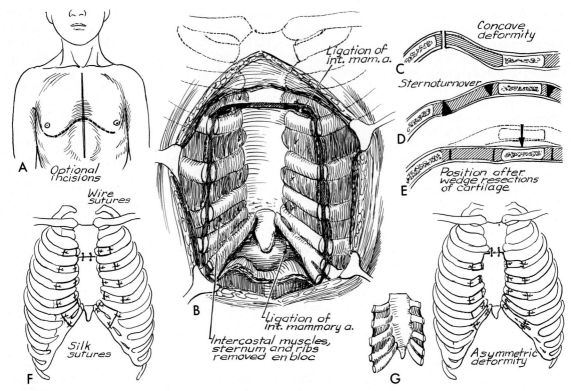

Figure 76–43. Sternoturnover procedure. *A,* Either a longitudinal and midline sternal incision or a transverse and inframammary incision may be used. *B,* The ribs and intercostal muscle bundles are transected bilaterally at the costal arches cephalad along the margin of the deformity. The internal mammary arteries are ligated and transected bilaterally. The sternum is ready for elevation and removal en bloc. *C to E,* The convex side of the sternum is flattened by wedge resections and trimmed to fit the defect in the thoracic wall. *F,* The sternum is sutured in place with stainless steel wire, and each costal cartilage or rib is sutured with heavy silk. *G,* In mild asymmetry, the reversed sternum is either shifted to one side parallel to the sternal axis or obliquely positioned after trimming. (After Wada, J., and Ikeda, K.: Clinical experience with 306 funnel chest operations. Int. Surg., *57*:707, 1972.)

is placed retrosternally in the mediastinal space, and 20 to 30 cm of water suction is applied. The subcutaneous tissue and skin are closed in layers.

On occasion, the sternum of a patient is so scaphoid that when the osteotomy has been performed and maintained by sutures, the distal end of the sternum projects forward, necessitating a transverse osteotomy in the distal portion of the sternum to allow it to fall downward in order to correct the exaggerated anterior curvature (Fig. 76–52*L, M*).

A chest radiograph is taken immediately after completion of the operation, and if a pneumothorax is present, it is aspirated. Some paradoxical motion of the anterior chest wall may be present in the first few postoperative days, but this is of little physiologic significance. Postoperative activity is not limited in the usual patient. Meticulous pulmonary toilet is necessary. Wound problems such as hematoma and infection are infrequent but may occur.

Sternum Turnover. The sternum turnover (sternoturnover) procedure is performed through a longitudinal or transverse inframammary incision (Fig. 76–43). Skin, subcutaneous tissue, and pectoralis muscle flaps are elevated. Blunt dissection separates the sternum from the mediastinal tissues. Likewise, the mediastinal tissues and ribs are elevated using blunt manual dissection. The ribs or cartilages and intercostal muscles are transected bilaterally at the costal arches and cephalad along the margin of the deformity.

The sternum is elevated, and both internal mammary arteries are ligated and divided. The sternum is transected just above the level of the beginning of the deformity, removed en bloc, and turned over; its convex side is flattened by the wedge resection and turned to fit the defect in the thoracic wall. The sternum is sutured in position with stainless steel wire, and each costal cartilage or rib is sutured with heavy silk. When there is mild asymmetry, the reversed sternum can be shifted to one side parallel to the sternal axis or obliquely positioned after trimming. It is important that the reversed sternum fits snugly in a suitable position. As noted by Ravitch (1965), the indications for the sternoturnover procedure are probably limited to patients with unusually wide defects in whom the required resections would not be tolerated. Infection in this large graft could be disastrous.

Costoplasty Technique. Wada and Ikeda (1972) developed the funnel chest costoplasty for asymmetric pectus deformity, usually involving the right side in adults (Fig. 76–44). In this procedure the deformed cartilages and ribs are mobilized by transecting their sternal attachments. Cartilages and ribs are straightened by multiple partial incisions or wedge resections and sutured to the sternum

anteriorly to form a new and elevated costal contour.

Internal and External Fixation. Various internal fixation devices have been used in an attempt to stabilize the sternum postoperatively and to prevent recurrence of pectus excavatum. These devices include stainless steel struts (Rehbein and Wernicke, 1957; Adkins and Gwathmey, 1958; Ravitch, 1965; Jensen and associates, 1970; Vidne and Levy, 1973), stainless steel wire mesh (May, 1961), Kirschner wires or Steinmann pins (Mayo and Long, 1962), and rib bone struts (Sweet, 1944; Brodkin, 1948; Adkins and Gwathmey, 1958).

Jensen and associates (1970) used a preformed stainless steel strut (Strib) manufactured especially for anterior chest wall stablization (Fig. 76–45). A transverse incision exposes the underlying deformed chest wall. Short incisions are made through the overlying pectoral muscles to expose each costochondral junction. Periosteal flaps are devel-

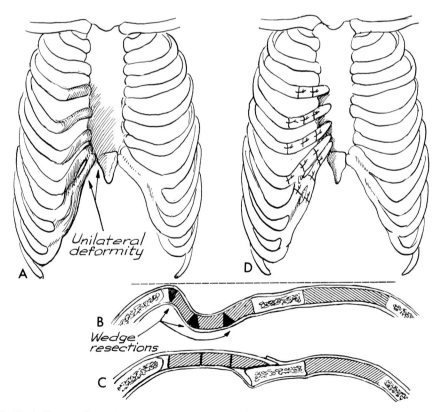

Figure 76–44. *A,* Deep, unilateral, asymmetric funnel chest. *B, C,* The deformed ribs and cartilages are straightened by multiple wedge resections and detachment of the cartilages from the sternum. *D,* The recontoured ribs are sutured to the sternum anteriorly. (After Wada, J., and Ikeda, K.: Clinical experience with 306 funnel chest operations. Int. Surg., 57:707, 1972.)

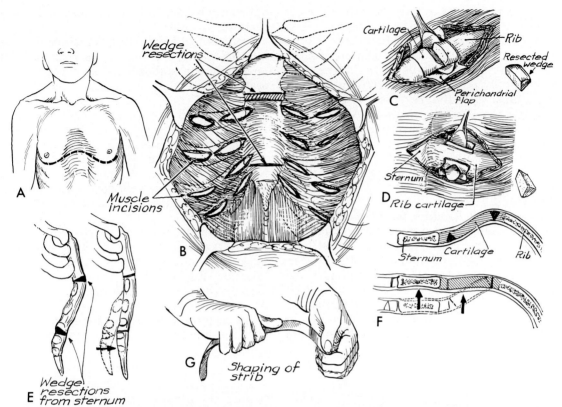

Figure 76–45. Stabilization of corrected pectus excavatum deformity using Strib internal fixation. *A,* Submammary incision extending from the anterior axillary line to the anterior axillary line, with the back of the incision turned up toward the axilla and the center curved cephalad to aid in exposure of the upper sternum. *B,* Skin, subcutaneous fat, and fascia flaps are elevated superiorly and inferiorly, exposing the pectoralis muscles. Short incisions through the muscles expose each costochondral junction. *C, D,* Subperichondral dissection exposes the cartilages, and wedges of cartilage are removed from each deformed cartilage as well as the web at the costal arch. The costochondral junction is not disturbed in children, as this is the growth line of the rib. *E,* The posterior aspect of the sternum is freed of all attachments up to the level of deformity. Wedge osteotomies of the sternum are performed, preserving the posterior periosteum to serve as a hinge. *F,* Reversed wedges are excised from the medial ends of the cartilages as they join the sternum, permitting straightening of the ribs. Cartilage wedges and lengths may be revised at this time to permit the desired positioning of the sternum. *G,* A Strib of the required length is selected by measuring the distance from one midaxillary line across the anterior chest to the opposite midaxillary line, and is hand bent.

oped, and a wedge of cartilage is removed from the web at the costal arch. The xiphoid process is freed from its rectus muscle attachments, and the sternum is divided with an osteotome. The sternum is retracted forward, and wedges of cartilage are removed from the posterior surfaces of the medial end of each cartilage where they join the sternum. If necessary, a second osteotomy of the sternum is performed. A stainless steel strut is placed from one midaxillary line to the other between the endothoracic fascia and the pleura posterior to the sternum; when adjusted in contour, it supports the sternum. The strut is removed after 12 to 18 months.

Vidne and Levy (1973) resected the deformed cartilages, performed an anterior cu-neiform osteotomy of the sternum, and placed a stainless steel strut retrosternally in a fashion similar to that of Jensen and his coworkers (1970). These authors removed the strut after approximately six months.

Barnard and DeWet Lubbe (1973) resected the deformed cartilages, mobilized the sternum, and performed an osteotomy through the posterior cortex of the sternum. A medium-sized Kirschner wire was bent slightly with an anterior convexity and inserted between the anterior and posterior tables of the sternum at the level of the fifth costal cartilage. The laterally protruding ends of wire partially overlapped the bony anterior thoracic wall to which they were fixed with silk sutures. The authors indicated that they do

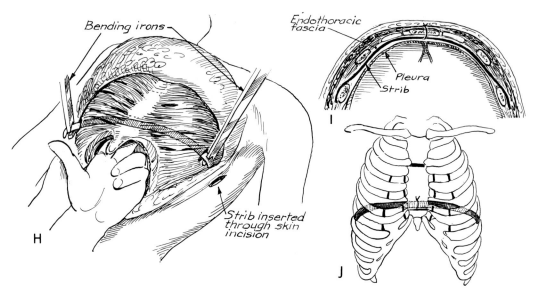

Figure 76–45 *Continued H* to *J,* Dissection is extended through the muscle bundles and endothoracic fascia to the pleura, and the Strib is guided across the mediastinum between the pleura and endothoracic fascia. Specially designed bending irons are used to form the ends of the strut around the adjacent ribs. Final contour adjustment is made by bringing the sternum and Strib into continuity and securing it in position with a heavy catgut suture. (After Jensen, K., Schmidt, R., Caramella, J., and Lynch, M.: Pectus excavatum: the how, when and why of surgical correction. J. Pediatr. Surg., 5:4, 1970.)

not remove the wire unless some need arises to do so.

Silicone Implant Reconstruction. Experience with silicone implants for breast augmentation stimulated the choice of this material for correction of purely cosmetic deformities in adults (Masson, Payne, and Gonzalez, 1970; Stanford and coworkers, 1972; Mendelson and Masson, 1977; Lavey and associates, 1982). Although standard breast implants may be helpful to fill out well-localized depressions, they are rarely used today because of variations in deformity and the unpredictable development of implant contractures. Custom implants are prefabricated from a plaster model of the deformity made in the surgeon's office. Such synthetic implants, however, should be used only in adult patients and only in patients without cardiopulmonary symptoms, as the anatomic deformity is not changed by this method. As with the use of all prosthetic materials, possible complications of bleeding, infection, and extrusion of the implant must be anticipated.

In the designing of the custom implants, it is important to recognize that the skeletal defect may be smaller than the external apparent defect. An implant that fills out the defect on the surface is likely to be larger than needed and may result in undesirable overcorrection (Fig. 76–46). It is generally preferable to slightly undercorrect in order to avoid protrusion of the implant. Such implants should also be made of moderately firm

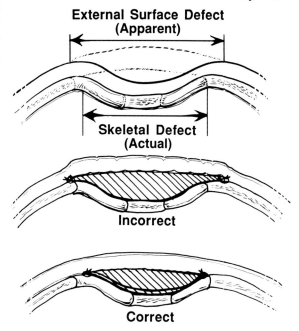

Figure 76–46. In planning custom implants, it is important to note the difference between the apparent surface defect versus the actual skeletal defect that needs to be corrected. Overcorrection is generally more troublesome than undercorrection.

consistency to augment the bony contour. Dacron patches on the back or suture tabs may be helpful to secure the implant in the desired position in the early postoperative period (Fig. 76–47).

Pectus Carinatum

Pectus carinatum (pigeon breast, chicken breast) is a protrusion deformity of the anterior chest wall and is regarded as the opposite of the pectus excavatum deformity. Pectus excavatum occurs approximately ten times more frequently than pectus carinatum. Hippocrates described the deformity and noted that patients in whom "the chest becomes sharply pointed and not broad become affected with difficulty of breathing and hoarseness; for the cavities which inspire and expire do not attain proper capacity" (Aston and Pickrell, 1977). In some patients a rigid chest develops: there is an increased anteroposterior diameter fixed in almost full inspiration, with insufficient respiratory efforts made only by the diaphragm and the muscles of respiration. There is alveolar hypoventilation and increased pulmonary circulatory resistance (Fishman, Turino, and Bergofsky, 1958; Bergofsky, Turino, and Fishman, 1959). The lungs lose compliance, and there is progressive emphysema with a tendency to pulmonary infection (Welch and Vos, 1947).

Etiology. The etiology of the deformity is unknown. Suggested theories include abnormal fusion of sternal segments (Currarino and Silverman, 1958), defective ossification (DeOliviera, Sambhi, and Zimmerman, 1958), rickets (Brodkin, 1958), and various influences of the diaphragm on chest wall development (Brodkin, 1949; Chin, 1957; Lester, 1961). Sweet's (1944) explanation of the overgrowth of the costal cartilages with forward protrusion of the manubrium, gladiolus, and xiphoid is reasonable and would explain to some extent how pectus carinatum is caused by an anterior growth of the cartilages and pectus excavatum by a posterior growth.

Types. Brodkin (1949) recognized and described two types of protruding chest deformities: *chondrogladiolar* (Fig. 76–48) and *chondromanubrial*. Chondrogladiolar prominence is characterized by forward projection of the lower anterior thorax and body of the sternum so that the level of the junction of the sternum and xiphoid is the most prominent point of the anterior chest wall. Associated

with the protrusion is the lateral depression of the anterior chest wall, which may be sufficiently deep to decrease the thoracic cavity and produce cardiorespiratory symptoms (Fig. 76–49) (Ravitch, 1960). This type of deformity is said to appear more often (Brodkin, 1949; Welch and Vos, 1973), although some reports do not agree (Lam and Taber, 1971). Chondromanubrial prominence is characterized by projection of the manubrium and the adjacent first and second cartilages, with a vertical or posteriorly directed gladiolus. Although he did not call the deformity "pectus carinatum," Ravitch (1952) reported correction of this type of defect in a patient with cardiac symptoms.

Robicsek and associates (1963) noted a third type of pectus carinatum—lateral pectus carinatum—either unilateral or bilateral. This deformity is rare.

Symptoms and Signs. Symptoms in most patients are vague and vary from retarded growth, exertional dyspnea, or chronic dyspnea to asthmatic attacks and palpitation (Robicsek and coworkers, 1963). Many patients, following surgical repair of the deformity, showed subjective improvement (Lester, 1953).

Surgical Techniques

Correction of Chondrogladiolar Deformity. Several operative methods of correction have been described, indicating that no single method is totally satisfactory. Lester (1953) resected approximately 2 cm of the sternal end of each cartilage below the second cartilage; the xiphoid was freed from the sternum, and subperiosteal resection of the sternum was extended from the level of the second rib. When necessary, the rib ends were also resected.

Chin (1957) detached the xiphoid from the sternum, leaving the rectus abdominis muscle attached to the xiphoid, and the sternal ends of the sixth and seventh ribs in children (the third to seventh ribs in adults) were resected superichondrially. A slot osteotomy was performed on the anterior sternum at the level of the fourth costal cartilage, and the detached xiphoid process was sutured into the slot osteotomy with the idea that the posterior pull of the xiphoid would correct the deformity.

Ravitch (1960) described a two-stage resection of the costal cartilages in one patient and a one-stage bilateral resection of cartilages, combined with a distal osteotomy, in

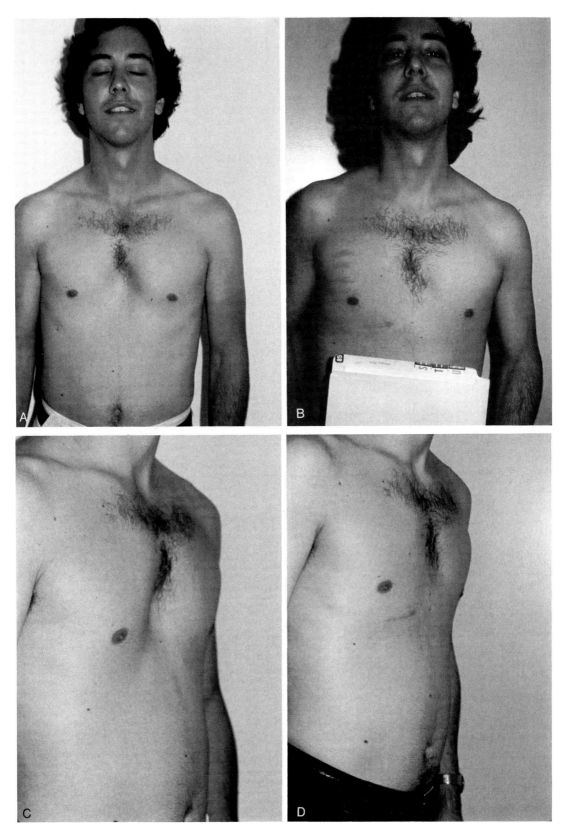

Figure 76–47. *A, C,* A male patient with typical pectus excavatum deformity. *B, D,* Appearance after correction with a custom-made silicone implant with synthetic polyester (Dacron) strips and suture loops (see Fig. 76–46).

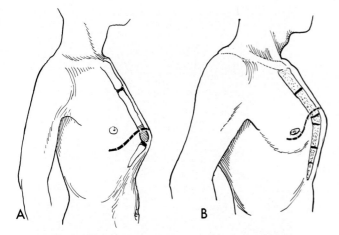

A

B

Figure 76–48. *A,* Chondrogladiolar type of pectus carinatum with forward projection of the lower anterior thorax and body of the sternum. The level of the junction of the sternum and xiphoid is the most prominent of the anterior chest wall. The broken line indicates the level of the incision for surgical correction. *B,* Chondromanubrial type of pectus carinatum of the manubrium and adjacent first and second ribs. The gladiolas may be directed vertically or posteriorly. The broken line indicates the level of the incision for surgical correction.

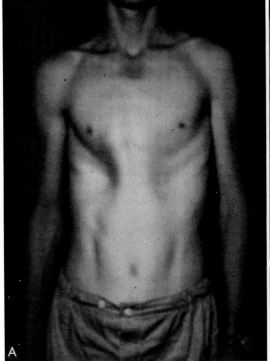

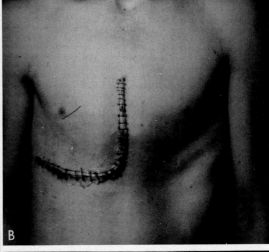

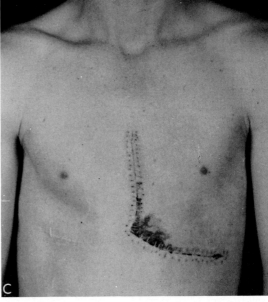

Figure 76–49. Pectus carinatum deformity. *A,* Chondrogladiolar type deformity with projection of the lower anterior thorax and body of the sternum. There is associated lateral depression of the anterior chest wall. The pectus carinatum correction in this patient was one of the first performed by Ravitch; the operation involved two stages. *B,* Patient in the postoperative period after correction of deformity of the right side of the thorax. *C,* Eight months later following correction of the deformity of the left side. (Courtesy of Dr. Mark M. Ravitch, Pittsburgh, PA.)

another patient to correct the manubriogladiolar type of deformity. In the patient undergoing the two-stage resection, the right pectoralis muscles and rectus muscles were reflected from the operative field; knobby lesions of the fourth to sixth costal cartilages, which were exaggerating the prominence of the sternum, were excised; and superiosteal resection of the fifth to ninth cartilages was performed. The redundant perichondrium was tightened with reefing sutures, and the pectoralis and rectus abdominis muscles were sutured in place. The left side was similarly repaired eight months later. The patient tolerated the one-sided operation so well that the next operation by Ravitch featured bilateral resection in one stage. In discussing the paper of Welch and Vos (1973), Ravitch noted that he performs all pectus carinatum deformities in one stage without sternal osteotomy (Fig. 76–50).

Robicsek and associates (1963) described correction of the sternal prominence by subperiosteal resection beginning at the third costal cartilage, transverse osteotomy of the sternum at the beginning of the abnormal forward sternum at the beginning of the abnormal forward curvature (usually just below the angle of Louis), resection of the lower protruding end of the sternum, and suture of the previously detached xiphoid process with stainless steel wire to the new end of the sternum (Fig. 76–51). The rectus muscles pulled the sternum downward, correcting the deformity.

Lam and Taber (1971) described correction of chondrogladiolar prominence by resection of the third to seventh cartilages and osteotomy of the anterior table of the upper portion of the sternum to permit the protruding sternum to be fractured backward. These procedures were combined with an osteotomy of the anterior table of the lower sternum at the level of the sixth cartilage, with removal of a wedge to allow elevation. The wedge of bone from the lower osteotomy line was used to maintain the new angulation.

Correction of Chondromanubrial Deformity. Ravitch (1952) reported correction of an unusual chondromanubrial type of deformity without calling it pectus carinatum (Fig. 76–52). Bilateral subperichondrial resection of five cartilages was done; the xiphisternal junction was divided and two osteotomies were performed. The superior os-

teotomy at the level of the greatest prominence of the convex deformity permitted the sternum to be lifted anteriorly, thereby fracturing the posterior cortical lamella and restoring normal alignment. This maneuver resulted in an anterior tilting of the lower portion of the body of the sternum, which was corrected by an osteotomy at the appropriate level to allow the sternum to be fractured posteriorly. The lower osteotomy was packed by fragments from the wedge osteotomy, and the corrected position was maintained without sutures. The manubrium and gladiolus were sutured together across the superior osteotomy. No traction or splinting was employed postoperatively.

Lam and Taber (1971) (Fig. 76–53) reported resection of the second to fourth cartilages subperichondrially and excision of a cuneiform segment 2 cm wide from the prominence of the convexity of the sternum. Transverse osteotomies above and below the resection permitted the sternum to be fractured into a flat position, which was maintained by sutures at the resection site.

Welch and Vos (1973) (Fig. 76–54) reported symmetric bilateral subperichondrial cartilage resection and double anterior table osteotomies at the first and third sternal segments. The pectoralis muscles were approximated to the sternum in the midline, and a triangular flap of the apex of the rectus fascia was placed into the corresponding pectoral defect anterior to the sternum.

Other techniques described for the correction of the chondromanubrial type of chest protrusion represent essentially only slight modifications of the Ravitch technique and are not detailed.

Sternal Clefts

Sternal clefts, described as early as 1772 by Sandifort, 1798 by Wilson, and 1818 by Weese, are rare but dramatic anomalies, often with a grotesque depression in the middle of the chest and the pulsating heart able to be seen through the thin skin (Fig. 76–55). The fascination with this group of deformities was partly stimulated by a patient, Herr Groux of Hamburg, who in the 1850's "traveled about the world exhibiting himself at universities, hospitals, and medical meetings, collecting a scrapbook of comments by

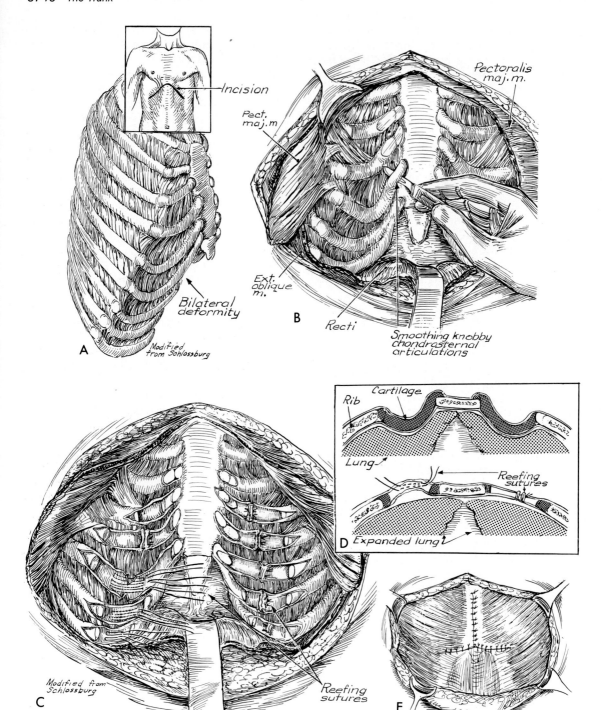

Figure 76–50. Ravitch technique for correction of chondrogladiolar type of pectus carinatum. *A, B,* A transverse curvilinear incision is used to elevate flaps down to and including the pectoralis muscles. The rectus muscle attachments are divided. Cartilaginous irregularities and knobby projections of the chondrosternal articulations are sharply smoothed out. *C, D,* The posteriorly curved, deformed cartilages are resected subperichondrially. The redundant perichondrium is tightened by mattress silk reefing sutures so that the new cartilage will grow in a straight line from the ribs to the sternum. *E,* The pectoralis muscles and recti are reattached to the sternum. (After Ravitch, M. M.: General Thoracic Surgery. Philadelphia, Lea & Febiger, 1972.)

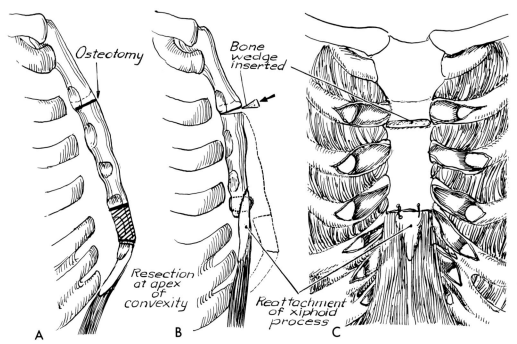

Figure 76–51. Correction of chondrogladiolar type of pectus carinatum with resection of the lower sternum. *A,* The costal cartilages have been resected subperichondrially; a transverse sternal osteotomy has been performed at the level of the second rib, leaving the posterior periosteum intact, and the protruding lower end of the corpus sterni had been resected. *B, C,* The lower end of the transected corpus sterni has been smoothed out and joined to the xiphoid with stainless steel wires. A bone wedge taken from the excised portion of the lower sternum is placed in the gap produced at the osteotomy by posteriorly directing the sternum. (After Robicsek, F., Sanger, P., Taylor, F., and Thomas, M.: The surgical treatment of chondrosternal prominence (pectus carinatum). J. Thorac. Cardiovasc. Surg., *45:*691, 1963.)

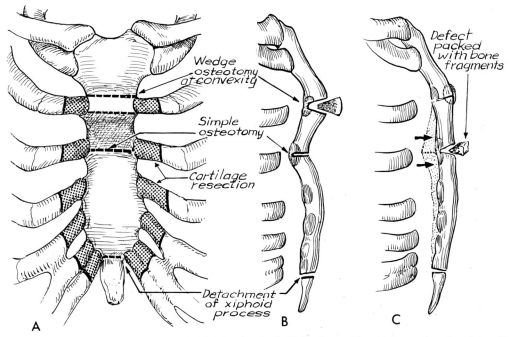

Figure 76–52. Correction of chondromanubrial deformity. *A, B,* Bilateral superichondrial resection of costal cartilages, division of xiphisternal junction, and two osteotomies. The superior wedge osteotomy at the level of greatest convexity allows the posteriorly directed sternal segment to be lifted anteriorly, thereby fracturing the posterior cortical lamella, restoring a more normal alignment. *C,* Anterior tilting of the lower portion of the corpus sterni thus produced is corrected by a simple osteotomy, with bone fragments used to splint the osteotomy site. The manubrium and gladiolus are stabilized by stainless steel sutures. (After Ravitch, M. M.: Unusual sternal deformity with cardiac symptoms. J. Thorac. Surg., 23:138, 1952.)

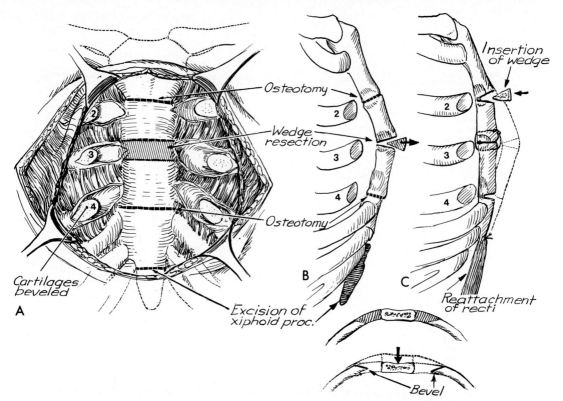

Figure 76–53. Correction of chondromanubrial deformity with resection of the center of convexity. *A, B,* Protruding costal cartilages of ribs, two, three, and four resected. Transverse osteotomies above and below the level of the deformity, a wedge resection at the level of the sternal prominence, and detachment of the xiphoid process permit the sternum to be straightened. *C,* Sternum stabilized by stainless steel wire at the site of sternal resection, bone wedge in upper osteotomy, and reattachment of xiphoid process. (After Lam, C., and Taber, R.: Surgical treatment of pectus carinatum. Arch. Surg., *103*:191, 1971.)

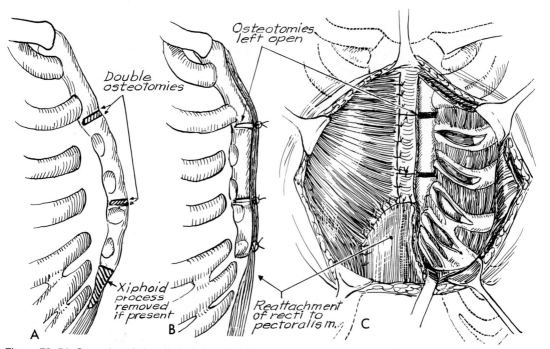

Figure 76–54. Correction of chondrogladiolar type of pectus carinatum with stabilization by rectus facia apex flaps. *A,* Following symmetric bilateral cartilage resection preserving the perichondrial sheaths, double anterior table osteotomies are made at the level of the first and third sternal segments and the xiphoid process is resected. *B, C,* The pectoralis muscles are reattached to the sternum in the midline and the rectus muscle apex flaps are advanced into the pectoralis defect anterior to the sternum. (After Welch, K., and Vos, A.: J. Pediatr. Surg., *8*:659, 1973.)

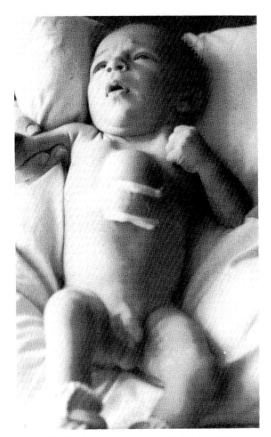

Figure 76–55. A newborn male with totally cleft sternum and large hernia covered by thin, pigmented skin. The lower swelling is the liver; the one above is the heart, visibly and palpably pulsating under the skin. The cleft above, between the upper sternal halves and clavicles on each side, showed striking respiratory paradox. The child could not tolerate compression of the chest sufficient to approximate the sternal halves. (From Ravitch, M. M.: Spectacular problems in surgery: congenital absence of sternum. Surg. Gynecol. Obstet., *116*:34, 1963. By permission of Surgery, Gynecology and Obstetrics.)

the distinguished physicians and surgeons who examined him . . . making a living by charging fees . . ." (Ravitch, 1977).

Because both the heart and sternum are formed embryologically from the fusion of bilateral mesodermal plates, a wide variety of deformities have been described both in terms of the clefts of the sternum and the location of the heart. Clinically, three groups can be identified:

1. *Cleft sternum without associated anomalies.* Because the fusion starts from above, the defects are either through the entire sternum or only the lower part, forming an inverted V.

2. *True ectopia cordis.* The heart is seen outside of the chest wall along with some degree of sternal cleft. There are frequently associated congenital heart malformations.

3. *Cantrell's pentalogy (thorocoabdominal ectopia cardis).* This deformity is characterized by absence or cleft of the lower sternum, crescentic ventral diaphragmatic defect, midline ventral abdominal defect or an omphalocele, defect of the apical pericardium with communication with the peritoneum, and a cardiac defect including either a ventriculoseptal defect or a ventricular aneurysm.

Treatment. With most major deformities, surgical intervention in early infancy or the neonatal period is necessary. Most sternal defects can be reapproximated and secured with wires. Selected osteotomies, chondrotomies, partial resections, or periosteal flaps are important to ensure union of the two halves of the sternum. During the closure, the cardiorespiratory status should be monitored closely in case of possible compromises (Fig. 76–56). Larger defects have been stabilized by transplanting segments of lower rib cartilages (Burton, 1947) or using Teflon felt reinforced with reverse rectus sheath (Ravitch 1977). Bilateral pectoralis major muscle mobilization can be used to cover the central defect. Ravitch reviewed 44 cases of surgical repairs reported in the literature from 1888 to 1975 with generally good to excellent result and only four deaths (Ravitch 1977). The parietal anomalies seen in Cantrell's pentalogy are usually repaired using adjacent muscles or flaps to restore thoracic and abdominal integrity. The cardiac malformation is corrected at the same time (Cantrell, Haller, and Ravitch, 1958; Miller and Mathew, 1973). Ectopia cordis is only infrequently operated on successfully.

Poland's Syndrome

Poland (1841), while still a medical student at Guy's Hospital in London, dissected an anomaly with absent pectoral muscle associated with hand deformities. Clarkson (1962), a plastic surgeon at the same hospital, upon being referred a similar patient, gave Poland credit for the earlier description and generated a wider interest in the deformity. Although Froriep (1839) had described a similar and more severe case in the non-English literature, this condition had become attached to the eponym of Poland's syndrome. More recently, Ravitch (1977, 1987) accu-

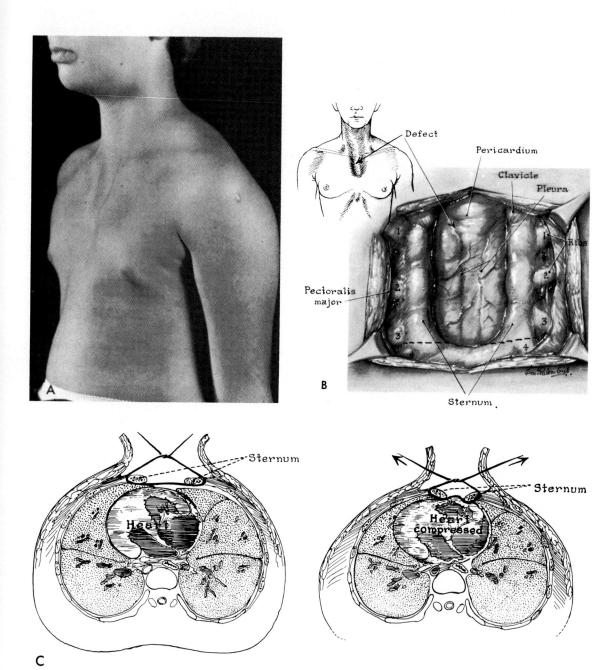

Figure 76–56. Cleft sternum in an older child; prosthetic repair. A 12 year old girl with sternum cleft of the third interspace. *A,* Preoperative photograph. Cardiac pulsations were visible, and the soft tissue in the cleft bulged with the Valsalva maneuver. (From Ravitch, M. M.: The Chest Wall. *In* Shields, T. W.: General Thoracic Surgery. Philadelphia, Lea & Febiger, 1972.) *B,* At operation the defect, thought clinically to be V-shaped, was found in fact to be a broad U. Transection of the sternal bars at the level indicated by the dotted line and sliding chondrotomies of cartilages I, II, and III allowed the sternal defect to be closed. However, each time the sternal halves were approximated (*C*), the patient developed hypotension and a profound bradycardia. It is obvious that the closure decreased the circumference of her chest, and the resultant decrease of lebensraum within the chest was intolerable. Therefore, the transected cartilages and sternal bars were resutured and the defect was covered with a prosthesis.

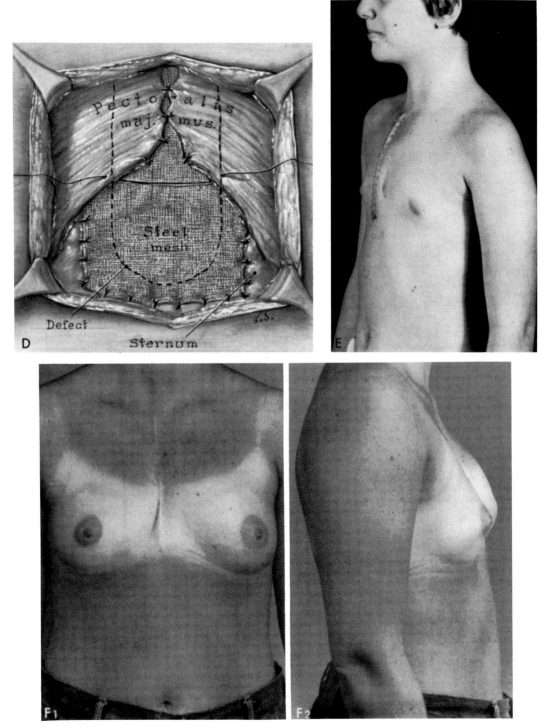

Figure 76–56 *Continued D,* Stainless steel wire mesh was all that was available. Doubled twice (i.e., four-ply), it seemed very satisfactory. (From Ravitch, M. M.: Disorders of the sternum and the thoracic wall. *In* Sabiston, D. C., and Spencer, F. C. (Eds.): Gibbon's Surgery of the Chest. 3rd Ed. Philadelphia, W. B. Saunders Company, 1976.) *E,* Immediately after operation the cleft has disappeared, the sternum is normally prominent, and the pulsation and paradox have disappeared. *F1, F2,* Twenty years later, the result remained excellent and the patient had no complaints.

Illustration continued on following page

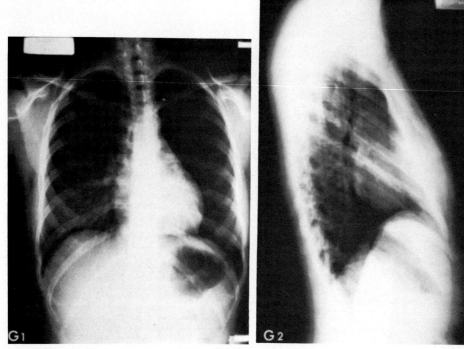

Figure 76–56 *Continued G1, G2,* X-rays faintly show the stainless steel mesh. (From Ravitch, M. M.: Congenital Deformities of the Chest Wall and Their Operative Correction. Philadelphia, W. B. Saunders Company, 1977.)

mulated considerable experience with this condition and clarified many of the issues related to diagnosis and treatment.

Clinical Description. The syndrome has been described with a variety of associated anomalies centered around the upper limb and torso; it is more common in males than females and rarely bilateral (Fig. 76–57). The absence of the sternal head of the pectoralis major muscle is considered the minimal expression of this syndrome. Involvement of adjacent muscles, such as the pectoralis minor, serratus, latissimus dorsi, and the external oblique, has been described. Skeletal deformities may involve *absence of portions of the ribs or costal cartilages* anteriorly. In severe cases, there may be significant paradoxical movement of the chest and even anterior lung herniation. The scapula may be smaller with winging (Sprengel's deformity). The *skin* of the area is hypoplastic with a thinned subcutaneous layer, and the axillary hair may be absent. The nipple is often higher in males and in females the *breast* is generally hypoplastic. The *hand deformities* may present as variable syndactyly, absent middle

phalanges, fusion of carpal bones, or shortened forearm.

Incidence and Associated Conditions. The syndrome is uncommon but not rare. Clinical series are generally small, and the exact incidence is difficult to determine. In a study of limb anomalies in newborns from Brazil, the overall incidence of Poland's syndrome is one in 30,000. Despite the low incidence, there is a slight suggestion of some degree of genetic transmission. There are several reports of family members and twins with the same diagnosis, although the presentations are generally different even in the same family. Chromosomal abnormalities have also been noted. A few cases of associated leukemia have also been reported. There are also some suggestions that maternal medication early in pregnancy may play a contributory role in some cases. Cases of Poland's syndrome associated with Mobius syndrome have been described, and it is unclear if this represents a different category than the isolated Poland's syndrome.

Surgical Corrections. The absence of the pectoral muscles has not been reported to

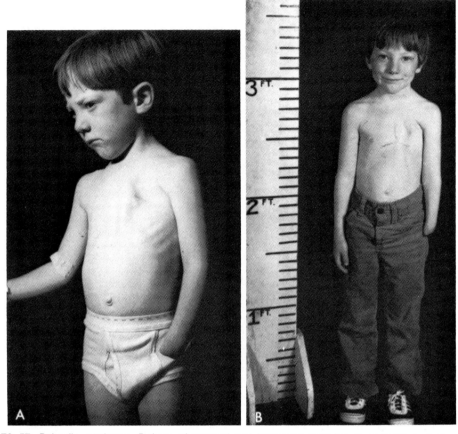

Figure 76–57. Poland's syndrome. Defects of pectoral and intercostal muscles, hypoplastic and elevated nipple, hypoplasia of subcutaneous tissue, absence of long portions of three costal cartilages, and ectromelia. Operation has stabilized the chest wall and corrected much of the abnormality. (From Ravitch, M. M.: Congenital Deformities of the Chest Wall and Their Operative Correction. Philadelphia, W. B. Saunders Company, 1977, p. 250.)

cause any functional problems. The deformities of the hand are corrected as may be indicated with any patients with syndactyly (see Chapter 128). The main concerns are usually the esthetic corrections, i.e., the absence of the anterior axillary fold, the pectoral depression in males, the hypoplastic breast in the female, and the occasional rib deformities.

Mild deformities presenting primarily as pectoral or breast asymmetries can be reasonably well corrected with either preformed or custom-made implants (Lavey and associates, 1982). Restoration of the anterior axillary fold, however, has been notoriously disappointing because of the inability of the implant to stretch and contract like normal muscle. The inelastic implant tends to protrude when the arm is down and leave a depression when the arm is elevated. Because of the simplicity and the minimal scar in-

volved, conservative custom implants should always be considered in the mild cases and satisfactory results can be obtained (Fig. 76–58). In general, a fixed solid implant is preferred for contour defects and soft breast implants should be used for breast volume restoration.

Ravitch recommended correction of the rib and sternal deformities by selective osteotomies or chondrotomies and the use of standard breast implants later (Fig. 76–59). The thin skin and axillary fold are frequent problems. Amoroso and Angelats (1981) and Hester and Bostwick (1982) used the latissimus dorsi muscle to provide coverage of the implants. The origin of the muscle is transposed from the posterior to the anterior aspect of the humerus to restore the anterior axillary fold. Urschel and coworkers (1984) used Marlex mesh covered with a synthetic dura mater graft to stabilize the rib defect and covered it

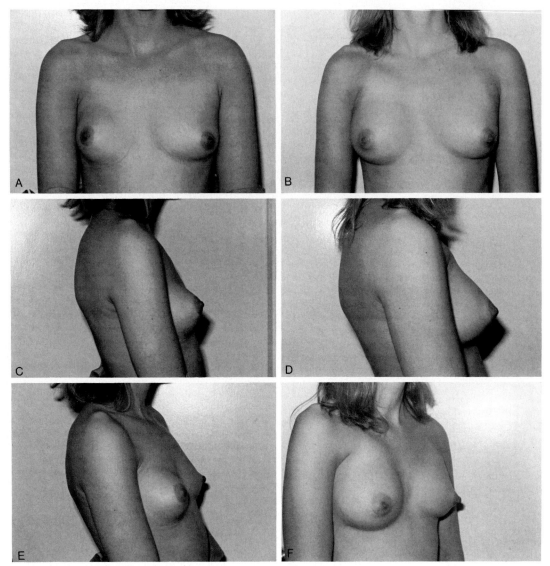

Figure 76–58. *A, C, E,* A 29 year old woman with Poland's syndrome inadequately reconstructed with a gel silicone breast implant. Note the asymmetric breast shapes and the infraclavicular depression. *B, D, F,* Following insertion of a small custom-made chest wall implant in the infraclavicular area (marked by ink), a larger breast implant (gel-saline combination), and a contralateral breast implant.

with a latissimus dorsi flap. A breast implant was placed between the layers as well. Haller and colleagues (1984) used autogenous rib struts to correct the anterior rib defect and covered them with latissimus dorsi muscle to achieve a permanent autogenous reconstruction in the older child or adult.

Ravitch expressed concern regarding the use of a major muscle in an area with existing muscle deficiency. In addition, the latissimus dorsi muscle may be hypoplastic in some of the patients. In a patient with previous failed implant reconstruction, Shaw (1989) utilized a tissue expander to lower the nipple and to develop the skin envelope. The hypoplastic breast and axillary fold were later reconstructed with an autogenous superior gluteal free flap (Fig. 76–60). In another patient with previous failure of implant reconstruction and associated absence of the anterior ribs, Marlex was used to strengthen the ribs (Fig. 76–61). A superior gluteal free flap was used as a living implant above the Marlex and behind the previously expanded thin skin. The use of autogenous tissue has the advantages of permanency, softness, and the ability to contour it secondarily.

ABDOMINAL WALL RECONSTRUCTION

The abdominal wall forms the barrier wall for several vital organs. Local incompetence or breakdown of the abdominal wall may become life-threatening by interfering with vital functions. The muscles of the abdominal wall participate in a variety of functions, such as posture, standing, walking, and bending. Other functions, such as lifting, straining during urination or defecation, and the labor of childbirth, require an increase in intra-abdominal pressure. In addition, the abdominal wall aids in vomiting and coughing and supports normal respiration.

To the extent that the integrity of the abdominal wall is maintained, normal activities take place unnoticed and are automatic. Defects, tumors, injuries, and infection interfere with the function of the abdominal wall, and diagnosis and therapy are required. Changes in fashion, along with the trend toward outdoor recreation and fitness, have made the esthetic appearance of the abdomen of importance to both women and men. Thus, an intimate knowledge of the anatomy of the abdominal wall, including its nerve and blood supply, is of special clinical concern to the reconstructive surgeon.

Dermolipectomies of the abdominal wall are discussed in Chapter 80.

Anatomy

The anterior abdominal wall is diamond-shaped. It is limited above by the lower rib margins and the xiphoid and below by Poupart's ligaments and the pelvic brim. It varies in appearance according to the sex, weight, and age of the individual, being slightly of convex contour in the average or normal person. In the thin individual it appears scaphoid, and in the obese person the convexity may be increased to a considerable extent so that the wall becomes pendulous, the lower portion overhanging in an apron-like fashion (Fig. 76–62). The protuberant and pendulous abdomen is the result of the accumulation of subcutaneous and intra-abdominal fat associated with relaxation of the abdominal wall.

UMBILICUS

The umbilicus is located below the abdominal midpoint, between the xiphoid process and the symphysis pubis. Situated over the disc between the third and fourth vertebrae, it is located approximately 2 to 4 cm above the line joining the crests of the ilia. Its position may vary considerably with the type of individual habitus. The vitelline duct, a fetal structure that passes through the umbilicus to the small intestine, is usually absent in the adult. If the proximal portion remains intact, it is known as Meckel's diverticulum, an appendage 2.5 to 7.5 cm long and located 60 cm from the ileocecal valve. If the duct persists in its entirety, a fistula, which discharges feculent material from the small bowel into the umbilical pit, results. Hernias involving the umbilicus usually contain properitoneal fat.

The linea alba extends from the xiphoid to the symphysis and is formed by the union of the aponeuroses of the abdominal muscles. In its upper portion it is approximately 0.5 cm wide, whereas below the umbilicus it becomes narrower and less distinct. Its fibers run transversely, longitudinally, and obliquely. Above the umbilicus some of the fibers enter the subcutaneous tissue and skin, producing

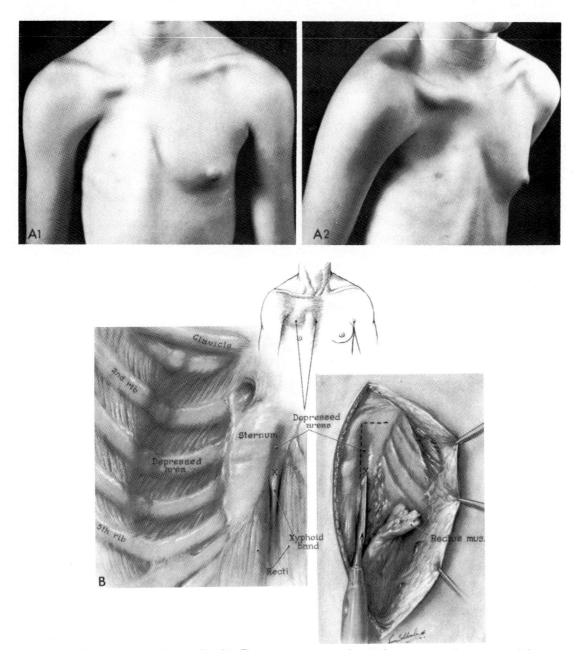

Figure 76–59. Poland's syndrome. *A1, A2,* The mammary, muscular, and cutaneous-subcutaneous defects are characteristic. *B,* Ribs and cartilages II, III, and IV were deeply incurvated. The left side of the sternum was depressed, and there was a lacuna in the manubrium.

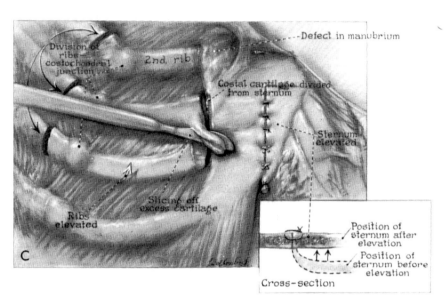

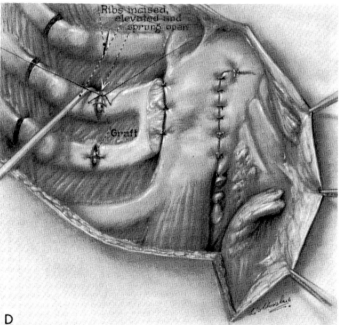

Figure 76–59 *Continued C,* Sectioning the sternum along the right-angled line shown allowed the left lower half to be elevated. The concave sections of cartilage and ribs were divided at either end and in the middle. *D,* Bone taken from osteotomies in the ribs was packed into the middle of the three chondrotomies of each cartilage, buckling the ribs forward.

Illustration continued on following page

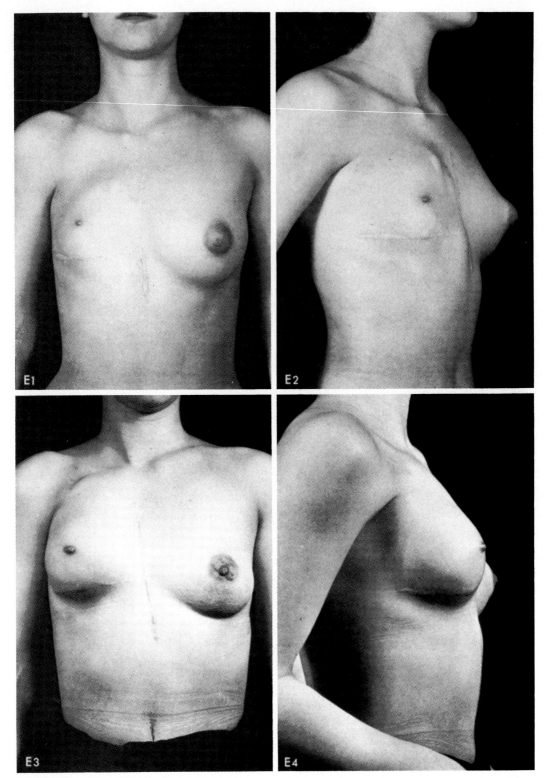

Figure 76–59 *Continued E1, E2,* Result six years after operation. The chest wall is solid and its configuration remarkably good, although the transverse limb of the incision should have been lower and curved. *E3, E4,* Ten years after operation and following insertion of a mammary implant. (From Ravitch, M. M.: Congenital Deformities of the Chest Wall and Their Operative Correction. Philadelphia, W. B. Saunders Company, 1977.)

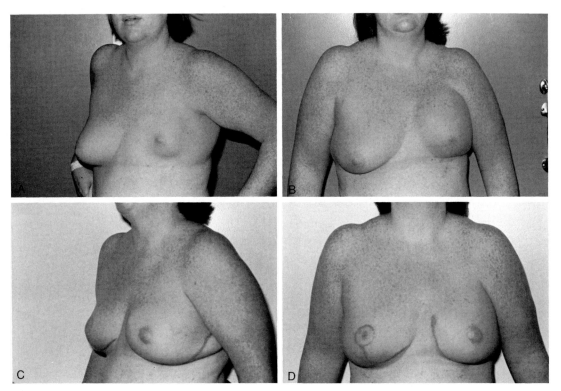

Figure 76–60. *A,* A 25 year old woman with Poland's syndrome and rupture of a previous saline breast implant. Note the position of the small nipple and the absence of the anterior axillary fold. *B,* A tissue expander was used to expand the upper chest skin, to create the breast envelope and to displace the nipple. *C, D,* A superior gluteal free flap was later placed under the preexpanded skin envelope, and a ptosis correction was done on the opposite breast later.

a slightly depressed groove. Occasionally, there are weak points between the transverse fibers through which properitoneal fat may herniate, i.e., epigastric hernias. They usually occur above the umbilicus.

The lineae semilunares form the lateral boundaries of the rectus muscles. They assume a slight lateral curve and extend from the pubic spines to the cartilages of the ninth ribs. They are formed by the union of the aponeuroses of the abdominal muscles as they join to form the sheaths of the rectus muscles. The upper extremity of the right semilunaris indicates the location of the fundus of the gallbladder. McBurney's point is located at the junction of the right semilunaris with a line drawn from the right iliac spine to the umbilicus.

The lineae transversae or transverse inscriptions are fibrous bands or grooves in the rectus muscles that are apparent on the abdomens of thin, muscular individuals. They are firmly adherent to the anterior sheath of the rectus muscles; posteriorly, the muscle is free of the sheath.

LAYERS OF THE ABDOMINAL WALL

The anterior abdominal wall is composed of the following layers: skin, superficial fascia, muscles and their aponeuroses, properitoneal fat, transversalis fascia, and peritoneum. The skin is lax and not adherent, except at the linea alba and the umbilicus. When stretched by subcutaneous fat, intra-abdominal tumors, or pregnancy, the skin may contain faint white or purplish lines, the lineae albicantes. The superficial fascia consists of a superficial fatty layer, Camper's fascia, and a deeper membranous layer, Scarpa's fascia. The latter is attached to the medial half of Poupart's ligament, and more laterally it is continuous with the fascia lata of the thigh.

MUSCLES AND FASCIAS

The *external oblique muscle,* the most superficial of the three muscles in the lateral aspect of the wall, arises from the lower eight ribs, where it interdigitates with the serratus

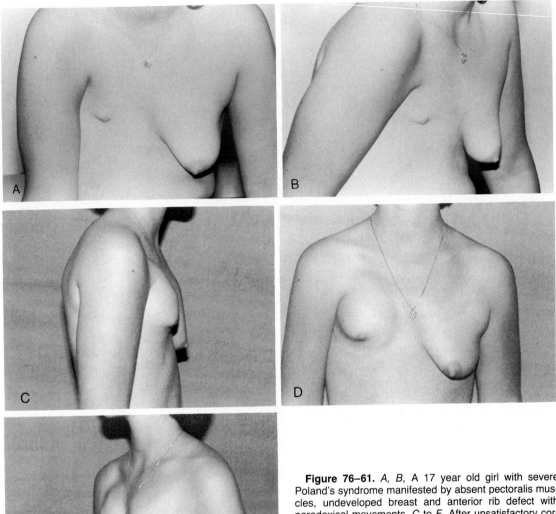

Figure 76–61. *A, B,* A 17 year old girl with severe Poland's syndrome manifested by absent pectoralis muscles, undeveloped breast and anterior rib defect with paradoxical movements. *C to E,* After unsatisfactory correction despite an attempted custom breast implant. The breast implant had apparently sunken partially into the chest.

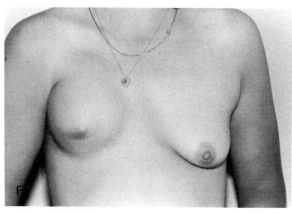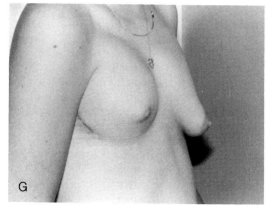

Figure 76–61 *Continued F, G,* The previous implant was removed, and an 800 ml expander was placed in the upper chest to lower the nipple and to create the breast skin envelope. A superior gluteal free flap was placed into the pocket created by the expander while the rib defect was reinforced by Marlex.

anterior and the latissimus dorsi. Its fibers fan out, extending upward and medially to be inserted into the anterior half of the iliac crest posteriorly, and by means of its broad aponeurosis they are thickened to form the inguinal (Poupart's) ligament, which passes between the anterosuperior iliac spines and the spine of the pubis. Just above and lateral to the pubic spine, the fibers of the aponeurosis are divided to form the external inguinal ring.

The *internal oblique muscle* lies beneath the external oblique and arises from the lumbodorsal fascia, the anterior two thirds of the iliac crest, and the lateral two thirds of the inguinal ligament. Its fibers radiate in a fanlike manner and pass upward and medially. The lower fibers join those of the transversus muscle to form the conjoined tendon, which is inserted into the crest and spine of the pubis and the ileopectineal line. The more superior fibers are inserted by a broad aponeurosis into the linea alba and the cartilages of the seventh to ninth ribs. The lower border

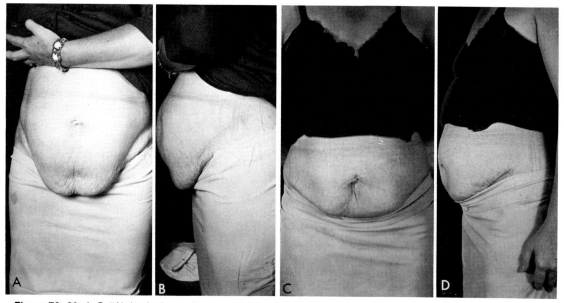

Figure 76–62. *A, B,* "Abdominal apron" with ventral hernia in a 41 year old multiparous housewife. Through a hammock incision that extended from the iliac spines to the crest of the pubis, the cutaneous abdominal wall and heavy panniculus were freed from the fascia of the external oblique superiorly to the umbilical hiatus. An imbrication repair of the large ventral hernia was performed using silk sutures. The heavy abdominal flap was drawn downward, an excess of more than 20 cm was discarded, and the wound was repaired in layers. *C, D,* Postoperative photographs four months following surgery.

of the internal oblique arches over the inguinal canal, and contraction and shortening of these fibers aid in preventing herniations by applying pressure against the canal.

The *transversus muscle* is located deep to the internal oblique and arises from the lower six ribs, the lumbodorsal fascia, the anterior two thirds of the iliac crest, and the lateral third of the inguinal ligament. It is inserted by an aponeurosis into the linea alba and by the conjoined tendon into the pubic spine and ileopectineal line.

The *recti abdomini* are long, broad muscles lying longitudinally in the medial aspect of the abdominal wall. Each arises from the front of the symphysis and the pubic crest and inserts into the xiphoid and the cartilages of the fifth to seventh ribs. Each is enclosed in a sheath.

The *pyramidalis* is a small triangular muscle superficial to the rectus muscle, arising from the front of the pubis and inserting into the linea alba approximately halfway between the symphysis and the umbilicus.

Muscle Functions

Unlike the muscles of the extremities with specific bony attachments and independent functions, the muscles of the abdomen are anatomically and functionally closely interdependent. The loss of one muscle function can interfere with the function of all adjacent muscles. The rectus abdominis muscle is anatomically formed by a series of individual muscle-nerve units. The loss of tone of one segment can render the remaining segments much less effective. Each of the abdominal muscles also contributes both to specific directional movements as well as to the general tone of the entire abdominal wall. The paired rectus abdominis muscles are the most effective ones for anterior flexion of the body and are important in rising out of bed or climbing. The external and internal oblique muscles are normally important in rotating the upper body against the lower body. The vertical component of their muscle forces, however, can substitute effectively for the rectus abdominis muscle function. All the muscles contribute together to increase intra-abdominal pressure such as in coughing or defecation.

Fascia and Ligaments

The *rectus sheath* is a fibrous envelope that encloses each muscle. The anterior layers are formed by the aponeurosis of the external oblique, together with the anterior half of the internal oblique aponeurosis. The posterior layer of the split aponeurosis of the internal oblique muscle passes beneath the rectus to form the posterior layer of the sheath in association with the aponeurosis of the transversus muscle. An important part of the stability of the abdominal wall is based on the unique system of static support provided by the fascial condensations and ligaments. The linea alba in the midline and the paired linea semilunaris on the sides extend from the ribs to the pubis. The attachments of the transverse inscriptions of the rectus abdominis muscle to the anterior rectus sheath (the linea semilunaris) and the linea alba complete the chain-link static network from which the muscles can contract. These keystone attachments should be preserved whenever feasible. Behind the lower fourth of the rectus muscle, the posterior layer of the sheath is absent. The inferior boundary of the sheath is called the linea semicircularis, the fold of Douglas, or the "arcuate line." The deep epigastric artery ascends anterior to this fold.

The *transversalis fascia* is the fascial lining of the abdominal cavity. It covers the deep surface of the transversus muscle and is separated from the peritoneum by extraperitoneal fat. Internal to this is the parietal peritoneum or serous lining of the anterior abdominal wall.

CIRCULATION

The abdominal wall is developed embryologically, is independent of the visceral organs, and has a distinctly different system of blood supply. The main sources of *arterial* supply are from the following:

1. The internal mammary artery through the upper rectus abdominis muscle to the upper central abdominal skin.

2. The segmental thoracic and lumbar intercostal arteries from the side between the external and internal oblique muscles with direct lateral skin perforators.

3. The external iliac artery giving off the deep inferior epigastric artery to the lower rectus abdominis muscle and skin and the deep circumflex iliac artery supplying the inner aspect of the ilium and terminating in the skin over the iliac crest.

4. The femoral artery giving off the superficial inferior epigastric artery to the lower

abdomen and the superficial circumflex iliac artery to the anterior iliac spine area.

Taylor and Palmer (1987) described extensive collateralization of these systems in well-defined patterns occurring both in the subcutaneous level and in the deeper muscular layer (see Chapter 10). A wide variety of regional arterialized skin or musculocutaneous flaps can be designed based on this anatomic concept.

Venous drainage of the abdomen parallels that of the arteries. The superficial veins that drain the upper abdomen are the superior epigastric, the intercostal, and the axillary veins. The lower abdomen is drained by the superior inferior epigastric, the superficial circumflex iliac, and the deep inferior epigastric veins. Enlarged veins occasionally are seen around the umbilicus and are called the caput medusae. A similar network of collateralization occurs between veins as in the arteries. Valves, however, do exist both in the superficial and deep systems, but retrograde flow against the valves can occur to some degree.

The superficial *lymphatics* drain into the groin nodes or the axillas. The deep lymphatics drain upward toward the internal mammary nodes in the mediastinum or the deep iliac nodes.

NERVES

The cutaneous nerve supply of the abdominal wall is predominantly from the sixth to the twelfth thoracic nerves, which pass into the subcutaneous layer laterally at the midaxillary line and anteriorly near the midline. The iliohypogastric and ilioinguinal nerves supply the inferolateral aspect of the abdomen. The intercostal nerves are both motor and sensory. Undermining of skin for abdominoplasty or skin flaps may result in areas of hypesthesia. Loss of muscle innervation may be observed in areas of abdominal wall weakness and bulging.

Principles of Abdominal Wall Reconstruction

INCISIONS AND CLOSURE

Despite improvements in suture material and surgical techniques, postoperative wound dehiscence, undesirable scars, and hernia

continue to occur. Surgeons should have a thorough knowledge of the factors important in the proper planning of abdominal incisions, the prevention of postoperative hernias, and the optimal methods of closure.

The making of any abdominal incision and its subsequent repair should follow the established surgical principles of wound healing and the anatomic facts previously outlined in terms of the blood and nerve supply, the fascial layers, and muscle tension. The normal anatomy should be disturbed as little as possible. Incisions placed across the blood and nerve supply or against the lines of tension are prone to postoperative complications of dehiscence or hypertrophic scars. Parallel incisions or T-incisions are generally undesirable because of compromise in circulation and denervation of muscles. Nonabsorbable material should be used because of the increased intra-abdominal pressure and the fact that the scar is not sufficiently strong until 8 weeks or more later. The sutures should not be tightened too tightly to avoid interruption of the circulation resulting in areas of focal necrosis.

The standard abdominal incision, however, is usually based on the ease of access to intra-abdominal lesions. It may be and is frequently inconsistent with anatomic and physiologic conditions inherent in the abdominal wall. This is one of the three major reasons for the relative frequency of postoperative hernias, the other two being inadequate suturing and infection. Placing abdominal incisions in a physiologic manner in order to guard against the pulling of sutures and the disruption of the wound is one of the cardinal principles of surgery. Sutures hold best when and where they pull across tissue fibers. This can be accomplished only by making the incision so that it runs parallel to the tissue fibers. Insofar as this applies to the skin of the abdomen, a knowledge of the lines of minimal tension is essential (see Chapter 1).

One of the objections raised concerning the transverse abdominal incision is the argument that it cuts across the abdominal muscles; as a matter of fact, however, this involves only one abdominal muscle, the rectus. During resuturing, the muscle sutures hold poorly and pull through easily, resulting in muscle diastasis. However, little or no attention is given to the fact that most vertical abdominal incisions, though sparing the recti physically, invalidate them physiologically by cutting the nerve supply. A paralyzed muscle is functionally a dead muscle. Any incision that cuts across the nerve supply of a muscle, even though the muscle heals, results in paralysis, lack of union, and eventually diastasis. Any incision that cuts across the main blood supply of a muscle results in delayed or absent healing with necrosis and retraction and so establishes a tissue void, which may ultimately lead to postoperative herniation. Of even greater importance is the meticulous repair of the investing fascia, because fascia is a strong binding tissue that provides satisfactory purchase for the sutures.

The upper abdominal wall is tense, firm, and strong owing to the costal attachment of the muscles and the fascia; the lateral pull of the muscles is the result of distribution of the fascial fibers. This anatomic finding is one of the main reasons for the difficulty in closing upper abdominal paramedian incisions. When such incisions open spontaneously following operation, it is usually found that the defect in the musculature runs in a transverse or horizontal direction. This is strictly in accordance with the normal lines of tension of the fasciae of the upper abdomen.

The aggregate of the lines of tension in the lower abdominal wall is generally in an oblique direction. Because of the lack of the prominent lineae transversae in the lower abdomen, as contrasted with the upper abdomen, the linea alba is much weaker. The rectus muscles, not having support of the transverse fibrous intersections, are more likely to bulge and separate after surgery or injury. However, in the lowermost portion of the abdomen, the rectus muscles and their investments are supported by the pyramidalis muscles and their fibrous fusion with the linea alba and by the reflections of the inguinal ligaments.

In general, the midline abdominal incision remains the most universally useful incision for exposure in a wide variety of intra-abdominal procedures. No muscle function, blood supply, or nerve innervation is disturbed. It has the added advantage of being able to be reused again and again. For limited exposure or localized procedures, incisions should be carefully planned to take advantage of the local anatomy. The McBurney incision for appendectomy is an elegant example of utilizing the muscle tensions to achieve a secure wound closure that has stood the test of time.

The sutures of the muscle are placed across the fibers, and contraction of the muscles serves to tighten the closure rather than pull it apart. A paramedian incision after previous midline incision, on the other hand, may be risky, in that the skin blood supply may not be reliable. Also, the denervated muscle may not hold sutures well.

GENERAL APPROACH TO RECONSTRUCTING DEFECTS OF THE ABDOMINAL WALL

Defects of the abdominal wall may result from tumor resection, radiotherapy, postoperative incisional hernia, massive infection, trauma, and congenital anomalies. The usual priorities in abdominal wall reconstruction are wound coverage or closure, protection of the visceral organs, fascial support, muscle function, and esthetics. While it may be impossible to achieve all of these goals in each case, an itemization of the goals helps the surgeon to plan reconstruction better. Often these goals are closely related so that achieving protection with a thicker flap may also provide better fascial support and an esthetic result. Decisions regarding the timing of reconstruction and selection of methods deserve some discussion.

Immediate closure or reconstruction of abdominal wall defects is always preferred to minimize the problems of massive fluid and protein loss, the likelihood of intraperitoneal infection, and the chances of undesirable scarring. Secondary dissection of the bowels from the operative scars is not only tedious but also risky. Occasionally, primary closure may not be feasible because of uncertain tumor margins, established residual local infection, excessive bulk of the bowels from edema or meconium, lack of available regional flaps, or the physiologic status of the patient. In such situations, the exposed bowels may be treated with sterile wet dressings for a few days until the conditions have improved sufficiently for closure. If closure is not possible, one can wait a few more days for granulation tissue to develop over the surface of the bowels and the communication of the peritoneal cavity to become sealed. This delay ensures the absence of deep-seated infection and reduces the urgency of the reconstructive procedures. If a flap is not available or suitable at this time, skin grafts may be sufficient to achieve the most important goal of wound closure, leaving the task of definitive reconstruction to a later and more opportune time.

Skin Grafts

Ferraro (1927) experimentally buried skin of unspecified size and thickness into lacerations in various abdominal organs. The growth of autogenous skin implanted inside the liver, spleen, and kidney was noted, whereas the skin allografts disintegrated. Butcher (1946) reported that full-thickness skin autografts lying loosely within the peritoneal cavity would survive, but growth of hair was retarded and the glandular structures underwent atrophy. Horton and associates (1953), studying the behavior of split-thickness skin and dermal grafts in the peritoneal cavity in dogs, found that they grew well in the abdominal cavity on both the parietal and visceral peritoneum. Mladick and associates (1969) successfully treated a patient in whom abdominal wall and peritoneum had been resected three weeks earlier by the application of split-thickness skin grafts to combat clostridial myonecrosis. Millard, Pigott, and Zies (1969) investigated skin grafting of full-thickness defects of the abdominal wall of the rat and dog. Grafts slightly smaller than the defect could be used, and the grafts were partially excised as the wound contracted.

Welch (1951), studying the use of allografts in the treatment of omphaloceles, found that lyophilized corium allografts are rapidly absorbed after transplantation. However, the grafts are not rejected if they are prepared in thimerosal (Merthiolate) prior to lyophilization. When allografts are treated with Merthiolate, they become nonviable or static and fail to produce significant immunologic reaction. Such grafts actually assume a supportive biomechanical function by acting as a framework for fibroblast ingrowth, collagen deposition, and formation of a firm replacement of the anterior abdominal wall (Prpic and associates, 1973). Prpic and associates (1974) used dermis autografts prepared in Merthiolate prior to lyophilization to repair surgically created full-thickness abdominal wall defects in rats.

Although the application of skin grafts is a relatively simple method for the closure of abdominal wall defects, the associated problem of lack of wall support is obvious. When the skin grafts are adherent to the surface of the gastrointestinal tract, the potential for massive adhesion formation is present. Subsequent surgery under such conditions is obviously treacherous.

In cases of massive fasciitis or enormous abdominal wounds, closure with normal tissue cannot be achieved. Skin grafts provide the only means of coverage. Dervin and Fischer (1982) treated six patients with massive fasciitis by aggressive debridement followed by topical wound care and nutritional support for 7 to 20 days. Skin grafts of 15 to 22 cm in diameter placed on the granulation tissue resulted in satisfactory healing in all patients. Follow-up of 12 to 26 months showed that all patients did well functionally by wearing external binders.

Flaps

Defects requiring full-thickness reconstructions were traditionally managed by multiple local flap delays, waltzing tube flaps, or even jump flaps carried via the wrist. Morgan and Zbylski (1972), for example, used an open jump flap carried from the contralateral side of the abdomen and flank on the forearm to reconstruct a full-thickness abdominal wall defect that had previously been covered with a split-thickness skin graft following radical resection for clostridial myonecrosis (Fig. 76–63). Five delays were performed before setting the flap into the arm. Three additional delays were performed prior to transferring the flap to the abdominal wall.

Aside from the multiple stages, these flaps were often not reliable and are now mostly of historic interest only. Instead of thinking of the abdomen as a large randomly supplied skin area, surgeons are now aware of the multiple specific sources of blood supply to the abdomen. This concept has provided abundant options in terms of regional skin flaps, muscles with skin graft, or musculocutaneous flaps. The reconstructive surgeon must be thoroughly familiar with the sources, directions, anatomic planes, distributions, and collaterals of the pertinent blood supply of the region.

The reader is encouraged to consult the following references: (1), Taylor and Palmer (1987) on angiosomes for the general concept of trunk blood supply, (2) Cormack and Lamberty (1982) for specific descriptions of the

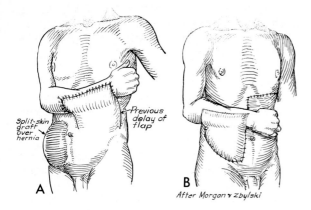

Split-skin graft over hernia

Previous delay of flap

A

B

After Morgan & Zbylski

Figure 76–63. *A,* Large ventral hernia covered by a split-thickness skin graft. Open jump flap set into arm carrier after five previous flap delays. *B,* Flap sutured to margin of defect after three more delays. Flap donor site covered by a split-thickness skin graft. (After Morgan, S. C., and Zbylski, J. R.: Repair of massive soft tissue defects by open jump flaps. Plast. Reconstr. Surg., *50:*265, 1972. Copyright © 1972, The Williams & Wilkins Company, Baltimore.)

blood supply of skin flaps and muscles of the region; (3) Mathes and Nahai (1982) for a systematic overview of the useful flaps; and (4) McCraw and Arnold's (1986) atlas for realistic color illustrations, which are helpful in preoperative planning (see also Chaps. 10, 11). Many of the flaps previously described for chest reconstruction are also suitable for upper abdomen reconstruction and are therefore not repeated. The *omentum with a skin graft over it* is also readily available in most of these cases to cover large surface areas. Its anatomy and usage were previously described in the chest section.

SKIN FLAPS

Full-thickness skin flaps may be elevated based medially on perforators from the rectus abdominis, laterally from the intercostal perforators, superiorly from the superficial superior epigastric vessels, or inferolaterally from the inferior epigastric vessels. Either rotation or transposition flaps may be used. The flap dissection should include the entire subcutaneous layer above the deep fascia, consistent with the concepts of fasciocutaneous flaps (Tolhurst and associates, 1983). Laterally, it may be convenient to include the thin fascia over the external oblique muscle. Bogart, Rowe, and Parsons (1976) used bilateral *groin flaps* to reconstruct a large full-thickness anterior abdominal defect after resection of a desmoid tumor. Primary closure of the donor defect is an important advantage in achieving a better overall esthetic result. A large area of the lower and lateral abdominal wall is suitable for design of the groin flap. Little, Fontan, and McCollough (1981) described an innervated *upper quadrant flap*

of the abdomen based on the intercostal neurovascular supply.

Deepithelized Skin Flaps

Deepithelized skin flaps were described by Poulard (1918) to correct scar craters in a manner similar to the technique of reduction mammaplasty of Strömbeck (1960), the treatment of lymphedema of Thompson (1962), and that described by Engdahl (1968) in reducing the extension of scars. Medgyesi (1972) described dermal skin flaps both as fascia substitutes and as a means of supporting fascial defects closed under tension (Fig. 76–64). The obvious primary advantage of flaps over free transplants is that they carry their own blood supply, making survival more certain. In one of Medgyesi's three patients in whom the technique was used as a fascia substitute, considerable bulging developed at the operative site but a recurrent hernia did not develop. Studies of the fate of skin placed in a subcutaneous position in this manner showed that epithelium, hair follicles, and sebaceous glands disappear but sweat glands are preserved (Thompson, 1960).

MUSCULOFASCIAL FLAPS

Farr (1922) used a flap of muscle and fascia from the lower thorax to close upper abdominal defects. Wangensteen (1934) described closure of large musculofascial defects of the abdominal wall by using the iliotibial tract of fascia lata as a flap. The fascia, suspended by the tensor fasciae femoris muscle with its nerve and blood supply intact, can provide closure of the abdominal wall defects below the umbilicus. However, Wangensteen (1946) pointed out that even in patients with long femurs, the longest iliotibial tract of fascia is usually too short for tension-free repair of defects beneath the costal margin. Therefore, a large upper abdominal defect may be reconstructed with a musculofascial flap of anterior rectus sheath and a part of the external oblique and aponeurosis. The lower abdominal musculofascial donor site is then repaired with the iliotibial tract. Bruck (1956) employed Wangensteen's technique in reconstructing the abdominal wall in a 3½ year old female following resection of the third recurrence of a fibrosarcoma. The bladder was sutured to a defect in the peritoneum; the musculofascial layer was closed with a fascia lata flap from the ipsilateral side, and a large skin defect was covered by a flap from the opposite lower extremity.

Lesnick and Davids (1953) described a technique of reestablishing integrity of the anterior abdominal wall by using a musculofascial flap from one area of the abdominal wall to close a defect in another area. A defect created by excision of the lower half of the rectus muscle and rectus sheath was reconstructed

with a flap of the external oblique muscle and aponeurosis detached from its costal origin and iliac insertion and transferred on its attachment to the anterior rectus sheath as a hinge.

Hershey and Butcher (1964) reported a one-stage closure of a large full-thickness defect of the abdominal and thoracic walls using flaps of external oblique and anterior rectus muscle fascia accompanied by the overlying skin and fat. Such flaps are broadly based laterally and posteriorly and may be made to extend across the midline. Elevation of the flaps into the axilla or lumbar region can be done, maintaining adequate blood supply and obviating the need for flap delay. However, Bekheit (1965) noted partial loss of such full-thickness flaps of skin and underlying muscle, which thus slowed wound healing. Although disruption or herniation does not usually occur following the elevation of full-thickness flaps, the donor or recipient site may subsequently bulge, necessitating the wearing of an abdominal support.

Gerber (1965) utilized a variation of Halsted's (1903) technique for repairing large in-

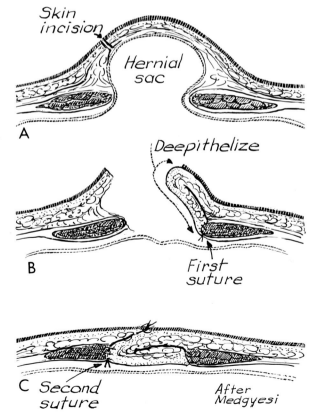

Figure 76–64. *A,* Eccentric skin incision over hernia sac provides more excess skin for shaping the flap. *B,* Hernia reduced and peritoneum closed. Skin flap has been deepithelized and inverted so that the shaved area covers the fascial defect. The first suture approximates the fascial edge to the free edge of the shaved skin flap. *C,* Flap sutured in position. At the junction of the skin and shaved flap, an incision may be made but not allowed to penetrate the full dermis. This permits approximation of the skin edges. (After Medgyesi, S.: The repair of large incisional hernias with pedicle skin flaps. Scand. J. Plast. Reconstr. Surg., 6:69, 1972.)

guinal hernias in order to restore abdominal wall integrity following the resection of desmoid tumors. The anterior rectus fascia was reflected to close one defect produced by resection of the contralateral rectus muscle and anterior fascia.

Rectus Abdominis Muscle and Myocutaneous Flap. The anatomy and variations of the long and paired muscles have been previously described in detail in the chest wall reconstruction section. Based either superiorly or inferiorly, they have the widest arc of rotation of any regional muscle for abdominal reconstruction. Bostwick, Hill, and Nahai (1979) used an inferiorly based rectus abdominis muscle to reconstruct the pelvic floor in a case of wide abdominoperineal resection.

Extra-abdominal Muscles and Musculocutaneous Flaps. Muscle from the proximal thigh provides a ready source of large muscle mass and wide skin territories for lower abdominal reconstruction. The morbidity is lower because the technique does not interfere with postoperative respiratory care. Such muscle can also potentially be dynamic substitutes for the lost abdominal muscle function in posture, can prevent hernia, and can assist in the expulsive efforts of bowel function. The most common muscles used are the rectus femoris, the tensor fasciae latae, and the vastus lateralis. The gracilis muscle medially is useful mainly for perineum reconstruction, but its muscle mass and width are limited.

Fascial Support

As a result of gravity and increased intra-abdominal pressure from daily activities, abdominal wall coverage without strong fascial or innervated muscular support is prone to develop weakness and herniation. When local fascial support is not available, distant autologous material or even synthetic material can be used.

FASCIAL GRAFTS

Gallie (1932) reported excellent results in repairing large abdominal wall incisional hernias by using a patch graft of fascia lata with the ends of the patch split into quarter-inch strips and woven into the wound margins. Two such patches sutured together with a fascial band were suggested for large defects.

McPeak and Miller (1960) noted that fascia lata was readily available and easily obtained. Because a minimal foreign body reaction, sufficiently strong to maintain the viscera within the abdominal cavity resulted, there was a smooth and glistening surface, similar to peritoneum, therefore reducing the chance of adhesions and intestinal obstruction. Thus, fascia lata grafts were strongly advocated to repair abdominal wall defects following tumor resection (Fig. 76–65). Likewise, fascia was favored over prosthetic materials, as recurrent tumors and especially fibrous and fascial tumors may grow along the latticework of the prostheses, making it difficult to differentiate recurrence of tumor from a fibrous scar reaction surrounding the prosthesis. In addition, the various metallic prostheses may interfere with postoperative radiation therapy, making it difficult to determine the amount of radiation delivered to the intra-abdominal contents. At the same time, a greater dose than desired is possibly delivered to tissues located superficial to the prosthesis.

On occasion, the wounds in children may be too large to close with autogenous fascia and the use of fascia allografts is indicated. Rehn (1911) documented experimentally that transplanted fascia allografts would survive, at least over a six-month period. Stephenson (1953) reported the repair of abdominal muscular agenesis in a 3 year old patient utilizing fascia lata from the mother. The repair was functionally intact, with palpable fascia bands providing support to the abdominal wall 13 months following transplantation. The transplantation of fascia is discussed in Chapter 14.

Sewell and Koth (1955) studied freeze-dried fascia xenografts and noted that they should not be used to reconstruct abdominal wall defects. The xenografts stimulated excessive foreign body reaction, which developed around the fascia grafts; at the same time, there was failure of ingrowth and replacement of the fascia by the host's fibroblasts. Koontz and Kimberly (1961) documented that in dogs, electron beam-irradiated ox fascia and lyophilized dura underwent graft resorption following transplantation in a manner similar to that of most allografts and xenografts. Their lack of usefulness for abdominal wall repair is therefore obvious.

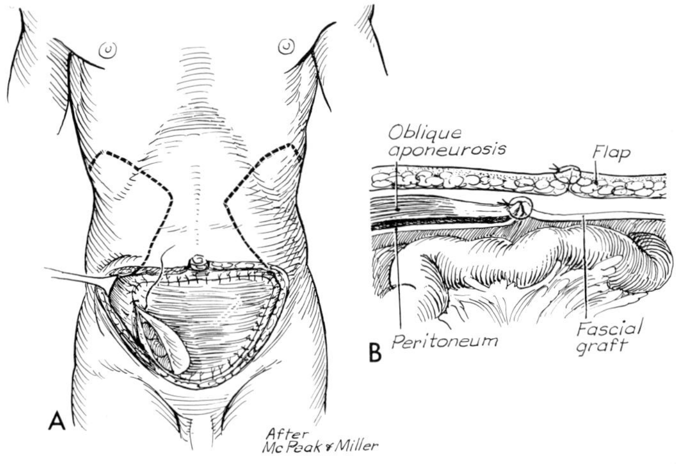

Figure 76–65. *A,* Lower abdominal defect with fascia lata sutured to the margins. Large thoracoepigastric flaps outlined. *B,* Transverse section showing fascia lata graft in place and under cover of flaps rotated medially and inferiorly. (After McPeak, C. J., and Miller, T. R.: Abdominal replacement. Surgery, 47:944, 1960.)

PROSTHETIC MATERIAL

Metal

Metallic prostheses are mainly of historic interest, having been replaced by various synthetics. Silver wire was used by Witzel (1900) for hernia repair. Goepel (1900), Meyer (1902), and Bartlett (1903) employed silver wire net. Wounds closed in this manner were rigid and prone to infection. Tantalum mesh became popular in the 1940's, as it was pliable and could be used successfully in the presence of infection (Throckmorton, 1948; Bussabarger, Dumouchel, and Ivy, 1950; Crile and King, 1951; Ye, Devine, and Kirklin, 1953; Cokkinis and Bromwich, 1954). Cantrell and Haller (1960) used tantalum in hernia repairs and reconstruction following resection of tumors of the abdominal wall. The dense fibrous reaction stimulated by the mesh was felt to be advantageous in the repair of large defects (Koontz and Kimberly, 1950; Flynn, Brant, and Nelson, 1951). However, tantalum mesh began to lose favor with reports of "work fracture" with fragmentation of the mesh, resulting in a weakened repair and associated pain in some patients (Pearce and Entine, 1952; McPeak and Miller, 1960).

Plastic

Numerous plastic materials have been considered, investigated, and used in the repair of abdominal wall defects: Nylon, Orlon, Teflon, Dacron, Marlex, and Mersilene. Marlex, a polyethylene derivative, has become one of the most popular synthetics. It was shown experimentally by Usher and Wallace (1958) to be well tolerated by tissues and to produce relatively little foreign body reaction.

Marlex net has been widely employed for reconstruction of postexcisional defects secondary to tumors, trauma, and massive infections with myonecrosis. Marlex provides adequate support and high resistance to infection (Usher, 1954; Usher and Wallace, 1958; Usher and Gannon, 1959; Schmitt and Grinnon, 1967). Markgraf (1972) reported the successful closure of infected abdominal wound dehiscence in three patients by suturing Marlex mesh to the edges of the wound and allowing several weeks to elapse before obtaining skin coverage by undermining and approximating the wound margins. The immediate wound cover with Marlex, or with any synthetic, in this fashion accomplishes several goals: (1) coverage of the viscera; (2) exteriorization of the necrotic wound margins, permitting effective drainage; (3) lessening of intra-abdominal pressure, causing less stasis in the vena cava; and (4) achieving increased capacity for the distended viscera and freer diaphragmatic excursions.

Various methods of skin closure can be achieved with Marlex. Military surgeons in Vietnam placed Marlex mesh within the abdominal cavity, sutured it to the peritoneum and posterior fasica of grossly infected abdominal war wounds, and allowed several days for the ingrowth of granulation tissue over the Marlex. Subsequently, split-thickness grafts were applied to the granulation tissue (Schmitt and Grinnon, 1967; Schmitt, Patterson, and Armstrong, 1967). However, when Marlex was placed in this fashion, it was necessary to prevent corrugation and irregularities of the mesh, mechanical factors that could delay the formation of granulation tissue and ultimate wound coverage by a skin graft.

Mansberger and associates (1973) reported the repair of massive (acute) abdominal wall defects by a series of planned operations. First, the peritoneal defect was closed by Silastic sheeting, with physiologic wet dressings placed on the surface of the sheeting. An endogenous membrane—"new peritoneum"—formed under the sheeting. Because of the inertness of the plastic sheeting, the new peritoneum formed without adhesions to the abdominal viscera. The plastic sheeting was removed at three to four weeks, and the endogenous membrane and granulating wound were covered with full-thickness skin flaps or a full-thickness skin graft. Six to eight weeks later, the flaps were elevated and Marlex was used to repair the fascial defect.

Wilson and Rayner (1974) used Mersilene net, a Dacron mesh, to repair large full-thickness postincisional defects of the abdominal wall. Mersilene mesh becomes firmly infiltrated with fibrous tissue, remains flexible and is minimally degenerative. The Mersilene net must be inserted under tension, and this is achieved by suturing the net to the intra-abdominal periphery of the wound, pulling it outward and suturing it to the external fascial sheath (Fig. 76–66). Studies in rats (Rayner, 1974) demonstrated that reperitonealization of the prosthetic net surface occurs simultaneously with the conversion of the fibrous coagulum that initially surrounds the net to the fibrous tissue. The abdominal cavity is truly sealed by the coagulum from 24 hours onward. At 96 hours, the coagulum has been converted into a cellular, loosely woven, fibrous tissue and the cavity surface of the net is uniformly covered with mesothelium, which, by histologic examination, shows a true peritoneal layer. These findings confirmed those of Ellis (1971) on the rate of reperitonealization.

Karakousis, Elias, and Douglas (1975) reconstructed large abdominal wall defects from tumor excision with Prolene mesh. This technique provided a strong and stable restoration of the fascial support. Adjacent skin flaps were mobilized to cover the mesh. When this is not possible because of the defect size, the mesh is left to granulate and later skin grafted. Voyles and associates (1981) reported 31 closures of abdominal defects with Marlex mesh with 29 being placed in heavily contaminated wounds. Although seven patients died from the primary illness, in no case was the Marlex a factor contributing to the intra-abdominal infection. In the patients who had undergone primary closure with adjacent skin or with flaps, the Marlex was retained in all. In 14 of the 15 patients treated with skin grafts or spontaneous granulation and epithelization, the Marlex had to be removed later. Stone and associates (1981) had somewhat better experience with Prolene mesh with 40 per cent of patients requiring subsequent removal of the implant.

Deficiencies and Defects of the Abdominal Wall

HERNIAS

Protrusion of a portion of the abdominal contents into or through a cleft or weak spot in the abdominal wall is one of the commonest of surgical abnormalities (see Fig. 76–62).

The term hernia is probably derived from the Greek *epvoo,* meaning a branch. It is probable that the Greek school of surgery in Rome, during the first centuries of the Christian era, practiced incision and some form of ligation of the inguinal hernial sac. In the Middle Ages, the brutal fireband and caustics were employed. The external limits of the hernia were apparently outlined with the

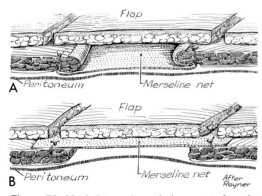

Figure 76–66. *A,* Intraperitoneal placement of synthetic mesh with sutures passing through the full thickness of the abdominal wall, producing an ischemic stimulus to adhesion formation. *B,* Onlay technique of securing the synthetic in order to avoid intraperitoneal suturing. (After Rayner, C. R. W.: Repair of full-thickness defects of the abdominal wall in rats avoiding visceral adhesions. Br. J. Plast. Surg., 27:130, 1974.)

patient in the standing position; after he was laid on his back and the sac emptied, the hot iron or stone was applied over its entire extent. When dissection was introduced during the sixteenth century by Vesalius and his followers, more rational methods began to appear. There was the "punctum aureum," the object of which was to pass a golden wire about the sac, twisting it tightly enough to prevent the intestine from passing through. This was later referred to as the "golden stitch" or "royal stitch."

During the eighteenth century, significant advances were made, especially in the anatomy of the inguinal and femoral canals, by Gimbernat, Camper, Cooper, Scarpa, and others. Cooper's work (1825) on the anatomy of hernias of the inguinal region is still current and classic. Bassini (1889) published his method of reconstructing the inguinal canal, ligating and excising the sac at its neck. Four years later in 1893, Halsted transplanted the cord anterior to the muscular and tendinous layers.

Today the repair of simple hernias is routine and considered one of the most satisfactory operations in surgery. Since this topic is adequately covered in detail in standard surgical texts, it is not dealt with further. Special problems of interest to plastic surgeons are discussed next.

Internal Hernias

Although plastic surgeons are generally not involved in intra-abdominal reconstructions, the possibilities of internal hernias should be considered in patients who underwent omental flaps or whose symptoms do not fit the nature of the surface reconstruction. Omentum is occasionally used as a flap for coverage of the chest. A potential internal hernia may exist, resulting in bowel hernia and obstruction. If not recognized promptly, this complication may be fatal.

When bowel mesentery is not closed properly, a similar hernia may result. Groce and Mehta (1979) reported a case of rupture of the diaphragm from the ninth rib, resulting in an "intercostal pleuroperitoneal hernia."

Ventral Hernia

The hernia that develops in an old operative incision often presents vexing problems in repair. The fascial defect has a tendency to enlarge with time, and closure with local tissue is difficult to impossible. When the neck is not too narrow, there is little danger of incarceration and most of these can be managed with external support. If surgical repair is desired, it is important to insist that the patient not be obese, a factor that might have contributed to the original occurrence of the hernia. Generally, it is best to excise the scar and dissect to healthy margins. The peritonial sac is dissected free, opened, excised, and repaired. The fresh healthy fascial edges are repaired with nonabsorbable suture under maximum muscle relaxation. If needed, adjacent fascial relaxing incisions are preferred. Artificial substitutes of metallic or synthetic meshes are used only when absolutely unavoidable.

Lumbar Hernia (Hernia after Latissimus Dorsi Flap)

Hernias from the abdominal cavity may develop through the posterior lateral wall, the so-called lumbar hernias. Most commonly, this hernia is due to posterolateral incisions for kidney surgery. The loss of the latissimus dorsi muscle also occasionally results in aggravating a potential weakness of the Petit's triangle. Petit's triangle is bounded by the external oblique anteriorly, the iliac crest inferiorly, and the latissimus dorsi posteriorly. The floor of the triangle is normally formed by the internal oblique muscle and a weakness or absence of it in this area is needed for the hernia to develop. When the latissimus dorsi muscle and the lumbar doral fascia are taken and the internal oblique is insufficient, a lumbar hernia may develop.

Hernia after TRAM Flap

Because of the large skin available and the ease of dissection of the muscle and its vascular pedicle, the rectus abdominis muscle is one of the most common flaps used by plastic surgeons for major reconstructions (see Chapter 79). It is used as a superiorly pedicled flap for breast reconstruction and for sternal dehiscence. It is also a popular free flap for reconstruction of the lower extremity and breast. A major disadvantage has been the occurrence of postoperative hernia and muscle weakness. Hartrampf (1984) emphasized strongly that unless the surgeon is able to avoid such complications consistently, this flap should not be used for elective procedures.

Because of the central role of the rectus muscle in abdominal wall competence, every effort should be made to repair the defect with adjacent normal muscle and fascia after a segment of the muscle is taken. The use of synthetic mesh is convenient but falsely reassuring to the surgeon. The presence in the central part of the abdomen of a patch of nonfunctioning material renders the adjacent oblique muscle less effective in substituting the vertical flexion function of the rectus abdominis muscle. When the abdomen is tensed during coughing or defecation, part of the force is lost on stretching this patch, which tends to bulge out paradoxically. Reapproximating the remaining working muscles toward the center, on the other hand, allows for more effective substitution of the lost muscle function. There is also less concern regarding the possibility of foreign body infection, particularly in the event of partial abdominal skin necrosis.

To be able to close the rectus sheath consistently after harvesting the TRAM flap, the most important factors are patient selection, conservation of the anterior rectus sheath, and maximum muscle relaxation during closure. Preexisting laxity of the abdominal wall, such as that from previous pregnancy, is helpful. Marked obesity, on the other hand, makes fascial closure a trying experience for the surgeon. Since the principal musculocutaneous perforators are concentrated in the periumbilical region, the lower half of the anterior sheath can be spared. The lateral 3 to 4 cm of the anterior sheath can also be left behind to facilitate fascial closure.

GAS GANGRENE

Although rare, clostridial myonecrosis of the abdominal wall is a devastating and highly lethal postoperative complication that requires prompt diagnosis and wide surgical debridement of all involved layers of the abdominal wall.

The clinical picture is characterized by wound swelling, tenderness, profuse serosanguineous drainage, and minimal wound discloration changing to a deep red or magenta hue within a few hours. A small amount of gas with crepitation, and toxemia out of proportion to the temperature elevation with tachycardia, hypotension, agitation, and delirium may be observed. Although bacteriologic wound examination usually reveals a number of aerobic and anaerobic organisms, at least one species of *Clostridium,* usually *C. oedematiens* or *C. septicum,* is also recovered. The organisms produce nearly a dozen exotoxins, the most important of which is lecithinase. Nonlethal toxins, among which are collagenase and hyaluronidase, play an important role in the pathogenicity of the organism. The main differential diagnosis is between anaerobic clostridial cellulitis and clostridial myonecrosis. The differentiating factor is the relationship of the gas to toxemia (Schwartz, 1969).

A wound containing a large amount of gas associated with mild toxemia is usually not gas gangrene. However, little or no gas associated with severe toxemia probably represents gas gangrene (clostridial myonecrosis).

Fear of not being able to close the abdominal wall defect should not limit the extent of the resection when a diagnosis of clostridial myonecrosis has been made. An area of residual infection may result in continued spread of the pathologic process or may serve as a source of fatal sepsis. Although oxygen administered at hyperbaric pressure, massive doses of antibiotics, and other adjunctive measures may help to decrease the extent of excision that is needed to control the clostridial infection, a massive forfeiture of skin, muscle, fascia, and peritoneum is usually necessary (Brummelkamp, Hogendijik, and Boerema, 1961; Sanders, 1963).

Reconstructive surgeons vary in their approach to closure of the massive defect usually produced in controlling this infection.

Mladick, Pickerell, Royer, and colleagues (1969) described resection of the entire anterior abdominal wall, the exposed viscera being allowed to form granulation tissue; full-thickness skin grafts were successfully applied three weeks later. McNally, Price, and MacDonald (1968) closed a defect with Marlex mesh, but they removed the prosthesis before applying skin grafts.

Morgan, Morain, and Eraklis (1971) reported a massive, anterior abdominal wall resection, including all of the right-sided muscles from the costal margin to the symphysis pubis and the entire left rectus muscle. The peritoneum was left in place and reinforced with Mersilene mesh. One month after resection, windows were cut from the Mersilene and split-thickness skin grafts were applied on the granulation tissue arising from the visceral peritoneum of the underlying organs. Several grafting procedures were required in order to obtain complete wound closure. The rationale for leaving the peritoneum intact was that it would act as a barrier to bacterial invasion of the abdominal cavity for approximately seven days before becoming necrotic. The authors preferred to resect the peritoneum when infected, as it is certain to slough, provide a nidus of infection, and delay skin graft or flap coverage of the wound. Gastrointestinal decompression and intravenous hyperalimentation can be of benefit in such patients when the viscera are exposed and split-thickness skin grafts are applied directly to their surface.

Eng, Casson, Berman and Slattery (1973) reported a case of full-thickness resection of the anterior abdominal wall for clostridial myonecrosis, which entailed suturing the greater omentum to the edges of the parietal peritoneum and covering the omentum with Marlex mesh, which was sutured to the external oblique aponeurosis between the remainder of the abdominal wall fascia and subcutaneous tissue (Fig. 76–67). By the third postoperative day, there was almost complete ingrowth of granulation tissue from the omentum through the Marlex mesh. Split-thickness skin grafts were applied to the wound on the eighth postoperative day.

Agenesis and hypoplasia in one or several of the muscular layers of the abdominal wall interfere with respiration, coughing, defecation, and urination. Congenital defects are commonly present where vessels or other structures penetrate the transversalis fascia. When the opening permits structures other than those normally present to leave the abdominal cavity, the defect is pathologic and results in herniation requiring surgical correction. The common sites of congenital defects are the internal abdominal ring, the

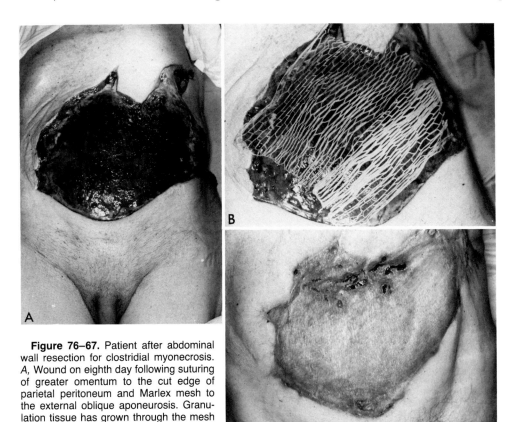

Figure 76–67. Patient after abdominal wall resection for clostridial myonecrosis. *A,* Wound on eighth day following suturing of greater omentum to the cut edge of parietal peritoneum and Marlex mesh to the external oblique aponeurosis. Granulation tissue has grown through the mesh and completely covers it. *B,* Meshed split-thickness skin graft applied to granulation tissue. *C,* Wound healing well eight weeks after application of skin grafts. (Courtesy of Phillip Casson, F.R.C.S., Institute of Reconstructive Plastic Surgery.)

esophageal hiatus, and the pelvic orifices through which the rectum, vagina, and urethra pass. Some of these latter abnormalities are discussed in a later section.

GASTROSCHISIS AND OMPHALOCELE

Congenital and acquired defects of the umbilical area are manifold and are related to its important embryonic roles as a conduit for blood and as a temporary extracoelomic reservoir for the midgut. Many of the defects are small, and only conservative care and observation are necessary. However, of lesser incidence but of far greater importance are other anomalous conditions that demand careful attention and often corrective surgical procedures in order to restore function to a level compatible with life, if not to improve the appearance of the area.

Gastroschisis and omphalocele are congenital defects of the anterior abdominal wall with different anatomic deficits and embryologic failures but with much in common in regard to surgical treatment.

Embryology

During the third week of embryonic life, closure of the body of the embryo is produced by a circumferential folding of four folds, which are the condensation of embryonic mesenchyma. The four folds—cephalic, caudal, and two lateral—have somatic and splanchnic layers. The somatic layers of the cephalic, caudal, and two lateral folds form the thoracic wall, epigastric wall, hypogastric wall, and lateral abdominal walls, respectively (Lewis, Kraeger, and Danis, 1973). The apex of the folds forms the future umbilical ring. Failure of differentiation of the mesenchyma forming the somatopleure of the lateral abdominal wall and resorption of the ectoderm adjacent to the somatopleure lead to a paraumbilical full-thickness defect in the anterior abdominal wall (Duhamel, 1963; Izant, Brown, and Rothmann, 1966; Lewis, Kraeger, and Danis, 1973). The midgut occupies the peritoneal cavity until the resorption appears.

An omphalocele (Fig. 76–68) is a perpetuation of the state existing at the sixth to 12th weeks of intrauterine life (12 to 40 mm), during which time the entire midgut passes from the abdominal cavity into the base of the yolk sac via the omphalomesenteric tract.

The umbilical cord is inserted into this sac of peritoneum-amnion. Normally, accelerated linear growth of bowel occurs during the extracoelomic phase as well as counterclockwise rotation through 270 degrees around the superior mesenteric vascular axis, prior to an orderly reduction of the bowel into the abdominal cavity. Failure of reduction of bowel and, therefore, continued extra-coelomic displacement of the viscera result in an omphalocele. With large defects, the liver and spleen may accompany the bowel outside the abdominal cavity.

An omphalocele is not a true hernia, since it has no peritoneum lining its sac and its contents have never been truly located within the abdomen. The cause of failure of reduction of the contents into the abdominal cavity is unknown. It may be related to failure of development of the abdominal wall, or it may be due to the presence of an abnormally small coelomic space that is inadequate to receive the viscera. The omphalocele sac containing the abdominal viscera may rupture prenatally or postnatally.

A hematoma or a cystic accumulation of Wharton's jelly in the base of the umbilical cord might be confused with a small omphalocele. However, the sac is usually considerably larger. It averaged 6 to 8 cm in size in a series of 19 patients (Soper and Green, 1961). The sac is usually thin and translucent immediately after delivery; however, within several hours it becomes lusterless and opaque, indicating dehydration and possible impending necrosis. Since the blood supply is poor, fissures are likely to develop, and this may be a sign of impending rupture. Sac rupture is a grave complication associated with a mortality rate of nearly 100 per cent (Mahour, Weitzman, and Rosenkrantz, 1973).

Gastroschisis (Fig. 76–69) is a full-thickness defect of the abdominal wall that occurs lateral to the insertion of the umbilical cord. Gastroschisis differs from an omphalocele in that there is lack of a covering sac or its remnant, the abdominal wall defect is lateral to the umbilicus, and there is a normal umbilical cord insertion (Moore and Stokes, 1953). Almost all patients with gastroschisis have in common nonrotation of the bowel, an abnormally short midgut, and a small peritoneal cavity (Hollabaugh and Boles, 1973). Nonrotation predisposes to volvulus and vascular infarction of the intestine.

Moore (1963) classified omphalocele into an

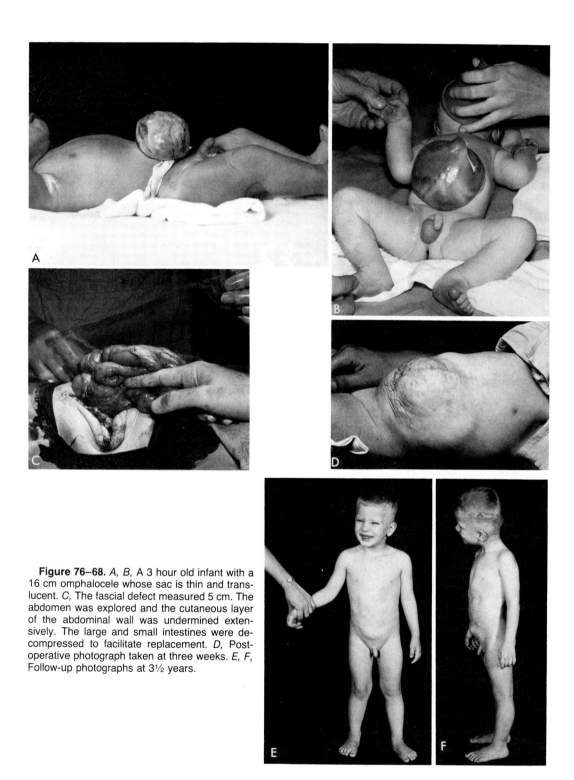

Figure 76–68. *A, B,* A 3 hour old infant with a 16 cm omphalocele whose sac is thin and translucent. *C,* The fascial defect measured 5 cm. The abdomen was explored and the cutaneous layer of the abdominal wall was undermined extensively. The large and small intestines were decompressed to facilitate replacement. *D,* Postoperative photograph taken at three weeks. *E, F,* Follow-up photographs at 3½ years.

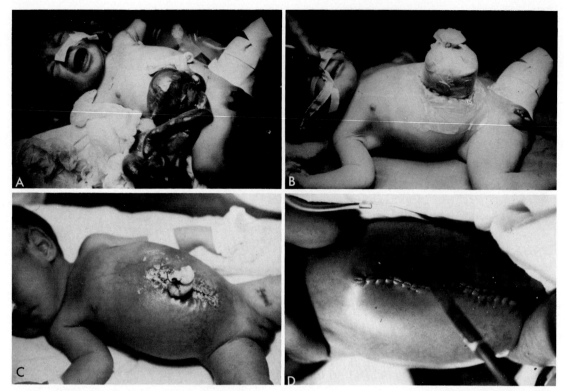

Figure 76–69. *A,* A 4 hour old infant with a 4 cm gastroschisis defect. The stomach and almost all of the intestinal tract protruded through the defect with the umbilical cord at its left edge. The intestines were shortened, malrotated, dilated, edematous, and purple. *B,* The abdominal cavity was too small to accommodate the gastrointestinal tract. A polyester mesh sack (Mersilene) lined with silicone rubber (Silastic) sheeting was sutured to the freshened edges of the defect. *C,* Beginning on the second postoperative day, a suture was tied approximately 1 cm proximal to the suture at the apex of the sack. This was continued every other day until the sack height was obliterated. Side to side plication sutures progressively narrowed the horizontal dimension of the defect. *D,* At 2 weeks of age, the abdominal defect was closed in layers, and a gastrostomy tube was placed.

antenatal type, in which the evisceration occurs early in pregnancy, the eviscerated intestines being distended, thickened, rigid, and covered with a gelatinous matrix, and a *perinatal type,* the evisceration presumably occurring late in pregnancy and possibly being induced by uterine contraction, with the bowel maintaining its elasticity and a minimal surface exudate.

In patients with gastroschisis or ruptured omphalocele of long duration, the eviscerated mass of bowel is thick, edematous, matted together, and covered with a fibrogelatinous membrane. Peristalsis is usually absent. However, most omphaloceles that rupture do so at or near term, and the bowel is not thick and matted (Wayne and Burrington, 1973).

Preoperative Management

An infant born with an omphalocele or gastroschisis constitutes a surgical emer-gency. The major causes of mortality in patients with omphalocele and gastroschisis have been sepsis, increased intra-abdominal pressure postoperatively, respiratory insufficiency, the catabolic state associated with prolonged intestinal ileus, and other associated congenital anomalies (Fig. 76–70) (Aitken, 1963; Rickham, 1963; Smith and Leix, 1966; Simpson and Lynn, 1968; Firor, 1971).

As outlined by Gross (1948, 1953), Soper and Green (1961), Wayne and Burrington (1973), and Mahour, Weitzman, and Rosenkrantz (1973), eviscerated organs or an intact sac should be covered with gauze sponges soaked in sterile saline or placed under a plastic bag to avoid heat, fluid, and electrolyte loss.

Preoperative management includes careful fluid volume control, parenteral administration of antibiotics, gastrointestinal intubation to prevent gastric distention and respiratory complications, preservation of body heat, blood gas determinations, and control of acid-base balance. Evacuation of meconium with rectal irrigations plays a significant role in reducing the mortality associated with these defects.

Postoperative mechanical respiratory assistance, when necessary, intravenous hyperalimentation until peristalsis returns, and tube feedings are major adjuncts in obtaining improved survival rates.

Roentgenograms of the abdomen and chest should be obtained, since they may show other malformations. The infant's blood should be typed and crossmatched for transfusion, and a venous cutdown should be performed in order to establish a relatively large caliber intravenous route for fluid administration.

Death rates, which were previously 70 to 80 per cent, have been reduced to 25 to 35 per cent (Lewis, Kraeger, and Danis, 1973; Hollabaugh and Boles, 1973; Wayne and Burrington, 1973).

Surgical Correction

The selection of the proper method of closure of each patient is difficult. Small defects are managed in a manner similar to that used for large umbilical hernias. The viscera are returned to the abdominal cavity, and the fascia and skin are closed in layers.

Major associated anomalies are not uncommon with gastroschisis and omphalocele and include intestinal atresia, malrotation, and volvulus, which may result in significant morbidity and mortality. Intestinal atresias occur in 20 to 25 per cent of patients (Moore

and Stokes, 1953; Schuster, 1967; Allen and Wreen, 1969; Hollabaugh and Boles, 1973; Lewis, Kraeger, and Danis, 1973). Such associated anomalies are ample reason for abdominal exploration and surgical correction (Gross, 1953; Grob, 1963; Aitken, 1963; Bill, 1969; Mahour, Weitzman, and Rosenkrantz, 1973), although one-stage closure or nonoperative management of large intact omphaloceles has been advocated (Drescher, 1963; Grob, 1963; Soave, 1963; Dorogi, 1964).

Failure to diagnose associated anomalies may result in severe complications and death following surgical closure of the abdominal wall defect (Cordero, Touloukian, and Pickett, 1969).

Soper and Green (1961) advocated a one-stage operation as the procedure of choice except when the fascial defect is too large to permit coaptation of its edges. If the sac contents are small and the coelomic cavity is large enough to receive the viscera without undue tension, the sac should be excised and closure of the wound layers accomplished with interrupted, nonabsorbable suture material. Depending upon the orientation of the defect, closure may be in a horizontal or vertical plane. The three umbilical vessels and the urachus should be individually divided and ligated at the periphery of the operative field. Careful inspection of the alimentary tract for associated anomalies is important, even at the expense of enlarging the fascial defect, which may be too small to allow such investigation through its natural confines. However, a one-stage operation is not safe when either the coelomic space is abnormally small or the eviscerated struc-

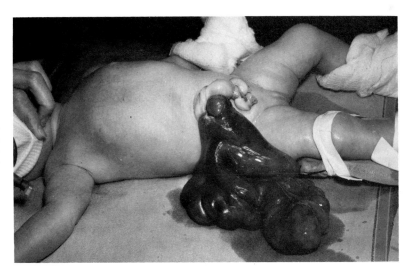

Figure 76–70. Antenatal rupture of an omphalocele sac with volvulus of exteriorized intestine. The infant was brought to the hospital four hours after birth. Postmortem examination disclosed dextroposition of the aorta, cor triloculare with common ventricle, and a small left atrium.

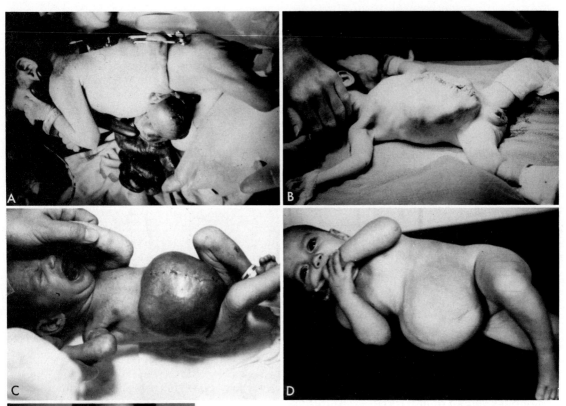

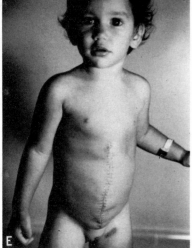

Figure 76–71. Gastroschisis treated by first-stage skin closure and second-stage fascial closure (method of Gross). *A,* Umbilical cord is located at the left edge of the gastroschisis defect. Almost all of the intestine and stomach and a portion of the liver protrude from the defect. The intestines were purple, matted, and hard. *B,* Skin flaps were elevated and approximated over the abdominal contents. *C,* At 2 weeks of age, the skin is tense, purplish, and shiny. *D,* At 6 months of age, the patient is healthy, but a large ventral hernia is present. *E,* The ventral hernia was repaired, and the rectus muscles were approximated with a prosthesis at 18 months of age.

tures are so large that reduction is accomplished only under tension. These factors result in elevation of intra-abdominal pressure and predispose to potentially fatal complications: intestinal kinking with obstruction, elevation of the diaphragm producing respiratory embarrassment, and compression of the inferior vena cava which may reduce venous return to the heart.

Operation may be performed in one or two stages, depending upon the ease with which the eviscerated structures can be reduced. Gross (1948) reported a two-stage method: the first stage consists of mobilizing the abdominal wall skin and subcutaneous tissues from the abdominal muscle fascia until sufficient coverage has been obtained to cover the intact amniotic sac. Several months later, when the mass can be reduced with ease, the sac is excised, and the abdominal wall is closed in layers (Fig. 76–71).

As emphasized by Soper and Green (1961), this method of management does not allow detection of coincidental alimentary tract abnormalities at the time of the initial operation; another extensive operation may be required during a period when diagnosis may be extremely difficult and the risks of delay or a second operation exceedingly high. Soper and Green (1961) presented an alternative to Gross's first-stage operation. The sac is excised to allow exploratory laparotomy and correction of whatever associated anomalies may exist. If the sharpness or narrowness of the fascial ring is such as to compromise circulation to the herniated viscera, relaxing incisions can be made. The skin is mobilized and closed directly over the viscera. The subsequent management is the same as that presented by Gross.

Early operative management should be performed in most cases of gastroschisis and omphalocele, with nonoperative management being reserved for the poor-risk premature patient or patients with other severe congenital anomalies (Mahour, Weitzman, and Rosenkrantz, 1973).

Closure

If primary closure produces significant abdominal cavity reduction, a staged procedure is indicated if a high chance of mortality is to be avoided. In some patients, flank-relaxing incisions and wide undermining may be sufficient to prevent increase in intra-abdom-

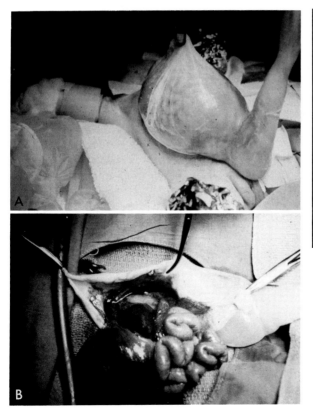

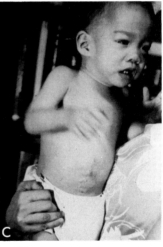

Figure 76–72. Omphalocele treated by the prosthetic silo technique similar to that shown in Figure 76–69B, C. *A*, Huge omphalocele measuring 15 × 20 cm with a fascial defect of 6 cm in an otherwise normal full-term female. *B*, Omphalocele opened showing intestines and almost the entire liver protruding through the defect. *C*, The child at 1 year of age with normal development following prosthetic silo technique closure.

inal pressure and skin flap necrosis (see Fig. 76–71). Manual stretching of the abdominal wall occasionally provides the necessary increase in the abdominal cavity to accommodate the bowel and allow closure without tension (Izant, Brown, and Rothmann, 1966).

Resection of normal bowel, liver, or spleen to allow primary closure is not indicated (Meltzer, 1956; Buchanan and Cain, 1956). Removal of the thick fibrinous peel from the surface of the bowel prolongs surgical time and increases bleeding and mortality (Moore and Stokes, 1953; Rickham, 1963).

Silon (Silastic-coated Dacron), polyethylene, and Teflon sheets sutured to the edges of the fascial defects reduce the complications of primary skin flap closure and provide an alternate method of staged abdominal wall reconstruction (Mahour, Weitzman, and Rosenkrantz, 1973).

Using a plastic pouch provides gradual return of the viscera into the abdominal cavity as the abdominal wall relaxes and the peritoneal cavity enlarges (see Figs. 76–69 and 76–72). It is surprising how rapidly the abdomen may accommodate the viscera (Shim, 1971).

Fonkalsrud (1975) raised a word of caution about the survival rate obtained using the various prostheses as part of the abdominal wall closure. His survival rate, using a two-stage closure, at the University of California, Los Angeles (UCLA), Medical Center over the past ten years was 94 per cent. Skin closure is initially followed by fascial closure after adequate growth and development have occurred.

Attention to meticulous sterile technique is absolutely necessary in managing patients with omphalocele or gastroschisis, particularly those treated in stages using prosthetic materials.

Spina Bifida

Barry M. Zide

During uterine life, closure of the neural groove begins in the thoracic region with fusion proceeding upward and downward. When fusion fails, spina bifida occurs, with resultant maldevelopment of the spinal cord and membranes. Spina bifida is the most common central nervous system (CNS) birth defect encountered by the pediatric neurosurgeon. The incidence varies from one in 200 in regions of Ireland (Elwood, 1972) to one in 1000 in North America (Amacher, 1989); it is rare in Scandinavians, blacks, and North American Indians. However, the mother of one child with overt spina bifida (as opposed to the occulta form) carries a one in 25 (4 to 5 per cent) chance of the second child being affected, and one in ten if two children already have the overt deformity (Thompson and Rudd, 1976). In some families it may be autosomal dominant in transmission (Fineman and associates, 1982). The above occurrences do not fit true mendelian transmission statistics. Thus, as in cleft lip and palate, the inheritance is considered *multifactorial* (Rudd, 1986).

In its least obvious presentation, the patient has spina bifida occulta. In this situation, abnormalities are noted on spine radiographs. Usually, one or more spinous processes are absent along with minimal evidence of the vertebral arch at the L5 and S1 levels. Incidental radiographs of the general population have documented this change in 20 to 30 per cent of cases (Boone and associates, 1985).

Local changes in the overlying skin, such as nevus, hair (Fig. 76–73), hemangioma, atrophy, dimple (Cheek and Laurent, 1985), or lipoma (Naidich, McLone, and Harwood-Nash, 1983) may be present in varying sizes in certain cases (Reigel, 1989). Parents or patients may request excision for esthetic reasons, but the surgeon must suspect an underlying pathology in which the cord and skin problem are contiguous. The disproportionate growth between the spinal cord and overlying tissues often causes a progressive neurologic malady. This entity, called *tethered cord*, is best treated by neurosurgical release before symptoms become manifest (Reigel, 1983; McLone and Naidich, 1989). Thus, the surgeon who sees children with cutaneous stigmata of spina bifida occulta should send them to be evaluated for cord tethering. Magnetic resonance imaging (MRI), ultrasonography, and computed tomography (CT) (Naidich, McLone, and Harwood-Nash, 1983) may demonstrate the low-lying terminal end of the spinal cord with limitation of movement in a cephalocaudal plane. Early intervention provides effective prophylaxis against later irreparable damage even in totally asymptomatic patients (Bruce

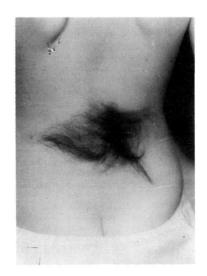

Figure 76–73. Spina bifida occulta. Note the tuft of hair. (From Mustardé, J. C.: Plastic Surgery in Infancy and Childhood. Edinburgh, Churchill Livingstone, 1971.)

and Schut, 1979; Chapman, 1982; McLone and associates, 1985; Hoffman and associates, 1985; Chapman and Beyerl, 1986). This type of pathologic fixation of the spinal cord does not occur only at birth, however. Previous inflammation (arachnoiditis) and even repaired meningomyeloceles may predispose to this distortion and stretching with growth and development. Thus, the neurosurgeon or plastic surgeon following a patient who has previously undergone myelomeningocele repair should remember that "retethering" of the cord definitely occurs (Heinz and associates, 1979). Correction of retethering may improve motor function and kyphoscoliosis. The most common signs of tethering in a patient with a repaired meningomyelocele are pain, ascending motor loss, progressive orthopedic problems, and scoliosis. To reiterate, if a patient presents in a plastic surgery office with, for example, sacral hypertrichosis, lipoma, dermal sinus (not to the coccyx), or hemangioma, there should be a high index of suspicion for a tethered cord. At the least, MRI or CT to exclude an underlying problem is mandatory. A referral to a pediatric neurosurgeon is appropriate even for asymptomatic patients.

The term *spina bifida cystica* includes *meningoceles*—the patient has a dorsal defect but no nerve involvement—or *meningomyeloceles* with varying degrees of neurologic involvement (e.g., paralysis, bladder and bowel incontinence).

The *meningocele* usually presents as a herniation of the cord coverings through the midline vertebral gap. The dorsal half of one or more vertebrae is absent and the contents of the bulge are limited to cerebrospinal fluid (CSF), meninges, and skin. This may occur anywhere along the cord, but most commonly in the lumbosacral area. The skin over this sac may be thinned (Fig. 76–74) or even prone to ulceration. The separate meningeal layers are indistinct and the entire bulge protrudes more with crying. Aberrant nerve elements may be noted in the excised tissue, but the patients do not demonstrate paralysis. Of the spina bifida cystica cases, meningocele (i.e., meninges alone) makes up approximately 10 to 15 per cent. Hydrocephalus is associated with meningocele, but is less common than the 80 to 90 per cent incidence expected with meningomyelocele (McLone and associates, 1985).

The more common form of spina bifida cystica, *meningomyelocele* (Fig. 76–75), denotes cord and meningeal dysplasia. In this situation there is a posterior midline mass of varying size. It may be covered by membrane that may or may not include nervous tissue and may or may not leak spinal fluid. The mass, which is most commonly in the thoracolumbar area, consists of meninges, CSF, cauda equina, and aberrant cord. Ten per cent are noted in the thoracic area and 5 per cent in the cervical region. Occasionally there are multiple lesions. All patients have Arnold-Chiari malformation (Park and associates, 1983), a congenital hindbrain anomaly in which the medulla and pons are posteriorly deviated. Varying degrees of lower extremity

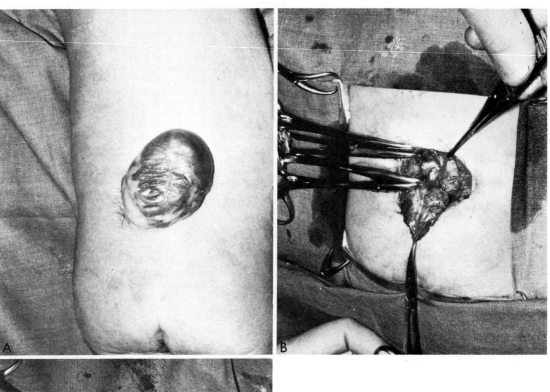

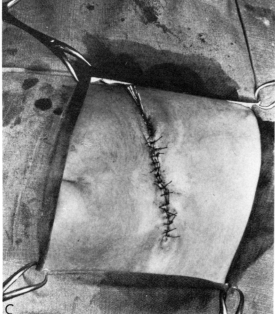

Figure 76–74. Lumbosacral meningocele. *A,* Preoperative appearance. *B,* Involvement of only a single spine; note the narrow meningeal pedicle. *C,* Closure of skin by direct approximation. (From Mustardé, J. C.: Plastic Surgery in Infancy and Childhood. Edinburgh, Churchill Livingstone, 1971.)

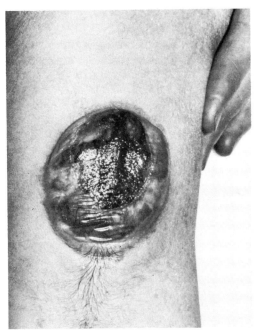

Figure 76–75. Lumbosacral meningomyelocele with exposed neural tissue. (From Mustardé, J. C.: Plastic Surgery in Infancy and Childhood. Edinburgh, Churchill Livingstone, 1971.)

weakness, anesthesia, bowel and bladder incontinence, and orthopedic problems commonly coexist. It is estimated that the average cost of caring for this type of patient with associated shunt, renal, and orthopedic problems ranges between $400,000 and $500,000 over the patient's lifetime (Amacher, 1989).

Urologic Update

In the past decade, dramatic therapeutic advances have occurred (Bauer, 1988). Ileal conduits have become obsolete. Clean intermittent catheterization is accepted even in the newborn period (Hannigan, 1979; Bauer and associates, 1984; Kaplan, 1986). Reliable artificial urinary sphincters are available. As long as the bladder can be emptied on a regular basis, competent antireflux surgery can result in a child who functions as if he has a normal bladder. Early testing has been feasible and even proved advisable, along with constant urologic surveillance.

After the meningomyelocele defect has been closed, a physical examination is performed to ascertain the innervation in the lower extremities and sacrum. The examination also includes (1) urine culture, (2) serum creatinine test, (3) excretory urogram,

(4) voiding cystourethrogram, and (5) urodynamic evaluation (Bauer and associates, 1984). The above studies provide a baseline value of the neurologic status of the urinary tract. Babies at risk for further deterioration of detrusor or external sphincter incoordination can be identified. Progressive denervation can be detected on subsequent studies. The data obtained allow correct parental counseling with regard to sexual and bladder function.

The above urodynamic and radiologic studies are performed as soon as the newborn can be safely moved and allowed on his back for an extended period. Urine cultures should be routinely taken every three to four months, or more often if infection is suspected. Long-term antibiotic prophylaxis (e.g., sulfa drugs) is often prescribed. Neonates with dyssynergic sphincter activity require intermittent catheterization as well as anticholinergic medication to treat or prevent the expected deterioration. When intermittent catheterization is not feasible, cutaneous vesicostomy is needed to provide appropriate bladder emptying. Annual urodynamic studies, as well as sonograms, are performed to evaluate the sphincter and upper tract drainage systems respectively. If reflux or infection develop, the child will require annual voiding cystourethrograms.

Parental Counseling

Parents of children with meningomyelocele should be informed that:

1. Ninety per cent or more of newborn children with meningomyelocele survive. The Chiari II hindbrain malformation is the principal cause of death (Park and associates, 1983).

2. Approximately 75 per cent have normal intelligence, but the frequency of learning disabilities is likely to be high (Hoffman and Epstein, 1986). In the absence of ventriculitis and intracerebral hemorrhage, children with meningomyelocele, *with or without hydrocephalus,* have a normal I.Q. Most mental retardation is acquired postnatally and is primarily due to CNS infection (McLone and associates, 1982).

3. Eighty-five per cent walk, with or without some form of assistance, by school age. This percentage decreases somewhat as adulthood is reached.

4. No therapy is available to restore neural

function, but chronic lifelong surveillance is necessary; evidence of worsening usually warrants aggressive treatment.

5. Eighty per cent of patients become socially continent with the use of drugs and intermittent catheterization.

6. Ten to 15 per cent of surviving children with meningomyelocele are not socially competitive and require some type of supportive care.

7. In the future, amniocentesis may be useful in detecting open neural tube defects in children (Seppala and Ruoslahti, 1973; Sever, 1978). Alpha-fetoprotein levels peak at 16 to 18 weeks after the last menses. Closed tube defects are not detectable by this method but ultrasonography may be helpful.

Timing of Closure

For a simple meningocele with resilient skin covering, the operation may be scheduled at three months or preferably earlier. The aim of surgery is to restore the continuity of the back. If the skin covering is at risk, surgery should be performed immediately after birth. The prognosis for normal development in these infants is good.

The timing of closure for meningomyelocele stirs controversy. Most surgeons tend to close the wound in the first 24 hours of life (Hoffman and Epstein, 1986). Charney and associates (1985) refuted this concept of urgency, seeing no evidence that a delay of even a few days is harmful as long as proper dressings are employed. They used the immediate postnatal period for parental briefing and "proper initial evaluation." Regardless of the timing, cord drying should not occur, otherwise lower limb function and sphincter tone may progress to complete paralysis. The exposed cord therefore must be protected, covered, and kept moist with saline, possibly with antibiotic solution and some type of film, in preparation for surgery. Constant moisture should be continued even during surgery while the cord is under the hot operating room lights. Through restoration of the cord to its normal CSF environment, intellectual, motor, and sensory function may be preserved. In addition, the normal back contour is preserved.

Surgical Management

The usual neurosurgical closure procedure, with or without a plastic surgeon, includes reconvolution of the cord with a five layer closure: (1) pia arachnoid, (2) dura, (3) iliocostal fascia, (4) subcutaneous tissue, and (5) skin. The larger defects may require coverage with a flap or graft, especially if adequate skin cover appears difficult to obtain. Patterson and Till (1959) suggested that 25 per cent of the patients may benefit from this plastic surgical aid, but Amacher (1989) set the figure considerably lower. Reigel (1989), however, reported that he was able to obtain primary skin coverage in all of 358 consecutive meningomyelocele patients without the use of any flaps.

The following outline details the methods currently practiced for the larger defects; wide skin undermining alone is unsafe and invariably leads to problems (Figs. 76–76, 76–77):

1. Local skin flaps
   a. Lumbosacral transposition flap (Davies and Adendorff, 1977)
   b. Limberg flap (Ohtsuka, Shioya, and Yada, 1979)
   c. Transposition flaps (Bajaj, Welsh, and Shadid, 1979)
   d. Double Z-rhomboid (Cruz and associates, 1983)
   e. Bilateral bipedicle flaps (Habal and Vries, 1977)
2. Latissimus musculocutaneous flap variations
   a. Latissimus advancement (McCraw, Penix, and Baker, 1978) without lateral incisions (Fig. 76–78)
   b. Latissimus bipedicle and relaxing incision with superficial gluteal fascia (Moore, Dreyer, and Bevin, 1984)
   c. Compound latissimus/gluteus flaps (Ramirez and associates, 1988)—no relaxing incision
3. Skin grafting—primary placement on turned-over muscle
   a. Delayed grafting, i.e., after watertight dural closure with the application of a porcine dressing (Luce and Walsh, 1985)

The mobility of skin on a baby's back suggests that most defects can be closed by simple undermining. For the larger and lower defects numerous flaps have been designed, some with and some without muscle. Local transposition of suprafascially dissected skin flaps can be done in numerous ways. Necrosis at the tips can occur in approximately 20 per cent of cases, but secondary healing tends to occur with appropriate care. The flaps can of

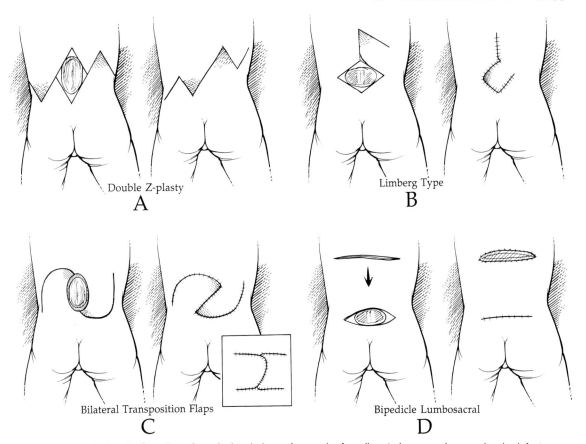

Figure 76–76. *A* to *D*, Overview of surgical techniques for repair of medium to large meningomyelocele defects.

course be evaluated with fluorescein (Venes, 1977). Most dog-ears disappear over time.

Davies and Adendorff (1977) transposed a large cross midline lumbosacral back flap with relative success. The donor defect required skin grafting. Double transposition flaps have been suggested (Bajaj, Welsh, and Shadid, 1979) and designed in the ying-yang pattern. One flap is based superiorly and the other inferiorly based, with "undermining near the base of the flap adjoining the defect kept to a minimum." These flaps may be approximated end to end or end to side to cover the dural repair. Skin grafts were used for resurfacing the secondary defects to "avoid tension." The defects in this series of ten patients ranged from 5.0 to 12.5 cm in diameter.

For lesions of medium to large size (up to 8 cm), Ohtsuka, Shioya, and Yada (1979) undermined Limberg-type flaps at the "level of the deep fascia" while attempting "to preserve the perforating vessels at the base of the flap as completely as possible." The au-

thors believed that this method was not indicated primarily for all defects. They preferred round or *wide oval* recipient sites, stating that "vertical spindle or [less] oval defects are better treated" by other methods.

Cruz and associates (1983) suggested the transposition of local fasciocutaneous flaps according to their double Z-plasty method. By using a four flap technique, the authors reduced tension on the final suture line. Although multiple flaps were "successfully" used in ten patients, the technique is probably not employed frequently, owing in part to the complexity of the design. The central suture line is often tight, lying immediately over the dural closure. The inferiorly based flaps tend to be more ischemic than those that are based superiorly.

When the lumbosacral meningomyelocele is large, simple medial advancement of the undermined skin often fails. Delay does not allow expeditious closure. Bipedicle skin flaps often require lateral relaxing incisions, which are repaired either by primary skin graft or

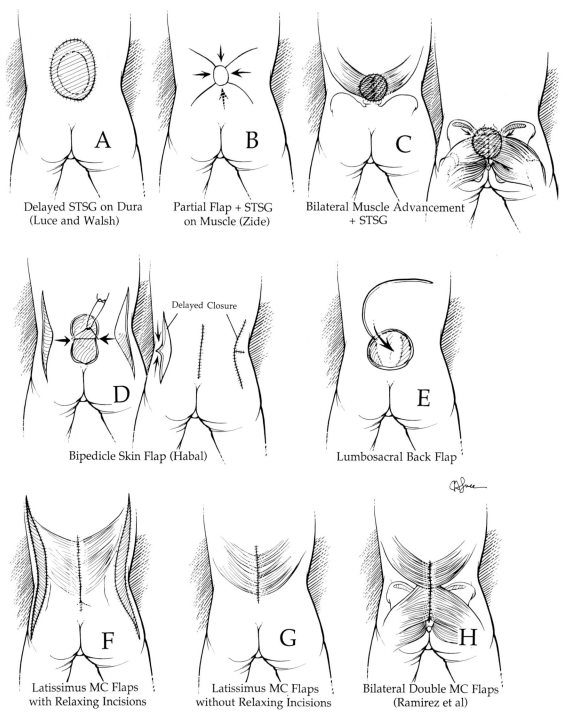

Figure 76–77. *A* to *H,* Overview of the techniques employed for the larger meningomyeloceles.

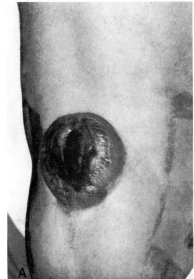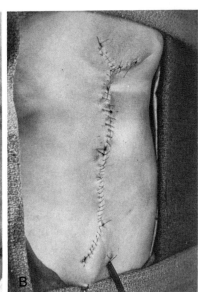

Figure 76–78. *A, B,* The latissimus dorsi musculocutaneous flap method to close a meningomyelocele defect without relaxing incisions. (Courtesy of J. McCraw, M.D.)

by secondary healing. The midline closure may still be tight, because bipedicle flaps are relatively immobile. Habal and Vries (1977) demonstrated a two stage bipedicle flap reconstruction that appeared to be tension free. Vertical flank incisions were used while the bipedicle flaps were mobilized medially. Some of the lateral defect was closed transversely in order to reduce the size of the donor defect on each flank. The lateral edges of the bipedicle flaps were sutured to the wound base. Ten days later, secondary closure of the lateral defects was accomplished with sutures or clips.

The advent of musculocutaneous flaps suggested that improved healing potential might be provided by dissecting at a deeper level. The tight closure could be less problematic because of the increased blood supply of the flap. Three variations have been proposed.

McCraw, Penix, and Baker (1978) and Moore, Dreyer, and Bevin (1984) described the use of bilateral latissimus musculocutaneous flaps used without and with relaxing incisions, respectively. By elevating the flaps in a submuscular plane, most of the lower flap skin was within the vascular territory of the latissimus dorsi muscle and its fascia. Distal to the iliac crest, however, the inferior portion of the bipedicle flap has a random blood supply. As shown in Figure 76–79, the fascial extension of the latissimus dorsi clearly ends in the lumbar region and joins to the lumbodorsal fascia before its insertion

onto the posterior iliac crest. This fascia, as well as the fascia over the gluteus, should be incorporated into the flap to provide additional strength to the deep layer of closure. The wound is approximated by closing fascia, subcutaneous tissue, and skin.

The technique of McCraw, Penix, and Baker (1978) differs from that of Moore, Dreyer, and Bevin (1984) in that the anterior flank skin is left intact in the former. The latissimus musculocutaneous flap is elevated away from all underlying structures, but the off-midline perforating vessels are left intact.

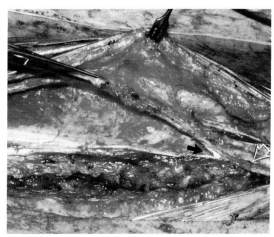

Figure 76–79. The retractor elevates the skin. The forceps grasp the latissimus fascial extension, which fuses *(black arrow)* inferiorly with the lumbodorsal fascia *(open arrow)*.

(The vessels are 8 cm from midline in the adult.) However, according to the authors, these vessels are divisible because the intact anterior skin acts as a buffer after loss of the perforators. In their case presentation of a massive lumbosacral meningomyelocele, they also reported detaching the external oblique fibers from the iliac crest. Inclusion of the external oblique fibers, according to Ramirez and associates (1988), restricts the advancement of the flap.

Musculocutaneous flap coverage of the large, low lumbosacral defects was associated with the highest incidence of problems. The latissimus musculocutaneous flaps, although superior to skin flaps, required extensive dissection and/or relaxing incisions, and the lower lumbar skin component was still random-pattern. Lehrman and Owen (1984) suggested using both latissimus muscles and/or both gluteus muscles for repair of large defects. In their patients, however, skin grafts were placed on top of the advanced muscles and no tension was placed on the closure line of the skin flaps. Ramirez and associates (1988) took this method one step further by using a "double" musculocutaneous technique. By elevating the gluteus maximus inferiorly and the latissimus superiorly (with overlying skin), the random intervening lumbar area could be adequately vascularized without relaxing incisions. Since elevation of the glutei in this way does not alter neurotization, ambulatory possibilities remain unchanged. Although this method offers many benefits, in particular more reliable advancement and blood supply, the dissection is more extensive. An adequate soft tissue pad, however, is placed over the repair.

How important is the overlying soft tissue pad? Owing to their inordinately high complication rate with skin flap repairs, Luce and Walsh (1985) suggested delayed grafting on dura after temporary porcine dressings. This technique would not seem to provide significant protection to the neural placode, but skin ulceration was not reported. Luce and Walsh actually stated that "primary closure has no role in the treatment of meningomyelocele." The vast majority of neurosurgeons, as well as the author, would disagree.

The author tends to rely on musculocutaneous flaps and skin grafts applied on muscle.

The author prefers turning or transposing local muscle whenever possible and applying skin grafts on top of that layer, as opposed to dura. The skin edges are advanced merely to reduce the overall size of the defect prior to skin grafting. The graft may be taken from the baby's back after insufflating the soft tissue with sufficient saline solution to allow the dermatome to work well. The 0.012 inch split-thickness skin graft is usually meshed 1½:1 and sutured into place with 5-0 chromic sutures.

In conclusion, the outlook for patients with meningomyelocele is not dismal. Most can be bright, sociable, and ambulatory. Closure of the meningomyelocele is performed primarily by neurosurgeons, who occasionally enlist assistance from plastic surgeons. For these lesions, the methods of repair vary from skin graft to skin flap to musculocutaneous flaps. The key is *infection-free* closure.

REFERENCES*

Adkins, P. C., and Gwathmey, C.: Pectus excavatum: surgical treatment. J. Thorac. Surg., 36:697, 1958.

Ahnfeldt, A. L., and Berry, F. B. (Eds.): Surgery in World War II. Thoracic Surgery. Washington, DC, Office of the Surgeon General, Department of the Army, Vol. 1, 1963; Vol. 2, 1965.

Aitken, J.: Exomphalos. Analysis of a 10-year series of 32 cases. Arch. Dis. Child., 38:126, 1963.

Alday, E. S., and Goldsmith, H. S.: Surgical technique for omental lengthening based on arterial anatomy. Surg. Gynecol. Obstet., 135:103, 1972.

Allen, R. G., and Wrenn, E. L., Jr.: Silon as a sac in the treatment of omphalocele and gastroschisis. J. Pediatr. Surg., 4:3, 1969.

Amoroso, P. J., and Angelats, J.: Latissimus dorsi myocutaneous flaps in Poland syndrome. Ann. Plast. Surg., 6:287, 1981.

Arnold, M.: The surgical anatomy of sternal blood supply. J. Thorac. Cardiovasc. Surg., 64:596, 1972.

Arnold, P. G.: Reconstruction of the sternum and anterior chest wall: aesthetic considerations. Clin. Plast. Surg., 8:389, 1981.

Arnold, P. G., and Pairolero, P. C.: Chondrosarcoma of the manubrium: resection and reconstruction with pectoralis major muscle. Mayo Clin. Proc., 53:54, 1978.

Arnold, P. G., and Pairolero, P. C.: Use of pectoralis major muscle flap to repair defects of anterior chest wall. Plast. Reconstr. Surg., 63:205, 1979.

Arnold, P. G., and Pairolero, P. C.: Chest wall reconstruction—experience with 100 consecutive patients. Ann. Surg., 199:725, 1984.

Arnold, P. G., and Pairolero, P. C.: Surgical management of the radiated chest wall. Plast. and Reconstr. Surg., 77:605, 1986.

Aston, S. J., and Pickrell, K. L.: Chest wall reconstruction. In Converse, J. M. (Ed.): Plastic and Reconstructive Surgery. 2nd ed. Philadelphia, W. B. Saunders Company, 1977.

Bakamjian, V. Y.: A two-staged method for pharngeal reconstruction with a primary pectoral skin flap. Plast. Reconstr. Surg., 36:173, 1965.

*References for spina bifida are on pages 3795–3796.

Bakamjian, V. Y., Culf, N. K., and Bales, H. W.: Versatility of the deltopectoral flap in reconstructions following head and neck cancer surgery. *In* Transactions of the International Congress of Plastic Surgeons, 4th Congress. Amsterdam, Excerpta Medica, 1967, p. 808.

Barnard, P. M., and DeWet Lubbe, J. J.: Pectus excavatum: a modified technique of internal fixation. S. Afr. Med. J., *47:*649, 1973.

Bartlett, W.: An improved filigree for the repair of large defects in the abdominal wall. Ann. Surg., *3:*47, 1903.

Bassini, E.: Nuovo methodo per la cura radicale dell'ernia. Atti Congr. Ass. Med. Ital. (1887) Pavia, 2:179, 1889.

Beardsley, J. M.: The use of tantalum plate when resecting large areas of the chest wall. J. Thorac. Surg., *19:*444, 1950.

Becker, J., and Schneider, K.: Indications for surgical treatment of pectus excavatum. J. A. M. A., *180:*22, 1962.

Beiser, D., Epstein, S., Stampfer, M., Goldstein, R., Noland, S., and Levitsky, S.: Impairment of cardiac function in patients with pectus excavatum, with improvement after operative correction. N. Engl. J. Med., *287:*267, 1972.

Bekheit, F.: Repair of defects after partial resection of the abdominal wall. J. Egypt. Med. Assoc., *48:*727, 1965.

Ben-Menachem, T., O'Hara, E., and Kane, H.: Paradoxical cardiac enlargement during inspiration in children with pectus excavatum: A new observation. Br. J. Radiol., *46:*38, 1973.

Bergofsky, E., Turino, G., and Fishman, A.: Cardiorespiratory failure in kyphoscoliosis. Medicine, *38:*263, 1959.

Bevegard, S.: Postural circulatory changes after and during exercise in patients with a funnel chest with special reference to factors affecting stroke volume. Acta Med. Scand., *171:*695, 1962.

Bill, A. H., Jr.: Omphalocele. *In* Mustard, W. T., Ravitch, M. M., Synder, W. H., Jr., Welch, K. J., and Benson, C. D. (Eds.): Pediatric Surgery. Vol. 1. 2nd Ed. Chicago, Year Book Medical Publishers, 1969, p. 685.

Bisgard, J. D., and Swenson, S. A., Jr.: Tumors of the sternum: report of a case with special operative technique. Arch. Surg., *56:*570, 1948.

Bogart, J. N., Rowe, D. S., and Parsons, R. W.: Immediate abdominal wall reconstruction with bilateral groin flaps after resection of a large desmoid tumor. Plast. Reconstr. Surg., *58:*716, 1976.

Bostwick, J. B., Hill, H. L., and Nahai, F.: Repairs in the lower abdomen, groin or perineum with myocutaneous or omental flaps. Plast. Reconstr. Surg., *63:*186, 1979.

Boyd, A.: Tumors of the chest wall. *In* Hood, R. M. (Ed.): Surgical Diseases of the Pleura and Chest Wall. Philadelphia, W. B. Saunders Company, 1986.

Boyd, A. D., Shaw, W. W., McCarthy, J. G., Baker, D. C., Trehan, N. K., et al.: Immediate reconstruction of full-thickness chest wall defects. Ann. Thorac. Surg., *32:*337, 1981.

Boyd, J. B., Taylor, G. I., and Corlett, R.: The vascular territories of the superior epigastric and the deep inferior epigastric systems. Plast. Reconstr. Surg., *73:*1, 1984.

Brewer, L. A.: Discussion of Welch, K. J.: Satisfactory surgical correction of pectus excavatum deformity in childhood. J. Thorac. Surg., *36:*697, 1958.

Brodkin, H. A.: Congenital chondrosternal depression (funnel chest) relieved by chondrosternoplasty. Am. J. Surg., *75:*716, 1948.

Brodkin, H. A.: Congenital chondrosternal prominence (pigeon chest): a new interpretation. Pediatrics, *3:*286, 1949.

Brodkin, H. A.: Pigeon chest: congenital chondrosternal prominence. A.M.A. Arch. Surg., *77:*261, 1958.

Brown, A. L.: Pectus excavatum (funnel chest). J. Thorac. Surg., *9:*164, 1939.

Brown, A. L., and Cook, O.: Cardiorespiratory studies in pre- and postoperative funnel chest (pectus excavatum). Dis. Chest, *20:*378, 1951.

Brown, J. B., Fryer, M. P., and McDowell, F.: Application of permanent pedicle blood-carrying flaps. Plast. Reconstr. Surg., *8:*335, 1951.

Brown, R. G., Fleming, W. H., and Jurkiewicz, M. J.: An island flap pectoralis major muscle. Br. J. Plast. Surg., *30:*161, 1977.

Bruck, H.: A method of reconstructing the whole abdominal wall. Br. J. Plast. Surg., *9:*108, 1956.

Brummelkamp, W. H., Hogendijik, J., and Boerema, I.: Treatment of anaerobic infections (clostridial myositis) by drenching the tissue with oxygen under high atmospheric pressure. Surgery, *49:*299, 1961.

Buchanan, R. W., and Cain, W. L.: A case of a complete omphalocele. Ann. Surg., *143:*552, 1956.

Burton, J. F.: Method of correction of ectopia cordis. Arch. Surg., *54:*79, 1947.

Bussabarger, R. A., Dumouchel, M. L., and Ivy, W. H.: Use of tantalum mesh to repair a large surgical defect in the anterior abdominal wall. J. A. M. A., *142:*984, 1950.

Butcher, E. O.: Hair growth and sebaceous glands in skin transplanted under skin and into the peritoneal cavity in the rat. Anat. Rec., *96:*101, 1946.

Campbell, D. A.: Reconstruction of the anterior thoracic wall. J. Thorac Surg., *19:*456, 1950.

Cantrell, J. R., and Haller, J. A.: Peritoneal reconstruction after extensive abdominal wall resection. Surg. Gynecol. Obstet., *110:*363, 1960.

Cantrell, J. R., Haller, J. A., and Ravitch, M. M.: A syndrome of congenital defects involving the abdominal wall, sternum, diaphragm, pericardium and heart. Surg. Gynecol. Obstet., *107:*602, 1958.

Carramenha e Costa, M. A., Carriquiry, C., Vasconez, L. O., Grotting, J. C., Herrera, R. H., and Windle, B. H.: An anatomic study of the venous drainage of the transverse rectus abdominis musculocutaneous flap. Plast. Reconstr. Surg., *79:*208, 1987.

Chang, N., and Mathes, S. J.: Comparison of the effect of bacterial inoculation in musculocutaneous and random pattern flaps. Plast. Reconstr. Surg., *70:*1, 1982.

Chin, E. F.: Surgery of funnel chest and congenital sternal prominence. Br. J. Surg., *44:*360, 1957.

Clarkson, P.: Poland's syndactyly. Guy's Hospital Report, *III:*335, 1962.

Clodius, L., Uhlschmid, G., and Hess, K.: Irradiation plexitis of the brachial plexus. Clin. Plast. Surg., *11:*161, 1984.

Cohen, M., Marshall, M. A., Silverman, N. A., and Levitsky, S.: Chest wall reconstruction for infected median sternotomy wounds. Contemp. Surg., *32:*13, 1988.

Cokkinis, A. J., and Bromwich, A. F.: Tantalum repair of very large incisional hernia. Br. J. Surg., *45:*623, 1954.

Colen, S. R., Romita, M. C., Godfrey, N. V., and Shaw, W. W.: Salvage replantation. Clin. Plast. Surg., *10:*125, 1983.

Cooper, A. P.: Lectures on the Principles and Practice of Surgery. Boston, F. Tyrell, 1825.

Cordero, L., Touloukian, R. J., and Pickett, L. K.: Staged

repair of gastrochisis with Silastic sheeting. Surgery, 65:676, 1969.

Cormack, G. C., and Lamberty, B. G.: The Arterial Anatomy of Skin Flaps. New York, Churchill Livingstone, 1982.

Crile, G., and King, D. E.: Successful use of tantalum mesh to repair an abdominal wall defect in the presence of massive faecal contamination. Surgery, 29:914, 1951.

Culliford, A. T., Cunningham, S. N., Zeff, R. H., Isom, O. W., Teiko, P., and Spencer, F. C.: Sternal and costochondral infections following open heart surgery. J. Thorac. Cardiovasc. Surg., 72:714, 1976.

Currarino, G., and Silverman, F.: Premature obliteration of sternal sutures and pigeon breast deformity. Radiology, 70:532, 1958.

de la Rocha, A. G., and Robertson, G. A.: Sealing the postpneumonectomy space: use of a pectoralis major myodermal flap. Ann. Thorac. Surg., 38:221, 1984.

DeLeon, A., Jr., Perloff, J., and Twigg, H.: The straight back syndrome: clinical cardiovascular manifestation. Circulation, 32:193, 1965.

DeOliviera, M., Sambhi, M., and Zimmerman, H.: The electrocardiogram in pectus excavatum. Br. Heart J., 20:495, 1958.

Dervin, A. S., and Fischer, R. P.: The reconstruction of defects of the abdominal wall with split thickness skin graft. Surg. Gynecol. Obstet., 155:413, 1982.

Dingman, R. O., and Argenta, L. C.: Reconstruction of the chest wall. Ann. Thorac. Surg., 32:202, 1981.

Dinner, M. I., and Dowden, R. V.: The L-shaped combined vertical and transverse abdominal island flap for breast reconstruction. Plast. Reconstr. Surg., 72:894, 1983.

Dormer, R., Keil, P., and Schissel, D.: Pectus excavatum. J. Thorac Surg., 20:444, 1950.

Dorogi, J.: Improved conservative treatment of exomphalos. Lancet, 2:888, 1964.

Drescher, E.: Observations on the conservative treatment of exomphalos. Arch. Dis. Child., 38:125, 1963.

Duhamel, B.: Embryology of exomphalos and allied malformations. Arch. Dis. Child., 38:147, 1963.

Dupont, C., and Menard, Y.: Transposition of the greater omentum for reconstruction of the chest wall. Plast. Reconstr. Surg., 49:263, 1972.

Ellis, H.: The cause and prevention of postoperative intraperitoneal adhesions. Surg. Gynecol. Obstet., 133:497, 1971.

Eng, K., Casson, P., Berman, I. R., and Slattery, L. R.: Clostridial myonecrosis of the abdominal wall. Resection and prosthetic replacement. Am. J. Surg., 125:368, 1973.

Engdahl, E.: Strengthening of scars with a buried dermal sheet. Scand. J. Plast. Surg., 2:109, 1968.

Fabricius, J., Davidsen, H., and Hansen, A.: Cardiac function in funnel chest: twenty-six patients investigated by cardiac catheterization. Dan. Med. Bull., 4:251, 1957.

Farr, R. E.: Closure of large hernial defects in the upper abdomen. Surg. Gynecol. Obstet., 34:264, 1922.

Feng, L. J., Berger, B. E., Lysz, T. W., and Shaw, W. W.: Vasoactive prostaglandins in the impending no-reflow state: evidence for a primary disturbance in microvascular tone. Plast. Reconstr. Surg., 81:755, 1988.

Ferraro, V.: Innesti auto-ed amoplastici di pelle in orgen: e nei muscoli. Arch. Sci. Med. (Torino), 51:149, 1927.

Firmin, R. K., and Wood, A.: Postoperative sternal wound infections. Infect. Surg., April 1987, p. 231.

Firor, H. V.: Omphalocele—an appraisal of therapeutic approaches. Surgery, 69:208, 1971.

Fish, H. G., Baxter, R. H., and Moran, R. E.: A conservative treatment of pectus excavatum in the young. Plast. Reconstr. Surg., 14:324, 1954.

Fishman, A., Turino, G., and Bergofsky, E.: Disorders of the respiration and circulation in subjects with deformities of the thorax. Mod. Concepts Cardiovasc. Dis., 27:449, 1958.

Flynn, W. J., Brant, A. E., and Nelson, G. G.: Four and one-half year analysis of tantalum gauze used in the repair of ventral hernia. Ann. Surg., 134:1027, 1951.

Fonkalsrud, E. W.: Personal communication, 1975.

Friedman, R. J., Argenta, L. C., and Andersen, R.: Deep inferior epigastric free flap for breast reconstruction after radical mastectomy. Plast. Reconstr. Surg., 76:455, 1986.

Froriep, R.: Beobachtung eines Falles von Mangel der Brustaruse. Notizen aus dem Bebiete der Naturund Heilkunde, 10(1):9, 1839.

Fuentes, C. E.: Total arm flap: an alternative method of chest wall reconstruction. Plast. Reconstr. Surg., 77:944, 1986.

Gallie, W. E.: Closing very large hernial openings. Ann. Surg., 96:551, 1932.

Gerber, A.: Plastic repair following the removal of large desmoid tumors of the abdominal wall. Calif. Med., 65:178, 1965.

Goepel, R.: Ueber die Verschilessung von Bruchpforten durch Einheilung geflochtener, fertiger Silberdrahtnetz. Verh. Dtsch. Ges. Chir., 29:174, 1900.

Graeber, G. M., Snyder, R. J., Fleming, A. W., Head, H. D., Lough, F. C., et al.: Initial and long-term results in the management of primary chest wall neoplasms. Ann. Thorac. Surg., 34:664, 1982.

Graham, E. V., Bigger, I. A., Churchill, E. D., and Eloesser, L.: Thoracic Surgery. Philadelphia, W. B. Saunders Company, 1943.

Grmoljez, P. F., Barner, H. H., William, V. L., and Kaiser, G. C.: Major complications of median sternotomy. Am. J. Surg., 130:679, 1975.

Grob, M.: Conservative treatment of exomphalos. Arch. Dis. Child., 38:148, 1963.

Groce, E. J., and Mehta, V. A.: Intercostal pleuroperitoneal hernia. J. Thorac. Cardiovasc. Surg., 77:856, 1979.

Gross, R. E.: New method for surgical treatment of large omphaloceles. Surgery, 24:277, 1948.

Gross, R. E.: The Surgery of Infancy and Childhood. Its Principles and Technique. Philadelphia, W. B. Saunders Company, 1953.

Hakelius, L.: Fatal complications after use of the greater omentum for reconstruction of the chest wall. Plast. Reconstr. Surg., 62:796, 1978.

Haller, A., Peters, G., Mazur, D., and White, J.: Pectus excavatum: a 20 year surgical experience. J. Thorac. Cardiovasc. Surg., 60:375, 1970.

Haller, J. A., Colombani, P. M., Miller, D., and Manson, P.: Early reconstruction of Poland's syndrome using autologous rib grafts combined with a latissimus muscle flap. J. Pediatr. Surg., 19:423, 1984.

Harii, K., and Ohmori, S.: Use of the gastroepiploic vessels as recipient or donor vessels in the free transfer of composite flaps by microvascular anastomosis. Plast. Reconstr. Surg., 52:541, 1973.

Hartrampf, C. R.: Abdominal wall competence in transverse abdominal island flap operations. Ann. Plast. Surg., 12:139, 1984.

Hartrampf, C. R.: The transverse abdominal island flap for breast reconstruction: a 7 year experience. Clin. Plast. Surg., *15:*703, 1988.

Hartrampf, C. R., Scheflan, M., and Black, P. W.: Breast reconstruction with a transverse abdominal island flap. Plast. Reconstr. Surg., *69:*216, 1982.

Hausmann, P. F.: The surgical management of funnel chest. J. Thorac. Surg., *29:*636, 1955.

Hershey, F. B., and Butcher, H. P.: Repair of defects after partial resection of the abdominal wall. Am. J. Surg., *107:*586, 1964.

Hester, T. R., and Bostwick, J.: Poland's syndrome—correction with latissimus muscle transposition. Plast. Reconstr. Surg., *69:*226, 1982.

Hidalgo, D. A.: Omentum free flaps. *In* Shaw, W. W., and Hidalgo, D. A. (Eds.): Microsurgery in Trauma. Mt. Kisco, NY, Futura Publications, 1987, p. 383.

Hill, H. L., Nahai, F., and Vasconez, L. O.: The tensor fascia lata myocutaneous free flap. Plast. Reconstr. Surg., *61:*517, 1978.

Hines, G. L., and Lee, G.: Osteoradionecrosis of the chest wall: management of postresection defects using Marlex mesh and a rotated latissimus dorsi myocutaneous flap. Ann. Surg., *49:*608, 1983.

Hodgkinson, D. J., and Arnold, P. G.: Chest wall reconstruction using the external oblique muscle. Br. J. Plast. Surg., *33:*216, 1980.

Hoffmeister, W.: Operation der angeboren en Trichterbrust. Beitr. Klin. Chir., *141:*214, 1927.

Holcomb, G. W.: Surgical correction of pectus excavatum. J. Pediatr. Surg., *12:*295, 1977.

Hollabaugh, R. S., and Boles, E. T.: The management of gastroschisis. J. Pediatr. Surg., *8:*263, 1973.

Hood, R. M.: Injuries involving the pleura and chest wall. *In* Hood, R. M. (Ed.): Surgical Diseases of the Pleura and Chest Wall, 1986, p. 213.

Horton, C., Georgiade, N., Campbell, F., Masters, F., and Pickrell, K.: The behavior of split-thickness and dermal skin grafts in the peritoneal cavity. An experimental study. Plast. Reconstr. Surg., *12:*269, 1953.

Hueston, J. T., and McConchie, I. H.: A compound pectoral flap. Aust. N. Z. J. Surg., *38:*61, 1968.

Humphrey, G. H., and Jaretzki, A.: Pectus excavatum: late result with and without operation. J. Thorac. Cardiovasc. Surg., *80:*686, 1980.

Hutchingson, J. E., Green, G. E., Mekhjian, H. A., and Kemp, H. G.: Coronary bypass grafting in 376 consecutive patients with three operative deaths. J. Thorac. Cardiovasc. Surg., *67:*7, 1974.

Ishii, C. H., Bostwick, J., Raine, T. J., Coleman, J. J., and Hester, T. R.: Double-pedicle transverse rectus abdominis myocutaneous flap for unilateral breast and chest wall reconstruction. Plast. Reconstr. Surg., *76:*901, 1985.

Izant, R. J., Brown, F., and Rothmann, B. F.: Current embryology and treatment of gastroschisis and omphalocele. Arch. Surg., *93:*49, 1966.

Jacobs, W. E., Hoffman, S., Kirschner, P., and Danese, C.: Reconstruction of a large chest wall defect using greater omentum. Arch. Surg., *113:*886, 1978.

Jaffe, H., and Lichtenstein, L.: Chondrosarcomas of bone. Am. J. Pathol., *19:*553, 1943.

Jensen, K., Schmidt, R., Caramella, J., and Lynch, M.: Pectus excavatum: the how, when and why of surgical correction. J. Pediatr. Surg., *5:*4, 1970.

Johnson, L. P.: Criteria for the management of moderate funnel chest deformities in children. Am. Surg., *38:*498, 1972.

Johnson, P., Frederiksen, J. W., Sanders, J. H., Lewis, V., and Michaelis, L. L.: Management of chronic sternal osteomyelitis. Ann. Thorac. Surg., *40:*69, 1985.

Julian, O. C., Lopez-Belio, M., Dye, W. A., Javid, H., and Grove, W. S.: The median sternal incision in cardiac surgery with extracorporeal circulation. Surgery, *42:*753, 1957.

Jurkiewicz, M. J., and Arnold, P. G.: The omentum: an account of its use in the reconstruction of the chest wall. Ann. Surg., *185:*548, 1977.

Jurkiewicz, M. J., Bostwick, J., Hester, T. R., et al.: Infected mediastinotomy wound. Ann. Surg., *191:*738, 1980.

Karakousis, C. P., Elias, E. G., and Douglas, H. O.: Abdominal wall replacement with plastic mesh in ablative cancer surgery. Surgery, *78:*453, 1975.

Koontz, A. R., and Kimberly, C. R.: Tissue reactions to tantalum mesh and wire. Ann. Surg., *131:*666, 1950.

Koontz, A. R., and Kimberly, C. R.: Electron irradiated ox fascia and lyophilized dura mater. Arch. Surg., *82:*318, 1961.

Lam, C., and Taber, R.: Surgical treatment of pectus carinatum. Arch. Surg., *103:*191, 1971.

Lambertsen, C. J.: The lung: physical aspects of respiration. *In* Mountcastle, V. (Ed.): Medical Physiology. St. Louis, C. V. Mosby Company, 1980.

Larsson, S., Pettersson, G., Eldh, J., and Eriksson, E.: Reconstruction of large anterior full thickness defect in the chest wall after resection of chondrosarcoma. Scand. J. Thorac. Cardiovasc. Surg., *18:*63, 1984.

Latham, W. D.: Operative treatment for postradiation defects of the chest wall. Ann. Surg., *32:*700, 1966.

Lavey, E., Apfelberg, D. B., Lash, H., Maser, M. R., Laub, D. R., and Gosain, A.: Customized silicone implants of the breast and chest. Plast. Reconstr. Surg., *69:*646, 1982.

Leonard, A. G.: Reconstruction of the chest wall using a de-epithelialised "turn-over" deltopectoral flap. Br. J. Plast. Surg., *33:*187, 1980.

LeRoux, B. T., and Sharma, D. M.: Resection of tumors of the chest wall. Curr. Probl. Surg., *20:*349, 1983.

Lesnick, G. N., and Davids, A. M.: Repair of surgical abdominal wall defect with pedicled musculofascial flap. Ann. Surg., *137:*569, 1953.

Lester, C.: Surgical treatment of funnel chest. Ann. Surg., *123:*1003, 1946.

Lester, C.: Pigeon breast (pectus carinatum) and other protrusion deformities of developmental origin. Ann. Surg., *137:*482, 1953.

Lester, C.: Surgical treatment of protrusion deformities of the sternum and costal cartilages (pectus carinatum, pigeon breast). Ann. Surg., *153:*441, 1961.

Lewis, J. E., Kraeger, R. R., and Danis, R. K.: Gastroschisis: Ten-year review. Arch. Surg., *107:*218, 1973.

Lindskog, G., and Felton, W.: Pectus excavatum. Surg. Gynecol. Obstet., *95:*615, 1952.

Little, J. W., Fontan, D. J., and McCullough, D. T.: The upper-quadrant flap. Plast. Reconstr. Surg., *68:*175, 1981.

Lyons, H., Zuhdi, M., and Kelly, J., Jr.: Pectus excavatum (funnel chest), a cause of impaired ventricular distensibility as exhibited by right ventricular pressure pattern. Am. Heart J., *50:*921, 1955.

Mahour, G. H., Weitzman, J. J., and Rosenkrantz, J. G.: Omphalocele and gastroschisis. Ann. Surg., *177:*478, 1973.

Maier, H. C.: Surgical management of large defects of the thoracic wall. Surgery, *22:*169, 1947.

The Trunk

Maisel, R. H., Liston, S. L., and Adams, G. L.: Complications of pectoralis myocutaneous flaps. Laryngoscope, 93:928, 1983.

Malangoni, M. A., Ofstein, L. C., Grosfeld, J. L., Weber, T. R., Eigen, H., and Baehner, R. L.: Survival and pulmonary function following chest wall resection and reconstruction in children. J. Pediatr. Surg., 15:906, 1980.

Mansberger, A., Kang, J. S., Beebe, H. G., and LeFlore, L.: Repair of massive acute abdominal wall defects. J. Trauma, 13:766, 1973.

Markgraf, W. H.: Abdominal wound deficiencies: a technique for repair with Marlex mesh. Arch. Surg., 105:728, 1972.

Marks, M. W., Argenta, L. C., and Lee, D. C.: Silicone implant correction of pectus excavatum: indications and refinement in technique. Plast. Reconstr. Surg., 74:52, 1984.

Maruyama, Y., Ohnishi, K., and Chung, C. C.: Vertical abdominal fasciocutaneous flap in the reconstruction of chest wall defects. Br. J. Plast. Surg., 38:230, 1985.

Masson, J. K., Payne, W. S., and Gonzalez, J. B.: Pectus excavatum: use of preformed prosthesis for correction in the adult. Plast. Reconstr. Surg., 46:399, 1970.

Mathes, S. J., and Nahai, F.: Clinical applications for muscle and musculocutaneous flaps. St. Louis, C. V. Mosby Company, 1982.

Matsuo, K., Hirose, T., Hayashi, R., and Senga, O.: Chest wall reconstruction by contralateral latissimus dorsi musculocutaneous flap. Plast. Reconstr. Surg., 82:994, 1988.

Mauer, E., and Blades, B.: Hernia of the lung. J. Thorac. Surg., 15:77, 1946.

May, A. M.: Operation for pectus excavatum using stainless steel wire mesh. J. Thorac. Cardiovasc. Surg., 42:122, 1961.

May, J. M., Toth, B. A., and Cohen, A. M.: Teres major latissimus dorsi skin-muscle flap for chest wall reconstruction. Plast. Reconstr. Surg., 69:326, 1982.

Mayo, P., and Long, G.: Surgical repair of pectus excavatum by pin immobilization. J. Thorac. Cardiovasc. Surg., 44:53, 1962.

McAfee, M. K., Pairolero, P. C., Bergstralh, E. J., Piehler, J. M., Unni, K. K., et al.: Chondrosarcoma of the chest wall: factors affecting survival. Ann. Thorac. Surg., 40:535, 1985.

McCormack, P., Bains, M. S., Beattie, E. J., and Martini, N.: New trends in skeletal reconstruction after resection of chest wall tumors. Ann. Thorac. Surg., 31:45, 1981.

McCraw, J. B., and Arnold, P. G.: McCraw and Arnold's Atlas of Muscle and Myocutaneous Flaps. Norfolk, VA, Hampton Press, 1986.

McCraw, J. B., Penix, J. O., and Baker, J. W.: Repair of major defects of the chest wall and spine with the latissimus dorsi myocutaneous flap. Plast. Reconstr. Surg., 62:197, 1978.

McGregor, I. A., and Jackson, I. T.: The extended role of the deltopectoral flap. Br. J. Plast. Surg., 23:373, 1970.

McNally, J. B., Price, W. R., and MacDonald, W.: Gas gangrene of anterior abdominal wall. Am. J. Surg., 116:779, 1968.

McPeak, C. J., and Miller, T. R.: Abdominal replacement. Surgery, 47:944, 1960.

Meade, R. H.: A History of Thoracic Surgery. Springfield, IL, Charles C Thomas, 1961.

Medgyesi, S.: The repair of large incisional hernias with pedicle skin flaps. Scand. J. Plast. Surg., 6:69, 1972.

Meltzer, A.: Huge omphalocele ruptured in utero. J. A. M. A., 160:656, 1956.

Mendelson, B. C., and Masson, J. K.: Treatment of chronic radiation injury over the shoulder with a latissimus dorsi myocutaneous flap. Plast. Reconstr. Surg., 60:681, 1977.

Mendelson, B. C., and Mason, J. K.: Silicon implants for contour deformities of the trunk. Plast. Reconstr. Surg., 59:538, 1977.

Meyer, L.: Zur chirurgischen Behandlung der angeboren en Trichterbrust. Verh. d. Berl. Med. Ges., 42:364, 1911.

Meyer, W.: Implantation of filigree of silver wire in the cure of hernia usually considered inoperable. 1902.

Millard, D. R., Jr., Pigott, R., and Zies, P.: Free skin grafting of full-thickness defects of abdominal wall. Plast. Reconstr. Surg., 43:569, 1969.

Miller, J. D., and Mathew, E. C.: Congenital cardiac diverticulum. Am. J. Dis. Child., 126:814, 1973.

Miller, L. B., Bostwick, J., Hartrampf, C. R., Hester, T. R., and Nahai, F.: The superiorly based rectus abdominis flap: predicting and enhancing its blood supply based on an anatomic and clinical study. Plast. Reconstr. Surg., 81:713, 1988.

Milloy, F. G., Anson, B. J., McAfee, D. K.: The rectus abdominis muscle and the epigastric arteries. Surg. Obstet. Gynecol., 122:293, 1960.

Mladick, R. A., Pickrell, K. I., Royer, J. R., McCraw, J., and Brown, I.: Skin graft reconstruction of a massive full-thickness abdominal wall defect. Plast. Reconstr. Surg., 43:587, 1969.

Moore, T. C.: Gastroschisis with antenatal evisceration of intestines and urinary bladder. Ann. Surg., 158:263, 1963.

Moore, T. C., and Stokes, G. E.: Gastroschisis. Surgery, 33:112, 1953.

Morgan, A., Morain, W., and Eraklis, A.: Gas gangrene of the abdominal wall: management after extensive debridement. Ann. Surg., 173:617, 1971.

Morgan, S. C., and Zbylski, J. R.: Repair of massive soft tissue defects by open jump flaps. Plast. Reconstr. Surg., 50:265, 1972.

Muhlbauer, W., and Olbrisch, R.: The latissimus dorsi myocutaneous flap for breast reconstruction. Chir. Plast. (Berlin), 4:27, 1977.

Nakao, K., Miyata, M., Ito, T., Ogino, N., Kawashima, Y., et al.: Omental transposition and skin graft in patients for advanced or recurrent breast cancer. Jap. J. Surg., 16:112, 1986.

Ochsner, A., and DeBakey, M.: Chone-chondrosternon. J. Thorac. Surg., 8:469, 1939.

Olivari, N.: The latissimus flap. Br. J. Plast. Surg., 29:126, 1976.

Ott, D. A., Cooley, D. A., Solis, R. T., et al.: Wound complications after median sternotomy: a study of 61 consecutive series of 9,279. Cardiovasc. Dis., 7:104, 1980.

Pairolero, P. C., and Arnold, P. G.: Chest wall tumors: experience with 100 consecutive patients. J. Thorac. Cardiovasc. Surg., 90:367, 1985.

Palmer, J. H. and Taylor, G. I.: The vascular territories of the anterior chest wall. Br. J. Plast. Surg., 39:287, 1986.

Parham, D. W.: Thoracic resections for tumors growing from the bony chest wall. Trans. S. Surg. Ass., II:223, 1899.

Pascuzzini, C. A., Dahlin, D. C., and Claggett, O. T.: Primary tumors of the ribs and sternum. Surg. Gynecol. Obstet., 390:104, 1957.

Pauson, D. L.: Carcinoma in the superior pulmonary sulcus. Ann. Thorac. Surg., 28:3, 1979.

Pearce, A. E., and Entine, J. H.: Experimental studies using tantalum mesh as a full-thickness abdominal wall prosthesis. Am. J. Surg., 84:182, 1952.

Pearl, S. N. and Dibbell, D. G.: Reconstruction after median sternotomy infection. Surg. Gynecol. Obstet., 159:47, 1984.

Pennington, D. G., and Pelly, A. D.: The rectus abdominis myocutaneous free flap. Br. J. Plast. Surg., 33:277, 1980.

Pers, M., and Medgyesi, S.: Pedicle muscle flaps and their applications in the surgery of repair. Br. J. Plast. Surg., 26:313, 1973.

Pickrell, K. L., Kelley, J. W., and Marzoni, F. A.: The surgical treatment of recurrent carcinoma of the breast and chest wall. Plast. Reconstr. Surg., 3:156, 1948.

Poland, A.: A deficiency of the pectoral muscles. Guy's Hospital Report, VI:191, 1841.

Ponten, B.: The fasciocutaneous flap—its use for soft tissue defects of the lower leg. Br. J. Plast. Surg., 34:215, 1981.

Poulard, A.: Traitement des cicatrices faciales. Presse Med., 26:221, 1918.

Prpic, I., Belmairic, J., Rosenberg, J. C., Sardesai, V., Walt, A. J., and Zamick, P.: Use of xenograft coverage for reconstruction of abdominal wall defect. Br. J. Plast., 27:125, 1974.

Prpic, I., Belamarie, J., Sardesai, V., Walt, A. J., and Zamick, P.: Lyophilised corium grafts for repair of abdominal wall defect. Br. J. Plast. Surg., 26:35, 1973.

Ramming, K. P., Holmes, E. C., Zarem, H. A., Lesavoy, M. A., and Morton, D. L.: Surgical management and reconstruction of extensive chest wall malignancies. Am. J. Surg., 144:146, 1982.

Ravitch, M. M.: Pectus excavatum and heart failure. Surgery, 30:178, 1951.

Ravitch, M. M.: Unusual sternal deformity with cardiac symptoms. J. Thorac. Surg., 23:138, 1952.

Ravitch, M. M.: The operative treatment of pectus excavatum. J. Pediatr., 48:465, 1956.

Ravitch, M. M.: The operative correction of pectus carinatum (pigeon breast). Ann. Surg., 151:705, 1960.

Ravitch, M. M.: Technical problems in the operative correction of pectus excavatum. Ann. Surg., 162:29, 1965.

Ravitch, M. M.: Congenital Deformities of the Chest Wall and Their Operative Correction. Philadelphia, W. B. Saunders Company, 1977.

Ravitch, M. M.: Poland's syndrome—a study of an eponym. Plast. Reconstr. Surg., 59:508, 1977.

Ravitch, M. M.: Poland's syndrome. Surgical Rounds for Orthopedics, Sept. 1987, p. 43.

Rayner, C. R. W.: Repair of full-thickness defects of the abdominal wall in rats avoiding visceral adhesions. Br. J. Plast. Surg., 27:130, 1974.

Rees, T. D., and Converse, J. M.: Surgical reconstruction of defects of the thoracic wall. Surg. Gynecol. Obstet., 121:1066, 1965.

Rehbein, F., and Wernicke, H. H.: The operative treatment of the funnel chest. Arch. Dis. Child. (Lond), 32:5, 1957.

Rehn, E.: Verh. Dtsch. Ges. Chir., I Teil, S.: 87:390, 1911.

Reusch, C. S.: Hemodynamic studies in pectus excavatum. Circulation, 24:1143, 1961.

Rickham, P. P.: Rupture of exomphalos and gastroschisis. Arch. Dis. Child., 38:138, 1963.

Robbins, K. T., and Woodson, G. E.: Chest wall metastasis as a complication of myocutaneous flap reconstruction. J. Otol., 13:13, 1984.

Robicsek, F., Sanger, P., Taylor, F., and Thomas, M.: The surgical treatment of chondrosternal prominence (pectus carinatum). J. Thorac. Cardiovasc. Surg., 45:691, 1963.

Robinson, D. W.: Surgical problems in the excision and repair of radiated tissue. Plast. Reconstr. Surg., 55:41, 1975.

Robinson, D. W.: The deltopectoral flap in chest wall reconstruction. Br. J. Plast. Surg., 29:22, 1976.

Roesler, H.: The relation of the shape of the heart to the shape of the chest: with special reference to the anteroposterior dimension and the morphology of various normal heart types. Am. J. Roentgenol. Radium Ther. Nucl. Med., 32:464, 1934.

Romero, L. H., Nagamia, H. F., Lefemine, A. A., Foster, E. D., Wysocki, J. P., and Berger, R. L.: Massive impalement wound of the chest: a case report. J. Thorac. Surg., 75:832, 1978.

Sanders, G. B.: Gas gangrene of the abdominal wall. XX Congrès de la Société Internationale de Chirurgie, 1963.

Sarr, M. G., Gott, V. L., and Townsend, T. R.: Mediastinal infection after cardiac surgery. Ann. Thorac. Surg., 38:415, 1984.

Sauerbruch, E. F.: Die Chirurgie der Brustorgane. 3rd Ed. Berlin, G. Springer, 1927.

Scheflan, M., Bostwick, J., and Nahai, F.: Chest wall reconstruction—management of the difficult chest wound. Ann. Plast. Surg., 8:122, 1982.

Schmitt, H. J., Jr., and Grinnon, G. L.: Use of Marlex mesh in infected abdominal war wounds. Am. J. Surg., 113:825, 1967.

Schmitt, H. J., Jr., Patterson, L. T., and Armstrong, R. C.: Re-operative surgery of abdominal wall wounds. Ann. Surg., 165:173, 1967.

Schuster, S. R.: A new method for the staged repair of large omphalocele. Surg. Gynecol. Obstet., 125:837, 1967.

Sewell, W. H., and Koth, D. R.: Homologous and heterologous freeze-dried fascia used to repair diaphragmatic and abdominal wall defects. Surg. Forum, 6:531, 1955.

Seyfer, A., Graeber, G., and Wind, G. (Eds.): Atlas of Chest Wall Reconstruction. Rockville, MD, Aspen Publishers, 1986.

Shaw, D., and Payne, R. L.: One stage tubed abdominal flaps. Surg. Gynecol. Obstet., 83:205, 1946.

Shaw, W. W.: Breast reconstruction by superior gluteal microvascular free flaps without silicone implants. Plast. Reconstr. Surg., 72:490, 1983.

Shaw, W. W.: Microvascular free flaps: the first decade. Clin. Plast. Surg., 10:1, 1983.

Shaw, W. W.: Discussion of "deep inferior epigastric free flap for breast reconstruction." Plast. Reconstr. Surg., 76:459, 1986.

Shaw, W. W.: Unpublished data, 1989.

Shaw, W. W., Baker, D. C., Klein, N. E., and Crais, T. F.: Microvascular transfer of living fascia lata: a new method of chest wall reconstruction. Plastic Surgery Forum, of the American Society of Plastic and Reconstructive Surgeons, 1980, p. 130.

Shaw, W. W., and Feng, L. J.: Unpublished data, 1988.

Shaw, W. W., and Hidalgo, D. A. (Eds.): Rectus abdominis free flaps. In Microsurgery in Trauma. Mount Kisco, NY, Futura Publications, 1987, p. 229.

Shim, W. K.: Surgical treatment of gastroschisis. Arch. Surg., *102:*524, 1971.

Simpson, T. E., and Lynn, H. B.: Omphalocele: results of surgical treatment. Mayo Clin. Proc., *43:*65, 1968.

Sisson, G. A., Straehley, C. J., and Johnson, N. E.: Mediastinal dissection for recurrent cancer after laryngectomy. Laryngoscope, *72:*1064, 1962.

Smith, W. R., and Leix, F.: Omphalocele. Am. J. Surg., *111:*450, 1966.

Soave, F.: Conservative treatment of giant omphalocele. Arch. Dis. Child., *38:*130, 1963.

Soper, R. T., and Green, E. W.: Omphalocele. Surg. Gynecol. Obstet., *112:*501, 1961.

Stahl, R. S., and Kopf, G. S.: Reconstruction of infant thoracic wounds. Plast. Reconstr. Surg., *82:*1000, 1988.

Stanford, W., Bowers, D., Lindberg, E., Armstrong, R., Finger, E. M., and Dibbell, D.: Silastic implants for correction of pectus excavatum. Ann. Thorac. Surg., *13:*529, 1972.

Stephenson, K. L.: A new approach to the treatment of abdominal muscular agenesis. Plast. Reconstr. Surg., *12:*413, 1953.

Stone, H. H., Fabian, T. C., Turkleson, M. L., and Jurkewicz, M. J.: Management of acute full-thickness losses of the abdominal wall. Ann. Surg., *193:*612, 1981.

Strömbeck, I. O.: Mammaplasty: report of a new technique based on the two pedicle procedure. Br. J. Plast. Surg., *13:*79, 1960.

Sweet, R.: Pectus excavatum: report of two cases successfully operated upon. Ann. Surg., *119:*922, 1944.

Tansini, I.: Sopro il mio nuovo processo di amputazione della mamella. Gas. Med. Ital., *57:*141, 1906.

Taylor, G. I.: Discussion of Miller, L. B., Bostwick, J. III, Hartrampf, C. R., Jr., Hester, T. R., Jr., and Nahai, F.: The superiorly based rectus abdominis flap: predicting and enhancing its blood supply based on an anatomic and clinical study. Plast. Reconstr. Surg., *81:*721, 1988.

Taylor, G. I., and Palmer, J. H.: The vascular territories (angiosomes) of the body: experimental study and clinical applications. Br. J. Plast. Surg., *40:*2, 1987.

Taylor, G. I., Corlett, R. I., and Boyd, J. B.: The versatile deep inferior epigastric (inferior rectus abdominis) flap. Br. J. Plast. Surg., *37:*330, 1984.

Throckmorton, T. D.: Tantalum gauze in the repair of hernias complicated by tissue deficiency. Surgery, *23:*32, 1948.

Tobin, G.: Muscle and myocutaneous flaps: refinements and new applications, *In* Current Problems in Surgery. Vol. 23, No. 5. May, 1986.

Tobin, G. R., Schusterman, M., Peterson, G. H., Nichols, G., and Bland, K. I.: The intermuscular neurovascular anatomy of the latissimus dorsi muscle: the basis for splitting the flap. Plast. Reconstr. Surg., *67:*637, 1981.

Tolhurst, D., Haeseker, B., and Zeeman, R. J.: The development of the fasciocutaneous flap and its clinical application. Plast. Reconstr. Surg. *71:*597, 1983.

Troisier, J., and Monnerot, D.: Thorax en entonnoir et doight Renté: deux tableaux généalogique. Bull. Mém. Soc. Med. Hop. Paris, *54:*311, 1930.

Trunkey, D. D.: Trauma. Sci. Am., *249:*28, 1983.

Tsur, H., Lieberman, Y., and Heim, M.: Diaphragm mobilization for closure of chest wall defects. Ann. Plast. Surg., *13:*234, 1984.

Tsur, H., Shafir, R., and Lieberman, Y.: Mobilization of both breasts for reconstruction of a midline anterior chest wall defect. Ann. Plast. Surg., *8:*314, 1982.

Urban, J. A.: Radical excision of the chest wall for mammary cancer, Lancet, *4:*1263, 1951.

Urschel, H. C., Byrd, H. S., Sethi, S. M., and Razzuk, M. A.: Poland syndrome: improved surgical management. Ann. Thorac. Surg., *37:*204, 1984.

Usher, F. C.: A new plastic prosthesis for repairing tissue defects of the chest and abdominal wall. Am. J. Surg., *97:*623, 1954.

Usher, F. C., and Gannon, J. P.: Marlex mesh: a new plastic for replacing tissue defects. Experimental studies. Arch. Surg., *78:*131, 1959.

Usher, F. C., and Wallace, S. A.: Tissue reactions to plastics. A. M. A. Arch. Surg., *76:*99, 1958.

Vidne, B., and Levy, M. J.: Surgical treatment for pectus excavatum. Israel J. Med. Sci., *9:*1565, 1973.

Voegele, L. D., Metcalf, M. M., Prioleau, W. H., and Hairston, P.: Median sternotomy infection—management and reconstruction. Am. Surg., *51:*645, 1985.

Voyles, C. R., Richardson, J. D., Bland, K. I., Tobin, G. R., Flint, L. M., and Polk, H. C.: Emergency abdominal wall reconstruction with polypropylene mesh. Ann. Surg., *194:*219, 1981.

Wachtel, F., Ravitch, M. M., and Grishman, A.: The relationship of pectus excavatum to heart disease. Am. Heart J., *52:*121, 1961.

Wada, J., and Ikeda, K.: Clinical experience with 306 funnel chest operations. Int. Surg., *57:*707, 1972.

Wada, J., Ikeda, K., Ishida, T., and Hasegaws, T.: Result of 271 funnel chest operations. Ann. Thorac. Surg., *10:*527, 1970.

Wangensteen, O. H.: Large defects of the abdominal wall employing the iliotibial tract of fascia lata as a pedicled flap. Surg. Gynecol. Obstet., *59:*766, 1934.

Wangensteen, O. H.: Repair of large abdominal defects by pedicled fascial flaps. Surg. Gynecol. Obstet., *82:*144, 1946.

Wayne, E. R., and Burrington, J. D.: Gastroschisis: a systemic approach to management. Am. J. Dis. Child., *125:*218, 1973.

Weg, J. G., Krumholz, R. A., and Harkleroad, L. E.: Pulmonary dysfunction in pectus excavatum. Am. Rev. Respir. Dis., *96:*936, 1967.

Welch, F., and Vos, A.: Surgical correction of pectus carinatum (pigeon breast). J. Pediatr. Surg., *8:*659, 1947.

Welch, K. L.: Use of homograft in the treatment of omphaloceles. Surgery, *29:*100, 1951.

Whalen, W. P.: Coverage of thoracic wall defect by a split breast flap. Plast. Reconstr. Surg., *12:*64, 1953.

Wilson, J. S. P., and Rayner, C. R. W.: The repair of large full-thickness post-excisional defects of the abdominal wall. Br. J. Plast. Surg., *27:*117, 1974.

Witzel, O.: Ueber den versenkte Silberdahtnets. Zentral Chir., *27:*257, 1900.

Woods, J. E., Arnold, P. G., Masson, J. K., Irons, G. B., and Payne, W. S.: Management of radiation necrosis and advanced cancer of the chest wall in patients with breast malignancy. Plast. Reconstr. Surg., *63:*235, 1979.

Ye, R. C., Devine, K. D., and Kirklin, J. W.: Extensive recurrent desmoid tumor of the abdominal wall: radical excision followed by reconstruction of abdominal wall with plastic procedure. Report of a case. Plast. Reconstr. Surg., *12:*59, 1953.

Spina Bifida

Amacher, A. L.: *In* Schmedek, H. H., and Sweet, W. H.: Operative Neurosurgical Techniques. Vol. 1. Orlando, New York, Grune & Stratton, 1989.

Bajaj, P., Welsh, F., and Shadid, E. A.: Versatility of lumbar transposition flaps in the closure of meningomyelocele skin defects. Ann. Plast. Surg., 2:103, 1979.

Bauer, S. B.: Early evaluation and management of children with spina bifida. *In* King, L. R. (Ed.): Urologic Surgery in Neonates and Young Infants. Philadelphia, W. B. Saunders Company, 1988, p. 252.

Bauer, S. B., Hallett, M., Khoshbin, S., Lebowitz, R. L., Winston, K. R., et al.: Predictive value of urodynamic evaluation in newborns with myelodysplasia. J.A.M.A., 252:650, 1984.

Boone, D., Parsons, D., Lachmann, S. M., and Sherwood, T.: Spina bifida occulta: lesion or anomaly? Clin. Radiol., 36:159, 1985.

Bruce, D. A., and Schut, L.: Spinal lipomas in infancy and childhood. Childs Brain, 5:192, 1979.

Chapman, P. H., and Beyerl, B.: The tethered spinal cord, with particular reference to spinal lipoma and diastematomyelia. *In* Hoffman, H. J., and Epstein, F. (Eds.): Disorders of the Developing Nervous System: Diagnosis and Treatment. Boston, Blackwell, 1986, p. 119.

Chapman, P. H.: Congenital intraspinal lipomas: anatomic considerations and surgical treatment. Childs Brain, 9:37, 1982.

Charney, E. B., Weller, S. C., Sutton, L. N., Bruce, D. A., and Schut, L. B.: Management of the newborn with myelomeningocele: time for a decision-making process. Pediatrics, 75:58, 1985.

Cheek, W. R., and Laurent, J. P.: Dermal sinus tracts. *In* Chapman, P. H. (Ed.): Concepts in Pediatric Neurosurgery. Vol. 6. Basel, S. Karger, 1985, pp. 63–75.

Cruz, N. I., Ariyan, S., Duncan, C. C., and Cuono, C. B.: Repair of lumbosacral myelomeningoceles with double Z-rhomboid flaps. J. Neurosurg., 59:714, 1983.

Davies, D., and Adendorff, D. J.: A large rotation flap raised across the midline to close lumbo-sacral meningomyelocoeles. Br. J. Plast. Surg., 30:166, 1977.

Elwood, J. H.: Major central nervous system malformations notified in Northern Ireland, 1964–1968. Dev. Med. Child Neurol., 14:731, 1972.

Fineman, R. M., Jorde, L. B., Martin, R. A., Hasstedt, S. J., Wing, S. D., and Walker, M. L.: Spinal dysraphia as an autosomal dominant defect in four families. Am. J. Med. Genet., 12:457, 1982.

Habal, M. B., and Vries, J. K.: Tension-free closure of large meningomyelocele defects. Surg. Neurol., 8:177, 1977.

Hannigan, K. F.: Teaching intermittent self-catheterization to young children with myelodysplasia. Dev. Med. Child Neurol., 21:365, 1979.

Heinz, E. R., Rosenbaum, A. E., Scarff, T. B., Reigel, D. H., and Drayer, B. P.: Tethered spinal cord following meningomyelocele repair. Radiology, 131:153, 1979.

Hoffman, H. J., and Epstein, F.: Disorders of the Developing Nervous System: Diagnosis and Treatment. Boston, Blackwell, 1986.

Hoffman, H. J., Taecholarn, C., Hendrick, E. B., and Humphreys, R. P.: Management of lipomyelomeningoceles. Experience at the Hospital for Sick Children, Toronto. J. Neurosurg., 62:1, 1985.

Kaplan, W. E.: Clear intermittent catheterization. *In* McLaurin, R. L. (Ed.): Spina Bifida: A Multidisciplinary Approach. New York, Praeger, 1986, pp. 274–276.

Lehrman, A., and Owen, M. P.: Surgical repair of large meningomyeloceles. Ann. Plast. Surg., 12:501, 1984.

Luce, E. A., and Walsh, J.: Wound closure of the myelomeningocele defect. Plast. Reconstr. Surg., 75:389, 1985.

McCraw, J. B., Penix, J. O., and Baker, J. W.: Repair of major defects of the chest wall and spine with the latissimus dorsi myocutaneous flap. Plast. Reconstr. Surg., 62:197, 1978.

McLaurin, R. L., Schut, L., Venes, J. L., and Epstein, F.: Pediatric Neurosurgery. 2nd Ed. Philadelphia, W. B. Saunders Company, 1989.

McLone, D. G., and Naidich, T. P.: The tethered spinal cord. *In* McLaurin, R. L., Schut, L., Venes, J. L., and Epstein, F. (Eds.): Pediatric Neurosurgery. Philadelphia, W. B. Saunders Company, 1989.

McLone, D. G., Czyzewski, D., Raimondi, A. J., et al.: Central nervous system infections as a limiting factor in the intelligence of children born with myelomeningocele. Pediatrics, 70:338, 1982.

McLone, D. G., Dias, L., Kaplan, W. E., et al.: Concepts in the management of spina bifida. *In* Humphreys, R. P. (Ed.): Concepts in Pediatric Neurosurgery. Vol. 5. Basel, S. Karger, 1985, pp. 97–106.

McLone, D. G., Hayashida, S. F., and Caldarelli, M.: Surgical resection of lipomyelomeningoceles in 18 asymptomatic infants. J. Pediatr. Neurosci., 1:239, 1985.

Moore, T. S., Dreyer, T. M., and Bevin, A. G.: Closure of large spina bifida cystica defects with bilateral bipedicled musculocutaneous flaps. Plast. Reconstr. Surg., 73:288, 1984.

Naidich, T. P., McLone, D. G., and Harwood-Nash, D. C.: Spinal dysraphism. *In* Newton, T. H., and Potts, D. G. (eds.): Computed Tomography of the Spine and Spinal Cord. San Anselmo, CA, Clavadel Press, 1983.

Naidich, T. P., McLone, D. G., and Mutluer, S.: A new understanding of dorsal dysraphism with lipoma (lipomyeloschisis): radiologic evaluation and surgical correction. Am. J. Neuroradiol., 4:103, 1983.

Ohtsuka, H., Shioya, N., and Yada, K.: Modified Limberg flap for lumbosacral meningomyelocele defects. Ann. Plast. Surg., 3:114, 1979.

Park, T. S., Hoffman, H. J., Hendrick, E. B., and Humphreys, R. P.: Experience with surgical decompression of the Arnold-Chiari malformation in young infants with myelomeningocele. Neurosurgery, 13:147, 1983.

Paterson, T. J., and Till, K.: The use of rotation flaps following excision of lumbar myelomeningocoeles: an aid to the closure of large defects. Br. J. Surg., 46:606, 1959.

Ramirez, O. M., et al.: A new surgical approach to closure of large lumbosacral meningomyelocele defects. Plast. Reconstr. Surg., 80:799, 1988.

Reigel, D. H.: Tethered spinal cord. *In* Humphreys, R. P. (Ed.): Concepts in Pediatric Neurosurgery. Vol. 4. Basel, S. Karger, 1983, pp. 142–164.

Reigel, D. H.: Spinal bifida. *In* McLaurin, R. L., Schut, L., Venes, J. L., and Epstein, F. (Eds.): Pediatric Neurosurgery. 2nd Ed. Philadelphia, W. B. Saunders Company, 1989.

Reigel, D. H., and McLone, D. G.: Myelomeningocele: operative treatment and results. *In* Marlin, A. E. (Ed.): Concepts in Pediatric Neurosurgery. Vol. 8. Basel, S. Karger, 1987.

Rudd, L. N.: Genetics. *In* Hoffman, H. J., and Epstein,

F. (Eds.): Disorders of the Developing Nervous System:
Diagnosis and Treatment. Boston, Blackwell, 1986, p.
47.

Seppala, M., and Ruoslahti, E.: Alpha-fetoprotein: physiology and pathology during pregnancy and application
to antenatal diagnosis. J. Perinatal Med., 1:104, 1973.

Sever, L. E.: Epidemiologic aspects of neural tube defects.
In Crandall, P. F. (Ed.): Proceedings of a Symposium.
The Prevention of Neural Tube Defects: The Role of
Alpha-Fetoprotein. New York, Academic Press, 1978,
pp. 75–89.

Thompson, M. W., and Rudd, N. L.: The genetics of
spinal dysraphism. In Morley, T. P. (Ed.): Current
Controversies in Neurosurgery. Philadelphia, W. B.
Saunders Company, 1976, pp. 126–146.

Venes, J. L.: The use of intravenous fluorescein in the
repair of large myelomeningoceles: technical note. J.
Neurosurg., 47:126, 1977.

77

Stephen R. Colen

Pressure Sores

The terms pressure sore, bedsore, and decubitus ulcer are frequently used interchangeably to describe ischemic tissue loss resulting from pressure, usually over a bony prominence. Bedsore and the term decubitus, which comes from the Latin *decumbere,* "to lie down," do not accurately describe the commonly seen pressure ulceration in the ischial region secondary to prolonged sitting. Pressure sore is the more accurate term, which reflects the current belief that the etiology is excessive pressure on the skin that results in tissue necrosis and ulceration. Sir James Paget (1873) was among the first to ascribe the etiology of bedsores to pressure, noting that such sores were "the sloughing and mortification" or death of a part produced by pressure. The spectrum of clinical presentation of pressure sores is broad, ranging from superficial skin loss to the progressive destruction of underlying fat, muscle, bone, and joints. If allowed to progress untreated, infection and sepsis may develop and death may ensue.

HISTORY

The period between the years 1749 and 1940 contains many theories on the etiology of pressure sores without much discussion of treatment. Charcot (1879) was of the opinion that nerve injury resulted in the release of a neurotrophic factor that caused tissue necrosis. Leyden (1874) and Munro (1940) believed that the loss of both sensation and autonomic control resulted in a decrease in peripheral reflexes that predisposed to skin ulceration. Munro (1940) further stated that ulceration was a sequela of paraplegia and should not be treated. These theories regarding etiology dominated the general thinking during this period and gave little hope for any successful treatment. Brown-Séquard (1853) strongly stated his beliefs that pressure and moisture were key etiologic factors. Comparing pressure sores in paraplegic and normal animals, he concluded that ulceration in the paralyzed animals healed at the same rate as that in normal animals as long as the ulcers were kept dry and free of contamination.

The assertions of Charcot and Munro, however, overshadowed other thinking during this period. Van Gehuchten (1908) proposed that muscle wasting and atony were more important causes of ulceration than loss of sensation. Küster (1908) was the first to focus attention on bacterial infection as an important etiologic factor in pressure sore development. Ascher (1928) pointed out the importance of secondary infection of damaged tissues in the extension of the necrotic process.

The era of surgical management was ushered in during World War II, when large numbers of paraplegics were being rehabilitated in an organized fashion. Cannon and associates (1950) stated that Scoville, at Cushing General Hospital, advocated surgical closure. Lamon and Alexander (1945) are credited with the first report of the surgical closure of a pressure sore with protective systemic antibiotic coverage using penicillin. Perhaps the development of antibiotics gave the surgeon the courage to close these potentially contaminated wounds. Most writers credit Davis (1938) with the concept of using flap replacement of scar epithelium in healed ulcers to provide bulky and well-padded skin coverage over the bony prominences. In 1943, Mulholland and associates pointed out the importance of nutrition and the restoration of positive nitrogen balance in treating patients with pressure sores. They reported rapid healing of pressure sores through the use of amino acid and dextrose dietary supplements, which restored positive nitrogen balance in a mixed group of general surgical and paraplegic patients.

Other reports of the surgical treatment of pressure sores in those wounded in World War II appeared in the literature. Among these were papers by Barker (1945); White, Hudson, and Kennard (1945); Gibbon and Freeman (1946); Croce, Schullinger, and Shearer (1946); Barker, Elkins, and Poer (1946); and White and Hamm (1946). The surgical treatment of bedsores developed quickly during this period until most surgeons favored the large, single pedicle type of flap for resurfacing the defect.

The efficacy and extent of ostectomy of the underlying bony prominence, particularly in the ischial area, received considerable attention. Removal of the tuberosity of the ischium was recommended (Kostrubala and Greeley, 1947). Operative success rates were increased from 47 per cent before the use of ischiectomy to 81 per cent after its adoption by Conway and associates (1951). Comarr and Bors (1958) cautioned against extensive ischiectomy, reporting an incidence of perineourethral diverticula in 46 per cent of patients with spinal cord injuries in whom the ischium had been removed as part of the operation. When bilateral total ischiectomy was performed the incidence was 58 per cent. Chase (1962) urged extreme caution in radical bone excision, and Guthrie and Conway (1969) admitted that there was a high incidence of perineal ulcer development after total ischiectomy.

Radical measures, such as bilateral high thigh amputation with the use of residual thigh skin flaps to cover large remaining defects, have been described (Georgiade, Pickrell, and Maguire, 1956; Chase and White, 1959; Berkas, Chesler, and Sako, 1961; Spira and Hardy, 1963; Royer and associates, 1969). Burkhardt (1972) reported the use of the skin of the entire lower leg, including the foot, by amputating at the mid-femoral area and filleting the distal part for coverage of extensive pressure sores.

In 1971, Ger introduced the principle of transposing adjacent muscle flaps into defects of the lower extremity with the application of split-thickness skin grafts over the muscle. More recently, musculocutaneous flaps have been described in which the overlying skin is supplied by perforating arteries through the muscle. The *Clinical Atlas of Muscle and Musculocutaneous Flaps* (Mathes and Nahai, 1979) helped to classify this concept of flap design. The ultimate role and value of muscle in the reconstruction of pressure sores remains to be defined by long-term clinical studies.

The possibility of providing sensory skin flaps in denervated regions was investigated by Dibbell in 1974 and Daniel, Terzis, and Cunningham in 1976. This concept holds great promise in the total rehabilitation of the paralyzed patient and the prevention of recurrences of pressure sores after surgical closure.

In the future the economic burden for the care of the spinal cord injured patient and the increasing population of chronically ill and elderly patients will put great pressures on physicians, hospitals, and the health budget. Consequently, early recognition of the patients at greatest risk, coordinated with treatment directed toward prevention and early definitive surgical care, must be the goal of the physician.

ETIOLOGY

Although neuropathic factors and shear have been implicated in the etiology of pressure sores, the single most important factor is excessive pressure. Unrelieved pressure for periods variously estimated at one to 12 hours is the major etiologic factor. Landis (1930), using a microinjection method to study capillary blood pressure, reported an average pressure of 32 mm Hg in the arteriolar limb, 20 mm Hg in the midcapillary bed, and 12 mm Hg in the venous side. Distribution of pressure points in man in the lying and sitting positions has been documented by Lindan, Greenway, and Piazza (1965) in their study using a "bed of springs and nails" (Fig. 77–1). In the supine position the sacrum, buttocks, heels, and occiput are subject to greatest pressures, in the range of 40 to 60 mm Hg. In the prone position the knees and chest sustain approximately 50 mm Hg. In the sitting position pressures up to 75 mm Hg develop over the ischial tuberosities. Pressures are transmitted from the surface to the underlying bone, compressing all the intervening tissues. Pressures are greatest over the bone, gradually decreasing toward the periphery. The greatest extent of tissue ischemia and necrosis would therefore be deep at the bony interface, and not at the skin surface. Husain (1953) demonstrated that by altering pressures, even for short periods lasting only five minutes, tissues are enabled to withstand much greater pressures.

The lowering of the nutritional status of the patient, whether by infection, starvation, or inanition, plays a role in the formation of pressure sores. Hubay, Kiehn, and Drucker (1957) considered a disturbed metabolic state to be necessary for both their formation and chronicity. While one might agree as regards chronicity, it is not essential that the metabolic state be altered for the formation of sores. Pressure sores have been known to develop in healthy young adult males suddenly immobilized because of accident or disease.

It has not been substantiated that neurotrophic factors are important in the etiology of pressure ulceration. Historically, Charcot in 1879 and Munro in 1940 placed great emphasis on the neurotrophic explanation for tissue ischemia and necrosis leading to ulceration.

Dinsdale (1974) concluded from pressure and friction studies on paraplegic pigs that friction was additive to pressure in producing skin ulceration. The shear theory postulates that stretching and compression of the muscle-perforating vessels to the skin results in subsequent ischemic necrosis. Dinsdale (1974) demonstrated that shear did not effect tissue injury by this mechanism, but instead contributed to skin ulceration by direct application of mechanical forces to the epidermis.

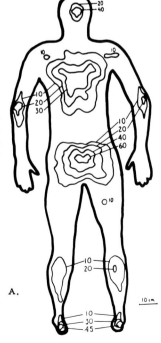
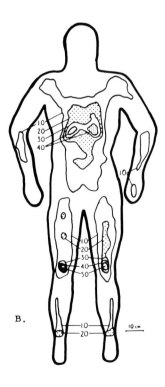

Figure 77–1. Comparison of pressure distribution in a healthy adult male supine (*A*) and prone (*B*) with his feet hanging over the edge of the bed. Values in mm Hg. (Redrawn from Lindan, O., Greenway, R. M., and Piazza, I. M.: Pressure distribution on the surface of the human body. Arch. Phys. Med. Rehab., *46*:378, 1965.)

A.

B.

From examination of all available data, it appears that pressure plays the key role in the formation of pressure sores. The critical questions clinically are how much pressure over what period of time is required to predictably produce ulceration, and which tissues are at greatest risk?

Research studies into the effects of pressure have been reported by Groth (1942), Kosiak (1959), and Dinsdale (1974). In a series of experiments in rabbits, Groth applied direct pressure to the posterior ischia. Pressure was transmitted by a single lever device for varying periods. The effect on the treated areas was examined both macroscopically and microscopically. Animals weighing 2 to 3 kg were exposed to a surface pressure of 143 mm Hg for three to four hours. Macroscopic changes were seen after a few days: slight swelling, redness, and small hemorrhages that progressed to well-circumscribed foci of necrosis, surrounded by a narrow reddish zone. At times, the well-circumscribed foci were missing and the changes appeared as distinct stripes, running in the direction of the muscle fibers. No changes were apparent in the nerves and larger blood vessels of the area. On microscopic examination there were capillary hemorrhages, waxy degeneration of Zenker, vacuolation, or loss of striation, followed by calcification in some of the necrotic muscle fibers. Phagocytosis with beginning interstitial proliferation, producing granulation tissue that formed a wall of demarcation around the necrotic musculature, was also observed. Seven days after the application of pressure a collagenous ground substance developed, leading to scar formation. Even in the animals that showed no macroscopic changes, there were microscopic alterations such as those described previously. As one might suspect, the longer the duration of pressure, the greater was the extent of the changes. Additional investigations on the role of sepsis and spinal transection were reported. Among the conclusions drawn by Groth (1942) were the following:

1. Pressure sores simulating those found in man can be produced experimentally.

2. They occur more frequently in flaccid paralytics than in spastic paralytics.

3. The larger the muscle mass, the greater is the ability to withstand pressure.

4. The effective pressure force increases toward the smaller surface. This phenomenon accounts for the greater destruction of tissue

found at the base of the inverted cone, typified by the small area of skin redness or destruction overlying a bony prominence. This condition is frequently observed in both ischial and trochanteric ulcers, and even to a lesser degree over the sacrum.

5. Generalized sepsis in an animal leads to local infection at the site of pressure, with abscess formation, extension of inflammation, thrombosis of the larger vessels, and consequently broader distribution of tissue necrosis. However, large vessel thrombosis per se is not a cause of ulceration because of the extensive collateral circulation usually present.

Kosiak (1959), in a well-controlled experiment using healthy dogs subjected to accurately controlled pressure ranging from 100 to 550 mm Hg for periods of one to 12 hours, came to the same conclusion, i.e., that prolonged pressure was the direct and main cause of pressure sores. Microscopic examination of tissue obtained 24 hours after the application of 60 mm Hg pressure for only one hour showed cellular infiltration, extravasation, and hyalin degeneration. Tissues subjected to higher pressures for longer periods showed, in addition, muscular degeneration and venous thrombosis. Kosiak concluded that intense pressure of short duration was as injurious to tissues as lower pressure of longer duration. The tissue ischemia in both situations led to irreversible cellular changes, producing ultimate necrosis and ulceration.

Kosiak (1959) disagreed with Groth (1942) in regard to the location and degree of severity of the changes, stating that they extended equally throughout the area under pressure instead of being most severe at the deepest part overlying the bony prominence. His conclusion was that skin and subcutaneous tissue act to provide a sling or suspension effect, with the result that only a fraction of the applied pressure is transmitted to the deep tissues.

Husain (1953) reported microscopic changes in rat muscle subjected to a pressure of 100 mm Hg for as little as one hour. His microscopic findings were essentially similar to those previously reported.

Keane (1979) noted that muscle is more susceptible to pressure injury than skin. As an example, he pointed out that body weight is borne on superficial weight-bearing bony prominences, these being covered with only skin and superficial fascia. Keane felt that in this way muscle was protected from the effects of pressure. Nola and Vistnes (1980) supported Keane by documenting significant areas of muscle necrosis noted histologically in rats when pressure was applied to a transposed muscle flap over bone. Daniel and Faibisoff (1982), in cadaver dissections, found that in normal human weight-bearing positions over bony prominences there is seldom, if ever, muscle interposed between bone and skin.

In 1974, Dinsdale analyzed the role of pressure and friction in the production of pressure sores in normal and paralyzed pigs. Pressure was mechanically applied with and without friction. Pressures of 160 to 1120 mm Hg were applied for three hours. Ulcerations extended into the dermis and were present after 24 hours. Dinsdale concluded that "friction is a factor in the pathogenesis of decubitus ulcers since it applies mechanical force in the epidermis." He cautioned against blindly accepting the pressure-ischemia relationship as the only cause for ulceration. Dinsdale concluded that a constant pressure of 70 mm Hg applied for more than two hours produced irreversible tissue damage. If the pressure was intermittently relieved, minimal changes occurred even at pressures of 240 mm Hg.

The above studies suggest that pressure equaling approximately twice the end-capillary arterial pressures (i.e., 70 mm Hg), unrelieved for between one and two hours, can produce ischemia.

Role of Paraplegia

Paraplegia may be caused by trauma or disease. Holdsworth (1954) made important observations on traumatic paraplegia that might explain the problem of ulcer development at certain sites and might influence the management of patients from the inception of the paraplegia. His study of 71 patients showed that correct nursing care, careful attention to simple bladder drainage, and proper rehabilitation measures resulted in an avoidance of all serious complications, maintenance of the general health of the patient, and a reduction in hospitalization time to an average of nine to ten months. In these patients not one serious bedsore developed, and in reviewing Holdsworth's paper one is impressed with the care exercised in the diagnostic assessment of the injury, a factor that must have been reflected in the notable results achieved.

Type and Level of Lesion

The level of the lesion must first be accurately determined. Since the spinal cord ends at the lower border of L1 (Fig. 77–2), any lesion below this level is purely a root lesion and regeneration after transection is possible, whereas in a true cord lesion there is no potential for regeneration. The prognosis in a root paralysis is better. The initial effect of a severe injury of the spinal cord is suppression of function below the level of the lesion. The suppression may be anatomic, in whole or in part, or physiologic. In the latter case, the capability of recovery exists. The extent of recovery is directly related to the severity and extent of the anatomic division. Partial recovery of power and sensation occurs with partial division. If the cord is completely divided, the isolated segments recover local reflex activity and the paralysis is of the upper motor neuron type, but anesthesia remains unchanged. When the anatomic division of the roots is complete, a flaccid paralysis eventually occurs.

During the period of suppression of function, it is impossible to determine the extent of anatomic damage to the cord, and as long as the condition persists the possibility of recovery of any cord function is uncertain. As a result, there is controversy about the initial treatment of these injuries:

1. If the cord is divided, no known form of treatment alters the prognosis. Therefore, in a complete transection of the cord, when the diagnosis is not in doubt, the patient can be started immediately on a routine of turning without fear of causing further damage.

2. If the cord is intact, there will be some recovery without treatment as long as it is protected from further injury. This means that a certain amount of immobilization is essential, a course that complicates the preventive therapy for pressure sores.

3. In partial lesions, decompression by laminectomy is indicated and should be done as soon as warranted; internal fixation allows routine turning of the patient.

During the initial period of spinal shock, the paralysis is flaccid in nature. As a result,

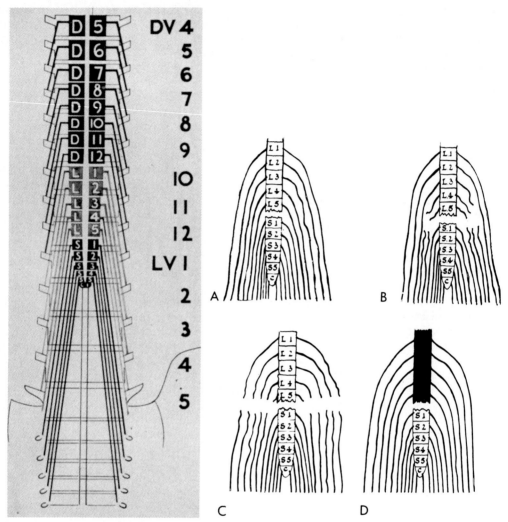

Figure 77–2. *Left,* The relationships of the vertebrae to the spinal cord and nerve roots. *Right,* Types of nerve damage. *A,* Cord divided; complete root escape. *B,* Cord divided; partial root escape. *C,* Cord and all roots divided. *D,* Cord divided; destruction of gray matter of lumbar segments. (From Holdsworth, F. W.: Traumatic paraplegia. Ann. R. Coll. Surg., *15*:281, 1954.)

many patients are left in the supine position in which undue pressure against the bony prominences of the occiput, thorax, sacrum, and heels may be allowed to develop. At these points, pressure sores may appear rapidly unless care is exercised to prevent prolonged pressure. In the patient who has injury without transection, some function may return after several weeks. Isolated cord segments may regain some function, and reflexes may reappear. The paralysis that was flaccid during the shock period becomes spastic or of the upper motor neuron type and may lead to the development of ulcers in quite different sites. If the patient is still restricted to bed, he may be turned on his side, incurring the risk of developing ulcers over the greater trochanters, or there may be spastic pressure of knee rubbing against knee or medial malleolus against medial malleolus. Combined with friction and maceration, such motion may result in ulcers in these areas. If the patient has been allowed to assume a sitting position and is not carefully instructed in how to avoid pressure, he may develop ischial ulcers as well as ulcers along the margins of the plantar surface of the heel and foot.

In spinal concussion, the initial effects are the same as in so-called spinal shock, but there is an eventual return to normal motor and sensory function. The latter shows some sign of recovery in a few hours, and Holdsworth (1954) noted that he had never seen total motor and sensory loss following concussion. Recovery begins with the appearance of sensation or motor power, or both. The return of any sensation in any segments, no matter how perverted, leads to the expectation of further recovery, and one can be certain that the cord is not transected. However, the failure of sensation to reappear or the occurrence of reflex activity of any kind (other than anal or bulbocavernous) without sensory or motor activity indicates that there has been a transection of the cord.

When there is complete paralysis and anesthesia due to a root lesion that is extensive, the root should be freed of pressure and protected from further injury.

Lesions above T10 are pure cord lesions with only a few unimportant roots involved, whereas fracture-dislocations below L1 are pure root lesions. If the cord lesion is partial and the vertebral fracture is stabilized without the need to resort to internal fixation, turning of the patient in bed is not dangerous. However, external fixation or splinting in a plaster bed, a treatment advocated in the past, is conducive to the development of pressure sores.

Effect of Spasticity

Spasticity, which not only contributes to the development of bedsores but also presents a serious surgical obstacle, has been reported as occurring in 40 per cent of the patients of Cannon and associates (1950) and in 54 per cent of the patients in the series of Pollock and associates (1951). The cord stump has been referred to by Scarff and Pool (1946) as a trigger zone upon which afferent stimuli from the posterior roots may fall, evoking a reflex response in the muscle masses below the lesion. Pollock and associates (1951) stated that the higher the cord lesion, the higher is the incidence of spasticity in mass reflex; e.g., 96 per cent in the cervical region, 40 per cent in the lumbar. An understanding of the neurologic factors involved is essential because the ability to predict the sites most likely to be involved may make it possible to prevent ulcers, and because such information guides the surgical treatment of pressure sores located in regions subject to considerable movement as a result of spasticity. The subject of spasticity relief will be discussed

further when such forms of treatment as alcohol washes, phenol injection (Griffith, 1966), and anterior and posterior rhizotomy are described, along with their physical and psychologic effects.

Clinical Studies Dealing With Production, Prophylaxis, and Therapy for Cord Injuries

Investigation of the histopathology of controlled spinal cord trauma in experimental animals has shown that spreading hemorrhage produces increasingly greater degenerative changes in the cord (Wagner and associates, 1969). This indicates the importance of the time factor to the effects of reversible and irreversible trauma, with progressive hemorrhagic necrosis of the spinal cord as the end result (Ducker and Assenmacher, 1969).

Ducker and Assenmacher (1969) also defined a 300 gm–cm concussion-contusion applied to animal spinal cord as a reversible force; i.e., the early paralysis caused may represent contusion to the neural element with associated conduction loss. Recovery is possible because the nutritional state of the spinal cord is maintained. However, irreversible trauma occurs with a 500 gm–cm force, and neuronal recovery is not possible because of inadequate spinal cord nutrition.

Circulatory changes seen after the initial trauma progress over the next 48 hours with marked inflammatory response in the vessel walls, increased leakage from the vascular system, and progressive hemorrhagic necrosis of the spinal cord. Cord edema is enhanced, and the combination leads to the development of an intramedullary hematoma. Under these circumstances the nutritional state of the spinal cord becomes irreversibly impaired, and neuronal recovery becomes an impossibility.

With these findings in mind, it follows that any factor that prevents or retards this progressively destructive mechanism must be investigated.

Steroid therapy by parenteral administration, as used by Ducker and Hamit (1969), has been shown to be of value in preventing permanent paraplegia in traumatized beagles, compared with untreated control animals subjected to the same force and left permanently paralyzed.

Drug therapy was the subject of considerable research by Osterholm and associates (1971). Their investigation, which offers the ultimate possibility of prevention or reduction of disability after cord trauma, has led to a technique of injecting alpha-methyltyrosine (AMT) within 15 minutes of the infliction of trauma.

Alpha-methyltyrosine, a highly toxic drug that has a deleterious nephrotoxic effect and can lead to uremia and death, has been used only in laboratory cats. It has the effect of providing chemical protection against hemorrhagic cord injury by acting against norepinephrine, a chemical essential for spinal cord function. After cord trauma, it accumulates in concentration in the tissues and leads to additional cord destruction by vasospasm, hemorrhage, sloughing, and major tissue destruction. Hemorrhage within the cat's cord begins about one hour after trauma; it increases in severity over the next few hours until necrosis begins in the fourth hour, and complete destruction results by 24 hours.

Alpha-methyltyrosine given to cats within 15 minutes of spinal trauma (500 gm–cm force) inhibits the destructive action of norepinephrine and prevents hemorrhagic necrosis. Approximately 75 per cent of the animals treated walk with normal gait or with minor extremity weakness. While the nephrotoxic effects of AMT cannot be controlled in humans, other norepinephrine antagonists are currently under study and offer promise of medical control of spinal cord injuries.

PATHOLOGY

Gross Pathology

Although there is an inclination to think of pressure sore lesions only in terms of their chronicity, it should be realized that there is an acute phase (Fig. 77–3). This may take the form of erythema or redness due to pressure, and pass through the stages of swelling, blistering, cyanosis, and beginning tissue necrosis. It is frequently found that the acute phase may be reversed by relief of pressure and other measures. Although Campbell (1959) recommended moderate heat to accompany the relief of pressure, Kosiak and associates (1958) believed it should not be used because it increases the metabolic requirements in an area already impoverished with regard to blood supply and thus may lead to additional tissue ischemia.

An incipient pressure sore may be mistaken for an ischiorectal or other form of

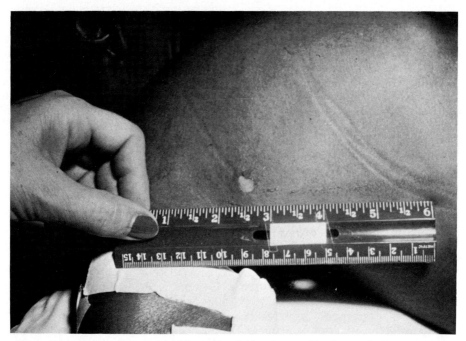

Figure 77–3. Early pressure sore of the axillary fold region resulting from a Stryker bed frame.

acute abscess and may be incised for drainage of pus that is not present. Instead of pus, grayish-yellow necrotic fat may be exposed. The site may become infected after incision, with resultant additional destruction of tissue. Occasionally, if there is an infection elsewhere in the body, organisms may settle in the traumatized area, even though the skin covering may be intact. In such cases, pus and necrotic fat may be apparent after incision of the area.

In the ulcers of the chronic form, there generally is deep destruction extending from skin and fat through fascia, muscle, and synovial membrane, if adjacent to a joint, and even into the joint. Osteitis or osteomyelitis with bone destruction may be present. In the most advanced cases, dislocations and pathologic fractures may be seen.

The ulcer of long standing that has passed through periods of repeated healing and breakdown may show considerable growth of marginal scar epithelium of a thin, shiny nature with wide surrounding zones of dense scar tissue. The granulation tissue may be pale and purulent. Some chronic ulcers show evidence of arrested epithelial ingrowth from the margin, resulting in turned-in, curled margins. This is especially seen in deep ulcers in which it is impossible for the epithelium to line the edges of the ulcer, owing to the failure of granulation tissue to grow upward and thus eliminate deep pockets.

The products of bacterial invasion and tissue breakdown form a foul-smelling, purulent discharge, which in itself is destructive of new epithelium. The continuous discharge of proteolyzed material leads to protein deficiency, anemia, temperature fluctuation, malaise, and a general lowering of the constitutional status.

Among the infecting organisms are staphylococci, streptococci, *Pseudomonas aeruginosa, Escherichia coli, Proteus mirabilis,* and others, often in combination. The character of the purulent exudate, i.e., its consistency and color, depends on the major infecting organism. Systemic administration of antibiotics, selectively matched to the infecting organism, is useful at times. However, their value is questionable in older chronic ulcers with heavy scarring and thrombosed vessels, factors that prevent access of the antibiotic to the ulcer.

The suppurative process may track great distances along fascial planes, establishing ramifying sinus tracts (Lopez and Aranha, 1974), penetrating bursae, entering joint cavities through the destruction of the joint capsule, and causing septic arthritis or joint destruction and dislocation (Fig. 77–4). Genitourinary complications, septicemia, and death may occur (Campbell, 1959).

In a retrospective autopsy study (Dalton, Hackler, and Bunts, 1965) of paraplegic patients, secondary amyloidosis was found in 40 per cent of those surviving the initial injury by at least one year. Seventy per cent of this subgroup died of renal failure secondary to renal amyloidosis. Chronic bedsores were a major factor in the development of amyloidosis in paraplegics.

In summary, pressure sore ulcers may take two major forms or may represent a combination of the two. They may start as superficial lesions involving skin alone or skin and fat. They may be treated in the early stages in a conservative fashion, because the condition is reversible if the ischemic tissue receives pressure relief and an enhanced oxygen supply. For the latter, serial transfusions (Matheson and Lipschitz, 1956; Kosiak, 1959)

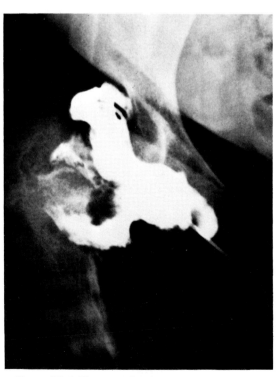

Figure 77–4. Sinogram showing communication between an ischial pressure sore and the hip joint.

increase the oxygen-carrying component. The use of hyperbaric oxygen for diabetic ulcers, stasis ulcers, and pressure sores of varying sizes was described by Fischer (1969), but follow-up reports are lacking. The second form may appear as an area of reddening of the skin with a small opening or no opening at all. Beneath the surface, however, there is widespread destruction in a cone-shaped area extending through all layers of tissue down to, and even including, bone. The second type invariably requires surgical resection and reconstruction.

Histopathology

The lesions are indistinguishable from other (nonspecific chronic) ulcers except in their extent. In the early stages of redness and swelling, there is vascular dilatation and interstitial edema, followed by epidermal separation, capillary clotting and hemorrhage, Zenker's waxy degeneration of muscle fibers, vacuolation, and death of tissue cells. There is cellular infiltration of the affected tissues by neutrophils and lymphocytes. Phagocytosis is increased, and a wall of demarcation formed by interstitial proliferation develops around the necrotic area.

Deposition of collagen in the granulation tissue at the base and margins of the ulcer may become so heavy that wound healing is seriously impaired. Thrombosis of larger vessels progresses, with the development of successively greater areas of tissue necrosis. Calcific deposits may be identified at times in the necrotic muscle fibers.

CLINICAL ASPECTS

Knowledge of the sites of predilection is useful from the standpoint of prophylaxis.

Yeoman and Hardy (1954), in a detailed analysis of 240 pressure sores in paraplegics, reported the following sites of involvement:

Site	Number	Percentage
Ischium	68	28
Sacrum	64	27
Heel	44	18
Trochanter	27	12
External malleoli	20	8
Tibial crest	10	4
Anterosuperior spine	5	2
Costal margin	2	1
Total	240	100

In a review of 1604 pressure sores in paraplegics, Dansereau and Conway (1964) reported the following anatomic distribution:

Ischial tuberosity	28%
Trochanter	19%
Sacrum	17%
Heel	9%
Malleolus	5%
Pretibial	5%
Patella	4%
Foot	3%
Anterosuperior spine	2.5%
Elbow	1.5%
Miscellaneous	6%
	100%

Petersen and Bittmann (1971), in a study of pressure sores in a region of Denmark, found that 63 per cent of patients developed them while in the hospital. Sacral, ischial and trochanteric sores were the most common; 10 per cent of the sores were found in ambulatory patients, 37 per cent in wheelchair patients, and 53 per cent in the bedridden.

The factors determining the site of involvement are many and include the state of paralysis (whether flaccid or spastic) and whether the patient is bedridden (and, if so, whether supine or prone). The patient may be in a wheelchair or may be wearing braces; if so, certain sites are more subject to pressure than others. The location of a patient's bed in relation to that of his roommates (Gelb, 1952) or to a television set or window view may determine the site of involvement, since he may spend long hours watching the television or facing away from a wall and conversing with roommates.

The early weeks after the onset of accident or disease are generally a period of flaccid paralysis and loss of vasomotor control, both factors that contribute to tissue breakdown. The patient generally lies supine, with changes of position to the side. Thus, it can be expected that sacral ulcers may develop, followed closely in frequency by trochanteric ulcers. Calcaneal, thoracic, and even occipital sores may also occur. Pressure sores involving the anterosuperior spine of the ilium, knees, tibial crests, elbows, and dorsum of the foot have a much smaller incidence, because the patient generally is not placed in the prone position. Even if he is, this position is tolerated so poorly by most patients that it is soon changed.

If spasticity develops, the bedridden patient

may develop medial condylar and medial malleolar sores with rapidity, owing to repeated rubbing of these parts against each other through spasm. There may also be associated trochanteric and sacral ulcers.

When the patient is finally allowed to sit up in bed, new sites are subjected to pressure, notably the ischial tuberosities, where a rapid breakdown of skin and subjacent tissues may follow the assumption of this position. Guttmann (1955) and Reichel (1958) both referred to shearing stress exerted on sacral and buttock skin by the elevation of the bed to a sitting position as a possible major cause of sacral pressure sores.

Sitting in a wheelchair may expose the thoracic or sacral regions to pressure, but more generally the pressure is exerted against the buttocks; thus, the ischial tuberosities, where a major portion of the weight is borne, may break down. It must also be emphasized that the dependent feet, which frequently become edematous and less able to withstand the pressure of resting on a foot piece, may show tissue necrosis on the plantar and posterior aspects of the heels and the lateral margins of the toes unless adequate protection is provided.

No surface of the body is immune to the development of ulcers. They have also been observed in soft tissue areas such as the midthigh, calf, upper arms, and forearms, and the situation is of course much worse in the quadriplegic population.

It is generally true that the lesions develop more quickly in a patient whose nutritional status is lowered. In long-standing ulcers the copious discharge of the products of proteolysis results in a nitrogen imbalance with a lowering of the serum proteins, anemia, and vitamin deficiency. When any or all of these conditions are present, there is a reduction in both the fat and lean body mass and a reduced ability to heal traumatized areas. Progression of the processes of breakdown is encouraged, and a vicious cycle may be instituted unless steps are taken to interrupt it.

TREATMENT

Treatment can be divided into two major categories: (1) systemic and (2) local, either conservative or surgical.

Systemic Treatment

NUTRITIONAL MEASURES

The prime concern after relief of pressure and wound toilet is the restoration of the patient's nutritional status. The measures undertaken vary according to the chronicity of the lesion and the general physical state. Of prime importance is the administration of a high protein, high calorie, high vitamin diet. In the presence of hypoproteinemia, the development of ulcers is rapid and healing is slow. By restoring a positive nitrogen balance, the healing of damaged tissue is facilitated.

Measures correcting the nutritional imbalance must be instituted early and must show results before any but life-saving surgery is attempted. In practice, it has been found that a daily intake of 135 gm of protein in the form of lean meats, cheese, skimmed milk, protein hydrolysate, and amino acids is effective. Vegetable protein is important, but animal protein is preferable. It may be necessary to supplement oral feedings by the use of a nasogastric tube or by hyperalimentation.

If fat occupies an excessive proportion of a patient's diet, he may be unable to ingest adequate protein. It may be wise to reduce the fat and increase the carbohydrate content of the menus.

If blenderized diets are impractical, high protein liquid diets are commercially available, but these are relatively more expensive and are hyperosmolar.

Intravenous hyperalimentation with a long-term, indwelling, centrally placed venous catheter is possible. Amino acid, glucose and fat emulsion are available for this purpose. The procedure for alimentation by this route has been standardized.

In general, it is less expensive, less complicated, and more effective to aliment the patient by the oral route whenever possible.

In the case of vitamin deficiency, some restoration occurs as a result of the dietary measures, but these should be supplemented by the administration of multivitamins. A geriatric formula type of vitamin compound has been found useful in these patients.

Unless there is a serum protein level above 6 mg per 100 ml, surgery should not be undertaken except as a life-conserving measure.

The inculcation of a psychologic desire to get the operation over with and thus start a rehabilitation program with the least possible delay may be of greater value than all the foregoing measures.

TREATMENT OF ANEMIA

The correction of anemia goes hand in hand with correction of the protein deficiency. A combination of diet, drugs, and blood transfusion may be required. Liver should be included as a regular item on the menu. Iron preparations, given by mouth or injection, may have an additional beneficial effect in that they reduce the frequency of loose stools, thus helping to maintain cleanliness in certain affected regions.

It may be necessary to give repeated transfusions of whole blood two or three times a week, not only preoperatively but also during and after surgery. By the judicious use of these measures, an effort is made to raise the hemoglobin level to a minimum of 12 gm, although some writers prefer a level of 15 gm (Matheson and Lipschitz, 1956). At any rate, the red cell mass should be raised as high as possible preoperatively and should be maintained at this level in the postoperative period.

COOPERATION WITH OTHER SERVICES

Infection, either at the site of the lesion or remote from it, must be eliminated as far as possible. This point requires no further elaboration except to emphasize the need for greater cooperation between hospital services, especially those covering the genitourinary, neurosurgical, dermatologic, and dental areas.

It is important in the handling and rehabilitation of the patient to secure the advice and assistance of other specialized services. The orthopedic service is consulted about the prevention or correction of flexion contractures, the treatment of septic joint fractures, and the stabilization of joints. The rehabilitation department can assess the patient's capabilities and outline a training program designed to make him as self-sufficient as possible, or even self-supporting. The psychologist and psychiatrist may be consulted regarding problems associated directly or indirectly with the general situation. The social service worker may be required to help settle the patient's family affairs or to enlist the aid of welfare or vocational agencies.

RELIEF OF SPASM

The presence of spasm in approximately 50 per cent of paraplegic patients must be of serious concern to all who treat them. Cannon and associates (1950) reported that spasm was serious enough to interfere with surgery in one-third of their spastic paraplegics. Consequently, it is necessary to consult the neurosurgeon when this condition exists.

When no ulcers are present, measures to correct spasm must be considered from the standpoint of prophylaxis. When there are sores, the continued spasmodic movement of the parts in most instances prevents healing. If surgical treatment is contemplated, it is essential that the spasm be controlled and eliminated, or the surgery almost without exception will fail.

Any consideration of the correction of spasm must also take into account the fact that such measures as anterior rhizotomy and alcohol injection may destroy reflex sexual activity and bladder control, thus greatly reducing the patient's psychologic sense of adequacy and social acceptance. As emphasized by Chase and White (1959), paraplegics have been robbed of so many functions that preservation of sexual function is an important aspect of rehabilitation. In connection with sexual ability, Talbot (1949, 1955), Munro (1954), and Zeitlin, Cottrell, and Lloyd (1957) reported complete erection in 66 to 74 per cent of male paraplegics. Talbot reported that anterior rhizotomy destroyed reflex sexual activity in six out of ten patients, and alcohol injection abolished erection in 28 out of 30 patients studied by Bors (1948). This argument was used by Chase and White (1959) to support the use of bilateral high-thigh amputation in paraplegics rather than subjecting these patients to neurosurgical intervention for spasm. Harding (1961) was of the opinion that intrathecal alcohol blocks and dorsal rhizotomy, which in his series yielded only temporary improvement in approximately half the cases, should be abandoned. He believed that procaine block, which Munro (1954) showed controlled mass reflex spasm permanently in selected patients, should be more widely used. When this fails, selective anterior rootlet rhizotomy and bilateral anterior dorsolumbosacral rhizotomy should be considered. Bors (1948) relieved spinal reflexes by peripheral obturator neurectomy combined with adductor myotomy.

Pharmacologic agents presently available to aid in the relief of spasm include diazepam, baclofen, dantrolene sodium, mephenesin carbonate, dimethothiazine, and orciprenaline. Specific medical contraindications must be carefully evaluated before these drugs are administered.

It will be realized, therefore, that the problem of spasm relief is not a simple one, there being many factors to consider. The merits and demerits of each method must be weighed carefully in the light of the overall situation. It is only after such deliberation and after discussion with the patient that a course of treatment permanently damaging to their physical status should be performed. However, a hard choice must often be made, because it is of little advantage to retain bladder and erectile function if by so doing it proves to be impossible to cover a large ulcer that may cause the patient to be totally incapacitated and bedridden and may possibly lead to his death.

RELIEF OF PRESSURE

Many developments in the field of pressure relief have occurred and are still being developed. The expense involved in this form of therapy is a major drawback in many instances and has prevented widespread adoption.

In the past the main method of pressure relief lay in the extensive application of bulky, nonabsorbent dressings to the affected parts. Reference was made to springy, synthetic, nonabsorbent fibers such as Acrilan and Dacron, encased in an absorbent cover of cotton. Their use was preferred to the type of flat, absorbent dressings frequently seen on the wards of many hospitals.

However, the work involved in changing the bulky dressings in a time of high labor costs, plus their overall inefficiency, led to a search for better and more efficient methods. Because the newer methods have not yet come into general use and because of the high cost involved, their adoption is likely to be slow; the older methods of pressure relief are still widely employed, and should be reviewed.

In practice, a dressing of sterile Acrilan or Dacron fiber, built up to a thickness of 5.0 to 7.5 cm over a regular absorbent gauze dressing and held in place by Elastoplast or Montgomery straps, produces a light, airy, resilient dressing that diffuses heat, allows air to circulate, and does not become sodden. It may be necessary to protect the skin under the Elastoplast or the straps by painting it with tincture of benzoin, collodion, or some of the aerosol sprays.

Other methods of pressure relief have been used, such as sheepskin (Ewing and associates, 1964; Nyquist and Bors, 1964) or easily removed bootees placed beneath the patient or applied to specific areas such as the foot (Butterworth and Golding, 1965). This was a step forward, but laundering posed certain difficulties, as the sheepskin either disintegrated or became so hard that it did not serve its purpose. Synthetic deep-piled pads were substituted successfully and were widely used because of the ease of laundering.

Another substitute material is silicone gel used in a cushion or pad (Spence, Burke, and Rae, 1967). The pads provide fairly good weight distribution but are quite expensive, and some patients find them hard to use. The Jobst Hydro-float flotation pad is somewhat cheaper and fits all sizes of wheelchair. The cost may be further reduced by using air cushions filled with water.

The water bed was first described by Arnott in 1838 and mentioned by Paget in 1873, but more or less remained in limbo until Weinstein and Davidson (1965) published a report of an updated modern version for the prevention and treatment of pressure sores. They described both a bed and a seat. Harris (1965, 1967) and Dewis, Caplan, and Pache (1968) reported favorably on the use of the bed with a plastic bladder to hold the water, which was contained in a Styrofoam form contoured to the body.

Pflandler in 1968 presented a comprehensive review of the whole subject of flotation for pressure relief, describing the principle (Archimedes), variations, and experience with its use at the University of Rochester Rehabilitation Center. A lifting device to make nursing care easier was incorporated into the contoured fiber glass bed, and the patient lies on a free-floating vinyl sheet called Staph-check, which is impregnated with a chemical formula designed to inhibit the growth of *Staphylococcus* organisms. The depth of the water varies from 1 foot at the shoulders to 2½ feet at the buttocks. This design allows the patient to assume a sitting position while still floating freely.

Thornhill and Williams (1968) reported their experiences with the water mattress in a large city hospital. They described ten patients who had satisfactory results from several points of view: (1) all ulcers showed signs of healing, (2) no new ulcers or lesions were observed in any patient while on the water mattress, and (3) the healing time was accelerated. Dewis, Caplan, and Pache (1968) reported that routine nursing care was continued, and only dry sterile dressings were applied to the ulcers. The patients were turned to increase their comfort and to aid pulmonary drainage. Frequent turning proved to be unnecessary, since the fluid support eliminated many of the pressure points.

Some of the commercial preparations that evolved during this period were the DePuy Flote-bed manufactured by DePuy, Inc.; Hydro-float manufactured by Jobst; and variations of these making use of such equipment as sports air cushions and camping mattresses filled with water in an attempt to reduce the expense. One of the great difficulties with the latter is the frequency of leaks. Although they can be patched, much water escapes before the leak is discovered.

One difficulty encountered was the inability of the patient to adjust to a jiggling, constantly moving surface. Another problem was observed when it came to changing position, and another involved difficulty in breathing because of limited movement or limited activity. An unexpected effect in many instances was the fact that once the patient became accustomed to the bed, he also became addicted to it and resisted being moved to a regular bed.

Kosiak and associates (1958) made a comparison of the pressures exerted at 12 points on the thigh, ischium, and coccyx when the patient was positioned on various materials. Kosiak found that pressure on a flat board varied from 50 to 500 mm Hg, on a wooden office seat from 97 to 200 mm Hg, and on a board with a 2 inch foam rubber pad from 53 to 160 mm Hg. These findings were recorded in 11 spinal injury patients, and the highest pressures were found to be exerted over the ischia and coccyx.

When these patients sat on an alternating pressure pad at ½ inch excursion, pressures in the inflated position ranged from 100 to 275 mm Hg. In the deflated position, pressures at critical sites were about equal to or below the level of the arterial diastolic pressure in all but four sites around the ischia and coccyx. Pressure greater than capillary pressure was exerted at least half the time at all sites, and constantly in four critical areas.

Weinstein and Davidson (1966) found water bed pressures of 18 mm Hg (average) against the heels, 19 mm Hg against the sacrum, and approximately 25 mm Hg against the trochanters when the patient was lying on his side. These pressures are below capillary pressures at heart level, which range from 20 to 30 mm Hg, so that the vicious circle of pressure producing vascular occlusion, anemia, and tissue necrosis is broken.

Baran and associates (1972), using a new mattress of a specially engineered polyurethane foam and a regular hospital mattress, compared various site pressures in five patients and noted that the pressures differed significantly. Another study of 16 patients by the same investigators, using a different method of recording pressures and adding an additional element of recommended support (the water mattress), yielded even stronger evidence in favor of the polyurethane mattress.

Although considerable improvement has been secured in the relief of pressure by these methods, the ultimate goal of weightlessness or total pressure relief remains elusive. The British Hoverbed, following the principle of the British Hovercraft in which jets of air are used to support a mass above ground or sea level, supports the body in reverse on jets of air directed upward. A disadvantage of this method is the noise produced by the powerful fans necessary to provide the supporting jets. The desiccating effect of blowing warm air over wounds is theoretically undesirable.

The noise factor was also encountered at first with the latest development in flotation therapy, the air-fluidized bed developed by Artz and Hargest (1971) and others at the Medical College of South Carolina. The use of this bed is well covered in a publication called *The Air Fluidized Bed, Clinical and Research Symposium,* edited by Artz and Hargest (1971).

The basic principle involves supporting the body on a bed whose fluid consists of air and ceramic spheres. According to Artz and Hargest (1971), the fluid is not to be confused with liquid, which is wet. The principle is simple, i.e., an object of any size or shape can be supported in an air stream if the volume and pressure of the stream are sufficient. By using hundreds of millions of ceramic spheres, 74 to 125 microns in size and made of crown optical glass with no free silica present, the density of the supporting medium is increased, and the volume of air necessary to support the body is markedly decreased. The volume of air is approximately 6 per cent of that required for the British Hoverbed. This results in a motor less powerful and much quieter than that of the Hoverbed. The patient is separated from direct contact with the spheres by a sheet of square-weave monofilament polyester woven to a controlled 37 micron porosity (Hargest, 1969). The design keeps the spheres in the bed, with the exception of an insignificant number of undersized spheres. The latter may cause a slight dust problem for a few days, while permitting free passage of warmed, humidified air that can be closely controlled to obtain the optimal temperature and humidity for the patient, creating an environment that inhibits bacterial growth (Sharbaugh and Hargest, 1971). The bed of spheres is approximately 12 inches deep at rest. When the blower is activated, the depth of the spheres is increased only ½ inch, and yet it provides the flotation equivalent to 17 inches of water for a 250 lb body. The body mass resting on the ceramic sphere and air bed penetrates to a distance of only 4 inches. Because of the penetration effect of the mass, there are surface pressures less than those obtained when the body rests on a foam mattress or water-filled bladder. Since the polyester sheet provides no support but moves freely to contour itself to the depression, no shearing forces are developed to damage the tissues.

Body wastes and secretions, which ordinarily would be considered sources of auto- and cross-contamination, have not been a problem. Studies by Sharbaugh and Hargest (1971) have shown that sequestration and desiccation of microorganisms within the air fluidized bed system constitute the main contributing factor in the bactericidal and fungicidal ability of the system, a factor making it of incalculable value in the hospital environment. Because of the very low pressures exerted on the body, the bed can be used for paraplegics and other decubitus-prone pa-

tients directly after surgery. Lying on skin grafts and flaps has not proved harmful, and dressing changes are simple (Hofstra, 1971).

Some disadvantages are that (1) active suction is sometimes necessary to maintain urinary drainage; (2) the noise may be annoying both to the patient and to others in the room; (3) the bed is heavy, necessitating some reinforcement at the corners; and (4) it is costly.

Favorable aspects, as reported by Hofstra (1971), are that (1) patient comfort is increased; (2) the need for medication to control restlessness and to aid sleep is greatly reduced; (3) the patient shows physiologic improvement, so that his appetite is improved; (4) the skin remains dry and does not become macerated; and (5) skin lesions are cleaner and healing is promoted.

The use of foam rubber rings is not satisfactory. They lead to a false sense of security on the part of the nursing staff, and a possible reduction in the frequency of position changes ordered by the doctor. In addition, while relieving pressure at one point, they may produce an annular area of pressure around this point that can lead to vascular constriction and disastrous results.

Blocks of foam rubber used as seats on wheelchairs may be either solid or cored. They afford some protection, but do not allow adequate circulation of air, and they tend to sag if laid on the canvas seat of the patient's chair. The sagging can be eliminated by the introduction of a piece of plywood across the canvas seat. It may be preferable to substitute as a seat pad one of the light, porous, foamed plastics in the form of a block 7.5 to 10 cm thick. These plastics have great resilience and shock absorption power, and form a protective pad beneath the ischial tuberosity for the patient in a wheelchair. A patient in a chair should be urged by all who see him to shift his position with great frequency until it becomes an ingrained habit. Houle (1969) evaluated a number of seat devices designed to prevent ischemia leading to ulceration. There are many types of seat cushions all aimed at the same objective, i.e., the reduction of pressure on the ischial tuberosities to the greatest degree possible.

For the bedridden patient, the foam rubber or plastic sectional mattress has properly replaced the usual types of inner springs. A more refined development is the alternating pressure mattress, which is, however, costly. The principle is sound, and these mattresses have proved helpful, but the support systems previously described are superior.

Too much reliance, however, must not be placed on any automatic instrument, which cannot be a substitute for human care and attention.

It must be kept in mind that, while pressure is being relieved in the area of an ulcer, other areas must not be subjected to undue pressure, especially during the postoperative period. Therefore, special care must be taken in the positioning and padding of the unaffected parts.

ROENTGENOGRAPHIC STUDIES

If there are sinus tracts and infected bursae, it is advisable to take roentgenograms using a contrast medium instilled into the tracts (see Fig. 77–4). The devious paths of the sinus tracts can thus be identified before surgery, and their presence may be an indication for more extensive surgery. The degree of involvement revealed by the roentgenogram is often quite astounding. An ischial ulcer may show osteomyelitis of the tuberosity, but in addition the suppurative process may track medially and anteriorly toward the pubis, especially in a patient who has been placed in the prone position. A trochanteric ulcer may show peripheral extensions around the thigh in the fascial and muscle planes. There may be extensions upward from the trochanter to the femoral neck and into the hip joint, producing a septic arthritis or pyarthrosis. A sacral decubitus may communicate with the hip joint (Lopez and Aranha, 1974).

Heterotopic bone can be demonstrated in many ulcers of long standing, and some deposits reach a large size. Although simple superficial periostitis is no contraindication to surgery when there is involvement of joints, the problem of treatment may be complex, and orthopedic consultation should be obtained. Resection of the femoral head may be indicated if there is a sinus tract communicating with the hip joint.

Local Treatment

CONSERVATIVE TREATMENT

Local treatment is aimed at securing a surgically clean wound. If the ulcer is not excessively large, it will fill in from below, and epidermal growth from the sides will produce a closed wound. However, coverage by scar epithelium is unsatisfactory because of associated vulnerability to the minimal trauma of daily activities.

Most pressure sores when first seen require surgical debridement of all the necrotic material, whether it be skin, fat, muscle, or all three. Fragments of dead bone at the base of the wound may be found lying free, and, if not removed, they continue to cause drainage. Fibrous septa are broken down, and unilocular or multilocular infected bursae are opened for free drainage. Devitalized fascia or tendons should be excised. Such simple surgical measures can generally be performed at the patient's bedside with only an occasional complication, such as mild bleeding. *Extensive debridement should be done in the operating room,* and the procedure may have to be repeated several times. The surgeon must be prepared to insert monitoring lines and to replace excessive blood loss by having cross-matched blood available in the operating room.

Surgical debridement is the most reliable technique, although some modest success with enzymatic debridement had been reported by Morrison and Casali (1957). Some patients have shown skin irritation after prolonged use of enzymatic debriding agents, but the irritation disappeared when these medications were stopped and saline dressings substituted. In addition to cleaning the wound, the associated foul odor was suppressed.

Frequent dressing changes are preferable, and wet to dry fluff gauze dressings are particularly suited to the rapid removal of necrotic material from the wound.

Irrigations of the depths of the ulcer, particularly those in the trochanteric and ischial areas, should be made daily or with each dressing change. The author's preference is a mixture of hydrogen peroxide and saline in equal parts. It is relatively bland, and the foaming action of the hydrogen peroxide provides a satisfactory mechanical flushing effect. Plain saline wet dressings and dilute acetic acid dressings have their advantages, and the use of 1.5 per cent Dakin's solution applied in the form of continuous moist dressings has shown good results (Griffith and Schultz, 1961). The surrounding skin may be protected by preparations such as a thick film of zinc oxide ointment or silicone cream to prevent maceration.

If an exceedingly large ulcer surface is moderately clean, a simple split-thickness skin graft is often applied to obtain a closed wound preparatory to carrying out a definitive flap procedure. This maneuver helps immeasurably in preventing inordinate protein loss and in restoring the hematocrit and the nutritional balance to levels that enhance the chances of surgical success.

It should be emphasized that at the start of local therapy, cultures of the ulcer drainage should be taken, the organisms identified, and their sensitivity to various antibiotics determined. The local use or application of antibiotics is usually ineffective, but it is thought that the systemic use of an effective drug matched to the organism may prove to be of value initially. It is used as a therapeutic measure when the organism has invaded other parts of the body. However, antibiotics are of little use in the older chronic ulcers with heavy scarring and thrombosed vessels in the area of inflammation, for the simple reason that these conditions prevent access of the therapeutic agent to the ulcerated sites.

The foregoing methods of conservative therapy may result in the healing of small or medium-sized ulcers after a period of time. It is unusual for a large ulcer to resurface itself, but this has sometimes been seen. In many instances, particularly when the level of the healed surface is below that of the surrounding skin and is not subject to pressure, healing may be adequate. As a general rule, however, the quality of the new skin covering is of a low grade without sebaceous or sweat glands or well-developed dermal and subdermal layers. Such scar epithelium is generally dry and thin with a poor blood supply and must be lubricated by the application of petrolatum, cocoa butter, cold cream, lanolin, or similar preparations. Areas thus healed are more subject to breakdown on slight trauma than is normal skin because of their poor vascularity and quality; healing is generally slower when there has been disruption of the continuity of such a skin surface.

With the conservative method of treatment, not only is the initial healing time lengthy, but also there may be repeated periods of morbidity due to minor trauma and tissue breakdown. Because of these factors, relatively early surgical therapy offers the best hope in the form of earlier closure and improved ability to withstand subsequent trauma. In addition, the achievement of the overall rehabilitation of the patient is a factor of the greatest importance economically, socially, and psychologically. There is no question that only a very small percentage of pressure sores can be treated adequately by conservative therapy.

SURGICAL TREATMENT

The history of the surgical closure of bedsores began with the report of four cases by Davis in 1938. The importance of the excision of the underlying bony prominence was also appreciated toward the end of World War II. This surgical concept was significant for several reasons. First, it eliminated an important element of infection, since it was demonstrated by microscopic studies that changes ranging from fibrosis to osteomyelitis were present in the affected bone. Second, it provided for the elimination of the projecting bony eminence, a significant factor in the recurrence of ulcers (Kostrubala and Greeley, 1947). Also in the same year, the Plastic Surgery Service at the Bronx (New York) Veterans Administration Hospital suggested the use of split-thickness skin grafts to resurface the donor defects created by the rotation of large flaps (Conway and associates, 1951). Bors and Comarr (1948), in a report on the treatment of ischial ulcers, advocated covering the open bony surface with flaps of nonfunctioning muscle. Georgiade, Pickrell, and Maguire (1956) reported bilateral high thigh amputation for the treatment of the "end stages" of pressure sores.

The gradual evolution in the surgical treatment of pressure sores has led to the presently accepted surgical objectives: (1) excision of the ulcerated area, including the underlying bursa and the usually infected scar tissue and/or undermined skin that encircles the defect; (2) resection of any existing bony prominence; (3) resurfacing of the defect with healthy skin, including adequate subcutaneous tissue padding; (4) designing the flaps as large as possible; and (5) obtaining additional padding by the use of muscle flaps if subcutaneous tissue is not adequate.

Timing

Elective reconstructive surgery should not be contemplated unless the general condition of the patient has stabilized and the ulcer shows the following signs of improvement: (1)

clearance of all necrotic tissue, (2) appearance of healthy granulation tissue, and (3) a tendency for the ulcer to decrease in size by diminution of the extent of the undermining and/or evidence of advancing epithelial margins.

General Principles

Preoperative Preparation of the Patient. Assumption of the prone position for increasing lengths of time preoperatively prepares the patient for the prolonged positioning required in the postoperative phase when surgery is planned for sacral, ischial, and in some instances trochanteric ulcers. Most patients initially find the position disagreeable to intolerable, but they can be persuaded to assume it. It is desirable that they do this preoperatively, so that they know what to expect after surgery and become accustomed to feeding themselves in this position. It is also a training period for bowel evacuation, which may pose a problem postoperatively.

Anesthesia. General endotracheal anesthesia is preferred to local infiltration and/or sedation alone, in order to avoid spasmodic reflex muscle movements. However, other surgeons find sedation alone acceptable provided that an anesthesiologist is in attendance to monitor the physiologic status.

A competent anesthesiologist, supervising fluid and whole blood replacement and capable of giving ample warning to the surgeon of the beginning of shock or the development of cardiac complications, is essential to the proper functioning of the surgical team. Paraplegic patients have wide fluctuations in blood pressure and pulse rate and lack the usual compensatory physiologic (sympathetic) responses to hypovolemia. There is often considerable blood loss despite the most exacting techniques. From a psychologic standpoint also, the conscious patient may be unduly worried or concerned about chance remarks made by the surgical team, or may become extremely restless through fear of lying too long in one position and incurring an additional pressure sore. Under general anesthesia these worries are eliminated, and the surgeon can devote himself totally to the problem of coverage.

Operating Room Conduct and Preparation. On the morning of surgery the ulcer is cleaned and a dry dressing applied. A new indwelling Foley catheter should be introduced to prevent changes in position while the patient's mobility is restricted during the postoperative period. The catheter is allowed to drain freely into a recipient closed system container.

Once the patient is in the operating room, anesthesia is induced and the endotracheal tube is placed while he is on the stretcher. The patient is positioned on the operating table, the surgeon being particularly careful to provide abundant cushioned support to the exterior bony prominences, anterior superior iliac spines, knees, tibial crests, and dorsum of the feet. The positioning of the patient is accomplished in such a way as to provide adequate exposure not only of the defect but also of the adjacent donor area.

The skin is prepared with the antiseptic solution of choice. Care is exercised to prevent the solution from running down and forming a pool on the dependent surface, possibly the groin, where signs of irritation develop in susceptible patients.

The entire area is draped to provide ample exposure, and no towel clips are used on the skin. If necessary, a few sutures may be placed for fixation of the surgical drapes.

The next step is to outline the extent of the ulceration, which is self-evident by external examination. However, in many patients a variable degree of undermining may be present around the periphery of the ulcer. It is important to determine the extent of the undermining by exploring with the finger or probing with a curved clamp in all directions. By applying slight upward pressure to the clamp, its tip may be felt or seen projecting through the skin; at this point a mark is made with ink (Fig. 77–5). In this manner a series of dots outline the extent of the undermining. This is a necessary maneuver because the above surfaces are covered by a pale, shiny granulation tissue, which is the source of serous drainage. The surface has the appearance of an endothelial type of lining. This tissue should be carefully removed either by including it with the ulcer if it is of limited extent, or by means of surface excision down to the normal-appearing tissue if the undermining is extensive. If any of the tissue of the undermined area is left behind, the risk of seroma formation under the flap, and its sequelae of delayed adherence or nonadherence of the flap to the undersurface, is considerably increased.

Postoperative Care. The postoperative

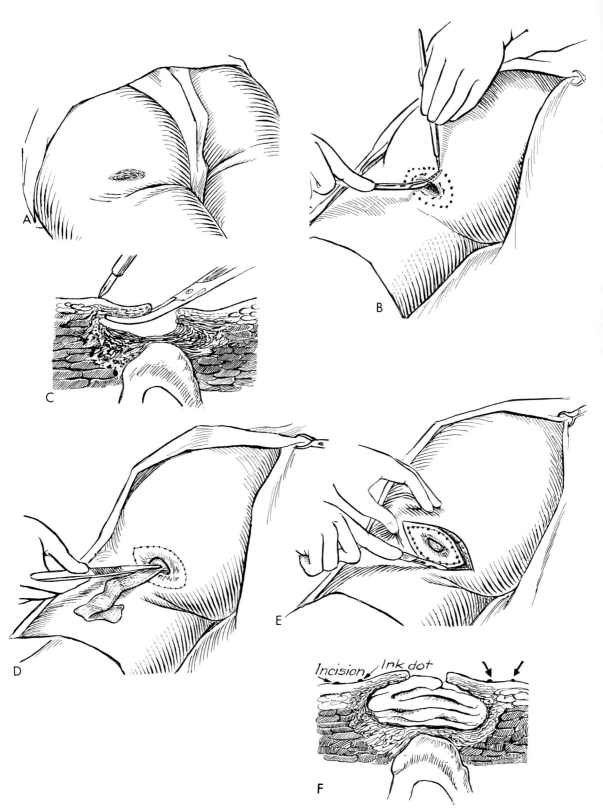

Figure 77–5. Ischial ulcer. *A* to *D,* The widest extent is demonstrated by a hemostat and marked on the skin surface with ink. The defect is filled with Betadine-soaked packing. *E, F,* Extent of soft tissue resection.

Illustration continued on following page

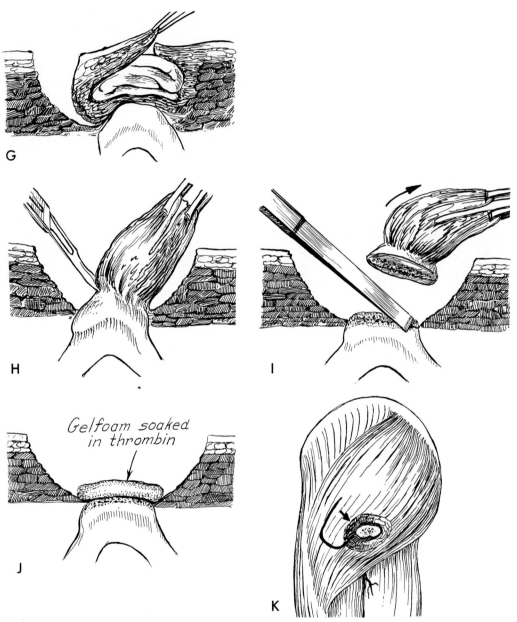

Figure 77–5 *Continued G* to *I,* Partial removal of ischial tuberosity. *J,* Hemostasis is facilitated by the application of Gelfoam (soaked in thrombin) on the bony surface. *K,* A flap of gluteus muscle may be rotated into the osseous defect; alternatively, a biceps femoris muscle flap may be employed.

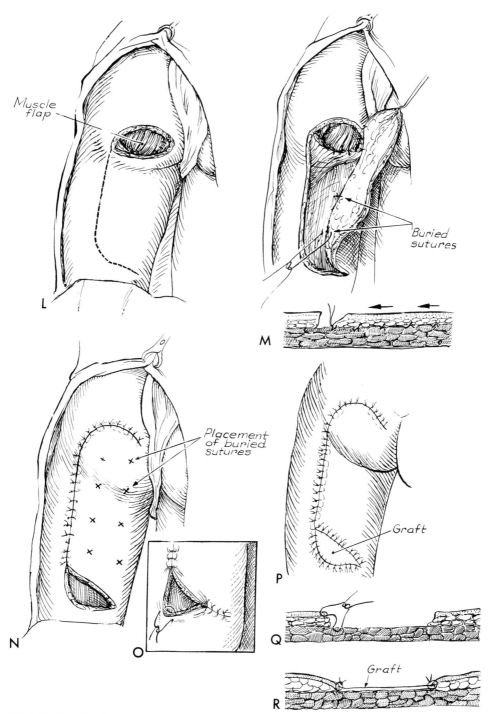

Figure 77–5 *Continued L,* Appearance after resection. Note the muscle flap applied to the osseous defect. The large rotation flap is outlined. *M,* "Creeping" advancement of the rotation flap by securing the undersurface of the flap to the deep muscles by catgut sutures. *N,* The flap has been rotated into the defect. *O,* The donor defect closed primarily by the V-Y principle. *P to R,* Technique of resurfacing the donor site by a split-thickness skin graft. Note that the skin surface of the flap is sutured to the defect before the application of the skin graft.

care in the treatment of a pressure sore is of the utmost importance. Beginning from the time the patient is transferred from the operating table, care must be exercised to prevent motion or shearing forces in the region of the flap. When the air fluidized bed is utilized the patient is allowed to lie supine for three weeks before being wedged into a semisitting position. He may be transferred to his regular bed by the end of the fourth week, requiring the usual frequent repositioning and turning. When the air fluidized bed is not available, the patient is placed on a regular bed in the prone position. Adequate padding with cushions, pillows, and foam rubber pads is used to make this position as comfortable as possible. The position can be changed from the prone slightly to the side position by the careful use of props inserted under the hips and chest. It is mandatory to control any residual spasms that may be present during the immediate postoperative period.

A check of the hematocrit for possible additional blood replacement is made in the recovery room, and again within the first 12 hours.

Closed suction drainage is maintained for seven to ten days, at which time it is removed if there is no significant drainage.

If the patient is having loose bowel movements that are soiling and contaminating the surgical area, an effort is made to constipate him. The use of low residue diets and codeine is helpful. However, when the stool is formed, it is not necessary to induce constipation.

The skin sutures, unless there is evidence of skin reaction, are left in place for approximately two weeks.

During the fourth postoperative week the patient may gradually be exposed to pressure on the repaired area, beginning with short periods of ten minutes and progressively increasing the time by daily increments of five to ten minutes or more. It must be emphasized to the patient in particular, as well as to the personnel involved with his care, that it is absolutely essential to establish a daily inspection routine, in the morning as well as after completion of each pressure period, for all areas that have been subjected to pressure. If there is any evidence of skin discoloration, pressure should be immediately relieved and discontinued until all redness disappears.

In addition to the daily inspection, the patient should be instructed that it is his responsibility to make frequent changes in position, whether in a wheelchair or a bed. This point is absolutely essential, and it should be constantly stressed to the patient that this is a lifelong concern whenever he is subjecting any area of his body to pressure, especially if it has been surgically repaired.

Surgical Therapy

An understanding of flap anatomy and physiology allows the treating surgeon several alternatives when faced with the task of reconstructing a patient with pressure sores. A carefully planned surgical strategy must be established. Future flap requirements must be considered when treating the initial pressure sore. Flap design must not violate other vascular territories or pedicles that would make future flaps impossible.

Each patient's rehabilitative potential must be considered from the outset. His potential for sitting, lying, and ambulating must be understood when planning the initial procedure for a pressure sore. The treatment of a sacral pressure sore in a quadriplegic with minimal use of the upper extremities is quite different from treating the same problem in a paraplegic with strong, well-functioning upper extremities. In the quadriplegic recurrent sacral, trochanteric, and ischial breakdown is far more common than in the paraplegic, and multiple flaps are therefore more likely to be required.

The development of the concept of myocutaneous, fasciocutaneous, and skin axial territories allows the treating surgeon many alternatives for flap design. The more complete this understanding is, the more creative and precise the surgeon can be when planning a flap to resurface a specific area.

The surgical principles in the treatment of pressure sores, described in 1956 by Conway and Griffith, have been modified and include:

1. Total excision of the ulcer, surrounding scar tissue bursae, and any soft tissue calcification that may be present.

2. Complete removal of all infected bone with recontouring of bony prominences to alleviate discrete pressure points. Removal of bone when treating an ischial pressure sore should redistribute pressure evenly over both ischia when the patient is sitting.

3. Careful hemostasis and appropriate suction drainage. Frequently, delaying closure

for 24 hours after an extensive debridement ensures hemostasis.

4. Obliteration of all potential "dead space" by use of either muscle flaps, myocutaneous flaps, or deepithelized skin flaps.

5. Closure of the wound with well-vascularized flaps, designed so that the suture line does not lie over areas of pressure and does not disturb the vascular supply to other flaps that may be required in the future.

6. The achievement of a primary, tension-free closure of the donor site, or the use of split-thickness skin grafts in the donor site.

Ulcer Excision. The extent of the excision should include all the scarred and discolored skin. It should be emphasized that in most cases all the undermined skin, if not extensive, should be excised. If the undermined area is double the size of the defect, the excision is restricted to abnormal-looking skin and the glistening covering on the surfaces of the undermined area. Excision of the bursa-like wall down to healthy-looking tissue must include the core of the ulcer, as well as the underlying bony prominence (see Fig. 77–5). The bone is removed with an osteotome, and any irregularities resulting from the ostectomy are smoothed with a rasp. Bleeding from the bony surface is controlled either by lightly tapping with the rounded head of a chisel so as to obliterate the open spaces, or by sparingly applying Gelfoam.

The bleeding from soft tissue surfaces is best controlled with an electrocautery and fine-pointed forceps for the small vessels; moderate-sized bleeding points are ligated with 4–0 catgut. To control rather extensive capillary oozing due to large areas of scarring and a deficient or absent vasomotor response, it is preferable to pack the cavity with a laparotomy pad soaked in warm saline solution.

At this point in the operation, a review of the excised area is undertaken to determine the completeness and adequacy of the resection. The surgeon must search for areas of undermining that may have been left behind, residual scar tissue that may prevent adequate healing, sharp bony edges, and so forth. The flap outline is planned as to size and orientation in relation to any possible changes in size or shape of the excised area.

Sacrum. Sacral pressure sores are frequently the first areas of breakdown in the acutely injured spinal cord patient. Prolonged bed rest in the supine position, which often accompanies the acute injury, will result in sacral breakdown if not carefully monitored with frequent repositioning. Sacral pressure sores are also seen in the rehabilitated patient who is forced to become bedridden by intercurrent illness, usually involving either respiratory or genitourinary infections. After complete excision of the ulcer and entire bursae, a conservative ostectomy should be aimed at removing the prominent spine over the sacrum, when present, and recontouring the posterior iliac crests. A smooth, evenly contoured sacrum is the object of the ostectomy.

The reconstructure options available for closure of sacral pressure sores are listed in Table 77–1.

Small, superficial ulcers can often be closed primarily. Skin grafts and reverse dermal grafts probably should be considered only in the ambulatory patient who develops a sacral pressure sore during an acute illness. They generally provide unstable coverage in the spinal cord injured patient.

The primary blood supply to the skin incorporated in the inferiorly based skin rotation flap is via musculocutaneous perforators from the superior and inferior gluteal arteries. The larger the area of skin elevated off the underlying gluteus maximus muscle, the greater is the number of skin perforators that must be divided, incrementally decreasing the arterial inflow to the elevated flap. For small sacral pressure sores a pure skin flap

Table 77–1. Closure of Sacral Pressure Sores

Primary closure (White and Hamm, 1946)
Skin graft
Reverse dermal graft (Wesser and Kahn, 1967)
Inferiorly based skin flap (Conway and Griffith, 1956)
Gluteus maximus myocutaneous flap (Minami, Mills, and Pardoe, 1977)
Gluteus maximus myocutaneous island flap (Maruyama and associates, 1980)
Gluteus maximus V-Y myocutaneous flap (Parry and Mathes, 1982)
Transverse lumbosacral flap (Hill, Brown, and Jurkiewicz, 1978)
Superior gluteus myoplasty (Ger, 1971; Ger and Levine, 1976)
Turnover gluteus myoplasty (Stallings, Delgado, and Converse, 1974)
Gluteal thigh flap (Hurwitz, Swartz, and Mathes, 1981)
Sensory island flaps (Snyder and Edgerton, 1965; Dibbell, 1974; Daniel, Terzis, and Cunningham, 1976)

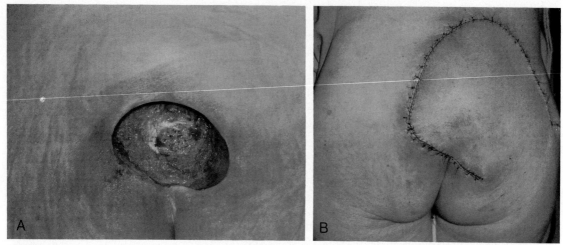

Figure 77–6. *A,* Preoperative view of a sacral pressure sore. *B,* The defect has been reconstructed utilizing a gluteus maximus myocutaneous flap. Only a small segment of muscle supplied by the superior gluteal artery is included in the flap.

design is sufficient, but for larger pressure sores a segment of gluteus maximus muscle should be incorporated, moving the superior gluteal artery vascular axis with the flap (a myocutaneous unit). This can be accomplished by dividing both the origin and insertion of the muscle at the sacrum and posterior iliac crests as well as the iliotibial tract. The more inferior fibers of the gluteus maximus muscle are left undisturbed, moving only that segment of muscle containing the superior gluteal artery (Figs. 77–6, 77–7). Modifications of this anatomic concept have resulted in the superior gluteal island myocutaneous flap (Fig. 77–8) and the V-Y gluteus maximus myocutaneous flap (Fig. 77–9). The latter flap

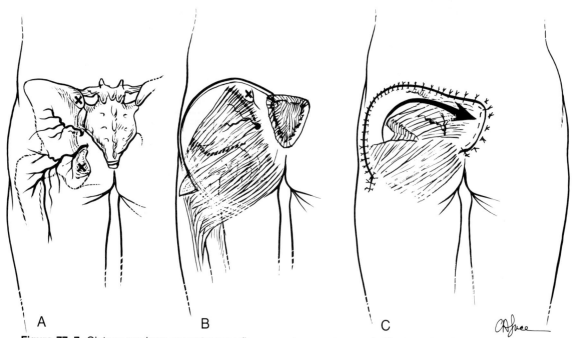

Figure 77–7. Gluteus maximus myocutaneous flap—sacral pressure sore. *A,* The superior gluteal artery is identified using the posterior iliac spine (*x*), the ischial tuberosity (*x*), and the sacrum as surface landmarks. *B,* A large rotation flap is designed. The superior gluteal artery myocutaneous distribution supports the gluteal skin component. The origin of the muscle is divided from the posterior iliac crest and sacrum. The muscle is divided between the superior and inferior gluteal arteries. *C,* The gluteus muscle fills the depths of the sacral pressure sore and the skin is closed without tension.

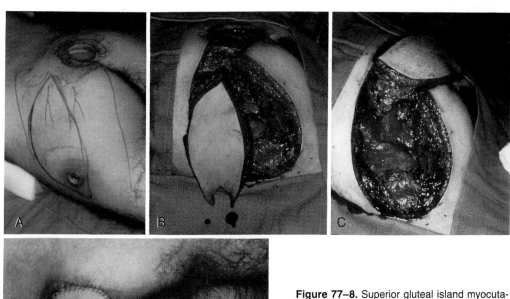

Figure 77–8. Superior gluteal island myocutaneous flap. *A*, Sacral pressure sore and a small trochanteric pressure sore. *B*, Excision of the trochanteric pressure sore and development of an island superior gluteal artery myocutaneous flap. *C*, The island flap transposed to the sacrum. *D*, Appearance after closure.

can be unilateral or bilateral, depending on the size and geometry of the defect. The potential disadvantage is that the resultant suture line lies directly over the sacral prominence, and this flap probably has its greatest use in the ambulatory patient.

The gluteal thigh flap (Fig. 77–10) based on posterior thigh extensions of the inferior gluteal artery has its primary role in the closure of pressure sores in the region of the ischium and trochanter, and should rarely be used except as a salvage procedure.

The transverse lumbosacral flap is based on contralateral lumbosacral perforators and is a secondary choice for closure of sacral pressure sores. This flap has a 20 per cent

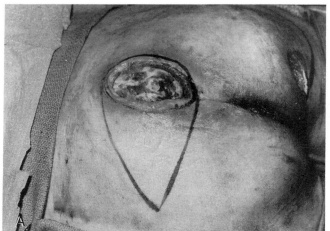

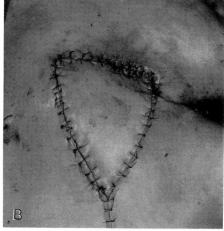

Figure 77–9. Sacral pressure sore repair utilizing a V-Y gluteus maximus myocutaneous flap. *A*, Sacral ulcer and design of flap. *B*, After flap coverage.

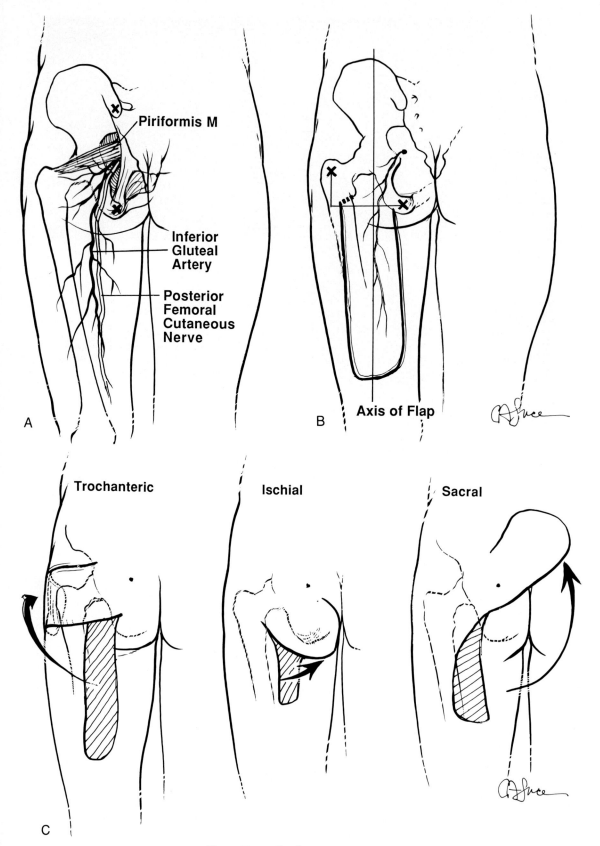

Piriformis M

Inferior Gluteal Artery

Posterior Femoral Cutaneous Nerve

Axis of Flap

A

B

Trochanteric

Ischial

Sacral

C

Figure 77–10 *See legend on oposite page*

viability complication rate, which makes its routine use unreliable.

The turnover gluteal myoplasty is technically difficult in that little useful flap is available for coverage when it is turned back upon itself. Its distal gluteal division must be quite low on the iliotibial tract. The low division of the gluteal fibers must violate other vascular territories that may be required in future flap design.

Dibbell in 1974 was the first to successfully transfer an innervated skin flap to the sacrum in a meningomyelocele patient in order to restore both soft tissue coverage and sensation. The procedure required multiple stages, and the resultant size of the soft tissue transferred was small. Daniel, Terzis, and Cunningham (1976) reported a technique of transferring intercostal neurovascular island flaps and free flaps to cover sacral and ischial pressure sores, in the expectation of restoring both soft tissue coverage and sensation. Its clinical usefulness has been limited since the cord level must be below T7 and the flap pedicle is quite short, barely reaching the sacrum. It must be hoped that in the future our knowledge of intrafascicular neural anatomy, sensory mapping, and nerve grafting will make these procedures clinically useful.

Ischium. This is the most common location of pressure sores, and despite successful flap closure, recurrence of ulceration often develops. Patients may require several flaps during their lifetime for closure of ischial pressure sores. The goal in bony resection is to balance the pressure exerted during sitting so that it is distributed equally over both ischia and posterior thighs. Spinal deformities can cause abnormal pressure on one ischium, and this must be considered when bony resection is planned. The argument for the so-called total prophylactic ischiectomy is not sound because of the high incidence of perineal ulcers and urethral complications following this procedure (Comarr and Bors, 1958; Guthrie and Conway, 1969). A more conservative ischiectomy accomplishes these goals without the associated perineal complications.

The reconstructive alternatives for closure

Table 77–2. Closure of Ischial Pressure Sores

Primary closure (Arregui and associates, 1965)
Gluteal thigh flap (Hurwitz, Swartz, and Mathes, 1981)
Inferior gluteus maximus myocutaneous flap (Minami, Mills, and Pardoe, 1977)
Hamstring myocutaneous flap (Hurteau and associates, 1981)
Biceps femoris myocutaneous flap (Tobin and associates, 1981)
Tensor fascia lata myocutaneous flap (Nahai and associates, 1978; Withers and associates, 1980; Krupp, Kuhn, and Zaech, 1983)
Gracilis myocutaneous flap (Wingate and Friedland, 1978)
Inferior gluteus maximus myoplasty (Ger and Levine, 1976)
Medially based posterior thigh skin flap ± biceps femoris (Conway and Griffith, 1956)

of ischial pressure sores are listed in Table 77–2.

To care for the patient who will potentially require multiple flap procedures for a lifetime, it is necessary to adopt a surgical strategy that is well thought out, so that vascular pedicles to future flaps are not injured when the initial procedure is performed. This principle is most important in the ischial region where the useful flaps encompass many vascular territories.

The first-line procedure for an ischial pressure sore is the gluteal thigh flap (Figs. 77–10, 77–11). Its design and elevation does not compromise other flap procedures. When the ischial pressure sore is large and deep, the biceps femoris can be turned back under the gluteal thigh flap to obliterate the large wound. Both the biceps femoris myocutaneous flap (Fig. 77–12) and the hamstring myocutaneous flap (Fig. 77–13) transect the inferior gluteal artery extensions to the posterior thigh. If these flaps are chosen initially, they make the use of a future posterior thigh flap unreliable. An inferior gluteus maximus myocutaneous flap (Fig. 77–14) can be successfully performed following a previous gluteal thigh flap. The gluteal thigh flap and the inferior gluteus maximus myocutaneous flap are the key procedures to reconstruct ischial

Figure 77–10. Gluteal thigh flap. *A,* A branch of the inferior gluteal artery extends down the posterior thigh in close association with the posterior femoral cutaneous nerve (S2). *B,* The surface landmarks used to design the flap are the midpoint between the ischial tuberosity (*x*) and the greater trochanter (*x*) proximally, and the medial femoral condyle and posterior border of the fascia lata distally. *C,* This flap can be transposed with the gluteus maximus muscle as an axial extension, or transferred alone as a skin-fascial flap. Its arc of rotation allows closure of trochanteric, ischial, and sacral pressure sores. The donor site can either be closed primarily or skin grafted.

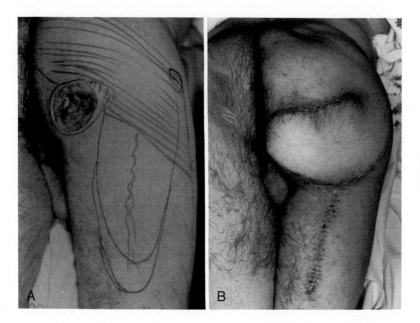

Figure 77–11. An ischial pressure sore repaired by gluteal thigh flap. *A,* Preoperative view with flap design. *B,* After closure.

Figure 77–12. An ischial pressure sore reconstructed utilizing a biceps femoris myocutaneous flap. *A,* Preoperative view with flap design. *B,* After closure.

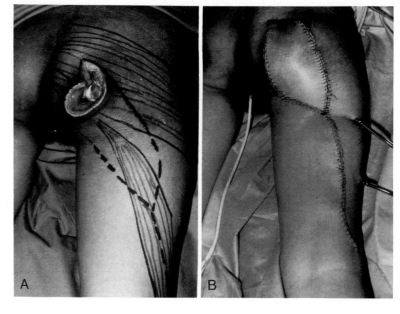

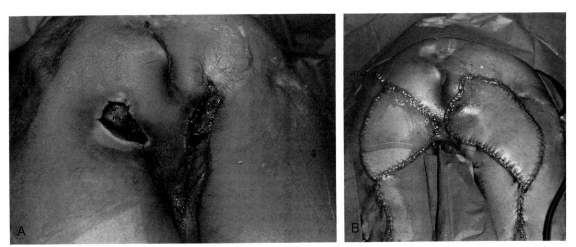

Figure 77–13. Bilateral ischial pressure sores reconstructed utilizing hamstring myocutaneous flaps. *A,* Preoperative view. *B,* After flap coverage.

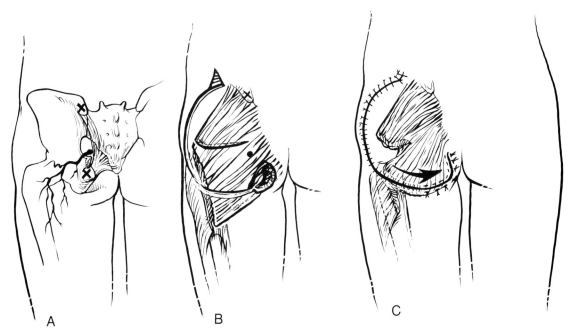

Figure 77–14. Gluteus maximus myocutaneous flap—ischial pressure sore. *A,* The inferior gluteal artery is identified using the posterior superior iliac spine (*x*), the ischial tuberosity (*x*), and the sacrum as surface landmarks. *B,* A large rotation flap is designed. The inferior gluteal artery myocutaneous distribution supports the entire skin component. The iliotibial insertion of the muscle is divided, and the muscle is split between the superior and inferior gluteal arteries. *C,* The gluteus muscle fills the depths of the ischial defect and the skin is closed without tension.

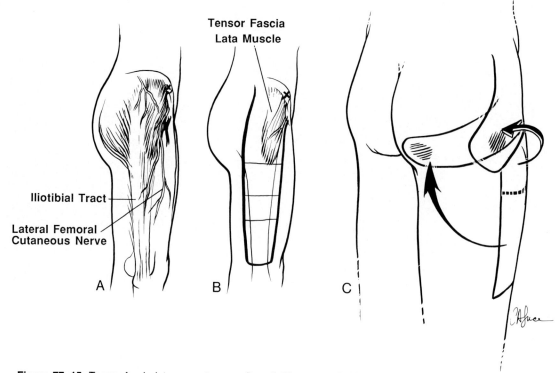

Figure 77–15. Tensor fascia lata myocutaneous flap. *A*, The tensor fascia lata muscle originates from the anterior 5 cm of the iliac crest. The muscle inserts into the iliotibial tract of the fascia lata in the thigh. The single dominant pedicle is a branch of the lateral femoral circumflex artery and enters the muscle 8 to 10 cm below the anterior superior iliac spine. The skin territory of this myocutaneous flap receives its sensory innervation from L2 and L3 via the lateral femoral cutaneous nerve and a lateral branch of T12. *B*, The anterior border of the flap is marked by drawing a line from the anterior superior iliac spine to the lateral condyle of the tibia. The greater trochanter of the femur is a useful landmark for the posterior border. The skin territory can usually be safely extended several centimeters both anterior and posterior to these landmarks. The length of the flap is marked according to the reconstructive needs. *C*, The posterior arc of rotation allows for reliable coverage of trochanteric and ischial pressure sores. The donor site can usually be closed primarily, but when a wide flap is elevated, the donor site may require skin grafting.

pressure sores. They are selected as primary procedures because they are reliable and do not compromise other flaps that may be required in the future. The tensor fascia lata myocutaneous flap (Fig. 77–15) is likewise a secondary choice because it violates the posterior thigh blood supply. The sensory innervation to the skin territory of this flap is primarily from the lateral femoral cutaneous nerve (L2, L3) and the lateral cutaneous branch of the iliohypogastric nerve (T12). If sensation is intact in this skin territory, it can be effectively used as a sensate flap. It is difficult to define the skin territory over the gracilis muscle accurately and therefore the gracilis myocutaneous flap is unreliable; it should be reserved as a salvage procedure. The inferior gluteus myoplasty or the medially based posterior thigh skin flap is rarely considered in the present-day treatment of ischial pressure sores.

Trochanter. Trochanteric pressure sores typically present with minimal skin involvement and extensive bursae formation. The mobile nature of the trochanter, especially when spasm is poorly controlled, predisposes these ulcerations to extensive undermining. Bony resection should remove the greater trochanter of the femur and create a smooth contour on its lateral surface.

The reconstructive alternatives are listed in Table 77–3.

The tensor fascia lata myocutaneous unit based on the lateral femoral circumflex artery is an extremely useful flap for reconstructing trochanteric pressure sores (Fig. 77–15). Its modifications as a V-Y flap, a bipedicle flap, and a sensory flap have been well described. The vastus lateralis muscle may be used in conjunction with the tensor fascia lata flap when a deep cavity must be filled, or it can be used independently either as muscle only

Table 77–3. Closure of Trochanteric Pressure Sores

Tensor fascia lata myocutaneous flap ± sensation (Nahai and associates, 1978; Dibbell, McCraw, and Edstrom, 1979; Nahai, Hill, and Hester, 1979; Schulman, 1980; Withers and associates, 1980; Cochran, Edstrom, and Dibbell, 1981; Lewis, Cunningham, and Hugo, 1981; Krupp, Kuhn, and Zaech, 1983)

Vastus lateralis myocutaneous flap (Minami, Hentz, and Vistnes, 1977; Dowden and McCraw, 1980; Bovet and associates, 1982; Hauben and associates, 1983)

Gluteal thigh flap (Hurwitz, Swartz, and Mathes, 1981)

Gluteus maximus, distally based (Becker, 1979)

Random bipedicle flap (Conway and Griffith, 1956)

Anteriorly based random thigh flap (Vasconez, Schneider, and Jurkiewicz, 1977)

---

or as a myocutaneous unit. The gluteal thigh flap described previously works well for trochanteric pressure sores but is probably best reserved for ischial ulcers (Fig. 77–16). The distally based gluteus maximus flap, the random bipedicle flap, and the anteriorly based random thigh flap are less useful in view of the large number of muscle and myocutaneous flaps presently available.

Other Anatomic Sites. The heel, knee, ankles, iliac crests, scapula, thoracic spine (Fig. 77–17), elbow, and occipital scalp are all sites that may develop pressure ulceration. The principles of treatment are the same as those described above. The reader is referred to the specific chapters in this text that deal with these anatomic sites for an in-depth discussion of the reconstructive alternatives.

Multiple Pressure Sores. Extensive recurrent ulcerations of the ischial, trochanteric, and sacral areas do not represent an uncommon problem (Fig. 77–18). These may be associated with extensive osteomyelitis of the ischium and femur and pyarthrosis of the hip. When the area of extensive ulceration is confined to the trochanter and ischium, it is best treated by proximal femoral resection with disarticulation of the joint. The resultant shortening of the leg allows for closure of these wounds with local tissues. The biceps femoris, rectus femoris, tensor fascia lata, and vastus lateralis muscles (Fig. 77–19) may be used to fill the depths of these wounds and eliminate potential "dead space." It is frequently best to delay closure of these wounds, after bony resection and debridement, for 24 hours so as to ensure complete hemostasis.

Total thigh flaps have been recommended for closure of massive recurrent combined ulcerations. Generally, this procedure should be reserved as a salvage procedure when all other techniques have been unsuccessful. This is a formidable surgical procedure, usually requiring 6 to 20 units of blood, with a prolonged operating time. If a unilateral total thigh flap is done, it is possible for the patient to sit in a wheelchair, but special attention is required. If bilateral thigh flaps are performed, the patient's center of gravity is changed and there is considerable difficulty with balance. A special bucket-type seat must be constructed. Despite this precaution the flaps continue to be subject to pressure and ulceration.

Although Conway and associates (1951) reported a case of hip disarticulation for a complicated trochanteric ulceration, it was Georgiade, Pickrell, and Maguire (1956) who first advocated the use of soft tissues of the amputated thigh as a total thigh flap for patients with trochanteric ulcers complicated by pyarthroses of the hip and osteomyelitis of the femur.

From a 16 year accumulated experience, Royer and associates (1969) presented a comprehensive study of the use of total thigh flaps for extensive decubiti. A careful urologic work-up is paramount in the preoperative evaluation of these patients because of the frequency of urinary complications. Urinary diversion by an ileal loop should be undertaken before surgical repair of the ulcers if there is evidence of severe urologic dysfunction with recurrent infections.

The surgical planning of the amount of soft tissue required determines the length of the flap. In a patient in whom a total thigh flap is required, the lower circumferential incision is made in the region of the popliteal space, as suggested by Georgiade, Pickrell, and Maguire (1956) (Figs. 77–20, 77–21). If a sacral defect is to be covered, a level approximately 9 inches below the knee should be chosen (Fig. 77–22). One variation of the flap is the island leg flap described by Weeks and Brower (1968). The entire length of soft tissue of the leg down to the level of the malleoli is used for coverage of extensive ulcers (Fig. 77–23).

In a follow-up of 41 thigh flaps performed on 28 paraplegics (Royer and associates, 1969), the most common complications were postoperative hemorrhage, infection, sinus

Text continued on page 3834

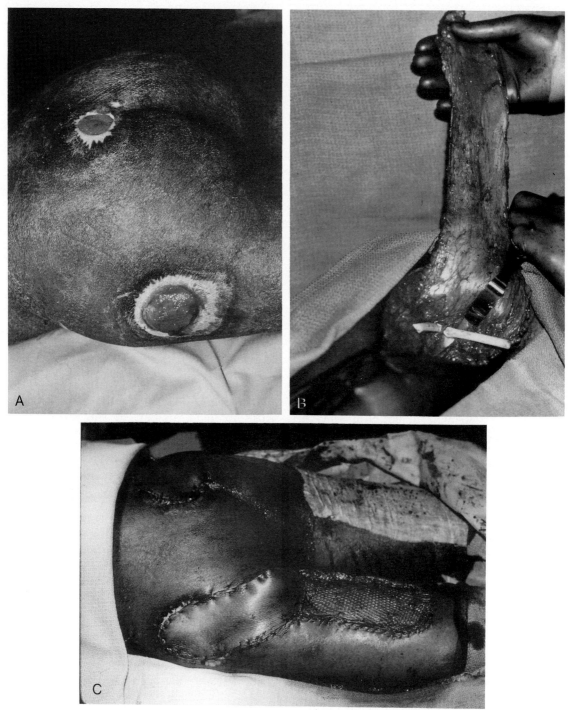

Figure 77–16. Gluteal thigh flap. *A,* A trochanteric and a small sacral pressure sore. *B,* A gluteal thigh flap elevated with the pedicle demonstrated, arising from the inferior gluteal artery. *C,* The trochanteric pressure sore reconstructed with the gluteal thigh flap. The donor site has been skin grafted. The sacral pressure sore has been reconstructed with a skin rotation flap.

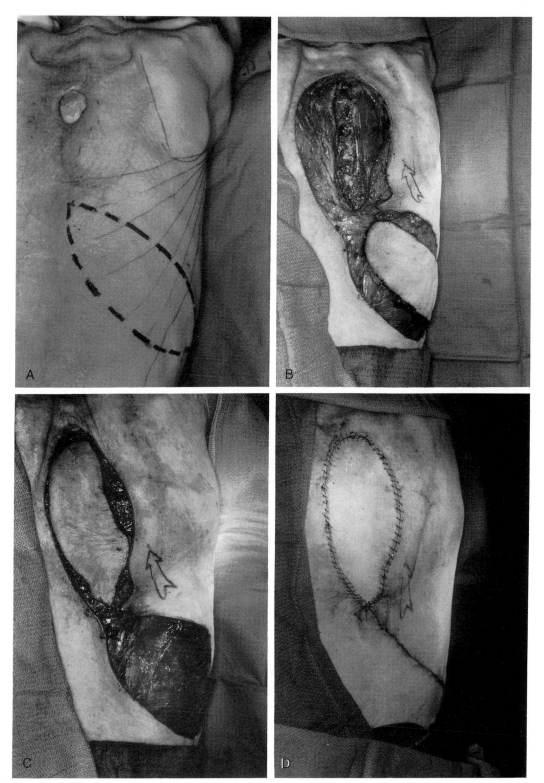

Figure 77–17. Thoracic spine pressure sore. *A,* A pressure sore in the region of the thoracic spine with the design of a latissimus dorsi myocutaneous flap outlined. *B,* Debridement and the flap elevated. *C,* Transposition of the flap into the defect. *D,* Reconstruction of the pressure sore.

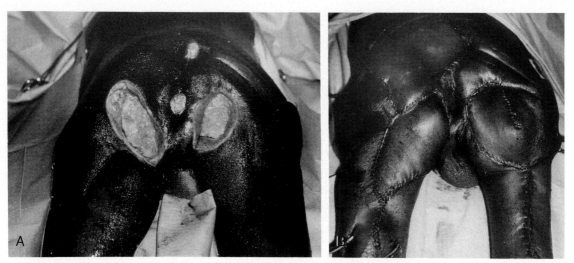

Figure 77–18. Bilateral ischial pressure sores and a sacral pressure sore. *A,* Preoperative view. *B,* Reconstruction completed utilizing a gluteal thigh flap, a V-Y hamstring flap, and a gluteus maximus myocutaneous flap.

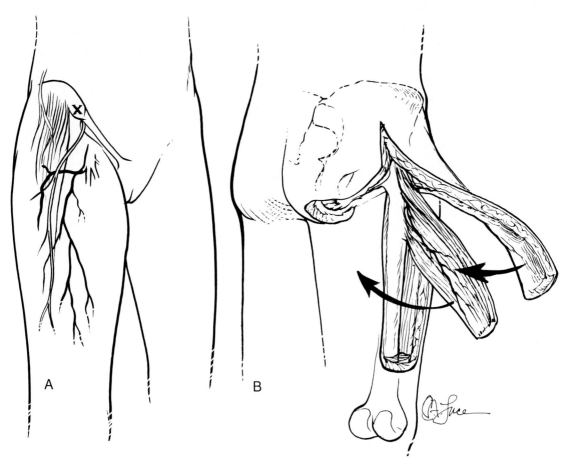

Figure 77–19. Tensor fascia lata myocutaneous flap including the vastus lateralis muscle. *A,* The tensor fascia lata and vastus lateralis muscles are supplied by branches of the lateral femoral cutaneous artery. They have an independent and wide arc of rotation. *B,* Utilizing the vascular axis of the tensor fascia lata and vastus lateralis, the two muscles can be used together when closing large, deep wounds in the trochanteric and ischial areas. The vastus lateralis can be used to close the depths of the wounds, and the tensor fascia lata used as external coverage.

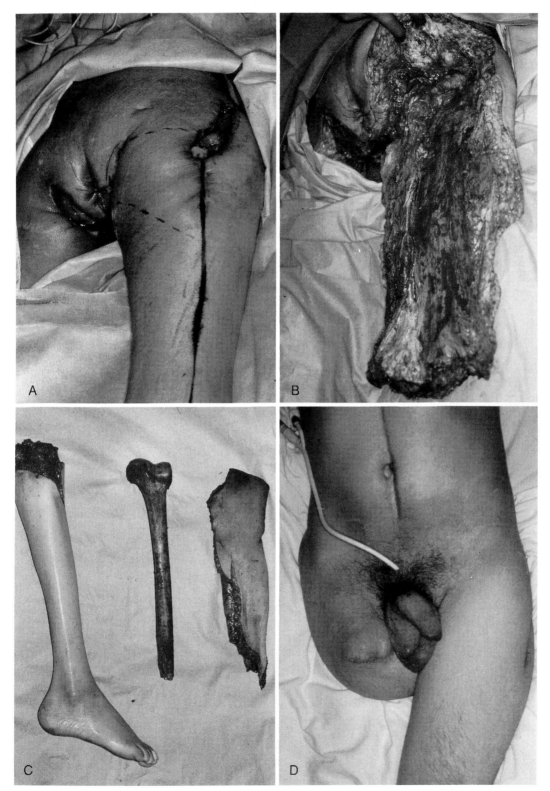

Figure 77–20. *A,* Recurrent bilateral ischial pressure sores in association with a large trochanteric pressure sore. *B,* *C,* A total thigh flap. *D,* Successful reconstruction of the trochanteric and bilateral ischial pressure sores.

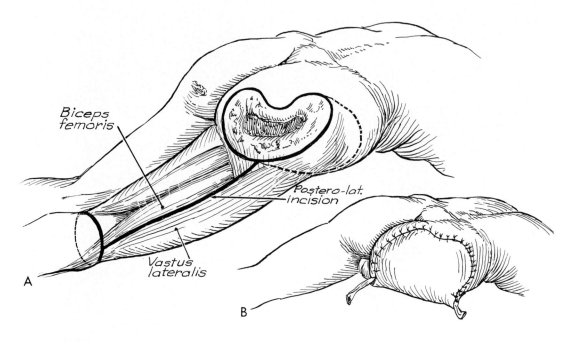

Biceps
femoris

Postero-lat.
incision

Vastus
lateralis

A

B

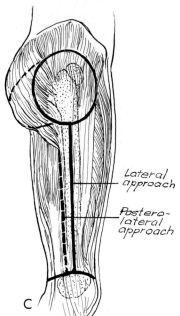

Lateral
approach

Postero-
lateral
approach

C

Figure 77–21. Total thigh flap, as suggested by Georgiade, Pickrell, and Maguire (1956), for large areas of compromised soft tissues and hip joint involvement. *A,* Lateral approach incision line between the biceps femoris and vastus lateralis muscles. *B,* The flap has been sutured in place after disarticulation of the extremity. *C,* The difference between the lateral and the posterolateral approach.

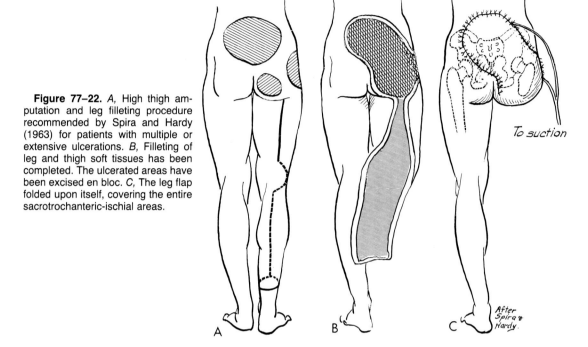

Figure 77–22. *A*, High thigh amputation and leg filleting procedure recommended by Spira and Hardy (1963) for patients with multiple or extensive ulcerations. *B*, Filleting of leg and thigh soft tissues has been completed. The ulcerated areas have been excised en bloc. *C*, The leg flap folded upon itself, covering the entire sacrotrochanteric-ischial areas.

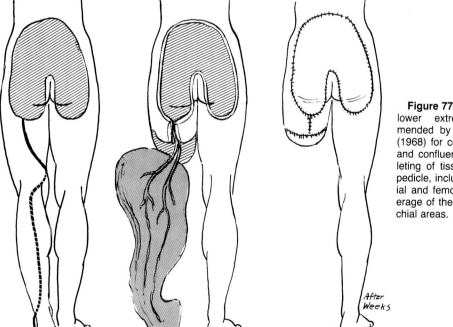

Figure 77–23. *A*, Outline of the lower extremity flap recommended by Weeks and Brower (1968) for coverage of extensive and confluent ulcerations. *B*, Filleting of tissues with a vascular pedicle, including the anterior tibial and femoral vessels. *C*, Coverage of the entire sacral and ischial areas.

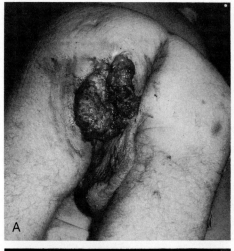

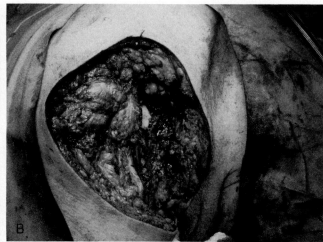

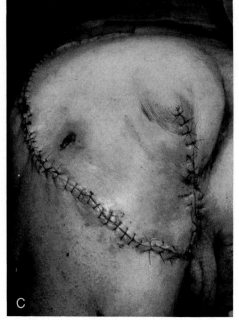

Figure 77–24. Squamous cell carcinoma arising in a long-standing ischial pressure sore. *A,* The lesion. *B,* Wide local excision. *C,* Reconstruction utilizing a superior gluteal myocutaneous flap.

tracts, wound dehiscences, acute pyelonephritis, and malrotation of the femoral stump. There was a total of 34 complications. It was significant that only five of the 28 patients (18 per cent) did not require additional surgery for recurrent ulcers or wound complications. Of the 17 survivors only nine were free of recurrent ulceration; of the 11 who died, only two were free of ulceration at the time of death. The total recurrence rate was approximately 60 per cent.

Malignant Degeneration. Malignant degeneration in chronic, long-standing pressure ulcers does occur. It is generally thought that a period of at least 10 to 15 years is required for this degeneration to occur (Fig. 77–24). The prognosis is poor. The condition should be suspected whenever the ulceration shows a cauliflower-type appearance. Treatment has generally involved radical excision and regional lymphadenectomy when possible (Bostwick, Pendergrast, and Vasconez, 1976).

Complications

Flap Necrosis. With an increased understanding of the regional blood supply and the almost routine use of muscle and musculocutaneous flaps, the incidence of flap loss and partial necrosis has markedly decreased. These are vigorous flaps compared with traditional skin flaps, and it is rare to experience flap necrosis when a major vascular pedicle is included in the flap design.

Hematoma. Hematomas are the most common complication and their presence often predisposes to other complications. Certainly flap necrosis, wound infection, bursa formation, and subsequent pressure sore recurrence can all be influenced by postoperative hematoma formation. When recognized in the postoperative period, all hematomas should be immediately evacuated. With extensive debridements and bony resections it is usually best to delay definitive flap closures for 24 hours to ensure adequate hemostasis.

Seroma. Seroma formation is common after flap closure of pressure sores. Residual "dead space" and inadequate patient immobilization with resultant shearing forces are usually responsible. Inadequate resection of the bursae can also predispose to seroma formation. Suction drainage should remain postoperatively for seven to ten days. If a seroma develops, the space established by the seroma has the potential to create a bursa unless remobilization of the patient is delayed so that adequate wound healing can be achieved.

Wound Infection. Despite appropriate preoperative wound cultures and adequate soft tissue and bony debridement, wound infections remain a significant postoperative complication. When diagnosed they should be aggressively treated with wide drainage and appropriate antibiotics. An unrecognized hematoma can predispose to wound infection.

Wound Separation. This occurs occasionally, particularly in the debilitated patient or when the flap is sutured under tension. When debilitation is a factor, extra efforts should be made to improve the nutritional status. Wound tension generally indicates improper planning of the flap design or an attempt to close the donor wound without using a skin graft.

Recurrence. The recurrence rate after surgical repair of pressure sores is high despite continued improvements in surgical technique. In a follow-up of 100 paraplegics, the recurrence rate was 44 per cent at four years after surgery (Harding, 1961). In the series reported by Griffith and Schultz (1961), 49 of the 73 ulcers surgically treated were recurrent; the three troublesome sites of recurrent ulceration were sacral (12), trochanteric (18), and ischial (19).

Despite the introduction of muscle and musculocutaneous flaps, the problem of recurrences remains unchanged. The main reasons for recurrence are the same as those for the initial ulceration. There often remains an underlying anger and self-destructive force that must be dealt with and controlled if these patients are to be truly rehabilitated. The pressure sore is most often a sign of underlying psychosocial problems rather than a disease itself. The clinician must always remember these complex issues when treating patients with pressure sores.

REFERENCES

Arregui, J., Cannon, B., Murray, J. E., and O'Leary, J. J., Jr.: Long-term evaluation of ischiectomy in the treatment of pressure ulcers. Plast. Reconstr. Surg., 36:583, 1965.

Artz, C. P., and Hargest, T. S.: Air-fluidized bed. *In* Artz, C. P., and Hargest, T. S. (Eds.): Clinical and Research Symposium. Medical University of South Carolina, Milton Roy Company, 1971.

Ascher, F.: Chirurgie der Haut und des Unterhautzellgewebes. *In* Kirschner M., and Nordmann, O. (Eds.): Die Chirurgie. Vol. 2. Part 1, 1928, p. 737.

Baran, E., Payandeh, A., Strax, T., Sokolow, J., and Grynbaum, B. B.: Deforming pressure measurements and a new type of mattress. Paper presented at American Congress of Rehabilitation Medicine, Denver, CO, Aug. 20–25, 1972.

Barker, D. E.: Surgical treatment of decubitus ulcers. J.A.M.A., 129:160, 1945.

Barker, D. E., Elkins, C. W., and Poer, D. H.: Methods of closure of decubitus ulcers in the paralyzed patient. Ann. Surg., 123:523, 1946.

Becker, H.: The distally-based gluteus maximus muscle flap. Plast. Reconstr. Surg., 63:653, 1979.

Berkas, E. M., Chesler, M. D., and Sako, Y.: Multiple decubitus ulcer treatment by hip disarticulation and soft tissue flaps from the lower limb. Plast. Reconstr. Surg., 27:618, 1961.

Blocksma, R., Kostrubala, J., and Greeley, P.: The surgical repair of decubitus ulcers in paraplegics. Plast. Reconstr. Surg., 4:123, 1949.

Bors, E.: Veterans Administration Technical Bulletin. TB 10–503, Washington, DC, Dec. 15, 1948.

Bors, E., and Comarr, A. E.: Ischial decubitus ulcer. Surgery, 24:680, 1948.

Bostwick, J., III, Pendergrast, W. J., Jr., and Vasconez, L. O.: Marjolin's ulcer: an immunologically privileged tumor? Plast. Reconstr. Surg., 57:66, 1976.

Bovet, J. L., Nassif, T. M., Guimberteau, J. C., and Baudet, J.: The vastus lateralis musculocutaneous flap in the repair of trochanteric pressure sores: technique and indications. Plast. Reconstr. Surg., 69:830, 1982.

Brown-Séquard, C. E.: Experimental Researches Applied to Physiology and Pathology. New York, H. Bailliere, 1853.

Burkhardt, B. R.: An alternative to the total-thigh flap for coverage of massive decubitus ulcers. Plast. Reconstr. Surg., 49:433, 1972.

Butterworth, R. F., and Golding, C.: A device for treating

pressure sores around the ankles. Geriatrics, *20*:413, 1965.

Campbell, R. M.: The surgical management of pressure sores. Surg. Clin. North Am., *39*:509, 1959.

Cannon, B., O'Leary, J. J., O'Neil, J. W., and Steinsieck, R.: An approach to the treatment of pressure sores. Ann. Surg., *132*:760, 1950.

Charcot, J. M.: Lectures on the Disease of the Nervous System. Delivered at La Saltpètrière. Translated from the 2nd Edition by G. Sigerson. Philadelphia, Henry C. Lea, 1879.

Chase, R. A., and White, W. J.: Bilateral amputation in rehabilitation of paraplegics. Plast. Reconstr. Surg., *24*:445, 1959.

Cochran, J. H., Jr., Edstrom, L. E., and Dibbell, D. G.: Usefulness of the innervated tensor fascia flap in paraplegic patients. Ann. Plast. Surg., *7*:286, 1981.

Comarr, A. E., and Bors, E.: Perineal urethral diverticulum—complications of removal of ischium. J.A.M.A., *168*:2000, 1958.

Conway, H., and Griffith, B. H.: Plastic surgery for closure of decubitus ulcers in patients with paraplegia; based on experience with 1000 cases. Am. J. Surg., *91*:946, 1956.

Conway, H., Stark, R. B., Weeter, J. C., Garcia, F. A., and Kavanaugh, J. D.: Complications of decubitus ulcers in patients with paraplegia. Plast. Reconstr. Surg., *7*:117, 1951.

Croce, E. J., Schullinger, R. N., and Shearer, T. P.: Operative treatment of decubitus ulcers. Ann. Surg., *123*:53,1946.

Dalton, J. J., Jr., Hackler, R. H., and Bunts, R. C.: Amyloidosis in the paraplegic; incidence and significance. J. Urol., *93*:553, 1965.

Daniel, R. K., and Faibisoff, B.: Muscle coverage of pressure points: the role of myocutaneous flaps. Ann. Plast. Surg., *8*:446, 1982.

Daniel, R. K., Terzis, J. K., and Cunningham, D. M.: Sensory skin flaps for coverage of pressure sores in paraplegic patients. A preliminary report. Plast. Reconstr. Surg., *58*:317, 1976.

Dansereau, J. G., and Conway, H.: Closure of decubiti in paraplegics. Report on 2000 cases. Plast. Reconstr. Surg., *33*:474, 1964.

Davis, J. S.: Operative treatment of scars following bed sores. Surgery, *3*:1, 1938.

Dewis, L. S., Caplan, H. I., and Pache, H. L.: Treatment of decubitus ulcers by use of a water mattress. Arch. Phys. Med., *49*:290, 1968.

Dibbell, D. G.: Use of a long island flap to bring sensation to the sacral area in young paraplegics. Plast. Reconstr. Surg., *54*:220, 1974.

Dibbell, D. G., McCraw, J. B., and Edstrom, L. E.: Providing useful and protective sensibility to the sitting area in patients with meningomyelocele. Plast. Reconstr. Surg., *64*:796, 1979.

Dinsdale, S. M.: Decubitus ulcers: role of pressure and friction in causation. Arch. Phys. Med. Rehab., *55*:147, 1974.

Dowden, R. V., and McCraw, J. B.: The vastus lateralis muscle flap: technique and applications. Ann. Plast. Surg., *4*:396, 1980.

Ducker, T. B., and Assenmacher, D.: The pathological circulation in experimental spinal cord injury. *In* Proceedings of the 17th V.A. Spinal Cord Injury Conference. Bronx, New York, Sept. 29, 30, Oct. 1, 1969.

Ducker, T. B., and Hamit, H. F.: Experimental treatments of acute spinal cord injury. J. Neurosurg., *30*:693, 1969.

Ewing, M. R., Garrow, C., Conn, B., Pressley, T. A., Ashley, C., and Kinsella, N. M.: Further experiences in the rise of sheep skins as an aid in nursing. Med. J. Aust., *2*:139, 1964.

Fischer, B. H.: Topical hyperbaric oxygen treatment of pressure sores and skin ulcers. Lancet, *2*:405, 1969.

Gelb, J.: Plastic surgical closure of decubitus ulcers in paraplegics as a result of civilian injuries. Plast. Reconstr. Surg., *9*:525, 1952.

Georgiade, N., Pickrell, K., and Maguire, C.: Total thigh flaps for extensive decubitus ulcer. Plast. Reconstr. Surg., *17*:220, 1956.

Ger, R.: The surgical management of decubitus ulcers by muscle transposition. Surgery, *69*:106, 1971.

Ger, R., and Levine, S. A.: The management of decubitus ulcers by muscle transposition—an eight year review. Plast. Reconstr. Surg., *58*:419, 1976.

Gibbon, J. H., and Freeman, L. W.: The primary closure of decubitus ulcers. Ann. Surg., *124*:1148, 1946.

Griffith, B. H.: Pressure sores. *In* Gibson, T. (Ed.): Modern Trends in Plastic Surgery. 2nd Ed. London, Butterworths, 1966.

Griffith, B. H., and Schultz, R. C.: The prevention and surgical treatment of recurrent decubitus ulcers in patients with paraplegia. Plast. Reconstr. Surg., *27*:248, 1961.

Groth, K. E.: Clinical observations and experimental studies of the pathogenesis of decubitus ulcers. Acta. Chir. Scand., *87* (Suppl. 76):207, 1942.

Guthrie, R. H., and Conway, H.: Surgical management of decubiti in paraplegics. *In* Proceedings of the 17th V.A. Spinal Cord Injury Conference. Bronx, New York, Sept. 29, 30, Oct. 1, 1969.

Guttmann, L.: The problem of treatment of pressure sores in spinal paraplegics. Br. J. Plast. Surg., *7*:196, 1955.

Harding, R. L.: An analysis of 100 rehabilitated paraplegics. Plast. Reconstr. Surg., *27*:235, 1961.

Hargest, T. S.: A ceramic application in patient care. Presented at a symposium on Use of Ceramics in Surgical Implants. Clemson University and South Carolina State Development Board, Jan. 31–Feb. 1, 1969.

Harris, C.: Decubitus ulcers in the sick aged. J. Am. Geriatr. Soc., *13*:538, 1965.

Harris, C.: Flotation as an aid in the treatment of decubitus ulcers. J. Am. Geriatr. Soc., *15*:605, 1967.

Hauben, D. J., Smith, A. R., Sonneveld, G. J., and Van der Meulen, J. C.: The use of the vastus lateralis musculocutaneous flap for the repair of trochanteric pressure sores. Ann. Plast. Surg., *10*:359, 1983.

Hill, H. L., Brown, R. G., and Jurkiewicz, M. J.: The transverse lumbosacral back flap. Plast. Reconstr. Surg., *62*:177, 1978.

Hofstra, P. C.: The air-fluidized bed for spinal injuries. *In* Artz, C. P., and Hargest, T. S. (Eds.): Clinical and Research Symposium. Medical University of South Carolina, Milton Roy Company, 1971.

Holdsworth, F. W.: Traumatic paraplegia. Ann. R. Coll. Surg., *15*:281, 1954.

Houle, R. J.: Evaluation of seat devices designed to prevent ischemic ulcers in paraplegic patients. Arch. Phys. Med., *90*:587, 1969.

Hubay, C. A., Kiehn, C. L., and Drucker, W. R.: Surgical management of decubitus ulcers in the post-traumatic patient. Am. J. Surg., *93*:705, 1957.

Hurteau, J. E., Bostwick, J., Nahai, F., Hester, R., and Jurkiewicz, M. J.: V-Y advancement of hamstring musculocutaneous flap for coverage of ischial pressure sores. Plast. Reconstr. Surg., *68*:539, 1981.

Hurwitz, D. J., Swartz, W. M., and Mathes, S. J.: The gluteal thigh flap: a reliable sensate flap for the closure of buttock and perineal wounds. Plast. Reconstr. Surg., 68:521, 1981.

Husain, T.: Experimental study of some pressure effects on tissues, with reference to bed-sore problem. J. Path. Bact., 66:347, 1953.

Keane, F. X.: The function of the rump in relation to sitting and the Keane Reciprocating Wheelchair Seat. Paraplegia, 16:390, 1979.

Kosiak, M.: Etiology and pathology of ischemic ulcers. Arch. Phys. Med., 40:62, 1959.

Kosiak, M., Kubicek, N. G., Olson, M., Danz, J. N., and Kottle, F. J.: Evaluation of pressure as a factor in the production of ischial ulcers. Arch. Phys. Med., 39:623, 1958.

Kostrubala, J. C., and Greeley, P. W.: The problem of decubitus ulcers in paraplegics. Plast. Reconstr. Surg., 2:403, 1947.

Krupp, S., Kuhn, W., and Zaech, G. A.: The use of innervated flaps for the closure of ischial pressure sores. Paraplegia, 21:119, 1983.

Küster, I.: Decubitus Eulenberg. Real Encyclopädie, 3:671, 1908.

Lamon, J. G., and Alexander, E. J.: Secondary closure of decubitus ulcer with aid of penicillin. J.A.M.A., 127:396, 1945.

Landis, E. M.: Micro-injection studies of capillary blood pressure in human skin. Heart, 15:209, 1930.

Lewis, V. L., Jr., Cunningham, B. L., and Hugo, N. E.: The tensor fascia lata V-Y retroposition flap. Ann. Plast. Surg., 6:34, 1981.

Leyden, E.: Klinik der Rückenmarkskrankheiten. Vol. 1. Berlin, A. Hirschwald, 1874, p. 156.

Lindan, O., Greenway, R. M., and Piazza, J. M.: Pressure distribution on the surface of the human body: 1. Evaluation in lying and sitting positions using a "bed of springs and nails." Arch. Phys. Med. Rehab., 46:378, 1965.

Lopez, E. M., and Aranha, G. V.: The value of sinography in the management of decubitus ulcers. Plast. Reconstr. Surg., 53:208, 1974.

Maruyama, Y., Nakajima, H., Wada, M., Imai, T., and Fujino, T.: A gluteus maximus myocutaneous island flap for repair of sacral decubitus ulcer. Br. J. Plast. Surg., 33:150, 1980.

Mathes, S. J., and Nahai, F.: Clinical Atlas of Muscle and Musculocutaneous Flaps. St. Louis, C. V. Mosby Company, 1979.

Matheson, A. T., and Lipschitz, R.: Nature and treatment of trophic pressure sores. S. Afr. Med. J., 30:1129, 1956.

Minami, R. T., Hentz, V. R., and Vistnes, L. M.: Use of vastus lateralis muscle flap for repair of trochanteric pressure sores. Plast. Reconstr. Surg., 60:364, 1977.

Minami, R. T., Mills, R., and Pardoe, R.: Gluteus maximus myocutaneous flaps for repair of pressure sores. Plast. Reconstr. Surg., 60:242, 1977.

Morrison, J. E., and Casali, J. L.: Continuous proteolytic therapy for decubitus ulcers. Am. J. Surg., 93:446, 1957.

Mulholland, J. H., Co Tui, F., Wright, A. M., Vinci, V., and Shafiroff, B.: Protein metabolism and bedsores. Ann. Surg., 118:1015, 1943.

Munro, D.: Care of the back following spinal cord injuries: a consideration of bedsores. N. Engl. J. Med., 223:391, 1940.

Munro, D.: The rehabilitation of patients totally paralyzed below the waist, with special reference to making them ambulatory and capable of earning their own living; end-result study of 445 cases. N. Engl. J. Med., 250:4, 1954.

Nahai, F., Hill, H. L., and Hester, T. R.: Experiences with the tensor fascia lata flap. Plast. Reconstr. Surg., 63:788, 1979.

Nahai, F., Silverton, J. S., Hill, H. L., and Vasconez, L. O.: The tensor fascia lata musculocutaneous flap. Ann. Plast. Surg., 1:372, 1978.

Nola, G. T., and Vistnes, L. M.: Differential response of skin and muscle in the experimental production of pressure sores. Plast. Reconstr. Surg., 66:728, 1980.

Nyquist, R. H., and Bors, E.: Useful appliances in spastic patients following spinal cord injury. Paraplegia, 2:120, 1964.

Osterholm, J. L., Mathews, S. J., Irvin, J. D., and Angelakos, E. T.: A review of altered norepinephrine metabolism attending severe spinal cord injury. Results of alpha-methyltyrosine treatment and preliminary studies. Personal communication, 1971.

Parry, S. W., and Mathes, S. J.: Bilateral gluteus maximus myocutaneous advancement flaps: sacral coverage for ambulatory patients. Ann. Plast. Surg., 8:443, 1982.

Petersen, N. C., and Bittmann, S.: The epidemiology of pressure sores. Scand. J. Plast. Surg., 5:62, 1971.

Pflandler, M.: Flotation, displacement and decubitus ulcers. Am. J. Nursing, 68:2351, 1968.

Pollock, L. J., Boshes, B., Finkelman, I., Chor, H., and Brown, M.: Spasticity, pseudospontaneous spasms, and other reflex activities late after injury to the spinal cord. Arch. Neurol. Psychiat., 66:537, 1951.

Reichel, S. M.: Shearing force as a factor in decubitus ulcers in paraplegics. J.A.M.A., 166:762, 1958.

Royer, J., Pickrell, K., Georgiade, N., Mladick, R., and Thorne, F.: Total thigh flaps for extensive decubitus ulcers. A 16 year review of 41 total thigh flaps. Plast. Reconstr. Surg., 44:109, 1969.

Rusk, H. A.: New horizons in rehabilitation medicine. *In* Proceedings of the 17th V.A. Spinal Cord Injury Conference. Bronx, New York, Sept. 29, 30, Oct. 1, 1969.

Scarff, J. E., and Pool, J. L.: Factors causing massive spasm following transection of cord in man. J. Neurosurg., 3:286, 1946.

Schulman, N. H.: Primary closure of trochanteric decubitus ulcers: the bipedicle tensor fascia lata musculocutaneous flap. Plast. Reconstr. Surg., 66:740, 1980.

Sharbaugh, R. J., and Hargest, T. S.: The effects of air-fluidized systems on microbial growth. *In* Artz, C. P., and Hargest, T. S. (Eds.): Clinical and Research Symposium. Medical University of South Carolina, Milton Roy Company, 1971.

Snyder, G. B., and Edgerton, M. T.: The principle of the island neurovascular flap in the management of ulcerated anesthetic weightbearing areas of the lower extremity. Plast. Reconstr. Surg., 36:518, 1965.

Spence, W. R., Burke, R. D., and Rae, J. W., Jr.: Gel support for prevention of decubitus ulcers. Arch. Phys. Med., 48:283, 1967.

Spencer, M. C.: Treatment of chronic skin ulcers by a proteolytic enzyme-antibiotic preparation. J. Am. Geriatr. Soc., 15:219, 1967.

Spira, M., and Hardy, S. B.: Our experience with high thigh amputations in paraplegics. Plast. Reconstr. Surg., 31:344, 1963.

Stallings, J. O., Delgado, J. P., and Converse, J. M.: Turnover island flap of gluteus maximus muscle for the repair of sacral decubitus ulcer. Plast. Reconstr. Surg., 54:52, 1974.

Talbot, H. S.: Report on sexual function in paraplegics. J. Urol., *61*:265, 1949.

Talbot, H. S.: Sexual function in paraplegics. J. Urol., *73*:91, 1955.

Thornhill, H. L., and Williams, M. L.: Experience with the water mattress in a large city hospital. Am. J. Nurs., *68*:2356, 1968.

Tobin, G. R., Pompi Sanders, B., Man, D., and Weiner, L. J.: The biceps femoris myocutaneous advancement flap: a useful modification for ischial pressure ulcer reconstruction. Ann. Plast. Surg., *6*:396, 1981.

Van Gehuchten, A.: Les centres nerveux cérébro-spinaux. Anatomie normale et éléments de neuropathologie générale à l'usage des médecins. Uystpruyst-Dieudonné, Louvain, 1908.

Vasconez, L. O., Schneider, W. J., and Jurkiewicz, M. J.: Pressure sores. Curr. Prob. Surg., *14*:1, 1977.

Wagner, C. W., Jr., Dohrmann, G. J., Taslits, N., Albin, M. S., and White, R. J.: Histopathology of experimental spinal cord trauma. *In* Proceedings of the 17th V.A. Spinal Cord Injury Conference. Bronx, New York, Sept. 29, 30, Oct. 1, 1969.

Weeks, P. M., and Brower, T. D.: Island flap coverage of extensive decubitus ulcers. Plast. Reconstr. Surg., *42*:433, 1968.

Weinstein, J. D., and Davidson, B. A.: A fluid support mattress and seat for the prevention and treatment of decubitus ulcers. Lancet, *2*:625, 1965.

Weinstein, J. D., and Davidson, B. A.: Fluid support in the prevention and treatment of decubitus ulcers. Am. J. Phys. Med., *45*:283, 1966.

Wesser, D. R., and Kahn, S.: The reversed dermis graft in the repair of decubitus ulcers. Plast. Reconstr. Surg., *40*:252, 1967.

White, J. C., and Hamm, W. G.: Primary closure of bedsores by plastic surgery. Ann. Surg., *124*:1136, 1946.

White, J. C., Hudson, H. W., and Kennard, H. E.: The treatment of bedsores by total excision with plastic closure. U.S. Naval Med. Bull., *45*:445, 1945.

Wingate, G. B., and Friedland, J. A.: Repair of ischial pressure ulcers with gracilis myocutaneous island flaps. Plast. Reconstr. Surg., *62*:245, 1978.

Withers, E. H., Franklin, J. D., Madden, J. J., Jr., and Lynch, J. B.: Further experience with the tensor fascia lata musculocutaneous flap. Ann. Plast. Surg., *4*:31, 1980.

Yeoman, M. P., and Hardy, A. G.: The pathology and treatment of pressure sores in paraplegics. Br. J. Plast. Surg., *7*:179, 1954.

Zeitlin, A. B., Cottrell, T. L., and Lloyd, F. A.: Sexology of the paraplegic male. Fertil. Steril., *8*:337, 1957.

78

Nicholas G. Georgiade
Gregory S. Georgiade
Ronald Riefkohl

Esthetic Breast Surgery

Contemporary concepts of female beauty and femininity necessitate that the breast be esthetically acceptable in all situations of dress and undress. The fact that the breasts represent a significant factor in acceptability as a female and in sexual attractiveness is another consideration. The complex physiologic responses in the breast further multiply the problems.

The continued advances in the plastic surgeon's ability to modify the female body image have resulted in an increased demand for this type of surgery. In the case of reduction mammoplasty, the motivation for surgical correction can be functional because of the intolerable size, which causes the patient not only severe shoulder and back pain, but also excoriations in the shoulder area. Excoriations in the inframammary area are a further source of patient distress.

The ability of the plastic surgeon to satisfy the patient undergoing esthetic surgery and to achieve a positive behavioral change depends on many factors. Sensitivity to the patient's complaints and problems, as well as effective communication and interaction, markedly increases the chances of positive patient reaction.

EMBRYOLOGY

The six week, 9 mm human embryo shows a linear ectodermal ridge (mammary ridge) extending from the axilla to the inguinal area bilaterally (Arey, 1974). This finding accounts for residual breast tissue and nipple being present occasionally in these areas (Fig. 78–1). Approximately two-thirds of these supernumerary areas are found in the anterior thorax and abdomen, and 20 per cent are

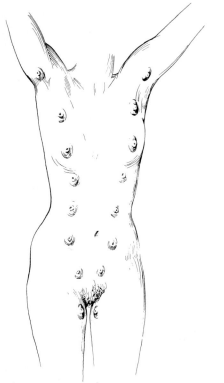

Figure 78–1. The possible locations of aberrant breast tissue and the nipple-areola areas.

observed in the axillary area. The remaining few may be found in other areas such as the groin, vulva, thighs, buttocks, back, face, and neck. The mammary ridges usually vanish rapidly with growth of the embryo, except those in the pectoral or midcranial areas (Deaver, 1917; Gray and Skandalakis, 1972).

By the fourth month the development of the mammary gland has continued with a downward thickening and growth of the ectoderm into the underlying mesoderm, and approximately 20 secondary outgrowths begin to form as solid cells. This early mammary tissue continues to bud, forming the lactiferous ducts, which continue to grow, branch, and canalize. By the seventh month the small duct acini have been formed. All the main ducts are concentrated together and open into what appears to be a depressed pit into the skin. This area demonstrates proliferation of the surrounding mesoderm with a formation of smooth muscle fibers arranged in circular and longitudinal fashion making up the nipple, through which the lactiferous ducts secrete. Soon after birth the flattened nipple becomes elevated. The smooth muscle

surrounding the nipple contracts on stimulation, causing the nipple to protrude even more because of the presence of the erectile tissue. The areola is created by the ectoderm and is recognizable by the fifth month. The areola contains apocrine glands (sebaceous glands) that are rudimentary mammary lobules (glands of Montgomery).

ANATOMY

Breast size and shape vary as a result of many anatomic and racial factors. The ideal breast, as perceived by the artist, is conical in shape. It should be positioned within the second and third ribs (superiorly), the seventh and eighth ribs (inferiorly), and the parasternal and anterior axillary lines. There is an extension of the breast into the axilla (tail of Spence). The breast rests mainly on the pectoral muscle, with some overhang over the serratus anterior muscle. There is some overlapping of the superior rectus sheath in the medial direction. The breast also overlaps the first digitation of the external oblique muscle. The nipple is located at the level of the fourth intercostal space and at a position slightly lateral to the midclavicular line. The location of the nipple may also be placed approximately 2 to 3 cm below the midhumeral position.

The breast is supported by surrounding connective tissue with fibrous attachments (Cooper's ligaments), which suspend and attach the breast to the pectoral major fascia as well as the overlying skin (Cooper, 1840). This allows some movement of the breast in the skin envelope and also serves as a support for the breasts. The breast is also surrounded by a layer of adipose tissue of varying thickness. The nipple is surrounded by the areola, which is lubricated by sebaceous glands (Montgomery). The nipple contains the orifices for the 16 to 24 mammary ducts of the breast.

The adult mammary gland is composed of multiple lobes, at least 20 of which are intimately associated with another lobe, so that these are not identifiable as separate lobes. All the lobes drain into main ducts that extend the distance of the breast and receive many contributories from the surrounding lobules forming the main duct for each lobe (Fig. 78–2).

As each main lobe comes in close approxi-

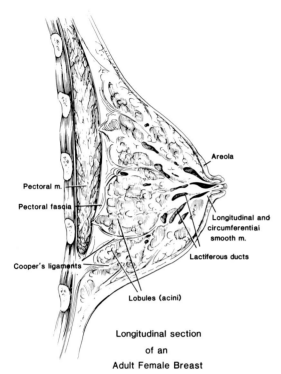

Figure 78–2. Longitudinal section of the breast. Note the various anatomic relationships to the breast parenchyma and the convergence of the ducts into the nipple. Cooper's ligaments attach the skin to the breast tissue.

mation to the nipple, it dilates, forming a lactiferous sinus that serves as a reservoir for milk storage (Fig. 78–2) (Testut, 1901; Claoué and Bernard, 1935; Handley, 1955; Hollinshead, 1971; Romanes, 1972; Montagna and MacPherson, 1974).

PHYSIOLOGY

There are three developmental phases of the breast.

The initial phase of breast development occurs between birth and puberty. During this period there is a gradual increase in the glandular tissue and surrounding stroma. The increase in glandular tissue is characterized by elongation of the smaller ducts with increased branching. Lobules are formed from these smaller ducts, which become canalized. These are all surrounded by a vascular stroma.

There are a number of hormones intimately involved in breast development (Haagensen, 1986). Estrogen, progesterone, adrenal corticoids, prolactin, insulin, thyroxine, and growth hormone have coordinating activities in breast development. The pituitary gland controls the endocrine system (estrogen and progesterone), which affects the development of the breast. Progesterone has its greatest effect on the alveolar system. Prolactin, which is a pituitary peptide hormone, effects major physiologic changes such as final differentiation of alveolar epithelial cells into mature milk-producing cells, as well as other morphologic changes (Fig. 78–3) (Gallagher and associates, 1978).

Predictable changes occur during the menstrual cycle in the epithelium of the ducts and acini as well as in the stromal tissue. The mature breast varies in density or consistency, depending on the phase of the menstrual cycle during which it is being examined. The resting phase of the breast is characterized by multiple ducts, lined with two layers of cuboidal cells, and the terminal alveolar ducts, which have a single layer of columnar cells, surrounded by myoepithelial cells. The main ducts are lined by pseudostratified epithelium. The stroma of the breasts varies, depending on its proximity to the ducts, with increased density occurring farther from the ducts and characterized by increased numbers of collagen fibers interspaced with fine elastic fibers. There is a higher ratio of fibroblasts, lymphocytes, plasma cells, mast cells, and histiocytes in a much less dense stroma of collagen but with a greater vascularity. During the proliferative phase or first days of the menstrual cycle (days 3 to 7) there is an increased level of estrogen, which causes epithelial proliferation, producing two to three layers of B cells that obscure the lumen. During this proliferative phase the stroma is dense and is characterized by an increased volume of fibroblasts and plasma cells. During the second week of the menstrual cycle (luteal phase) there is follicular differentiation, which occurs with an increase in progesterone production. At this time, three types of epithelial cells may be distinguished. The first cell type consists of the myoepithelial cells in the most basal layer, which have small dense nuclei with clear cytoplasms. The B cells are first found in the proliferative phase, which persists with characteristically round cell nuclei, prominent nucleoli, and homogeneous pale eosinophilic cytoplasm with polygon-shaped B cells. The third type of epithelial cell is the A cell, which has a columnar shape that

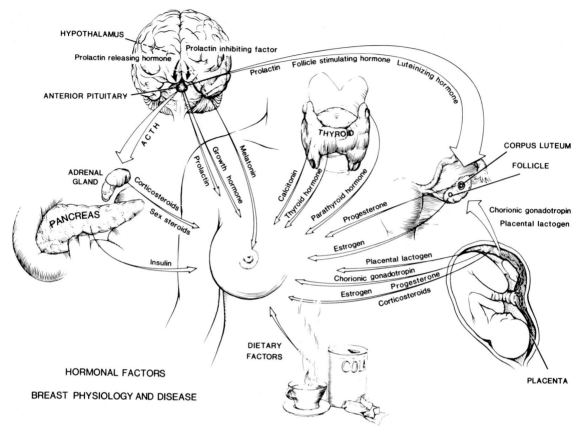

Figure 78–3. The various hormones and glands affecting breast function. Exogenous factors such as caffeine also affect breast physiology.

circumscribes the lumen, as well as a dense basal nucleus, a basophilic cytoplasm, associated with higher ribonucleic acid (RNA) and ribosome content. This follicular stage has less of an inflammatory infiltrate than the proliferative phase.

The secretory phase occurs during days 21 to 27 and is under the influence of estrogen, progesterone, and prolactin. The level of prolactin increases in conjunction with steroid production. Metabolic hormones cause lipid droplets to appear in the alveolar cells. During this stage, breast volume increases 15 to 30 ml, with associated water retention in the stroma. This appears to be caused by a histamine effect on the microcirculation as a result of estrogen activity. More recently, prolactin has been targeted as a predominant factor in premenstrual tension. Apocrine secretion from the luminal epithelial cells occurs with the progesterone exposure, as does apical budding with dilatation of the acinar lumen. There is a significant increase in the

RNA and ribosome content of the luminal epithelial cells. The stroma in this phase changes from the dense compactness of the proliferative phase to an edematous tissue with prominent, fluid-filled spaces and venous congestion.

The final phase of the menstrual cycle (days 28 and beyond) is associated with withdrawal of estrogen and progesterone. Apocrine budding ceases, but the lumina remain distended with eosinophilic granular secretion. The basal cells remain engorged with glycogen. The stroma then returns to its previous compact, well-demarcated state with an increased plasma cell infiltrate.

During the menopause there is diminution of estrogen and marked decrease in progesterone. Menopause is associated with breast involution and with gradual atrophy of the glandular tissue. There is an incomplete regression of the glandular epithelium associated with decreased cellularity and vascularity of the stroma.

In the postmenopausal breast there is replacement of the epithelium and stroma by fat, but some increase in elastic fibers in the connective tissue stroma. Remains of fragmented ducts are seen with only a vestigial duct system. There is decreased vascularity and some lymphocytic infiltration around the periductal remnants (McCarty and associates, 1983).

BLOOD SUPPLY

Arterial

There are three main arterial routes supplying the breast (Fig. 78–4).

The internal thoracic (internal mammary) artery lies just lateral but in close proximity to the sternum, in a position deep to the chondral areas of ribs one to six. The important branches are the perforators through the intercostal spaces, which provide 60 per cent of total breast blood flow, mainly to the me-

dial portion. The mammary branches extend to the nipple area; there are extensive anastomoses with branches from the lateral thoracic artery, and also some with the intercostal vessels.

The lateral thoracic artery from the subclavian artery, usually a direct branch from the axillary artery, is occasionally a branch from the thoracoacromial or subscapular artery. Thirty per cent of the blood flow of the upper-outer and lateral portions of the breast is supplied by the lateral thoracic artery, which approaches the breast along the anterolateral thoracic wall. The mammary branches approach the breast tissue from the deep portion of the upper-outer quadrant of the breast.

The lower lateral aspect of the arterial supply of the breast is from the branches of the third, fourth, and fifth posterior intercostal arteries.

Some minor sources of arterial supply are branches from the axillary artery, the thoracic artery, the subscapular artery, and the thoracodorsal pectoral branches of the thoracoacromial artery.

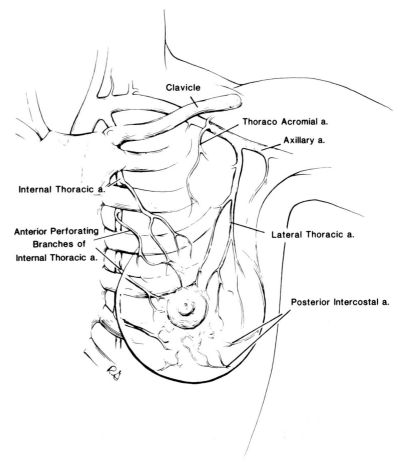

Figure 78–4. Blood supply of the breast. The internal mammary branches pass through the intercostal spaces and provide most of the blood supply to the breast. The lateral thoracic artery supplies the upper and lateral vascularity. The posterior intercostal vessels are the least important source of blood to the breast.

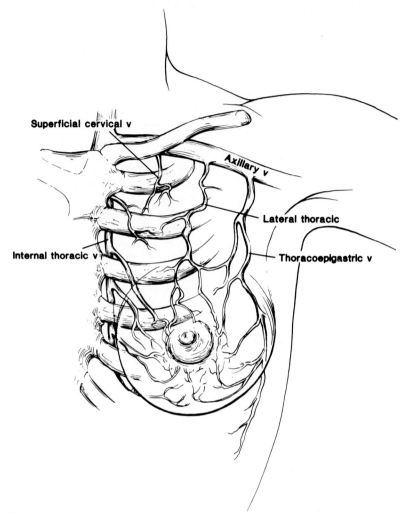

Figure 78–5. Venous supply of the breast. The venous system has superficial transverse and longitudinal drainage components that empty into the internal thoracic veins and the lower neck venous supply. The axillary vein drains the upper and lateral chest area.

Venous

The venous drainage of the breast has two main avenues (Fig. 78–5).

The first is the superficial and deep venous system. The superficial system has both a transverse and a longitudinal network. The transverse vessels, located subcutaneously along the medial aspect of the breast, empty into the internal thoracic veins. The longitudinal venous system drains in a cephalad direction into the lower neck veins.

The second, the deep drainage system, is located within the chest wall in the intercostal veins that drain into the vertebral veins, azygos vein, and superior vena cava. The largest venous system consists of the perforating branches of the internal thoracic vein, which drains into the innominate vein. The lateral breast, chest wall, and pectoral muscle area are drained into the axillary vein.

LYMPHATIC SUPPLY

The four main lymphatic routes of the breasts are the cutaneous, the internal thoracic, the posterior intercostal, and the axillary areas (Fig. 78–6). The lymphatics follow the vascular pathways and have valves that guide the lymph flow in the direction of the venous flow. The skin lymphatics usually empty into the axillary lymph nodes. The superficial lymphatics of the medial aspect of the breast empty into the internal mammary chain and may cross the midline. The inferior portion of the breast may drain to the lymphatics on the rectus abdominis muscle sheath and into the subdiaphragmatic lymphatics and the intra-abdominal nodes.

The areola of the breast has a subareolar plexus (Sappey) of lymphatics that drain into the anterior pectoral lymph nodes. The retroareolar mammary lymphatics pass into the arteriopectoral lymph nodes (Rotter's nodes) and into the deep axillary nodes (Grozzman's pathway).

Most of the lymph flow is from the breast stroma that surrounds the mammary tissues, and most of the lymph nodes flow into the axillary lymph nodes. The lymphatic vessels empty into the regional lymph nodes, which are aggregates of lymphocytes that filter the lymph flow. The axillary nodes have the greatest volume of lymph flow and have valves to continue the lymph flow in the direction of the venous flow. These nodes are divided into six groups. Those underneath the lateral pectoral muscle are called the external mammary nodes. The interpectoral nodes (Rotter's) lie between the pectoralis major and minor muscles and infiltrate the pectoralis major, necessitating muscle removal when these nodes are excised. The scapular nodes lie in close approximation to the subscapular vessels and intercostobrachial nerve; removal of these nodes usually involves sacrifice of the nerve. The axillary vein lymph nodes lie on the lateral, caudal, and ventral aspects of the vein, and are sep-

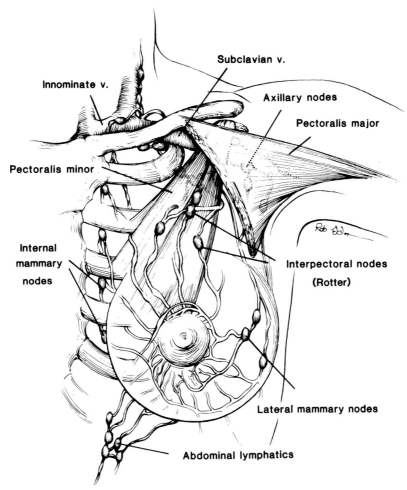

Figure 78–6. Lymphatic system. The lymphatics follow the vascular supply to the breast. The largest amount of lymph flow is to the axillary lymph nodes. Lymph nodes are found in all systems. Note the lymph nodes (Rotter's) between the pectoralis major and minor muscles in the upper outer quadrant.

arated from it by a fascial layer. Ten to 12 central axillary nodes lie embedded in the central axillary fat. The axillary nodes eventually drain into the third or fourth subclavicular nodes, which are the highest and most medial group along the ventrocaudal surface of the axillary vein, extending from the apex of the axilla medially to the thoracoacromial vein. One or more large lymphatic trunks conduct subclavicular lymph node drainage medially to the junction of the jugular and subclavian veins. They are continuous with the deep cervical nodes located in the supraclavicular area.

The medial breast tissue lymphatics flow into the internal mammary lymph nodes and from there into the mediastinal lymph nodes.

The lymphatics in the inferior portion of the breast drain into the subdiaphragmatic lymphatics and on into the subpectoral and intra-abdominal lymph nodes, and also to the liver.

INNERVATION

The breast receives sensory and sympathetic autonomic innervation (Fig. 78–7). The sensory innervation to the upper breast is by the supraclavicular nerves from the third and fourth branches of the cervical plexus. The anterior cutaneous divisions of the intercostal nerves (two to seven) emerge through the chest wall as perforating branches with the internal thoracic artery. The small medial branches of the anterior cutaneous nerves supply the medial and inferior aspects of the breast. The lateral branches travel subcutaneously to the areola and midclavicular area. The lateral cutaneous nerve from T4 appears to be the dominant innervation to the nipple (Goldwyn, 1976). Sympathetic beta-adrenergic stimulation causes contraction of the smooth muscle of the nipple and blood vessels. Although myoepithelial cells of the alveoli lack innervation, they respond indirectly to

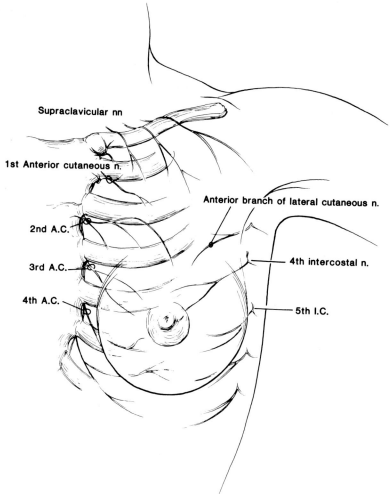

Figure 78–7. Nerve supply of the breast. Innervation of the breast is superiorly from the supraclavicular nerves, the intercostal nerves supplying the innervation to the medial aspect of the breast. The lateral cutaneous nerves provide anterior branches to supply the lateral mammary area up to and including the nipple via the fourth anterior branch. The lateral branches of the anterior cutaneous nerves accompany the branches of the internal thoracic area; they supply innervation of the medial aspect of the breast.

nervous excitation such as manipulation and nipple sucking. Beta-adrenergic stimulation releases norepinephrine, causing relaxation of the myoepithelial cells of the nipple.

Krause's end bulbs and Ruffini's corpuscles, sensitive to touch, stretch, and warmth, are located in the dermis of the areola and nipple. Their presence appears to contribute greatly to the response of the nipple and areola to stimulation.

BREAST REDUCTION SURGERY

The concepts and techniques utilized in esthetic breast surgery are refinements of techniques initially described approximately 60 years ago. Although the techniques of breast surgery were sporadically recorded hundreds of years ago, the state-of-the-art practice is more recent (Paulus, 1846; Leclerc, 1861; Schultze, 1892; Morestin, 1905; Aubert, 1923; Holländer, 1924; Campbell, 1926).

Three presentations in the past 60 years have been the most significant contributions. The procedure of breast amputation and free nipple graft was described by Thorek in 1922 and is still used today, particularly for patients with severe hypermastia. The technique has been modified by others (Bames, 1948; Wise, Gannon, and Hill, 1963; McCormack and Bales, 1976; Rubin, 1983).

The Biesenberger technique (1928) involved extensive undermining of the overlying skin and severing of the suspensory ligaments (Cooper's). Wedge excisions of breast tissue in an inverted "S" shape involving the lateral aspect of the breast were carried out, and resulted in a subsequent high risk of associated tissue loss including the breast and skin. This was a more popular technique in the 1930's and 1940's, but it has now been largely abandoned for more up-to-date procedures.

The next significant improvement in the management of the areolar complex during a reduction mammoplasty was described by Schwarzmann (1930), who utilized a superiorly and medially positioned dermal pedicle upon which the nipple-areola complex was attached. From this basic concept of maintaining skin vascularity to support the viability of the nipple-areola complex, a number of surgical procedures using dermal pedicles have evolved. The horizontal dermal pedicle described by Strömbeck (1960) was one of the

earlier techniques (Fig. 78–8A). This was followed by Skoog (1963) with a superior lateral dermal pedicle (Fig. 78–8B). At approximately the same time, in the late 1950's, Arie (1957) and Pitanguy (1962) utilized a superior dermal pedicle. This was similar in concept to the later modifications by others (Weiner and associates, 1973; Cramer and Chong, 1976; Hugo and Bauer, 1983) who used this technique also (Fig. 78–8C) for superior dermal nipple-areola pedicle flaps.

An inferior, oblique dermal technique was described by Dufourmentel and Mouly in 1961 (Fig. 78–8D). In 1972, McKissock described the vertical dermal pedicle. In the later 1970's, an inferior dermal pedicle technique was described by Robbins (1977), Courtiss and Goldwyn (1977), and Ribeiro and Backer (1983), and modified by Georgiade and associates (1979a, 1983).

The current state of the art for correction of hypermastia utilizes the concept described previously, with modifications preferred by some plastic surgeons, such as the reduction technique of Galvao (1983) (Fig. 78–9), with preservation of the superior, medial, lateral, and inferior pedicles. The "B" technique, reported by Regnault (1974) (Fig. 78–10), with further improvement by Meyer and Kesselring (1983), who described a closure with an "L"-shaped suture line, is still a popular procedure.

At the present time, four techniques appear to be used most often: (1) the superiorly based dermal pedicle, (2) the vertical bipedicle dermal flap, (3) the free nipple graft, and (4) the inferior pyramidal dermal flap.

Superiorly Based Dermal Pedicle. The superiorly based dermal pedicle as described by Pitanguy (1962), Weiner and associates (1973), Cramer and Chong (1976), and Hugo and Bauer (1983) is particularly well suited for reduction mammaplasty of less than 500 gm. The standard marking method is carried out with the patient in an upright position (Fig. 78–11).

A superiorly based dermal pedicle is designed and elevated with the incision extending approximately 1 cm into the keyhole area in order to facilitate positioning and insetting of the nipple areola in the new superior position (Fig. 78–12). Resection of the inferior portion of the breast is then carried out. The areola is maintained in position with 5-0 Vicryl intradermal sutures and 5-0 nylon skin sutures to approximate the skin edges. The vertical portions of the flap are closed

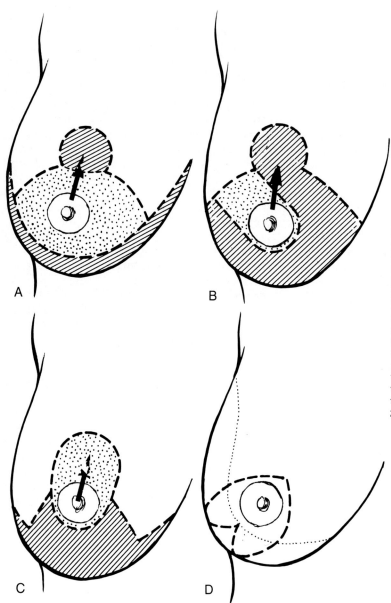

Figure 78–8. Types of dermal pedicles. *A,* The classic bipedicle lateral dermal pedicle with the nipple-areola complex in the midposition (Strombeck). Superior movement is difficult in the larger, ptotic breast. *B,* The lateral dermal areola flap (Skoog). This type of flap can be easily rotated superiorly. The vascularity of the nipple-areola complex is challenged with this technique. *C,* The superiorly based dermal nipple-areola flap. *D,* The markings and placement of the inferior, oblique dermal flap. This technique should be restricted to the smaller breast (hypertrophy of 200 to 300 gm).

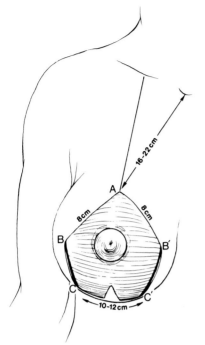

Figure 78–9. The modified vertical dermal pedicle (Galvao).

with interrupted 4-0 Vicryl intradermal sutures, and the inferior portions of the flap are closed, care being taken not to extend the incision into the midline (Figs. 78–12*C,D*, 78–13).

At the completion of the procedure, a suction drain is inserted through the lateral aspect of the incision and maintained for one to two days. The sutures are removed on the 10th day, and on the 12th day the subcuticular sutures are removed from the periareolar area.

The initial measurements for the eventual size of the breasts and location of the nipple are carried out in an upright position in the Pitanguy procedure. With the patient in a semi-upright position under general oroendotracheal anesthesia and after suitable skin preparation, two heavy sutures (one placed in the clavicular notch and the other at the midline of the manubrium) are used to outline the new position of the nipple-areola area (Fig. 78–14).

Points C and C′ are marked at the level of the inframammary crease. Points A and A′

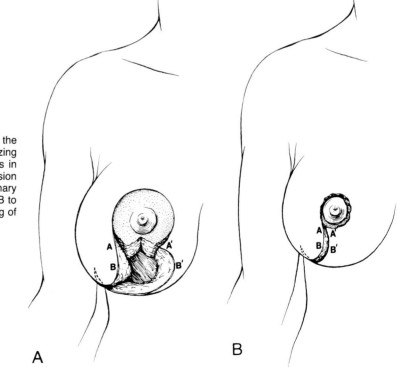

Figure 78–10. The design of the reduction mammoplasty, utilizing the configuration shown, results in placement of the lateral extension of the scar in the inframammary area. A is approximated to A′, B to B′ for proper closure and coning of the breast.

A

B

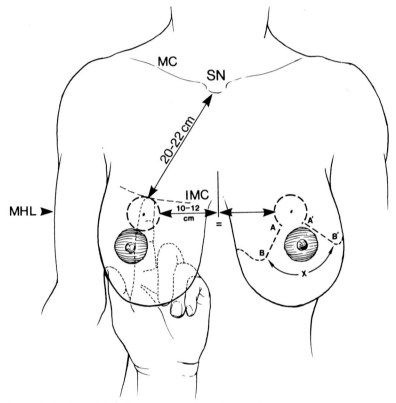

Figure 78–11. The standard procedure for preoperative markings of the hypertrophic breast. Note the key points including the location of the nipple areola at the level of the inframammary crease (slightly higher in the younger patient). The width of the resection *(×)* is individually tailored, as is the base of the dermal pedicle. A width of 8 cm results in a small breast cup. A 9 cm dermal base width yields a B cup breast. The distance from the midsternum to each areola should be the same and will vary between 10 and 12 cm, depending on the size of the patient. The areola is marked with a circular wire either 3.5 or 4.0 cm in diameter. Lines AB and A′B′ are 5 cm in length. The distance between B and B′ is determined by the size of the estimated resection and will vary from 8 to 10 cm in a 500 gm resection and up to 14 cm in a resection of 1500 gm of breast tissue. Note the height of the areola in relation to the midhumeral line (MHL). MC = midclavicular; SN = sternal notch; IMC = inframammary crease.

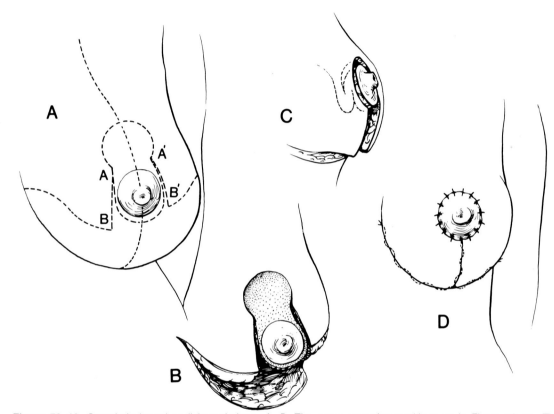

Figure 78–12. Superiorly based pedicle technique. *A, B,* The same operative markings as in Figure 78–11. The superior pedicle is deepithelized with a 1.5 cm deepithelized circumareolar area. The incisions extend approximately 1 to 2 cm into the keyhole. The resection of breast tissue is carried out. *C,D,* The pedicle is folded on itself and the medial and lateral flaps are approximated.

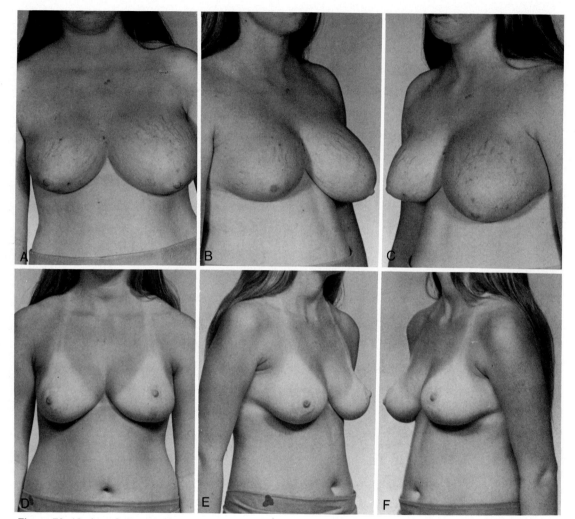

Figure 78–13. *A,* to *C,* Preoperative photos of a 13 year old patient with asymmetric and hypertrophic breasts and with associated ptosis. *D* to *F,* Patient is shown three years after reduction mammoplasty of approximately 800 gm utilizing a superiorly based dermal pedicle on the right breast and a vertical dermal pedicle for reduction of the left breast.

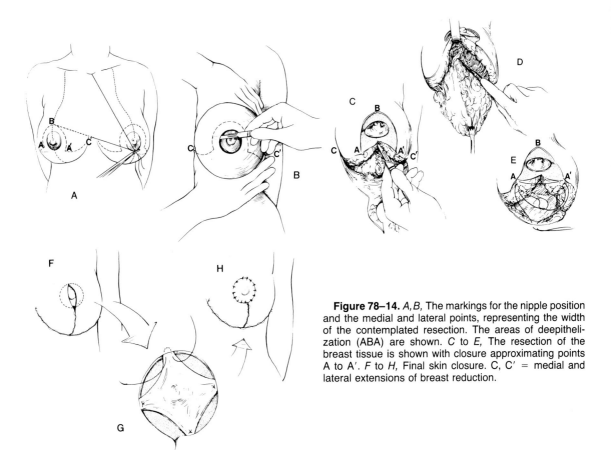

Figure 78-14. *A,B,* The markings for the nipple position and the medial and lateral points, representing the width of the contemplated resection. The areas of deepithelization (ABA) are shown. *C* to *E,* The resection of the breast tissue is shown with closure approximating points A to A'. *F* to *H,* Final skin closure. C, C' = medial and lateral extensions of breast reduction.

are placed at the widest points of the estimated reduction. Points A and B and A' and B can be up to 7 cm in length. Points C to A and A' to C' are the estimated lines of the medial and lateral extension of the excision (Fig. 78–14*A,B*).

The areas of A,B and A' are deepithelized following a partial-thickness incision placed around the areola, approximately 4.5 cm in diameter.

The resection of skin and breast tissue is carried along the lines of C, AA', C'. A keel-shaped glandular resection is accomplished with preservation of the adipose layer that remains in the superior portion of the breast tissue (Fig. 78–14*C,D,E*).

Closure is facilitated by first approximating points A and A' to evaluate the final size and shape of the breast. At the same time, adjustments are made: the deeper sutures are used to bring together the lateral and medial remaining segments, and the opposite breast is reduced in the same manner.

The new position of the nipple is determined and approximated at point B. Using a template, the predetermined size of the areola, usually 4.0 to 4.5 cm in diameter, is marked on the skin, and the area is deepithelized. The nipple-areola complex is transposed to its new position, using "U"-type sutures passing only through the dermis to avoid postoperative suture scars (Figs. 78–14 *F,G,H,* 78–15).

Vertical Bipedicle Dermal Flap. The vertical dermal pedicle technique for mammary reduction was first reported by McKissock in 1972 and 1976. The measurements are carried out with the patient in an upright position (see Fig. 78–11). The vertical lines of the keyhole should be acute, with the length of lines AB and A'B' not exceeding 5 cm. The lateral and medial flaps are marked as horizontal "lazy-S" lines for better projection of the breast and avoidance of the "boxy" appearance. Following deepithelization of the vertical dermal pedicle, excision of the lateral and medial horizontal triangles of skin, fat, and glandular tissue is achieved. The vertical pedicle is incised along its vertical line, freeing it from the remaining breast (Fig. 78–

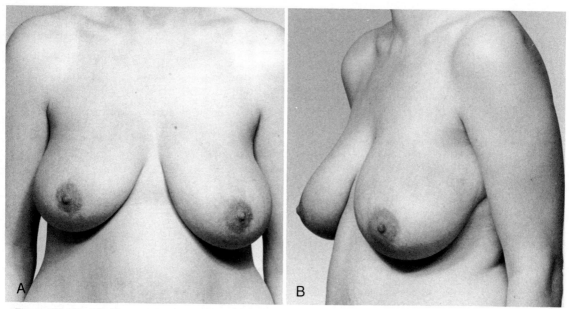

Figure 78–15. *A,B,* Preoperative frontal and lateral views of a 25 year old patient with moderate breast hypertrophy and associated ptosis.

16). The flap is extended superiorly into the keyhole bilaterally for a distance of 1.5 cm, allowing the flap to be folded on itself at the time of closure. The desired amount of breast tissue is excised, leaving at least a 1.0 cm thickness of the vertical pedicle with the base thicker.

The breast tissue from under the lateral and medial flaps is also excised (Fig. 78–16B). After suitable tailoring, the flaps are approximated in the usual fashion, using inverted 4-0 Vicryl subcuticular sutures; suction drains are inserted, and continuous 3-0 subcuticular nylon pull-out sutures are used to approximate the skin. The areola is positioned with 5-0 inverted Vicryl dermal sutures and interrupted 5-0 nylon skin sutures. Sterile paper tapes are used to reinforce the closure of the skin edges. A bulky mechanic's waste dressing is applied over 4 × 3 cotton sponges and maintained in position with an 8 inch stockinette cut on a bias and applied as a figure-of-eight dressing (Fig. 78–17).

Free Nipple Graft. The free nipple graft technique used most commonly for massive hypertrophy is the one described and modified by Bames (1930, 1948), Wise, Gannon, and Hill, (1963), and McCormack and Bales (1976), and further modified by Rubin (1983). This technique, which appears to be particularly advantageous when more than 2000 gm of breast tissue are resected, combines a partial breast amputation with free nipple-areola grafts.

The measurements for the surgical correction of this type of hypermastia are shown in Figure 78–18A. The dermal pedicle of the midportion of the breast, which will become the inferior portion of the breast, is marked. The distance from the projected superior areola border is usually 20 to 23 cm from the clavicular notch. The point to be marked will be higher by 2 to 3 cm after the mammary reduction because of traction on the skin of the hypertrophied breast. The length of each arm (AB and AC) is measured at 8 cm. The distance between C and B will vary with the amount of breast tissue to be resected; it is usually 18 to 20 cm or more, and up to 160 degrees between each arm of the flap (Fig. 78–18AB). The skin between points B and C is deepithelized (Fig. 78–18A). At this time, before amputation of the inferior breast, the nipple-areola complex is removed at the predetermined size (usually 4.5 cm) and stored on moistened gauze sponges. Excision of the breast is carried out along CX,BY lines, but left intact along the inferior portion of the specimen which is left attached to allow for sufficient blood supply if any of this tissue is needed for additional bulk to contour the breast suitably at the time of closure. The skin of the lower flap may also be deepithelized and left attached to the pectoral muscle

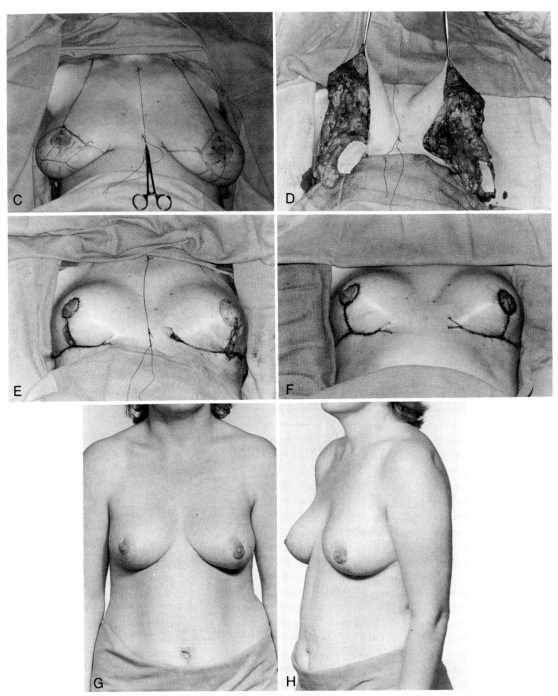

Figure 78–15 *Continued C,* The operative markings are shown after the method of Pitanguy, Ribeiro, and Backer. The suture placed in the midline at the clavicular notch and manubrium is used to place the areola in its new position. *D,* The heel type of resection is shown bilaterally. *E,* The right nipple areola is shown in its new position. The new deepithelized position for the left nipple-areola is shown. *F,* The completed breast closure. *G,H,* Six months postoperative frontal and lateral views of the same patient. 520 gm of tissue were removed from the left breast and 476 gm from the right breast.

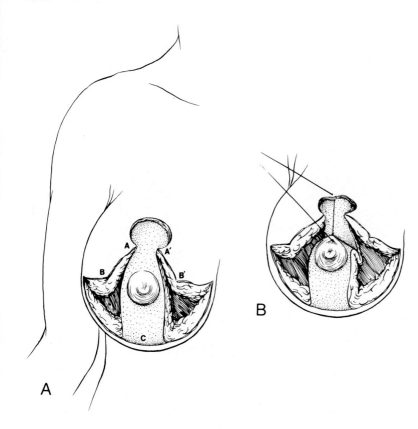

Figure 78–16. Vertical bipedicle dermal flap technique. *A,* The breast markings are made (see Fig. 78–11). The vertical dermal pedicle is deepithelized. The breast tissue has been excised along previous markings, with the lateral and medial flaps incised along modified S-type lines in order to minimize the "boxy" appearance. *B,* The line of incision is extended into the keyhole medially and laterally for a distance of 1.5 cm to assist in the mobilization of the nipple-areola complex.

at the level of the third interspace along with the underlying tissue as needed for contouring purposes (Fig. 78–18C). The position of the nipple-areola complex is determined with the patient in an upright position. Some surgeons prefer to determine the new position utilizing two 3-0 sutures attached to the midclavicular notch, the second suture at the manubrium. The two sutures can be positioned at the same location on each breast. A 4.5 cm circular area is deepithelized. The free nipple-areola graft is trimmed of excess tissue and placed on its new position with interrupted 5-0 black silk sutures, which are tied over a bolus dressing (Figs. 78–18D, 78–19).

Inferior Pyramidal Dermal Flap. A reduction mammoplasty utilizing this technique (Georgiade and associates, 1979a, 1983) is versatile for breasts of varying sizes (300 to 2000 gm resection of breast tissue). This technique has had uniformly satisfactory results, with maintenance of sensation to the nipple and minimal decrease in the blood supply to the skin flaps or nipple-areola complex.

Measurements are carried out as described previously with the patient in a standing position (see Figs. 78–11, 78–20A). The patient is then placed in a slightly elevated position and the procedure is carried out under general oroendotracheal anesthesia and with suitable skin preparation.

The skin is deepithelized over what will be the dermal pedicle, leaving a dermal width of 2 cm in the periareolar area. The pyramidal dermal pedicle flap is created with the sides slanting obliquely away from the dermal pedicle, creating a wide-based pyramid (Fig. 78–20B). Note the thickness of the breast parenchyma beneath the nipple-areola area, which increases to the base of the flap pedicle.

The breast parenchyma and the previously marked skin area are excised, usually starting at a point lateral to the pedicle but not extending into the medial or lateral inframammary areas. The excision is extended along the lines A'B' and around the keyhole, removing the tissue with a uniform thickness of overlying skin flap of approximately 1.5 cm (Fig. 78–20A). The weight of the tissue removed is compared with the opposite breast for a better estimation of comparative resection.

The new breast mound is contoured, utilizing 4-0 Vicryl sutures intradermally for the flaps and 5-0 Vicryl for positioning the areola.

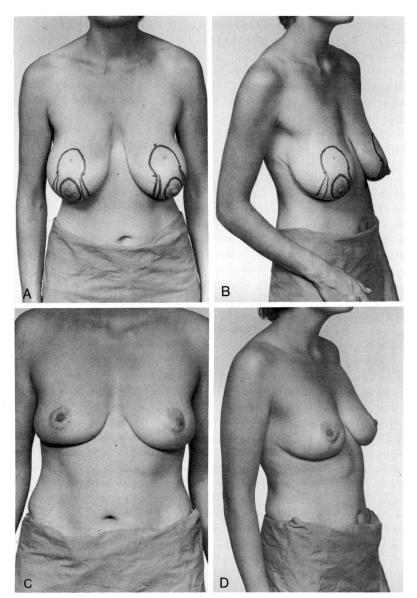

Figure 78–17. *A,B,* Preoperative frontal and oblique views of a 22 year old patient with the markings for a reduction mammoplasty utilizing the vertical pedicle technique (see Fig. 78–16). *C,D,* two years after reduction of approximately 600 gm of breast tissue.

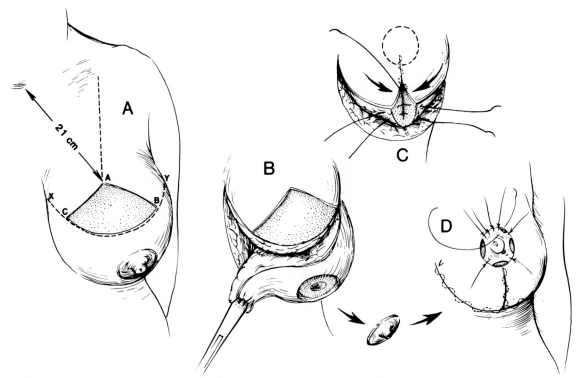

Figure 78–18. The free nipple graft technique. *A,* The angle ABC may vary, up to 160 degrees. Point A is the estimated position of the new areola. The area between CAB is deepithelized. *B,* The nipple areola is excised as a full-thickness graft. The excess breast tissue is excised leaving the inferior portion attached until it is determined whether any additional bulk is required for satisfactory contour. *C.* Points C to B are approximated and the breast is appropriately coned. *D,* The new position of the nipple areola is marked, the full-thickness nipple-areola graft is applied in its new position, and the graft is tied under a bolus. Subcuticular sutures are used to approximate the skin edges.

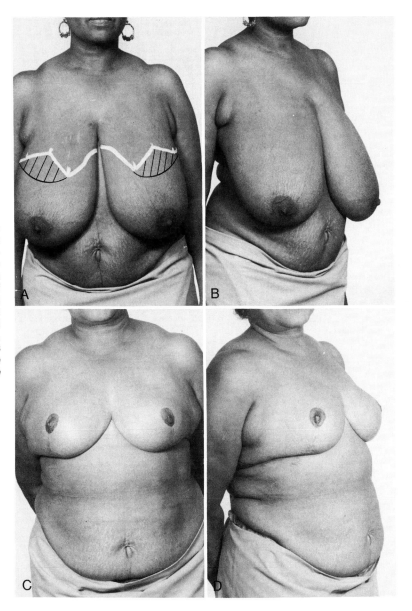

Figure 78–19. *A,B,* Preoperative frontal and oblique views of a 52 year old patient with massive hypertrophied breasts. A Rubin reduction mammoplasty with a free nipple graft was performed. 2200 gm of breast tissue were removed from the right breast and 2300 gm from the left breast. Note the shaded areas marked on the frontal view, which represent the areas of dermis to be infolded. *C,D,* Postoperative (seven years) frontal and oblique views.

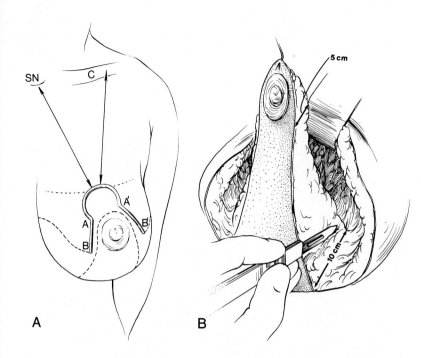

Figure 78–20. Inferior pyramidal dermal technique. *A,* The markings (as in Fig. 78–11) are made according to the width of the resultant flaps. The inferior dermal pedicle and the lines of medial and lateral excision are marked. The lateral and medial inferior areas of redundant tissue are resected and tailored to the individual breasts. Note that the dermal periphery of 2 cm is maintained around the areola. *B,* Following deepithelization of the inferior aspect, the pedicle is developed as an inferior-based pyramidal flap. The base of the flap is maintained at least 10 cm in thickness. The nipple base is also maintained at least 5 cm in thickness. SN = sternal notch.

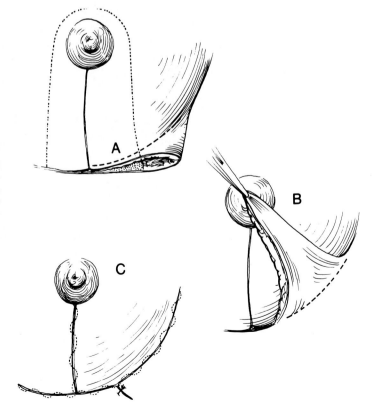

Figure 78–21. *A,* The lateral and medial flaps are approximated over the dermal pedicle. The dotted line shows the extent of the skin excision, which is never extended to the midline. *B,* The redundant skin is directed medially and laterally and tailored. *C,* Subcuticular sutures approximate the skin edges.

The lateral and medial aspects of the redundant breast skin and underlying tissue are adjusted (Fig. 78–21). The incisions are never extended to the midline area. Running 3-0 Prolene subcuticular sutures are used to approximate the skin edges (Figs. 78–22, 78–23, 78–24).

BREAST PTOSIS

Ptosis of the breasts probably can be best assessed by study of the relationship of the nipple to the inframammary crease.

The classic works of Lexer (1912) and Kraske (1923) first described a technique for correction of ptosis with elevation of the nip-

ple-areola complex and resection of excess tissue in the nipple-areola area. Modifications of this technique are now commonly used. Three categories of breast ptosis are described by Regnault (1973) and are probably the most accurate methods of categorizing breast position (Fig. 78–25). In the simple Class A type of breast ptosis, a simple elliptic deepithelization superior to the areola can be carried out, bringing the nipple areola into a slightly higher position (Fig. 78–26). In Class B ptosis, it is usually necessary to carry out a deepithelization superiorly and also an advancement technique, with excision of the redundant skin in a V-type fashion inferiorly and laterally (Figs. 78–27, 78–28). The most severe type of ptosis, Class C, is corrected

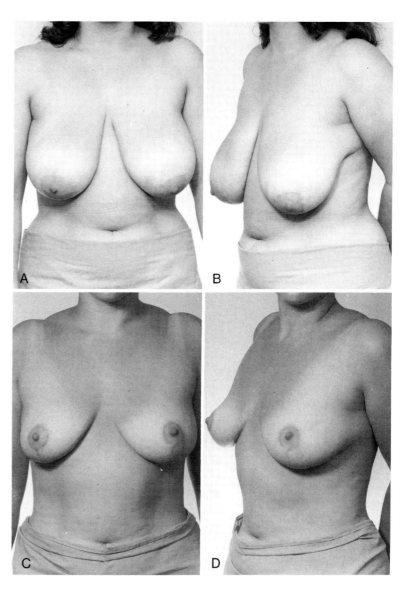

Figure 78–22. *A,B,* Preoperative frontal and oblique views of a 25 year old patient. A reduction mammoplasty was performed utilizing the inferior pyramidal pedicle technique. 700 gm of breast tissue were removed from the right breast and 800 gm from the left breast. *C,D,* Three-year postoperative views.

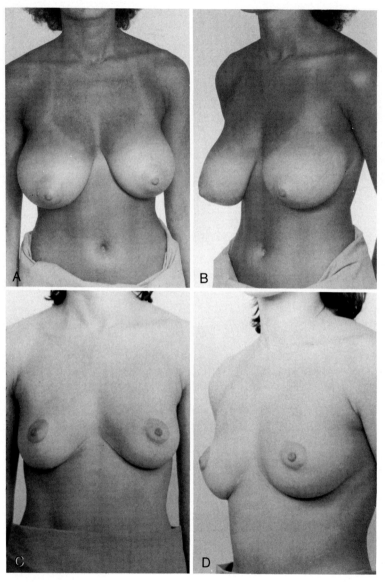

Figure 78–23. *A,B,* Preoperative frontal and oblique views of a 23 year old patient. Note the asymmetry of the breasts, the right breast being larger than the left. An inferior pyramidal pedicle reduction mammoplasty was performed. 775 gm of breast tissue were removed from the right breast and 600 gm from the left breast. *C,D,* 2½-year postoperative views.

Figure 78–24. *A,B,* Preoperative frontal and oblique views of a 17 year old patient with breast hypertrophy. *C,D,* 2½-year postoperative views of the same patient (inferior pyramidal technique with 1200 gm resection).

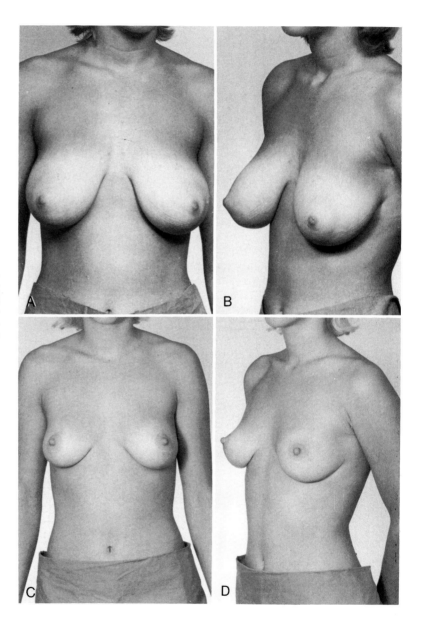

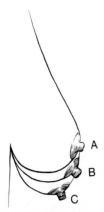

Figure 78–25. Breast ptosis classification. *A,* Minimal ptosis. The position of the nipple is located at or just inferior to the inframammary crease. *B,* Moderate ptosis. The position of the nipple is approximately 3 cm below the inframammary crease. *C,* Severe ptosis. The nipple is greater than 3 cm below the inframammary crease.

with the same procedure as described for Class B, or with an inferior or vertical dermal pedicle when there is an excess of breast skin (Fig. 78–29). Often an augmentation mammoplasty must be performed at the same time if there is also a loss of breast substance. It is preferable that the markings be made preoperatively with the patient in an upright position, but the augmentation should be carried out first, since the augmentation alters

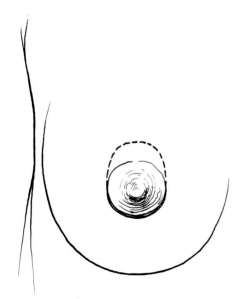

Figure 78–26. The area within the dotted line is deepithelized and the areola is elevated. Medial and lateral periareolar incisions can be extended to provide better contour.

the height of the nipple-areola complex (Fig. 78–30). It may not be necessary to elevate the nipple-areola complex as high as originally estimated before the augmentation. Various other techniques for mastopexy have been described by Pousson (1897), Dartigues (1925), Noel and Lopez-Martinez (1928), da Silva (1964), Regnault (1973), Goulian (1976), and Pitanguy (1983).

NIPPLE HYPERTROPHY

Nipple hypertrophy can be corrected by a number of techniques. The simplest is that described by Regnault (1973), which involves removing a portion of the periphery of the nipple through to the dermis and collapsing the distal portion to the new position (Fig. 78–31). A portion of the nipple can be excised in a vertical manner, and the nipple can be turned on itself as described by Pitanguy (Fig. 78–32). Excision of a portion of the nipple is possible in certain situations, but blockage of the lactiferous ducts may be a problem (Fig. 78–33).

NIPPLE INVERSION

A number of useful techniques have been described (Teimourian and Adham, 1983). The simplest was reported by Hauben and Mahler (1983). The technique is based on the assumption that the inverted nipple, compared with the normal nipple, has less fibrous muscular tissue present, thus giving less bulk and less tissue for nipple projection. This technique does not divide the lactiferous ducts, but mobilizes the tissue to create a greater bulk and a thicker nipple pedicle (Fig. 78–34). The Pitanguy technique (1983) involves actual release of the fibrous tissue between the ducts with a direct approach made through a transnipple-areola incision. The ducts are dissected free from the surrounding fibrous muscular tissue and released. The tissues are then approximated, the deep layers first, to provide more bulk to the nipple-areola complex (Figs. 78–35, 78–36).

The Broadbent and Woolf technique (1976) utilizes a similar direct approach through the transnipple-areola incision. According to the authors, the ducts have always been found to be short and hypoplastic, maintaining the

Text continued on page 3873

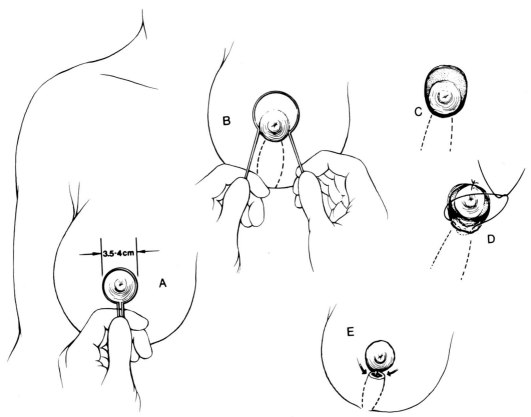

Figure 78–27. *A,* The size of the presenting areola is determined utilizing a previously shaped steel wire constructed in various diameters. *B,* The new position of the areola is determined with the patient standing preoperatively. The same wire is opened in order to fit around the areola, which when closed will be the same size as the presenting areola. *C,* The surrounding area is deepithelized with the inferior periareolar area incised to allow movement of the areola superiorly. *D,* The amount of movement superiorly is determined and the inferior portion of the defect is closed proportionately. *E,* The skin excess is obvious after closure *(D).*

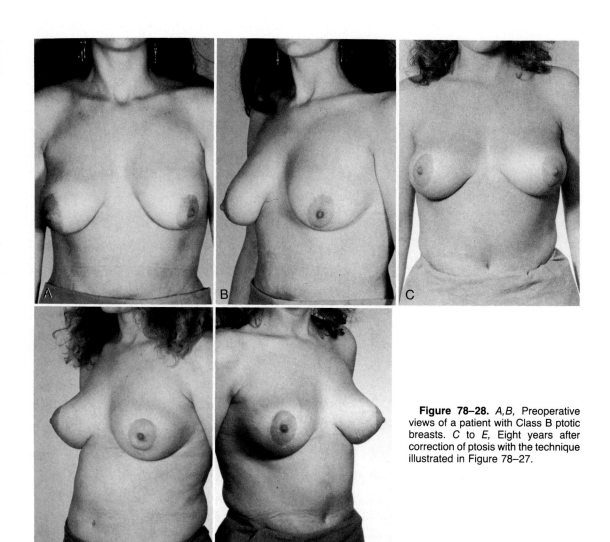

Figure 78–28. *A,B,* Preoperative views of a patient with Class B ptotic breasts. *C* to *E,* Eight years after correction of ptosis with the technique illustrated in Figure 78–27.

Figure 78–29. *A,B,* A 57 year old patient with severe ptosis and redundant breast skin corrected by a vertical dermal pedicle flap (see Fig. 78–27A). *C,D,* Two years after ptosis correction.

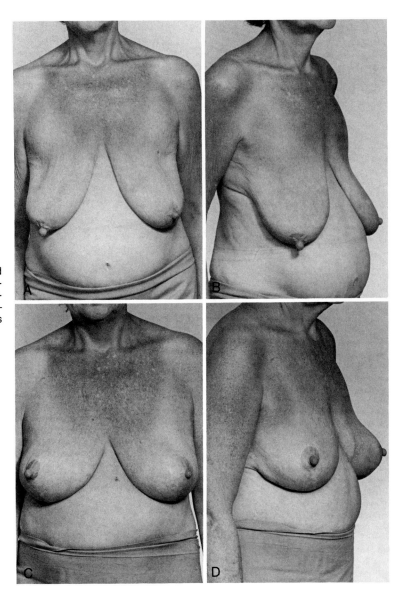

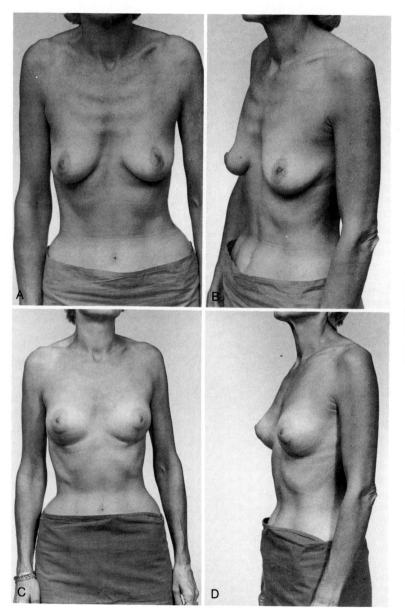

Figure 78–30. *A,B,* Preoperative frontal and oblique views of a 47 year old patient with moderate atrophy of the breast tissue and associated Class A-B ptosis. *C,D,* Four months after ptosis correction and augmentation with a 165 ml gel prosthesis placed in the submammary position.

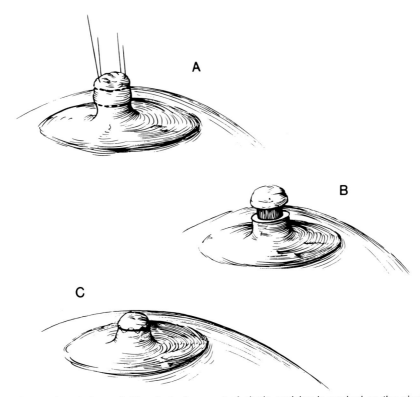

Figure 78–31. Regnault technique. *A,* The desired amount of nipple excision is marked on the nipple. *B,* The area within the markings is deepithelized. *C,* Small, buried 5-0 Vicryl sutures and a 4-0 nylon subcuticular suture approximate the nipple at its new height.

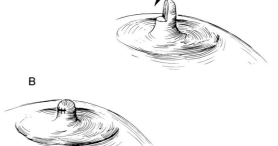

Figure 78–32. Pitanguy technique. *A,B,* A simple "L"-type nipple excision of one-half of the nipple with the remaining portion of the nipple turned as a flap, decreasing the nipple height.

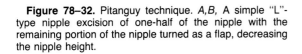

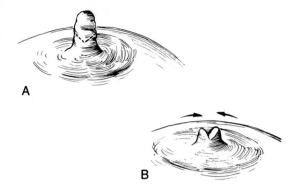

A

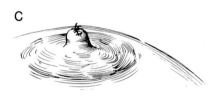

B

Figure 78–33. *A* to *C,* A V-type nipple excision at any level can decrease the nipple projection but causes some ductal obstruction.

C

Figure 78–34. Nipple inversion. *A, B,* The inverted nipple is isolated and retracted superiorly with two 4-0 nylon sutures. At the point of great protrusion an incision is made. *C,D,* The perinipple area is undermined as shown and a pursestring suture is inserted around the base to give greater nipple projection. *E,* The redundant tissue in the areola is trimmed slightly to the base of the new nipple, leaving some of the residual "dog-ears" to minimize postoperative tension on the areola.

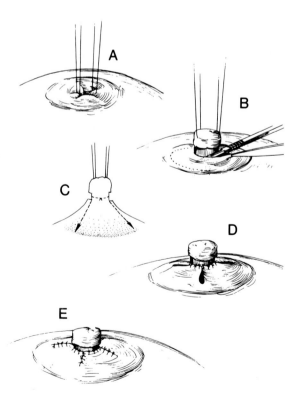

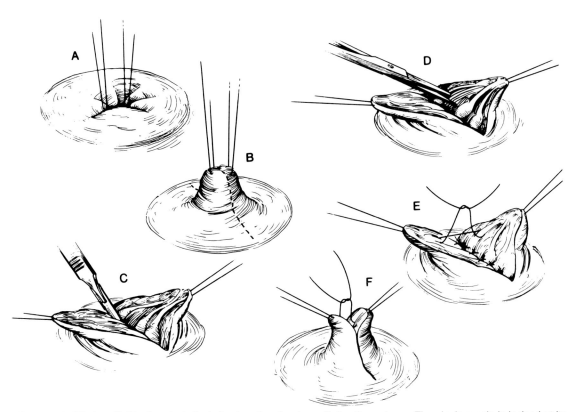

Figure 78–35. *A to C,* The inverted nipple is placed on tension with traction sutures. The nipple areola is incised at its midline through the entire thickness of the nipple into the breast itself. *D,* The fibrous and muscular tissue between the ducts is incised. *E,F,* The breast tissue and nipple are approximated, maintaining the nipple in a projecting position.

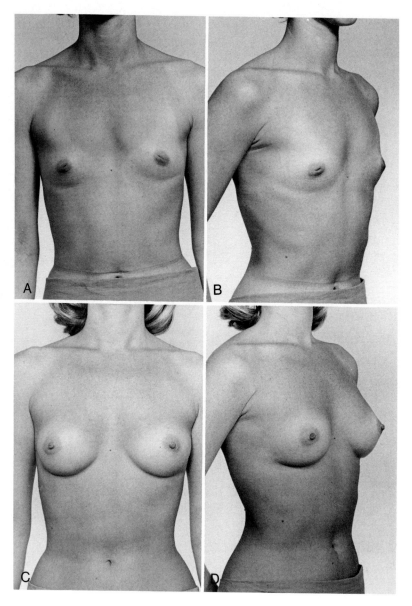

Figure 78–36. *A,B,* Preoperative frontal and oblique views of a 30 year old patient with mammary hypoplasia and inverted nipples. *C,D,* One-year postoperative views. Note that the nipple inversion has been corrected by the Pitanguy technique. Gel-filled prostheses were used for augmentation.

nipple in an inverted position. There is also an associated deficiency of fibrous and collagenous bulk beneath the nipple. In this technique the ducts and connective tissue are severed at right angles, releasing the shortened ducts. Closure is carried out in layers as illustrated (Figs. 78–37, 78–38).

Schwager and associates (1974) described a technique that made a periareolar incision along the inferior half of the areola. The areola and nipple tissue is separated from the underlying breast tissue, care being taken to preserve as much of the ductile tissue as possible. The nipple is everted and maintained in position with a buried pursestring suture.

PROLIFERATIVE BREAST DISEASE

The term "fibrocystic disease" has been largely abandoned in recent years as a greater understanding of this condition has resulted in differentiation between significant and physiologic changes in the breast. Emphasis is now placed on the presence of proliferative disease of the breast rather than on the nonproliferative or simple cystic components.

Studies by Dupont and Page (1985) have clarified the risk factors in women with benign proliferative breast lesions. Women with a family history of breast cancer appear to be at only a slightly greater risk of developing breast malignancy when they are found to have nonproliferative lesions such as cysts, fibroadenomas, apocrine changes, or mild hyperplasia without a tendency for cellular bridging or space distention, sclerosing adenosis, epithelium-related calcification, or papillary apocrine disease. In women having proliferative breast disease without atypical hyperplasia there appears to be an increased cancer risk almost twice that of women with nonproliferative disease. The addition of atypical hyperplasia (atypia) increases the risk to almost five and one-half times that in nonproliferative disease.

The most striking finding of Dupont and Page (1985) in their evaluation of over 10,000 consecutive breast biopsies was that women with atypical lobular or ductal hyperplasia and a positive family history have an 11 times greater risk of developing breast cancer. Other pertinent findings were that the presence of calcification in a patient with proliferative breast disease also increases the risk of malignancy. It was also noted that patients with cysts and positive family history have almost a three times increased risk factor. Women over 55 years of age with proliferative disease have an increased risk factor of 2.2.

It would appear from these studies that a breast biopsy may be indicated in patients with dense, nodular breasts and a positive family history. A diagnosis of atypical hyperplasia with a positive family history in properly selected patients appears to identify them as valid candidates for consideration of a subcutaneous mastectomy.

The patient whose breast examination is difficult owing to extensive benign nodular disease with nonspecific mammographic findings and marked breast density provides the greatest degree of complexity in the early detection of breast neoplasia.

Subcutaneous Mastectomy

The amount of breast tissue excised in the techniques to be discussed is approximately 90 to 95 per cent (Jarrett, Cutler, and Teal, 1978; Woods, Irons, and Arnold, 1980; Georgiade and associates, 1982). This appears to be a reasonable goal in maximizing the specimen for adequate pathologic evaluation. Removal of the nipple is not routinely carried out at the time of the mastectomy. Careful tagging of the nipple base is done at the time of breast extirpation; this maneuver minimizes the need for nipple excision to approximately 1 per cent of the surgical cases. If the histologic examination reveals atypical epithelial hyperplasia or dysplastic changes in the nipple area, the nipple is excised under local anesthesia as a secondary procedure, usually by the fifth postoperative day.

TECHNICAL ASPECTS OF SUBCUTANEOUS MASTECTOMY

The actual location of the incision for the mastectomy depends on the size of the breast as well as the location of the nipple-areola complex and the degree of ptosis. Most patients can be managed by means of an inframammary incision lying approximately 5.5 cm inferior to the areola. This is a curvilinear incision extended laterally for a distance of 8 to 10 cm depending on the size of the breast

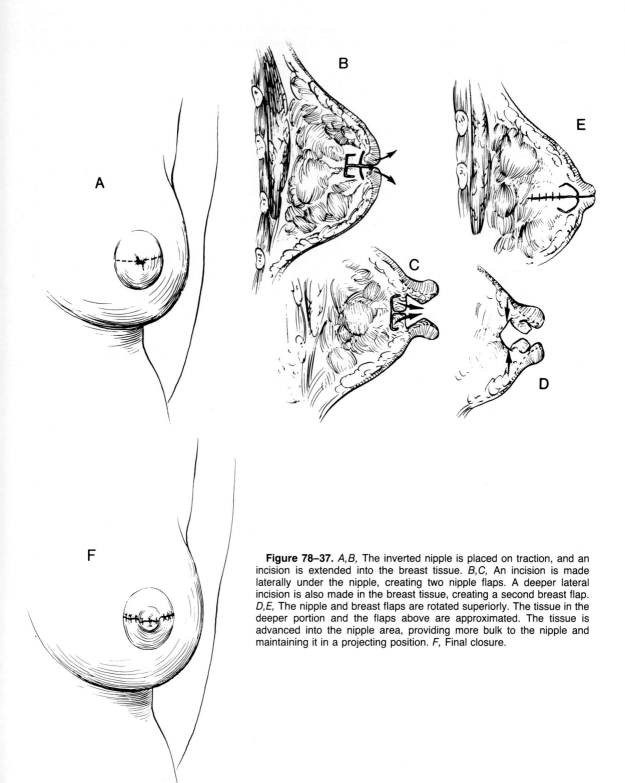

Figure 78–37. *A,B,* The inverted nipple is placed on traction, and an incision is extended into the breast tissue. *B,C,* An incision is made laterally under the nipple, creating two nipple flaps. A deeper lateral incision is also made in the breast tissue, creating a second breast flap. *D,E,* The nipple and breast flaps are rotated superiorly. The tissue in the deeper portion and the flaps above are approximated. The tissue is advanced into the nipple area, providing more bulk to the nipple and maintaining it in a projecting position. *F,* Final closure.

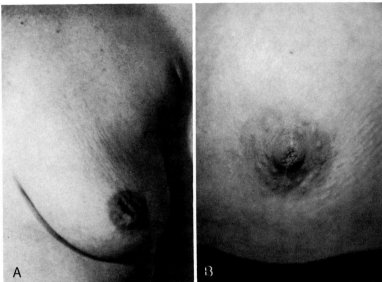

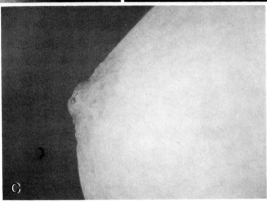

Figure 78–38. *A,* Preoperative appearance of a patient with inverted nipples. *B,C,* Frontal and oblique views one year postoperatively. (Photos courtesy of Drs. Broadbent and Woolf.)

and the volume of tissue to be removed (Fig. 78–39). The dissection is then carried to the serratus muscle and extended along the fascial plane over the pectoral musculature, separating the breast mass from its inferior fascial attachments (Fig. 78–40). The second plane of excision is initiated medially, separating the breast tissue and utilizing sharp dissection, which is extended in the fatty cushion layer between the breast tissue and the subdermal vascular plexus (see Fig. 78–39). A thicker layer of tissue is left at the nipple-areola base, and the specimen is marked for ease of identification. The dissection is also performed laterally and superiorly. The tail of Spence is included in the specimen. Removal of this distal portion of the breast is facilitated by retraction of the superior aspect of the pectoral muscle. Extension of this dissection also allows sampling of the inferior axillary lymph nodes.

A submuscular pocket is created. The in-

cision for the pocket is made over the seventh rib and through the serratus anterior muscle (see Fig. 78–40). Sharp dissection releasing the serratus muscle allows continuation of the dissection superiorly beneath this muscle and the pectoralis major (but above the pectoralis minor muscle). The dissection is extended medially, cauterizing the lower perforating branches of the internal mammary vessels, and inferiorly releasing the superior attachments of the rectus fascia. The wound is irrigated with bacitracin solution (50,000 units per 500 ml sterile saline). Hemostasis is obtained, a suction drain is inserted in the submuscular pocket, and another drain is inserted in the subcutaneous pocket.

A double-lumen, high profile prosthesis of suitable size (Fig. 78–41) is inserted, with adjustment for disparity on either side by the addition of sterile saline into the outer pocket of the prosthesis.

The serratus muscle layer is approximated

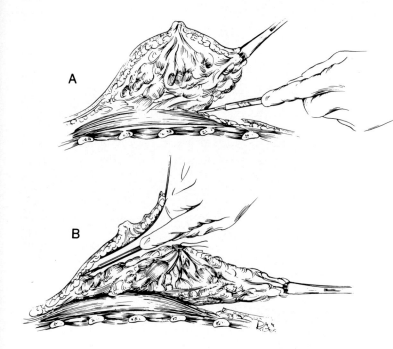

Figure 78–39. *A,* Excision of the breast tissue is on the pectoral fascia and is extended to the axillary area. *B,* Sharp dissection separates the breast tissue from the subdermal adipose layer. The base of the nipple is identified with a suture, as is the axillary tail of the specimen for orientation by the pathologist.

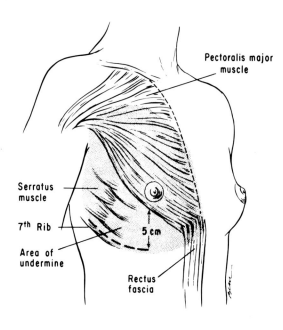

Figure 78–40. The skin incision is made in the inframammary fold. The incision through the serratus anterior muscles is at the level of the sixth or seventh ribs. Sharp dissection is carried under the pectoralis major, but above the pectoralis minor muscle, which is incised along the anterior axillary line. The dissection is extended medially and inferiorly beneath the rectus fascia and medially over the perforating internal mammary vessels.

rotary arm motions and large sweeping circles in both directions.

Management of Moderately Hypertrophied and Ptotic Breasts

Reduction of the breast and skin envelope at the time of subcutaneous mastectomy necessitates careful preoperative planning in order to minimize the frequency of nipple-areola necrosis. In these situations, a wide dermal pedicle is designed and used to carry the nipple areola to its new position at the time of ptosis correction (Figs. 78–43, 78–44). The prosthesis is inserted in the subpectoral-subserratus position as in a routine subcutaneous mastectomy. The less severe type of ptosis can be improved by utilizing superiorly based nipple-areola flaps (see Fig. 78–12).

Massively Hypertrophied Breasts

Resection of breast tissue in excess of 700 gm often necessitates consideration of repositioning of the nipple-areola complexes as free grafts. The grafts are placed over a dermal bed at the time of breast recontouring after insertion of the prosthesis in the submuscular position. The markings are the same as for a reduction mammoplasty, except that the keyhole area is not deepithelized. However, the same area is deepithelized after creation of the breast mound, and the nipple-areola graft is positioned in the new area (Fig. 78–45).

Complications

In spite of the surgeon taking all the necessary precautions, untoward results occasionally occur.

Hematoma Formation. This is usually manifest within the first 24 hours, and every effort should be made to evacuate the hematoma, preferably in the operating room under optimal conditions. Preoperatively, all medications such as aspirin or aspirin products that affect platelet aggregation should be eliminated. If the hematoma has caused ischemia to the overlying tissues in the nipple-areola complex, it may be preferable at this time to remove the prosthesis and replace it

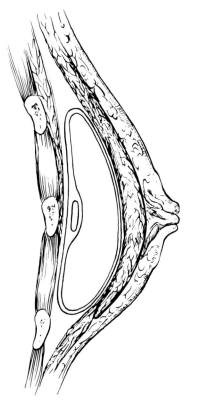

Figure 78–41. The position of the double-lumen prosthesis in the subpectoral-subserratus pocket. It is important to maintain the position of the prosthesis inferiorly to minimize fullness in the superior portion of the chest area.

using 4-0 nylon sutures placed between the inferior portion of the underlying fascia closer to the skin surface, to allow the prosthesis to be at a slightly lower level when the serratus muscle is reattached to its original location (see Fig. 78–40). An additional layer of 4-0 Vicryl is used to approximate the dermal layer. A 4-0 subcuticular running suture further approximates the skin edges and is followed by the application of sterile paper strips (Fig. 78–42).

The use of a bulky mechanic's waste dressing over the sterile dressing immobilizes the breast tissues and prostheses in the proper position. It is important that the breast mounds be examined within 24 hours to minimize possible damage by a hematoma, which should be evacuated.

The drains are usually removed by the fourth or fifth postoperative days, the submuscular drain being removed approximately one day before the subcutaneous drain.

Breast exercises are started on the tenth postoperative day. They usually consist of

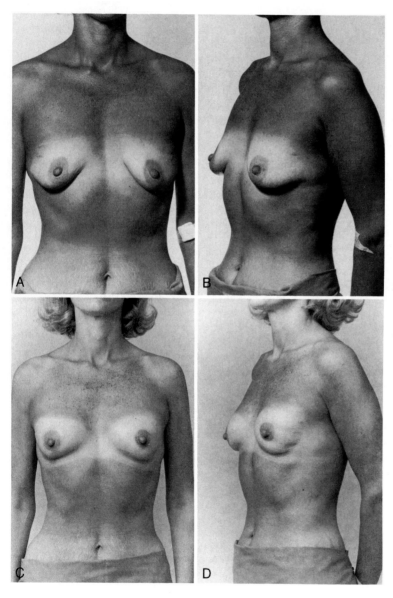

Figure 78–42. *A,B,* Preoperative frontal and oblique views of a 32 year old female with fibrocystic disease and ptosis. *C,D,* Six years after subcutaneous mastectomy and immediate reconstruction with subpectoral-subserratus double-lumen prostheses.

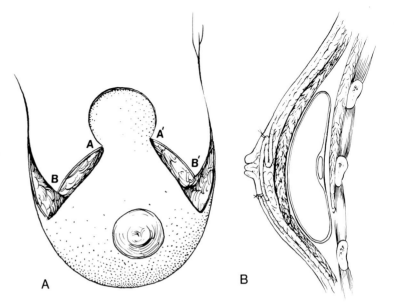

Figure 78–43. *A,* A wide dermal pedicle is important in order to maintain the vascularity of the nipple-areola complex. *B,* A cross sectional view of the superiorly based nipple-areola pedicle with the prosthesis in the subpectoral-subserratus position.

A

B

a few days later if the blood supply to the skin appears to be improved.

Tissue Ischemia. Tissue ischemia may occur particularly in the region of the nipple-areola complex. Unless this is marked, it usually is not necessary to remove the prosthesis if it has been placed in the subpectoral-subserratus position. The blood supply to the muscle usually provides additional vascularity to the ischemic area, and although a small area of tissue loss may occur, this area normally reepithelizes rapidly over a period of a few weeks.

Skin Redundancy or Persistent Ptosis. These may be present postoperatively and may be of concern initially to patients who had large, ptotic breasts before surgery. Secondary revision of the redundant tissue and correction of the nipple-areola ptosis can be carried out under local anesthesia a few months after the initial surgery.

AUGMENTATION MAMMOPLASTY

Ronald Riefkohl

The overwhelming majority of women who request an augmentation mammoplasty feel inadequate because of their small breasts (Baker, Kolin, and Bartlett, 1974). Most patients do not want excessively large breasts that would attract attention, but rather want to be "normal" and have a well-proportioned figure.

Breast enlargement has been accomplished by one of three approaches (Letterman and Schurter, 1978):

1. Materials have been injected within the breast, such as paraffin or silicone. However, this method has been condemned because of the severe complications that arise (Gurdin, 1972).

2. Numerous materials have been used to construct implants, such as polyvinyl alcohol, polyether, polyurethane, polypropylene, and silicone. An alloplastic implant (see Chap. 20) should be chemically inert, nonirritating, easy to construct, and noncarcinogenic. Silicone is available in fluid, gel, or solid forms, depending on the degree of polymerization and the amount of free silica added (Cronin and Gerow, 1964). Although silicone probably fulfills the requirements of an ideal breast implant, it may be minimally soluble and it causes a foreign body reaction. There are also reports of systemic illnesses, human adjuvant disease, and granulomas in regional lymph nodes associated with silicone implants (Riefkohl, Roberts, and McCarty, 1985).

3. Finally, attempts to enlarge the breasts with autogenous tissue such as lipoma, fat, dermal-fat grafts, and omentum have had unacceptable and unpredictable results.

Preoperative Evaluation

Most patients seeking breast enlargement have healthy motives, but many have a distorted understanding of the procedure and the limitations involved.

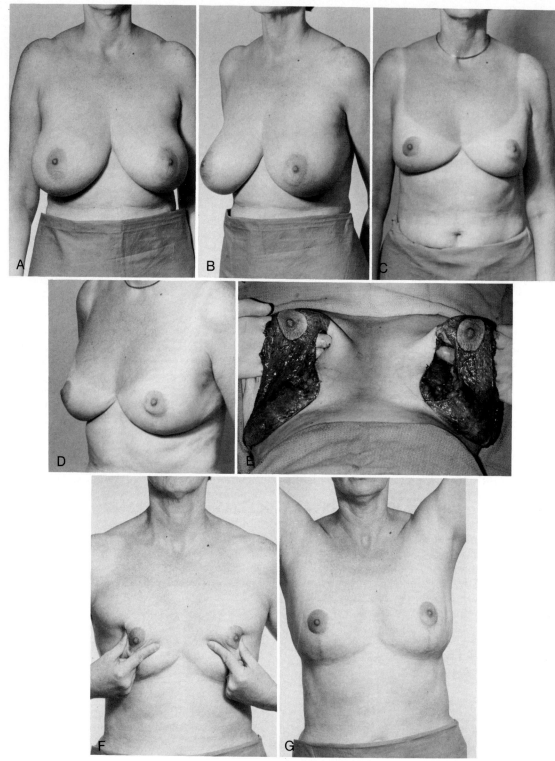

Figure 78–44. *A,B,* Preoperative frontal and oblique views of a 43 year old patient with extensive proliferative breast disease and associated ptosis and hypertrophy. *C,D,* Appearance 18 months after subcutaneous mastectomy and reduction mammoplasty, with resection of 1840 gm of breast tissue and insertion of a double-lumen prosthesis in the subpectoral-subserratus position. *E,* Intraoperative view showing the wide, vertical dermal pedicle flaps. *F,G,* Postoperative appearance revealing soft breast mounds without capsular contracture or deformity.

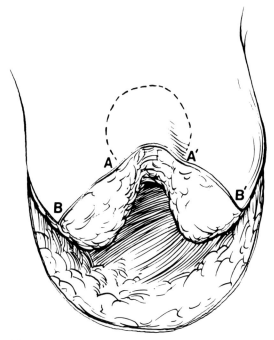

Figure 78–45. Flaps AB and A'B' are approximated following the subpectoral-subserratus insertion of the prosthesis. The new position of the nipple-areola complex is deepithelized and the graft is applied under a bolus.

The history taking should include a discussion of (1) previous breast problems, particularly if biopsies were obtained; (2) pregnancies and their effects on the breasts; (3) changes associated with menstruation, such as pain, swelling, enlargement, or nipple discharge; (4) a personal or family history of abnormal bleeding; (5) current medications; (6) drug allergies; and (7) past surgical procedures with any associated complications. Any family history of breast cancer should also be obtained.

The physical examination should focus on the general body build, particularly the dimensions and shape of the chest wall. The breast examination must be meticulous, noting the size of the breasts and nipple-areola complexes, the position of the breasts on the chest wall, any asymmetry in breast position or shape, the presence or absence of stretch marks or scars, the presence or absence of ptosis, and the type and degree of nodularity.

A candid discussion of any unusual finding is frequently enlightening in that some women are totally unaware of even markedly abnormal aspects. This is an appropriate time to review any unusual problems that will have a bearing on the result, such as tubular breasts, a chest wall abnormality, or a significant degree of ptosis.

Many patients have difficulty describing the breast size they desire. Numerous techniques to assist this selection have been described (Regnault, 1977; Brody, 1981). Patients frequently request a certain brassiere size, but unfortunately different brands of the same size vary in the fit. It is not prudent to promise a particular size, but rather one should obtain a general idea of the patient's wishes. One must temper this with surgical judgment as to the optimal size of implants that the patient can accommodate.

There are few contraindications to augmentation mammaplasty in a healthy patient who is otherwise a good surgical candidate. However, individuals who have inappropriate motives and goals or a serious psychologic disorder, or those who may have difficulty tolerating potential complications or limitations, should not be accepted for surgery.

Major preparations are unnecessary for this type of surgery, although patients should avoid aspirin in the preoperative period and should be free of concurrent infection. It probably is not feasible to avoid scheduling surgery during the last two weeks of the menstrual cycle, although this may be desirable for some patients. Preoperative oral antibiotics are unnecessary, although administration of an antibiotic intravenously 30 to 60 minutes before surgery is recommended. Frontal, lateral, and oblique photographs of the breasts should be obtained.

There is controversy regarding preoperative mammography. It probably should be performed in patients over 40 years of age, those with a family history of breast cancer, or those in whom significant nodularity is evident. Since there will be distortion and interference with interpretation of mammograms postoperatively (Smahel, 1978), a baseline study has little value.

Operative Technique

Regardless of whether the implants will be placed in a subglandular or a submuscular pocket, the inframammary folds should be marked with the patient in the upright position. The type of incision selected depends on several variables.

The advantage of the inframammary incision (Fig. 78–46) is its simplicity. However,

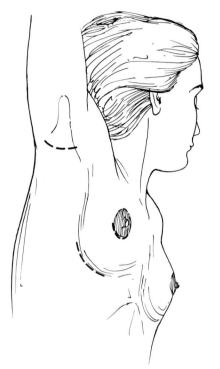

Figure 78–46. Incision sites employed for augmentation mammoplasty: transaxillary, periareolar, and inframammary.

tissue, which may confuse the mammographic interpretation. However, it is technically easier to incise directly through the breast tissue, and a much smaller periareolar incision is necessary. With the subcutaneous dissection, there is often induration and nodularity in the inferior aspect of the breasts, which usually resolves after several months. There is also more bruising in the inferior aspect of the breasts with the subcutaneous dissection. The incision is placed inferiorly at the junction of the areola with the skin. Medial shifting may preserve branches of the fourth intercostal nerve (Farina, Newby and Alani, 1980).

The transaxillary incision avoids placement of a scar on the breast (Höhler, 1977), but provides the worst exposure. An incision is made transversely in the center of the axilla, and either submuscular or subglandular dissection is done bluntly with a urethral sound (Fig. 78–47) (Höhler, 1977). It is difficult to obtain symmetric pockets with this technique, and damage to the intercostalbrachial nerve and subclavian vein thrombosis have been reported (Höhler, 1977).

If a concomitant abdominoplasty is planned, implants may be inserted through a

a well-defined inframammary crease is necessary, and usually the scars are more conspicuous than periareolar or transaxillary scars. Scar revision is frequently necessary (McKinney and Gilbert, 1983). The incision should be made just above the inframammary crease; a length of 4 cm is sufficient.

The periareolar incision results in the least conspicuous scar (Jones and Tauras, 1973; Courtiss and Goldwyn, 1976). The disadvantages are that the deep dissection is more difficult and the operative time is increased. Patients with small nipple-areola complexes or with areolae of light color may not be ideal. The deep plane of dissection may be reached by incising vertically through the breast tissue (Courtiss and Goldwyn, 1976; Wilkinson, 1983), or by dissecting subcutaneously to the inframammary crease (Jones and Tauras, 1973; Rees, Guy, and Coburn, 1973), thus not transversing breast tissue. There are several possible problems associated with incising through breast tissue, such as bacterial contamination of the wound; cicatricial blockage of breast tissue that could lead to cyst formation, particularly during pregnancy; and microcalcification within scar

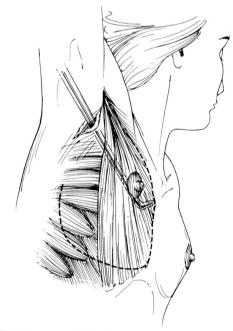

Figure 78–47. Although the submuscular dissection is depicted as done through a transaxillary incision, the principle of widely releasing the pectoralis major and serratus anterior muscles applies for any incision. The muscle attachments are bluntly avulsed inferiorly and medially.

tunnel from the abdominoplasty wound (Hinderer, 1975; Regnault, 1983).

LOCATION OF IMPLANT

Implants have been classically placed beneath the gland (Fig. 78–48A), the advantages being the ease of the dissection, more predictable sizing and contouring, and satisfactory results, provided that capsular contracture does not occur (Hetter, 1979). Submuscular placement may be necessary, however, for the very thin patient with minimal breasts (Courtiss and Goldwyn, 1976; Regnault, 1977).

The rationale for submuscular placement (Fig. 78–48B) is based on problems associated with subglandular placement, especially capsular contracture (Dempsey and Latham, 1968; Griffiths, 1969; Regnault, 1977; Scully, 1981; Mahler, Ben-Yakar, and Hauben, 1982; Tebbetts, 1984), although sensory changes in the nipple, the potential for communication with breast parenchyma, and interference with the interpretation of mammograms are also avoided.

The submuscular dissection is easier and relatively avascular (Truppman and Ellenby, 1978), and there is no communication with breast parenchyma, thus, theoretically, there is no contamination from breast bacteria (Fig. 78–48B). Minimal sensory changes in the nipple occur, but are usually temporary (Tebbetts, 1984). Pathologic breast conditions are easier to detect mammographically (Bostwick, 1983), and a biopsy will not endanger the implant. There are also fewer complications such as hematoma, infection, and extrusion of the implant (Truppman and Ellenby, 1978). However, submuscular placement is undesirable if there is any significant degree of ptosis (Tebbetts, 1984) or if a distinct inframammary fold exists (Maxwell, 1984). The implants may ride upward or shift laterally over time, causing an asymmetry in implant position (Tebbetts, 1984). In addition, the inframammary folds will be less distinct and a double fold deformity may be present in some patients. It is also difficult to perform closed capsulotomies in the 5 to 10 per cent of patients who develop capsular contractures (Truppman and Ellenby, 1978; Tebbetts, 1984). Muscular contraction over the implant can be unattractive, and "cleavage" is not as easily obtained (Regnault, 1977). Finally, there is more postoperative pain than in the subglandular dissection (Regnault, 1977).

DISSECTION OF POCKET

The subglandular dissection should be as large as possible, but dissection in the lateral aspect is minimized to avoid injury to the lateral cutaneous nerves.

A submuscular implant may be either partially or completely covered by muscle (Regnault, 1983). The implant is positioned beneath the pectoralis major but above the pectoralis minor muscle. If the implant is completely submuscular, dissection of the pocket must extend 1 to 2 cm below the inframammary crease; thus, the pectoralis major muscle must be detached inferiorly. The degree of medial detachment of the pectoralis major muscle varies from only stretching of the sternal attachments to complete transection. The intercostal nerves laterally must still be preserved (see Fig. 78–40).

A transaxillary approach to the breast is considerably more difficult and hemostasis may become a problem, particularly along the inferior and medial muscle attachments (see Fig. 78–47).

Before insertion of the implant, the wound should be carefully inspected and thorough

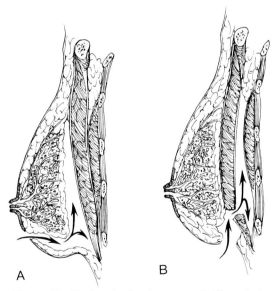

A   B

Figure 78–48. Prosthesis placement. *A,* The subglandular dissection is depicted as approached through a periareolar incision, with additional subcutaneous dissection to the inframammary region. *B,* The submuscular dissection is depicted as approached through an inframammary incision. Either subglandular or submuscular dissection may be done through any incision.

hemostasis secured. The pockets should be irrigated either with normal saline or with an antibiotic solution.

IMPLANTS

Most implants are disc shaped, although teardrop or modified teardrop configurations are also popular. Orienting of the latter two types may be difficult and, because of the recommendations to dissect a large pocket and massage the breasts postoperatively, late deformity due to rotation of implants within the capsule may occur.

Several types of implants are currently available. The gel-filled silicone implant was first introduced by Cronin and Gerow (1964) but it no longer has Dacron patches or seams. The main problem associated with this type of implant is leaching of silicone gel through the shell.

The inflatable implant is reputedly associated with softer capsules because of the absence of silicone leaching. However, few studies support this contention (McKinney and Gilbert, 1983), and hard breasts still occur (Regnault and associates, 1972; Asplund, 1984). In experimental studies there is no difference between capsules associated with gel-filled and inflatable implants. The advantages are the greater ease of implant insertion through a smaller incision, and the ability to correct an asymmetry by placing different volumes in the implants (Regnault and associates, 1972). Medications may also be added to the saline solution, as the silicone shell is an osmotic membrane (Rees, Guy, and Coburn, 1973). The main disadvantage of inflatable implants is a deflation rate ranging from 1.2 to 76 per cent (Williams, 1972; Rees, Guy, and Coburn, 1973; McKinney and Gilbert, 1983). The cause of this deflation was leakage from valves and seams in earlier models, but the newer models apparently perforate at a crease or fold where stress fatigue of the silicone shell occurs. Thus, many surgeons do not recommend underfilling these implants; however, capsular contracture may still produce folds in a normally filled or overfilled implant. Other reported problems are a "sloshing" effect due to air bubbles left within the implants (Courtiss, Webster, and White, 1974), and palpable valves with earlier models.

The main rationale for the double-lumen implant is that it prevents leaching of silicone gel into the surrounding tissues. Another advantage is the additional security provided if the inner shell breaks: the gel will be contained by the outer shell. In addition, if the outer shell perforates, the implant does not totally deflate. Slight breast asymmetry may be corrected and, as with inflatable implants, medications may be added to the outer compartment. One model also has a percutaneous valve through which medication or saline may be added or removed (O'Keeffe, 1981). The disadvantage of the double-lumen implant is possible perforation of the outer shell. Thus, a significant breast asymmetry should be corrected with different-size implants so that only a minimal amount of fluid is added to the outer compartment to obtain symmetry.

The polyurethane-covered silicone gel implant currently remains clouded with controversy. The first such implant was introduced by Ashley (1970, 1972), who reported no significant problems. The rationale for this implant is minimal capsule formation (Ashley, 1970, 1972; Capozzi and Pennisi, 1981; Herman, 1984); however, hard breasts have still been reported (Slade and Peterson, 1982). It is postulated that the ingrowth of scar tissue into the polyurethane surface breaks up the vector forces of scar contracture, and thus the capsule of scar is not able to contract in unison into a sphere, as occurs around a silicone implant (Capozzi and Pennisi, 1981; Brand, 1984). However, this theory has not been supported by scientific study (Brody, 1984).

There are, moreover, many disadvantages associated with polyurethane implants. A longer incision is necessary for insertion; it is difficult to insert and position the implant; it is difficult to remove at the time of reoperation (Slade and Peterson, 1982; Eyssen, von Werssowetz, and Middleton, 1984; Brand, 1984); and an allergic reaction, which appears to be self-limiting, occurs in a small percentage of patients (Eyssen, von Werssowetz, and Middleton, 1984). Another problem is that blood collects between the polyurethane shell and the silicone implant (Sterling, 1985). One major concern is that the polyurethane shell is degraded (Smahel, 1978; Slade and Peterson, 1982), but precisely what happens to this material is not known (Lilla and Vistnes, 1976). Studies reveal that polyurethane undergoes microfragmentation and phagocytosis, but it may also be broken down and dissolved within the tissues. There is an intense foreign body reaction with numerous macrophages and multinucleated giant cells (Brand, 1984), which may be so intense that severe cellulitis necessitating removal of the implant has occurred (Cocke, Leathers, and Lynch, 1975). Late problems include a high infection rate, which may be difficult to resolve because all the polyurethane particles cannot be easily removed (Barker, Retsky, and Schultz, 1978; Capozzi and Pennisi, 1981; Slade and Peterson, 1982; Brand, 1984; Nagel, 1985; Sterling, 1985). In addition, the breasts lack "bounciness"; axillary lymphadenopathy may occur; and with vigorous manipulation of the breasts, there may be late hematomas (Jervis, 1985).

Three types of polyurethane implants have been used: the Ashley (Ashley, 1970); the Natural-Y (Eyssen, von Werssowetz, and Middleton, 1984); and the Meme (Herman, 1984). The Meme does not have the Y septum present in the Natural-Y and it also is reported to be softer. The polyurethane coat in the Meme implant has a different pore size and density. All these implants are easily damaged during insertion or removal at the time of surgery.

IMPLANT PLACEMENT AND WOUND CLOSURE

Regardless of the type of implant selected, it should be carefully handled and inserted. Glove powder or lint should be removed from the implant surface.

The use of drains is controversial (Cronin and Greenberg, 1970), but they are probably unnecessary if thorough hemostasis is achieved.

The installation of steroids or antibiotic solutions within the pocket or within the implant has many advocates.

The wound should be closed with meticulous technique and without damaging the implant.

Postoperative Management

The type of dressing varies from a brassiere to a large, bulky, occlusive bandage. Postoperative antibiotics are probably unnecessary. The restrictions on postoperative patient activities vary considerably, but most surgeons today believe that early activity combined with a vigorous massage program is preferable (Courtiss, Webster, and White, 1974).

The follow-up regimen also varies; however, it probably is prudent to see the patients frequently to reinforce the importance of massage programs and to examine the breasts. It has been observed that forbidding the wearing of brassieres may reduce the incidence of difficult capsular contractures (Cole, 1985). "Prophylactic" compression capsulotomies should also be performed routinely, rather than when needed, since release of adhesions is frequently achieved even with soft breasts (Cole, 1982).

Mammograms should be obtained as indicated. There is controversy about the interpretation of these studies (Pennisi, 1978), and it was reported that only 25 per cent of the breast parenchyma is visible with the gel implant (Wolfe, 1978). However, calcification or consolidation associated with breast pathology can still be visualized (Rintala and Svinhufvud, 1974; Pennisi, 1978). Inflatable implants have been reported to be opaque (Cohen, Goodman, and Theogaraj, 1977; Wolfe, 1978), but others reported that the breast parenchyma is still well visualized (Snyder, 1978). With a subglandular implant insertion the breast tissue is compressed, thus altering the pattern ordinarily seen (Rintala and Svinhufvud, 1974).

Complications

Fluid Accumulation. Fluid accumulation was a common problem with the older implants and apparently was treated with simple aspiration (Cronin and Greenberg, 1970; Williams, 1972; Gurdin, 1972).

Hematoma. The frequency of hematomas in some studies is less than 2 per cent (Cronin and Greenberg, 1970; Williams, 1972). The associated symptoms are pain, swelling, and occasionally fever. Hematomas may develop slowly without symptoms or rapidly with symptoms. They should be drained surgically unless they are very small; immediate drainage is not always necessary. After several days the blood clot liquefies, facilitating removal, and there will be no active oozing within the pocket. However, if the hematoma is painful or large, surgical drainage should be carried out immediately.

Sensory Changes. Changes in nipple-areola sensation probably occur temporarily in most patients, but in 15 per cent dysesthesia and anesthesia may be permanent (Courtiss and Goldwyn, 1976). The type of incision has no bearing on this complication (Courtiss and Goldwyn, 1976; Hetter, 1979; Farina, Newby, and Alani, 1980). Apparently, sensory changes are unlikely with submuscular implants, but it is still possible to damage the lateral intercostal nerves before they course upward over the breast parenchyma and pass subcutaneously to the nipple-areola complex (Courtiss and Goldwyn, 1976; Farina, Newby, and Alani, 1980).

Infection. The incidence of infection is approximately 2 to 4 per cent (Cronin and Greenberg, 1970; Courtiss, Goldwyn and Anastasi, 1979; Biggs, Cukier, and Worthing, 1982; McKinney and Gilbert, 1983). Infection is evident an average of 10 days postoperatively, but may occur at any time (Courtiss, Goldwyn, and Anastasi, 1979). It is manifested by swelling, discomfort, drainage, and occasional exposure of the implant. After routine cultures have been obtained, the wound should be drained and irrigated. Removal of the implant may not always be necessary, particularly if a periareolar incision was used with the original surgery (Courtiss, Goldwyn, and Anastasi, 1979). However, if the implant is not removed, severe capsular contracture usually follows. If the implant is removed, it may be replaced in three to six months (Biggs, Cukier, and Worthing, 1982). Most infections are caused by *Staphylococcus aureus, S. epidermidis* being the next most common organism (Courtiss, Goldwyn and Anastasi, 1979; McGrath and Burkhardt, 1984).

Scars. Hypertrophic scars are distinctly uncommon with periareolar incisions, but are not infrequent with inframammary incisions.

Asymmetry. Asymmetry in implant position may be attributed to the dissection of unequal pockets and/or capsular contracture. The problem may be resolved by either extension or plication of the pocket. When submuscular implants have shifted superiorly, additional pectoralis major muscle attachments usually need to be divided inferiorly and medially. Ptosis of implants has been reported with the use of steroids placed either in the pocket or in the prosthesis.

Implant Extrusion. Implant extrusion may occur through the overlying scar or normal skin (Gurdin, 1972). The usual cause is infection, but implant folds (Derman, Argenta, and Grabb, 1983), steroid instillation, or the wearing of a tight brassiere may be causative (Gurdin, 1972). The causative factors should be resolved and the implant replaced in a submuscular pocket.

Contour Irregularities. Palpable or visible contour irregularities were common with the older implants that had valves and seams (Cronin and Greenberg, 1970). They also occur after incomplete compression capsulotomy, or with rupture of a gel implant and consequent encapsulation of the extruded silicone gel. A breast cyst or tumor may be present and could be confused with a ruptured gel implant. A tight capsular contracture is probably the most common cause of an unattractive breast contour.

Capsular Contracture. Capsular contracture remains the most frustrating complication of augmentation mammoplasty and is the most common reason for both patient and physician dissatisfaction. It is one of the most challenging problems in esthetic surgery today.

A capsule of scar tissue forms around any nondegradable material that is too large to be engulfed by macrophages, and yet is so inert that a foreign body reaction does not occur. A contracture of the capsule results in spherical compression of the implant, and thus the loss of its pliability. Capsular contracture should not necessarily be considered a complication, but should be regarded as an exaggeration of normal wound healing. There is no well-circumscribed time interval during which capsular contracture occurs, but it is usually observed around four to eight months postoperatively. It may arise slowly or precipitously (Gayou and Rudolph, 1979).

The frequency of capsular contracture has been reported to be between 0 and 74 per cent (Hipps, Raju, and Straith, 1978; Gayou and Rudolph, 1979), but interpretation of the reported data is difficult because there are so many variables involved. In many studies it is not clear whether the incidence reflects the number of patients or the number of breasts. Classification of capsular contracture is also highly subjective, but the Baker system appears to be the most reproducible (Table 78–1) (Little and Baker, 1980).

The thickness of the capsule is not directly proportional to the palpable firmness (Gayou and Rudolph, 1979); however, studies on patient capsules suggest a relationship. Other studies imply that inflatable implants are associated with thinner capsules (Rudolph and associates, 1978).

Numerous factors have been proposed to be

Table 78–1. The Baker Classification of Capsular Contracture

Grade I	The augmented breast feels as soft as an unoperated breast
Grade II	Minimal—the breast is less soft; the implant can be palpated but is not visible
Grade III	Moderate—the breast is firmer; the implant can be palpated easily and it (or distortion from it) is visible
Grade IV	Severe—the breast is hard, tender, painful, and cold; distortion is present

associated with an increased likelihood of capsular contracture. There is suggestive evidence that leaching of silicone gel initiates contracture formation (Rudolph and associates, 1978; Barker, Retsky, and Schultz, 1978; McKinney and Gilbert, 1983; Ksander and Vistnes, 1985). However, the presence of silicone in the capsule is not always related to the degree of clinical hardness. Newer, low-bleed implants seem to cause less foreign body reaction (Gayou and Rudolph, 1979; Barker, Retsky, and Schultz, 1981), but long-term clinical studies are not available at this time. There is no correlation with the type of cutaneous scar formed (Gayou and Rudolph, 1979). Improperly managed hematomas often precede the development of firmness (Hipps, Raju, and Straith, 1978; Gayou and Rudolph, 1979). There is controversy as to whether rupture of a gel implant precipitates capsular contracture. Several studies (Rudolph and associates, 1978; Gayou and Rudolph, 1979) suggest that rupture is not a factor, and in fact satisfactory results were obtained by intentionally rupturing gel implants to treat capsular contracture (Freeman, 1972). However, this practice has been condemned because of experimental studies (Vistnes, Bentley, and Fogarty, 1977). Other studies suggest that free silica present in the shell is associated with capsular contracture (Rudolph and associates, 1978). Foreign bodies such as dust, lint, glove powder, or implant impurities may initiate the process. An inadequately sized pocket, in which the implant is tight when inserted, does not result in a soft breast.

Subclinical infection has been proposed to cause contracture. In experimental animals, *Staphylococcus epidermidis* inoculation is associated with thicker capsules than in controls (Shah, Lehman, and Tan, 1981; Shah, Lehman, and Stevenson, 1982). Several studies report culturing *S. epidermidis* from the wound during surgical capsulotomy (Shah, Lehman, and Tan, 1981; Burkhardt and associates, 1981). However, similar positive culture rates have also been reported at the time of augmentation mammoplasty (Courtiss, Goldwyn and Anastasi, 1979; Burkhardt and associates, 1981). Hence, interpretation of the role of this organism is difficult. On the other hand, frank infection definitely leads to capsular contracture (Hipps, Raju, and Straith, 1978).

There may be poorly understood physical and geometric properties of implants that influence contracture (Ksander and Vistnes, 1985). Finally, both postoperative management and patient compliance may also affect the incidence of capsular contracture.

The myofibroblast may be responsible for contracture, as capsules respond to smooth muscle stimulants and relaxants (Baker, Chandler, and LeVier, 1981). Myofibroblasts have been reported in both contracted and noncontracted capsules (Gayou and Rudolph, 1979) and are observed in 80 per cent of hard capsules. However, they are also present in soft capsules (Rudolph and associates, 1978).

There are numerous recommendations to modify or treat capsular contracture. Some writers suspect that small, unrecognized hematomas are a factor and suggest placing drains at the time of surgery (Hipps, Raju, and Straith, 1978; Gayou and Rudolph, 1979). Drains would also remove the steroids or antibiotic solutions placed within the wound. The design, size, and shell thickness of implants probably have an influence, and it is not entirely clear if inflatable or gel implants should be used. Both under- and overinflating of the implants have been recommended. Steroids, probably the most effective means of reducing the incidence, may be instilled within the wound or within the prosthesis (Peterson and Burt, 1974; Perrin, 1976; Vinnik, 1976). Steroids ameliorate the inflammatory response, reduce the activity and number of fibroblasts, and inhibit wound contracture (Baker, 1981). Placed within the wound, steroids reduced the capsule rate from 74 to 58 per cent. When "expansion exercises" were added to the regimen, the rate was further reduced to 28 per cent (Vinnik, 1976). However, the instilling of steroids within the wounds did not eliminate capsular contracture (Hipps, Raju, and Straith, 1978; Gayou and Rudolph, 1979; Carrico and Cohen, 1979). Also, there is dependent pooling of the steroids in an inferior position, and the period of time that steroids remain within the tissues is unknown. It is apparently more effective to place steroids within the prosthesis, but the intraluminal steroid concentration has a bearing on both the incidence of capsular contracture and steroid-related problems (Carrico and Cohen, 1979; Ellenberg and Braun, 1981; Cucin, Guthrie, and Graham, 1982; Caffee, 1984). If methylprednisolone is given, only 20 mg or less should be used per implant. The half-life of intraluminal methylprednisolone is 30 days (Perrin, 1976), but with double-lumen implants, less steroid diffuses into the tissues because some of the drug diffuses into the gel (Cucin, Guthrie, and Graham, 1982). Steroids are associated with a distinct set of problems, which occur more often with triamcinolone than with methylprednisolone (Ellenberg, 1977; Ellenberg and Braun, 1981): mainly thinning and atrophy of the overlying soft tissues (Ellenberg, 1977; Carrico and Cohen, 1979; Ellenberg and Braun, 1981; Oneal and Argenta, 1982). Steroid-related problems may occur as early as five months postoperatively (Ellenberg and Braun, 1981). The implants may shift inferiorly; there may be thinning of the surgical scars and striae; and bluish discoloration of the skin may occur (Hipps, Raju, and Straith, 1978; Carrico and Cohen, 1979; Gayou and Rudolph, 1979). Implants rarely may become exposed by erosion of the thin, overlying soft tissues (Carrico and Cohen, 1979), or may need to be removed because of impending erosion (Oneal and Argenta, 1982). If the steroid-containing implants are removed, the soft tissue atrophy usually reverses (Oneal and Argenta, 1982).

Another recommendation is percutaneous injection of steroids within the capsule (Baker, Bartels, and Douglas, 1976), but this maneuver risks damage to the implant and could produce undesirable tissue atrophy or skin pigment changes.

Antibiotics are beneficial if subclinical infection proves to be a factor in capsular contracture (Gayou and Rudolph, 1979; Burkhardt and associates, 1981). Studies have shown that cephalothin or gentamicin pass through the silicone shell and are still active 12 months postoperatively (Burkhardt and associates, 1981).

Pulsed electromagnetic energy treatment in association with a two-stage augmentation mammoplasty has been recommended (Silver, 1982). Defined as "diapulse" treatment, short bursts of nonthermal electromagnetic energy are administrated postoperatively.

Vitamin E, a series of related tocopherols with analogous biologic action (Baker, 1981), stabilizes lysosomal membranes, inhibits inflammation, reduces the number of fibroblasts, and retards collagen accumulation. Experimental studies showed no benefit after the second postoperative week (Peters, Shaw, and Raju, 1980). Clinical studies indicated that, by adjusting the dose as the clinical situation dictates, the number of severe contractures may be reduced substantially (Baker, 1981).

Many types of massage programs have been advocated and probably do help to minimize firmness, although patient compliance remains a significant problem.

Compression capsulotomies (Baker, Bartels, and Douglas, 1976; Nelson, 1981), accomplished by several different manual means to tear the capsule, are reasonably successful, although there are numerous possible complications: contour distortion due to an incomplete capsular tear, implant displacement or rupture, hematoma, infection, and various upper extremity injuries to surgeons (Laughlin, Raynor, and Habal, 1977; Nelson, 1980, 1981; Derman, Argenta, and Grabb, 1983). Implant rupture is an important risk; one study reported that 16 per cent of implants were found to be ruptured at open capsulotomy, although only 60 per cent of the patients had had closed capsulotomies (Derman, Argenta, and Grabb, 1983). Thus, many of these implants apparently ruptured from other causes. Unfortunately, implant rupture may also occur with high pressure injection of silicone into surrounding tissues (Nelson, 1980). The recurrence rate is also distressingly high (Baker, Bartels, and Douglas, 1976; Vinnik, 1976; Hipps, Raju, and Straith, 1978; Little and Baker, 1980), most recurrences being noted within the first six months. Some patients may require periodic compression capsulotomies indefinitely. However, if the breasts remain soft for one year, recurrences are unlikely (Little and Baker, 1980).

Surgical capsulotomy involves circumferential and radial division of the capsule and extension of the pocket (Fig. 78–49). The recurrence rate is approximately 30 per cent (Hipps, Raju, and Straith, 1978; Little and Baker, 1980). Complications include hema-

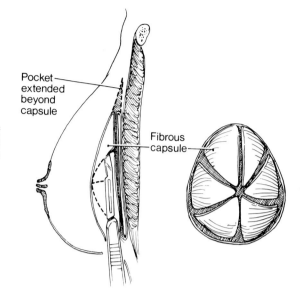

Figure 78–49. Surgical capsulotomy requires division of the fibrous spherical capsule with both circumferential and radial incisions. The size of the pocket should also be extended beyond the extent of the capsule.

toma formation, infection, and exposure of the implant (Nelson, 1981).

Capsulectomy has been recommended, but is unnecessary unless the capsule is calcified, in which case it should be completely removed. The recurrence rate is approximately 35 per cent (Hipps, Raju, and Straith, 1978).

Another recommendation is dissection of one side of the capsule and replacement of the implant in the new pocket (Mladick, 1977; Gayou and Rudolph, 1979).

Other methods advocated include exchanging the implant for a double-lumen type with steroids instilled in the outer compartment, and replacement of a subglandular implant into a submuscular pocket. If a tight capsule forms around a submuscular implant, surgical capsulotomy must be performed, and replacement with a double-lumen implant with steroids is probably indicated.

Loss of Cleavage. Loss of cleavage between the two breasts occurs if the pockets communicate (Georgiade, Riefkohl, and Georgiade, 1983). Treatment includes capsulotomy, medial plication to close the communication, and pocket extension superiorly and laterally.

Lactation Fistula. An internal lactation fistula has been reported (Georgiade, Riefkohl, and Georgiade, 1983). Augmentation mammoplasty should always be postponed until all the postpartum lactational changes in the breast have subsided.

Implant Rupture. Implant rupture may occur because of trauma, shell fatigue, or weakening from "fold friction" (Schmidt, 1980). There is always the possibility that an unrecognized injury to the implant may have occurred at the time of surgery. A ruptured gel bag implant is not always clinically apparent, but may be visualized by mammography.

Mondor's Disease. Mondor's disease (Georgiade, Riefkohl, and Georgiade, 1983), or thrombophlebitis of the inframammary veins, is not an uncommon postoperative problem. It usually is self-limiting and asymptomatic; however, a tender cord rarely may be palpated, particularly when the arm is elevated. No treatment is necessary.

Pneumothorax. Pneumothorax is a rare complication that may occur as a consequence of infiltration of local anesthetic or the performance of intercostal nerve blocks.

Other Issues

There is no evidence that silicone implants lead to breast carcinoma or sarcomatous changes (Hoopes, Edgerton, and Shelley, 1967). It is puzzling why so few cases of breast carcinoma have been reported in women who have had augmentation mammoplasty, but it may be that the group at risk has not aged sufficiently. However, several cases have been reported (de Cholnoky, 1970; McKinney and Gilbert, 1983; Gottlieb and associates, 1984).

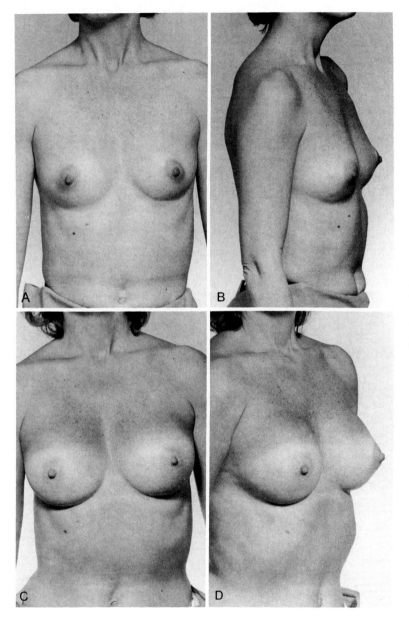

Figure 78–50. *A,B,* Preoperative frontal and oblique views of a 33 year old patient with small breasts. *C,D,* Appearance three years after augmentation utilizing a 5 cm infra-mammary incision and 185 ml gel-filled prostheses.

Figure 78–51. *A,B,* Frontal and oblique views of a 29 year old patient with hypoplastic breasts. Note the presence of supernumerary nipples. *C,D,* Four months after an inframammary incision and subpectoral muscle augmentation with double-lumen prostheses.

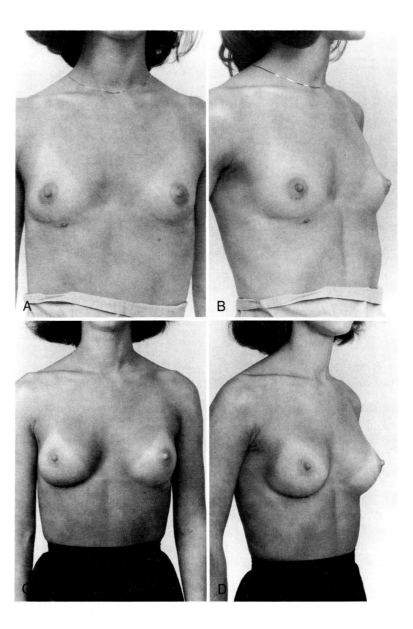

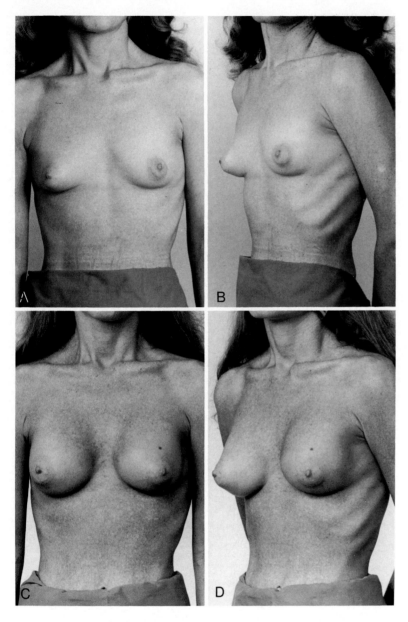

Figure 78–52. *A,B,* Preoperative frontal and oblique views of a 27 year old patient with moderate-sized areolae and small breasts. *C,D,* Postoperative views seven months after augmentation mammoplasty by means of a periareolar incision. Round gel prostheses were inserted.

Pregnancy and nursing are still possible after augmentation mammoplasty. There should be no difficulty unless there is blockage of ducts from the surgical scarring. Another relatively common problem related to pregnancy is capsular contracture, apparently because the patients temporarily abandon the massage programs.

Preexisting stretch marks on the breast are usually improved by augmentation mammoplasty, but rarely they are amplified and may become erythematous (Figs. 78–50, 78–51, 78–52).

REFERENCES

Arey, L. B.: Developmental Anatomy. 7th Ed. Philadelphia, W. B. Saunders Company, 1974.

Arie, G.: Una nueva tecnica de mastoplastia. Rev. Lat. Am. Cirurg. Plast., *3*:22, 1957.

Ashley, F. L.: A new type of breast prosthesis: preliminary report. Plast. Reconstr. Surg., *45*:421, 1970.

Ashley, F. L.: Further studies on the Natural-Y breast prosthesis. Plast. Reconstr. Surg., *49*:414, 1972.

Asplund, O.: Capsular contracture in silicone gel and saline–filled breast implants after reconstruction. Plast. Reconstr. Surg., *73*:270, 1984.

Aubert, V.: Hypertrophie mammaire de la puberté. Resection partielle restauratrice. Arch. franco-belg. de Chir., *26*:284, 1923.

Baker, J. L., Jr.: The effectiveness of alpha-tocopherol (vitamin E) in reducing the incidence of spherical contracture around breast implants. Plast. Reconstr. Surg., 68:696, 1981.

Baker, J. L., Jr., Bartels, R. J., and Douglas, W. M.: Closed compression technique for rupturing a contracted capsule around a breast implant. Plast. Reconstr. Surg., 58:137, 1976.

Baker, J. L., Jr., Chandler, M. L., and LeVier, R. R.: Occurrence and activity of myofibroblasts in human capsular tissue surrounding mammary implants. Plast. Reconstr. Surg., 68:905, 1981.

Baker, J. L., Jr., Kolin, I. S., and Bartlett, E. S.: Psychosexual dynamics of patients undergoing mammary augmentation. Plast. Reconstr. Surg., 53:652, 1974.

Bames, H.: The correction of pendulous breasts. Am. J. Surg., 10:80, 1930.

Bames, H.: Reduction of massive breast hypertrophy. Plast. Reconstr. Surg., 3:560, 1948.

Barker, D. E., Retsky, M. I., and Schultz, S.: "Bleeding" of silicone from bag-gel breast implants, and its clinical relation to fibrous capsule reaction. Plast. Reconstr. Surg., 61:836, 1978.

Barker, D. E., Retsky, M., and Schulz, S. L.: The new low bleed mammary prosthesis: an experimental study in mice. Aesth. Plast. Surg., 5:85, 1981.

Biesenberger, H.: Eine neue Methode der Mammaplastik. Zentralbl. f. Chir., 55:2382, 1928.

Biesenberger, H.: Eine neue Methode der Mammaplastik. Zentralbl. f. Chir., 57:2971, 1930.

Biesenberger, H.: Deformitäten und Kosmetische Operationen der Weiblichen Brust. Vienna, Verlag von Wilhelm Maudrich, 1931.

Biggs, T. M., Cukier, J., and Worthing, L. F.: Augmentation mammaplasty: a review of 18 years. Plast. Reconstr. Surg., 69:445, 1982.

Bostwick, J.: Aesthetic and Reconstructive Breast Surgery. St. Louis, C. V. Mosby Company, 1983.

Brand, K. G.: Polyurethane coated silicone implants and the question of capsular contraction (letter). Plast. Reconstr. Surg., 73:498, 1984.

Broadbent, T. R., and Woolf, R. M.: Benign inverted nipple: trans-nipple-areolar correction. Plast. Reconstr. Surg., 58:673, 1976.

Brody, G. S.: Breast implant size selection and patient satisfaction. Plast. Reconstr. Surg., 68:611, 1981.

Brody, G. S.: Discussion of Herman, S.: The Meme implant. Plast. Reconstr. Surg., 73:420, 1984.

Burkhardt, B. R., Fried, M., Schnur, P. L., and Tofield, J. J.: Capsules, infection, and intraluminal antibiotics. Plast. Reconstr. Surg., 68:43, 1981.

Caffee, H. H.: The effects of intraprosthetic methylprednisolone on implant capsules and surrounding soft tissue. Ann. Plast. Surg., 12:348, 1984.

Campbell, D.: Arabian Medicine and Its Influence on the Middle Ages. Vols. 1,2. London, Kegan Paul, French, Trubner, 1926.

Capozzi, A., and Pennisi, V. R.: Clinical experience with polyurethane-covered gel-filled mammary prostheses. Plast. Reconstr. Surg., 68:512, 1981.

Carr, B., Bishop, W., and Anson, B.: Mammary arteries. Q. Bull., Northwestern Univ. M. School, 16:150, 1942.

Carrico, T. J., and Cohen, I. K.: Capsular contracture and steroid-related complications after augmentation mammaplasty. A preliminary study. Plast. Reconstr. Surg., 64:377, 1979.

Claoué, C., and Bernard, I.: Données Anatomiques en Vue de la Chirurgie Réparatrice Mammaire. Paris, Librairie Maloine, 1935.

Cocke, W. M., Leathers, H. K., and Lynch, L. B.: Foreign body reactions to polyurethane covers of some breast prostheses. Plast. Reconstr. Surg., 56:527, 1975.

Cohen, I. K., Goodman, H., and Theogaraj, S. D.: Xeromammography—a reason for using saline-filled breast prostheses. Plast. Reconstr. Surg., 60:886, 1977.

Cole, N.: Personal communication, 1982.

Cole, N.: Personal communication, 1985.

Cooper, A. P.: On the Anatomy of the Breast. Vol. 2. London, Longmans, 1840, pp. 1–89.

Courtiss, E. H., and Goldwyn, R. M.: Breast sensation before and after plastic surgery. Plast. Reconstr. Surg., 58:1, 1976.

Courtiss, E. H., and Goldwyn, R. M.: Reduction mammaplasty by the inferior pedicle technique. An alternative to free nipple and areola grafting for severe macromastia or extreme ptosis. Plast. Reconstr. Surg., 59:500, 1977.

Courtiss, E. H., Goldwyn, R. M., and Anastasi, G. W.: The fate of breast implants with infections around them. Plast. Reconstr. Surg., 63:812, 1979.

Courtiss, E. H., Webster, R. C., and White, M. F.: Selection of alternatives in augmentation mammoplasty. Plast. Reconstr. Surg., 54:552, 1974.

Cramer, L., and Chong, J.: Unipedicle cutaneous flap: areola nipple transposition on an end-bearing, superiorly based flap. In Georgiade, N. G. (Ed.): Reconstructive Breast Surgery. St. Louis, C. V. Mosby Company, 1976, p. 143.

Cronin, T., and Gerow, F.: Augmentation mammoplasty: a new "natural feel" prosthesis. In Broadbent, T. R. (Ed.): Transactions of the Third International Congress of Plastic Surgery. Amsterdam, Excerpta Medica Foundation, 1964.

Cronin, T. D., and Greenberg, R. L.: Our experiences with the Silastic gel breast prosthesis. Plast. Reconstr. Surg., 46:1, 1970.

Cucin, R. L., Guthrie, R. H., and Graham, M.: Rate of diffusion of Solu-Medrol across the Silastic membranes of breast prostheses—an in vitro study. Ann. Plast. Surg., 9:228, 1982.

Dartigues, L.: Traitment chirurgical du prolapus mammaire. Arch. Franco-Belges Chir., 28:313, 1925.

da Silva, G.: Mastopexy with dermal ribbon for supporting the breast and keeping it in shape. Plast. Reconstr. Surg., 34:403, 1964.

Deaver J. B.: The Breast: Its Anomalies, Its Diseases and Their Treatment. Philadelphia, Blakiston, 1917.

de Cholnoky, T.: Supernumerary breast. Arch. Surg., 39:926, 1939.

de Cholnoky, T.: Augmentation mammaplasty: survey of complications in 10,941 patients by 265 surgeons. Plast. Reconstr. Surg., 45:573, 1970.

Dempsey, W. C., and Latham, W. D.: Subpectoral implants in augmentation mammaplasty: preliminary report. Plast. Reconstr. Surg., 42:515, 1968.

Derman, G. H., Argenta, L. C., and Grabb, W. C.: Delayed extrusion of inflatable breast prosthesis. Ann. Plast. Surg., 10:154, 1983.

Dufourmentel, C., and Mouly, R.: Plastie mammaire par la méthode oblique. Ann. Chir. Plast., 6:45, 1961.

Dupont, W. D., and Page, D. L.: Risk factors for breast cancer in women with proliferative breast disease. N. Engl. J. Med., 312:146, 1985.

Ellenberg, A. H.: Marked thinning of the breast skin flaps after the insertion of implants containing triamcinolone. Plast. Reconstr. Surg., 60:755, 1977.

Ellenberg, A. H., and Braun, H.: A 3½ year experience with double-lumen implants in breast surgery. Plast. Reconstr. Surg., 65:307, 1981.

Eyssen, J. E., von Werssowetz, A. J., and Middleton, G.

D.: Reconstruction of the breast using polyurethane-coated prostheses. Plast. Reconstr. Surg., *73*:415, 1984.

Farina, M. A., Newby, B. G., and Alani, H. M.: Innervation of the nipple-areola complex. Plast. Reconstr. Surg., *66*:497, 1980.

Freeman, B. S.: Successful treatment of some fibrous envelope contractures around breast implants. Plast. Reconstr. Surg., *50*:107, 1972.

Gallagher, H., Leis, H., Snyderman, R., and Urban, J.: The breast. *In* Reyniak, J. (Ed.): Physiology. St. Louis, C. V. Mosby Company, 1978, p. 23.

Galvao, M.: Reduction mammoplasty with preservation of the superior, medial, lateral and inferior pedicles. *In* Georgiade, N. G. (Ed.): Aesthetic Breast Surgery. Baltimore, Williams & Wilkins Company, 1983, p. 175.

Gayou, R., and Rudolph, R.: Capsular contraction around silicone mammary prostheses. Ann. Plast. Surg., *2*:62, 1979.

Georgiade, N. G., and Georgiade, G. S.: Reduction mammaplasty utilizing the inferior pyramidal dermal pedicle flap. *In* Georgiade, N. G. (Ed.): Aesthetic Breast Surgery. Baltimore, Williams & Wilkins Company, 1983, p. 291.

Georgiade, N. G., Riefkohl, R., and Georgiade, G. S.: Problems in aesthetic breast surgery and their management. *In* Georgiade, N. G. (Ed.): Aesthetic Breast Surgery. Baltimore, Williams & Wilkins Company, 1983, p. 365.

Georgiade, N. G., Serafin, D., Morris, R., and Georgiade, G.: Reduction mammaplasty utilizing an inferior pedicle nipple-areolar flap. Ann. Plast. Surg., *3*:211, 1979a.

Georgiade, N. G., Serafin, D., Riefkohl, R., and Georgiade, G. S.: Is there a reduction mammaplasty for "all seasons"? Plast. Reconstr. Surg., *63*:765, 1979b.

Georgiade, N. G., Serafin, D., Georgiade, G. S., and McCarty, K. S., Jr.: Subcutaneous mastectomy: an evolution of concept and technique. Ann. Plast. Surg., *8*:8, 1982.

Goin, J. M., Goin, M. K., and Gianini, M. H.: The psychic consequences of a reduction mammaplasty. Plast. Reconstr. Surg., *59*:530, 1977.

Goldwyn, R.: Plastic and Reconstructive Surgery of the Breast. Boston, Little, Brown and Company, 1976.

Gottlieb, V., Muench, A. G., Rich, J. D., and Pagadala, S.: Carcinoma in augmented breasts. Ann. Plast. Surg., *12*:67, 1984.

Goulian, D.: Modified dermal mastopexy operation for resection of breast tissue allowing simultaneous reconstruction. *In* Georgiade, N. G. (Ed.): Reconstructive Breast Surgery. St. Louis, C. V. Mosby Company, 1976, p. 202.

Gray, S. W., and Skandalakis, J. E.: Embryology for Surgeons. Philadelphia, W. B. Saunders Company, 1972, p. 405.

Griffiths, C. O.: The submuscular implant in augmentation mammoplasty. *In* Sanvenero-Rosselli, G. (Ed.): Transactions of the Fourth International Congress of Plastic Surgery. Amsterdam, Excerpta Medica Foundation, 1969.

Gurdin, M.: Augmentation mammoplasty. *In* Goldwyn, R. M., (Ed.): The Unfavorable Result in Plastic Surgery—Avoidance and Treatment, Boston, Little, Brown and Company, 1972.

Haagensen, C. D.: Diseases of the Breast. 3rd Ed. Philadelphia, W. B. Saunders Company, 1986.

Handley, R. S.: The anatomy of the breast. *In* Breast Cancer and Its Diagnosis and Treatment. Baltimore, Williams & Wilkins Company, 1955, p. 8.

Hauben, D. J., and Mahler, D.: A simple method for the correction of the inverted nipple. Plast. Reconstr. Surg., *71*:556, 1983.

Herman, S.: The Meme implant. Plast. Reconstr. Surg., *73*:411, 1984.

Hetter, G. P.: Satisfactions and dissatisfactions of patients with augmentation mammaplasty. Plast. Reconstr. Surg., *64*:151, 1979.

Hinderer, U. T.: The dermolipectomy approach for augmentation mammaplasty. Clin. Plast. Surg., *2*:359, 1975.

Hipps, C. J., Raju, D. R., and Straith, R. E.: Influence of some operative and postoperative factors on capsular contracture around breast prostheses. Plast. Reconstr. Surg., *61*:384, 1978.

Höhler, H.: Further progress in the axillary approach in augmentation mammaplasty: prevention of encapsulation. Aesth. Plast. Surg., *1*:107, 1977.

Holländer, E.: Die Operation der Mammahypertrophie und der Hängebrust. Dtsch. Med. Wochensch., Leipz. u. Berl., *1*:1400, 1924.

Hollinshead, W. H.: Anatomy for Surgeons. Vol. 2. New York, Harper & Row, 1971, p. 17.

Hoopes, J. E., Edgerton, M. T., Jr., and Shelley, W.: Organic synthetics for augmentation mammaplasty: their relation to breast cancer. Plast. Reconstr. Surg., *39*:263, 1967.

Hugo, N. E., and Bauer, B.: Reduction mammoplasty, single superiorly based pedicle. *In* Georgiade, N. (Ed.): Aesthetic Breast Surgery. Baltimore, Williams & Wilkins Company, 1983, p. 235.

Jarrett, J. R., Cutler, R. G., and Teal, D. F.: Subcutaneous mastectomy in small, large, or ptotic breasts with immediate submuscular placement of implants. Plast. Reconstr. Surg., *62*:702, 1978.

Jervis, W.: Experience with polyurethane covered implants. Presented at The American Society for Aesthetic Plastic Surgery, Boston, 1985.

Jones, F. R., and Tauras, A. P.: A periareolar incision for augmentation mammaplasty. Plast. Reconstr. Surg., *51*:641, 1973.

Kallius, E.: Ein Fall von Milchleiste bei einem menschlichen Embryo. Anat. Hefte, Wiesb., *8*:153, 1897.

Kraske, H.: Die Operation der atrophischen und hypertrophischen Hängebrust. Munch. Med Wochenschr., *70*:672, 1923.

Ksander, G. A., and Vistnes, L. M.: The incidence of experimental contracture varies with the source of the prosthesis. Plast. Reconstr. Surg., *75*:668, 1985.

LaLardrie, J.: Reduction mammoplasty: the "dermal vault" technique. *In* Georgiade N. G. (Ed.): Aesthetic Breast Surgery. Baltimore, Williams & Wilkins Company, 1983, p. 166.

Lamont, E.: Congenital inversion of the nipple in identical twins. Br. J. Plast. Surg., *26*:178, 1973.

Laughlin, R. A., Raynor, A. C., and Habal, M. B.: Complications of closed capsulotomies after augmentation mammoplasty. Plast. Reconstr. Surg., *60*:362, 1977.

Leclerc, L.: La Chirurgie D'Abulcasis. Paris, J. B. Bailliere, 1861, p. 128.

Letterman, G., and Schurter, M.: History of augmentation mammoplasty. *In* Owsley, J. Q., and Peterson, R. A. (Eds.): Symposium on Aesthetic Surgery of the Breast. St. Louis, C. V. Mosby Company, 1978, pp. 243–249.

Lewis, J.: Mammary ptosis. *In* Georgiade N. G. (Ed.):

Aesthetic Breast Surgery. Baltimore, Williams & Wilkins Company, 1983, p. 130.

Lewison, E. F.: Breast Cancer. Baltimore, Williams & Wilkins Company, 1985, p. 28.

Lexer, E.: Hypertrophie bei der Mammae. Munch. Med. Wochenschr., 59:2702, 1912.

Lilla, J. A., and Vistnes, L. M.: Long-term study of reactions to various silicone breast implants in rabbits. Plast. Reconstr. Surg., 57:637, 1976.

Little, G., and Baker, J. L.: Results of closed compression capsulotomy for treatment of contracted breast implant capsules. Plast. Reconstr. Surg., 65:30, 1980.

Mahler, D., Ben-Yakar, J., and Hauben, D. J.: The retropectoral route for breast augmentation. Aesth. Plast. Surg., 6:237, 1982.

Maxwell, G. P.: Discussion of "transaxillary subpectoral augmentation mammaplasty: long-term follow-up and refinements." Plast. Reconstr. Surg., 74:648, 1984.

McCarty, K. S., Jr., Glaubitz, L. C., Thienemann, M., and Riefkohl, R.: The breast: anatomy and physiology. In Georgiade, N. G. (Ed.): Aesthetic Breast Surgery. Baltimore, Williams & Wilkins Company, 1983, p. 1.

McCormack, R., and Bales, H.: Natural contour reduction mammaplasty for huge breasts. In Georgiade, N. G. (Ed.): Reconstructive Breast Surgery. St. Louis, C. V. Mosby Company, 1976, p. 212.

McGrath, M. G., and Burkhardt, B. R.: The safety and efficacy of breast implants for augmentation mammaplasty. Plast. Reconstr. Surg., 74:550, 1984.

McKinney, P., and Gilbert, T.: Long-term comparison of patients with gel and saline mammary implants. Plast. Reconstr. Surg., 72:27, 1983.

McKissock, P. K.: Reduction mammaplasty with a vertical dermal flap. Plast. Reconstr. Surg., 49:245, 1972.

McKissock, P. K.: Reduction mammaplasty by the vertical bipedicle flap technique: rationale and results. Clin. Plast. Surg., 3:309, 1976.

Meyer, R., and Kesselring, U.: Reduction mammoplasty (twelve years' experience with the L-shaped suture line). In Georgiade, N. G. (Ed.): Aesthetic Breast Surgery. Baltimore, Williams & Wilkins Company, 1983, p. 219.

Mladick, R. A.: Treatment of the firm augmented breast by capsular stripping and inflatable implant exchange. Plast. Reconstr. Surg., 60:720, 1977.

Montagna, W., and MacPherson, E. E.: Proceedings: some neglected aspects of the anatomy of human breasts. J. Invest. Dermatol., 63:10, 1974.

Morestin, H.: Hypertrophie mammaire. Bull. Mem. Soc. Anat., Paris, 80:682, 1905.

Mouly, R., and Bodin, B.: Reduction mammoplasty, lateral technique. In Georgiade, N. G. (Ed.): Aesthetic Plastic Surgery. Baltimore, Williams & Wilkins Company, 1983, p. 205.

Nagel, G. P.: Augmentation mammaplasty with the polyurethane prosthesis. Presented at The American Society for Aesthetic Plastic Surgery, Boston, April, 1985.

Nelson, G. D.: Complications of closed compression after augmentation mammaplasty. Plast. Reconstr. Surg., 66:71, 1980.

Nelson, G. D.: Complications from the treatment of fibrous capsular contracture of the breast. Plast. Reconstr. Surg., 68:969, 1981.

Noel, M., and Lopez-Martinez, M.: Nouveaux procédés chirurgicaux de correction du prolapsus mammaire. Arch. Franco-Belges Chir., 31:138, 1928.

O'Keeffe, P. J.: The steroid adjustable mammary implant. Aesth. Plast. Surg., 5:129, 1981.

Oneal, R. M., and Argenta, L. C.: Late side effects related to inflatable breast prostheses containing soluble steroids. Plast. Reconstr. Surg., 69:641, 1982.

Page, D. L., Dupont, W. D., Rogers, L. W., and Rados, M. S.: Atypical hyperplastic lesions of the female breast: a long-term follow-up study. Cancer, 55:2698, 1985.

Passot, R.: Mon procédé de correction esthétique de la ptose mammaire. Hôpital (Paris), 13:162, 1925.

Paulus, Ægineta, F.: On male breasts resembling the female. In Adams, F. (Transl.): The Seven Books of Paulus Æginata. Vol. 2, Book 6, Sect. 46. London, Sydenham Society, 1846, p. 334.

Penn, J.: Breast reduction. Br. J. Plast. Surg., 7:357, 1954.

Pennisi, V. R.: Discussion of "xeromammography—a reason for using saline-filled breast prostheses." Plast. Reconstr. Surg., 61:107, 1978.

Perrin, E. R.: The use of soluble steroids within inflatable breast prostheses. Plast. Reconstr. Surg., 57:163, 1976.

Peters, C. R., Shaw, T. E., and Raju, D. R.: The influence of vitamin E on capsule formation and contracture around silicone implants. Ann. Plast. Surg., 5:347, 1980.

Peterson, H. D., and Burt, G. B., Jr.: The role of steroids in prevention of circumferential capsular scarring in augmentation mammaplasty. Plast. Reconstr. Surg., 54:28, 1974.

Pitanguy, I.: Une nouvelle technique de plastie mammaire. Étude de 245 cas consécutifs et présentation d'une technique personnelle. Ann. Chir. Plast., 7:199, 1962.

Pitanguy, I.: Aesthetic Plastic Surgery of Head and Body. New York, Springer Verlag, 1981, p. 63.

Pitanguy, I.: Breast reduction and ptosis. In Georgiade, N. G. (Ed.): Aesthetic Breast Surgery. Baltimore, Williams & Wilkins Company, 1983, p. 247.

Pousson, M.: De la mastopexie. Bull. Mem. Soc. Chir., Paris, 23:507, 1897.

Rees, T. D., Guy, C. L., and Coburn, R. J.: The use of inflatable breast implants. Plast. Reconstr. Surg., 52:609, 1973.

Regnault, P.: Breast ptosis: definition and treatment. Clin. Plast. Surg., 3:193, 1973.

Regnault, P.: Reduction mammaplasty by the "B" technique. Plast. Reconstr. Surg., 53:19, 1974.

Regnault, P.: Nipple hypertrophy. A physiologic reduction by circumcision. Clin. Plast. Surg., 2:391, 1975.

Regnault, P.: Reduction mammaplasty by the "B" technique. In Goldwyn, R. (Ed.): Plastic and Reconstructive Surgery of the Breast. Boston, Little, Brown & Company, 1976, p. 269.

Regnault, P.: Partially submuscular breast augmentation. Plast. Reconstr. Surg., 59:72, 1977.

Regnault, P.: Partially subpectoral breast augmentation. In Georgiade, N. G. (Ed.): Aesthetic Breast Surgery. Baltimore, Williams & Wilkins Company, 1983, p. 87.

Regnault, P., Baker, T. J., Gleason, M. C., Gordon, H. L., Grossman, A. R., et al.: Clinical trial and evaluation of a proposed new inflatable mammary prosthesis. Plast. Reconstr. Surg., 50:220, 1972.

Ribeiro, L., and Backer, E.: Inferior based pedicles in mammaplasties. In Georgiade, N. G. (Ed.): Aesthetic Breast Surgery. Baltimore, Williams & Wilkins Company, 1983, p. 260.

Riefkohl, R., Roberts, T. L., 3rd, and McCarty, K. S., Jr.: Lack of adverse effect of silicone implant on sarcoidosis of the breast. Plast. Reconstr. Surg., 76:296, 1985.

Rintala, A. E., and Svinhufvud, U. M.: Effect of augmentation mammaplasty on mammography and thermography. Plast. Reconstr. Surg., *54*:390, 1974.

Robbins, T. H.: A reduction mammaplasty with the areola-nipple based on an inferior dermal pedicle. Plast. Reconstr. Surg., *59*:64, 1977.

Romanes, G.: Cunningham's Textbook of Anatomy. 11th Ed. London, Oxford University Press, 1972, p. 552.

Rubin, L. R.: The surgical treatment of the massive hypertrophic breast. *In* Georgiade, N. G. (Ed.): Aesthetic Breast Surgery. Baltimore, Williams & Wilkins Company, 1983, p. 322.

Rudolph, R., Abraham, J., Vecchione, T., Guber, S., and Woodward, M.: Myofibroblasts and free silicon around breast implants. Plast. Reconstr. Surg., *62*:185, 1978.

Sattin, R. W., Rubin, G. L., Webster, L. A., Huezo, C. M., Wingo, P. A., et al.: Family history and the risk of breast cancer. J.A.M.A., *253*:1908, 1985.

Schmidt, G. H.: Mammary implant shell failure. Ann. Plast. Surg., *5*:369, 1980.

Schultze, O.: Milchdrüsenentwickelung und Polymastie. Sitzungsb. d. Phys.-Med. Gesellsch. zu Würzburg, *26*:77, 1892.

Schwager, R. G., Smith, J. W., Gray, G. F., and Goulian, D., Jr.: Inversion of the human female nipple, with a simple method of treatment. Plast. Reconstr. Surg., *54*:564, 1974.

Schwarzmann, E.: Die Technik der Mammaplastik. Chirurgica, *2*:932, 1930.

Scully, S. J.: Augmentation mammaplasty without contracture. Ann. Plast. Surg., *6*:262, 1981.

Shah, Z., Lehman, J. A., Jr., and Stevenson, G.: Capsular contracture around silicone implants: the role of intraluminal antibiotics. Plast. Reconstr. Surg., *69*:809, 1982.

Shah, Z., Lehman, J. A., and Tan, J.: Does infection play a role in breast capsular contracture? Plast. Reconstr. Surg., *68*:34, 1981.

Silver, H.: Reduction of capsular contracture with two stage augmentation mammaplasty and pulsed electromagnetic energy (diapulse therapy). Plast. Reconstr. Surg., *69*:802, 1982.

Skoog, T.: A technique of breast reduction; transposition of the nipple on a cutaneous vascular pedicle. Acta Chir. Scand., *126*:453, 1963.

Slade, C. L., and Peterson, H. D.: Disappearance of the polyurethane cover of the Ashley Natural-Y prosthesis. Plast. Reconstr. Surg., *70*:379, 1982.

Smahel, J.: Tissue reactions to breast implants coated with polyurethane. Plast. Reconstr. Surg., *61*:80, 1978.

Snyder, R. E.: Discussion of "xeromammography—a reason for using saline-filled breast prostheses." Plast. Reconstr. Surg., *61*:107, 1978.

Sterling, H. E.: Two-year experience with the Meme implant. Presented at The American Society for Aesthetic Plastic Surgery, Boston, April, 1985.

Strömbeck, J. O.: Mammaplasty: report of a new technique based on a two-pedicle procedure. Br. J. Plast. Surg., *13*:79, 1960.

Tebbetts, J. B.: Transaxillary subpectoral augmentation mammaplasty: long-term follow-up and refinements. Plast. Reconstr. Surg., *74*:636, 1984.

Teimourian, B., and Adham, M. N.: Congenital anomalies of nipple and areola. *In* Georgiade, N. G. (Ed.): Aesthetic Breast Surgery. Baltimore, Williams & Wilkins Company, 1983, p. 347.

Testut, L.: Traité D'Anatomie Humaine. Paris, Octave Doin, 1901, pp. 808, 907, 915, 920.

Thorek, M.: Possibilities in the reconstruction of the human form. N.Y. Med. J., *116*:572, 1922.

Thorek, M.: Plastic Surgery of the Breast and the Abdominal Wall. Springfield, IL, Charles C Thomas, 1942.

Truppman, E. S., and Ellenby, J. D.: A 13-year evaluation of subpectoral augmentation mammoplasty. *In* Owsley, J. Q., and Peterson, R. A. (Eds.): Symposium on Aesthetic Surgery of the Breast. St. Louis, C. V. Mosby Company, 1978.

Vinnik, C. A.: Spherical contracture of fibrous capsules around breast implants. Prevention and treatment. Plast. Reconstr. Surg., *58*:555, 1976.

Vistnes, L. M., Bentley, J. W., and Fogarty, D. C.: Experimental study of tissue response to ruptured gel-filled mammary prostheses. Plast. Reconstr. Surg., *59*:31, 1977.

Vogel, P. M., Georgiade, N. G., Fetter, B. F., Vogel, F. S., and McCarty, K. S., Jr.: The correlation of histologic changes in the human breast with the menstrual cycle. Am. J. Pathol., *104*:23, 1981.

Vor Herr, H.: The Breast: Morphology, Physiology and Lactation. New York, Academic Press, 1974.

Weiner, D. L., Aiache, A. E., Silver, L., and Tittiranonda, T.: A single dermal pedicle for nipple transposition in subcutaneous mastectomy, reduction mammaplasty or mastopexy. Plast. Reconstr. Surg., *51*:115, 1973.

Wellings, S. R., Jensen, H. M., and Marcum, R. G.: An atlas of subgross pathology of the human breast with special reference to possible precancerous lesions. J. Natl. Cancer Inst., *55*:231, 1975.

Wilkinson, T. S.: Breast augmentation for periareolar incision. *In* Georgiade, N. G. (Ed.): Aesthetic Breast Surgery. Baltimore, Williams & Wilkins Company, 1983, p. 71.

Williams, J. E.: Experiences with a large series of Silastic breast implants. Plast. Reconstr. Surg., *49*:253, 1972.

Williams, W. R.: Polymastism, with special reference to mammae erraticae and the development of neoplasms from supernumerary mammary structures. J. Anat. Physiol. (Lond.), *25*:225, 1897.

Wise, R. J., Gannon, J. P., and Hill, J. R.: Further experience with reduction mammaplasty. Plast. Reconstr. Surg., *32*:12, 1963.

Wolfe, J. N.: On mammography in the presence of breast implants (letter). Plast. Reconstr. Surg., *62*:286, 1978.

Woods, J. E., Irons, G. B., Jr., and Arnold, P. G.: The case for submuscular implantation of prostheses in reconstructive breast surgery. Ann. Plast. Surg., *4*:2, 1980.

79

John Bostwick III

Breast Reconstruction

A woman's breasts are a primary symbol of her femininity and the loss of a breast can be a major impairment to her body image and feelings of attractiveness. This loss can have devastating sequelae, causing a marked impact on the woman's emotional stability and social adjustment. When the loss of the breast is a result of the local treatment of breast cancer, the woman not only has to confront the reality of the tumor prognosis but also must face a constant reminder of the mastectomy deformity. An external breast prosthesis worn to simulate the missing breast is not incorporated into the woman's body image and therefore does not alleviate her sense of deformity.

Women with missing breasts after the local treatment of breast cancer have encouraged reconstructive surgeons to develop techniques that can provide attractive, symmetric breasts. For breast reconstruction to be properly utilized to help the woman with carcinoma, it must be incorporated into a comprehensive rehabilitation plan. The esthetic and psychologic goals can be addressed while the oncologic aspects of the treatment plan are carried out. Most patients seen by the plastic surgeon for breast reconstruction have had mastectomy for breast cancer, but the surgical techniques are also useful for breast reconstruction of congenital deformities and acquired conditions such as those resulting from burns and trauma.

The plastic surgeon who is involved in breast reconstruction after breast cancer should have a comprehensive understanding of the biology, natural history, risk factors, and treatment of breast cancer. He should also be familiar with the psychologic factors associated with breast cancer as well as those associated with any major deformity. The actual breast reconstruction requires a working knowledge of the full range of esthetic surgical procedures of the breast as well as the spectrum of breast reconstruction techniques from the placement of a silicone breast implant beneath the available tissue, to tissue expansion, to the transfer of musculocutaneous flaps.

BREAST CANCER

Breast cancer is the most common major cancer in women. The American Cancer Society estimated that 130,000 women would develop breast cancer in 1988. The current biologic concept of breast cancer postulates that it is a systemic disease that begins as a

Table 79–1. Factors Associated with Increased Risk of Breast Cancer

Category	Risk Factor
Demographic	White
	Higher socioeconomic class
Anthropometric	Increased weight
Dietary	Increased fat and calorie consumption
Menstrual	Earlier age at menarche
	Later age at menopause
	Decreased frequency of artificial menopause
Reproductive	Never married
	Late age at first full-time delivery
Hormonal	Prolonged use of exogenous estrogens at menopause; prolonged use of oral contraceptives (?)
Other	History of benign breast disease
	Family history of breast cancer

Table 79–3. Risks to Sisters of Patients with Unilateral Breast Cancer

Risk to Unaffected Sisters by Age	By Age of Patient at Diagnosis		By Family Type	
	≤50 (N = 276)	≥51 (N = 322)	Type I (N = 226)	Type II (N = 215)
30–40	2	1	1	1
40–50	5	5	6	7
50–60	6	4	3	8
60–70+	2	4	4	4
Lifetime	14	13	14	20

Data from Anderson, D. E., and Badzioch, M.: Risk of familial breast cancer (letter). Lancet *1*:392, 1984.

focus in the breast and spreads by the lymphatics and the bloodstream. Breast cancer must be regarded as a chronic disease and, while many women live for many years after the diagnosis of breast cancer, most die with detectable breast cancer cells in their bodies (Harris and associates, 1987). The etiology of breast cancer remains unknown although there are a number of important factors and determinants (Table 79–1). Breast cancer has a definite genetic component and its incidence is particularly increased in first degree maternal relatives, in mothers and especially in sisters (Tables 79–2, 79–3) (Anderson, 1977).

The complexity of the overall management of the woman with breast cancer is such that treatment is enhanced by the established breast management team. The team is directed by the oncologic surgeon and the radiation therapist; the pathologist, the medical oncologist, and the plastic surgeon are contributing members of this team.

The early diagnosis of breast cancer increases the ten year survival rate, and is

Table 79–2. Effect of Family History* on Relative Risk of Breast Cancer

	Relative Risk
Affected first degree relative	2.3
Affected mother *and* sister	14
Affected second degree relative	1.5

*First degree relative denotes mother or sister; second degree indicates aunt or grandmother.

From Barton, F. E., Jr.: Breast cancer, subcutaneous mastectomy, and breast reconstruction. Selected Readings Plast. Surg., 3:4, 1986.

facilitated by breast self-examination and surveillance by the primary physician. The breast imaging specialist adds significant information, particularly regarding early diagnosis and localization. The oncologic surgeon provides the definitive diagnostic evaluation and staging. The pathologist determines the specific diagnosis with the tissue provided by the surgeon. The radiation therapist and medical oncologist supply both adjunctive treatments and systemic therapies (Holleb, 1986). The reconstructive surgeon can provide breast reconstruction to support the emotional, psychologic, and esthetic rehabilitation of the woman. Peer support groups, psychologists, clinical nurse specialists, and social workers also contribute to the overall management of the woman with breast cancer.

The oncologic management of breast cancer focuses on both the local and the systemic aspects of the disease. The first effective improvement in local control of breast cancer was developed by Halsted (1894) in 1889 with the introduction of the radical mastectomy. Until that time there were no effective operations for local control of breast cancer, and women often succumbed to large, ulcerative, bulky breast tumors. The halstedian concept of the treatment of breast cancer and metastasis was that the cancer spread in an orderly fashion from the original focus of breast cancer to become trapped in the regional nodes by direct endolymphatic extension. En bloc resection of the breast, underlying chest wall musculature, and axillary nodes was designed to contain and control the tumor locally before its systemic spread (Haagensen, 1986). Because of the major deformity associated with the radical mastectomy, many women encouraged their surgeons to perform

Table 79–4. Carcinoma of the Breast, Columbia Clinical Classification Stages A and B. Size of Primary Tumor Correlated with Axillary Metastasis. Personal Series of Radical Mastectomies, 1935–1968

Size of Primary Tumor (Clinical Measurement)	No. of Patients	Patients with Involved Axillary Nodes	
		No.	%
No palpable tumor	26	5	19.2
Less than 10 mm	22	5	22.7
10–19 mm	119	29	24.4
20–29 mm	223	68	30.5
30–39 mm	180	84	46.7
40–49 mm	147	68	46.3
50–59 mm	101	61	60.4
60–79 mm	77	40	51.9
80 mm and over	27	14	51.9
Total	922	374	40.6

From Haagensen, C, D., and Bodian, C.: A personal experience with Halsted's radical mastectomy. Ann. Surg., *199*:143, 1984.)

Table 79–5. Breast Cancer Clinical Staging

T1	<2 cm diameter	
	T1a	Not fixed to pectoralis
	T1b	Fixed to pectoralis
		i. Tumor <0.5 mm
		ii. Tumor >0.5 cm, <1.0 cm
		iii. Tumor >1.0 cm, <2.0 cm
T2	>2 cm, <5 cm	
	T2a	Not fixed to pectoralis
	T2b	Fixed to pectoralis
T3	>5 cm	a & b as above
T4	Direct extension to chest wall or skin	
	T4a	Fixed to chest wall
	T4b	Edema, ulceration, satellite nodules on breast
	T4c	Both
N0	No worrisome nodes	
N1	Mobile nodes thought to contain tumor	
N2	Nodes thought positive and fixed to one another or to axilla	
N3	Supra/infraclavicular nodes, arm edema	
M0	No metastasis	
M1	Distant metastasis	

less aggressive breast and chest wall resections. As some surgeons gained experience with less than radical mastectomies, they found that the same level of local control could be obtained with no lowering of the survival rate. The total mastectomy is now the most commonly recommended local treatment for the woman with breast cancer and it is usually combined with an axillary dissection (DeVita, Hellman, and Rosenberg, 1985).

Breast cancer involves a complex host-tumor relationship, and the axillary lymph nodes can reflect the patient's immunologic status relative to the breast tumor. The pathologic evaluation of breast cancer metastasis to the regional lymph nodes continues to be an important prognostic factor for breast cancer both systemically and locally. There is a direct relationship between the number of axillary lymph nodes containing tumor and the incidence of local recurrence and ultimate survival (Tables 79–4, 79–5, 79–6). The axillary lymph node status along with the hormonal receptivity of the breast tumor provides important information for the planning of systemic treatment.

Radiation has been used for many years for the adjunctive treatment of breast cancer and is effective in reducing local recurrences after surgical resection. Adjunctive radiation therapy has not been shown to increase or prolong survival; however, there has been some lowering of the local recurrence rate. The sequelae of radiation therapy to the chest wall, including breast necrosis, osteoradionecrosis, coronary atherosclerosis, brachial plexitis, lymphedema, and secondary tumor induction, have made physicians reluctant to administer it routinely to patients after mastectomy. The management of such postradiation problems must also be incorporated into the field of breast reconstruction (Sando and Jurkiewicz, 1986). The potential long-term harmful effects of total breast irradiation in survivors for 20 years and more must also be considered. This information is needed when women under 40 years of age are receiving this type of treatment.

There continues to be controversy over the

Table 79–6.

	Stage I	
T1	N0	M0
	Stage II	
T2	N0	M0
T1–T2	N1	M0
	Stage IIIA	
T3	N0–N2	M0
T1–T3	N2	M0
	Stage IIIB	
T1–T3	N3	M0
T4	N1–N3	M0
	Stage IV	
T1–T4	N1–N3	M1

optimal local treatment for the woman with breast cancer. Patient selection factors are important and include the following: the size and location of the tumor, the size and consistency of the breast, the age of the patient, and the status of the axillary nodes (Fisher and associates, 1985). Controlled clinical trials are under way to help define the best approach for each combination of stage of disease and for each specific patient. Total mastectomy and axillary dissection continue to be the most common approach to controlling local disease as well as staging of the breast cancer, although there is a trend toward less than total breast removal: i.e., lumpectomy, axillary dissection, and radiation therapy. Regardless of the local treatment of the breast cancer, women now expect to have a breast after the local treatment either by lumpectomy-radiation or total mastectomy and breast reconstruction.

The clinical and pathologic stage of the breast cancer is a major determinant of the application of systemic therapies. These programs, including adjuvant chemotherapy and hormonal therapy, are also focused on the treatment of metastatic disease. Palliation is the primary goal of management of metastatic breast cancer. Hormonal sensitivity is the single most important determinant of prolonged survival. Cytotoxic chemotherapy is used to treat systemic disease when hormonal treatment does not produce a remission.

Adjuvant chemotherapy trials indicate that cure rates can be improved by sequential hormonal and cytotoxic chemotherapy. Adjuvant chemotherapy is administered for a duration of six months or less. Breast reconstruction is usually initiated after the chemotherapy program is completed, although reconstruction before or during treatment is not contraindicated. When the patient undergoes immediate breast reconstruction, the adjuvant chemotherapy is begun as soon as there is satisfactory healing of the mastectomy wound. Because of the chronic nature of systemic breast cancer and the induction of successful remissions with systemic therapy, breast reconstruction for a woman with systemic disease can be extremely helpful for her overall outlook. Generally these patients must be carefully selected with full input from all members of the breast management team.

Since breast cancer strikes many women in the prime of their life, and is a chronic disease without a definitive cure for many patients, it is important for the treating physicians to consider the relationship of palliation to quality of life. Psychologic rehabilitation and other measures to enhance the quality of life must be considered with a sensitivity to the patient's emotional and esthetic concerns. Since there remains controversy over local and systemic therapy, the patient should be aware of the options of local therapy available to her and the potential of breast reconstruction before a decision is made regarding local treatment. Breast reconstruction can provide a major support to the psychologic adjustment of the woman after local (surgical) treatment of breast cancer (Berger and Bostwick, 1984).

BREAST RECONSTRUCTION

The goal of breast reconstruction is to follow the principles of oncologic management and to reconstruct breasts that meet the patient's expectations both psychologically and esthetically. Breast symmetry is a major factor for a woman in achieving satisfaction after breast reconstruction. In order to ensure symmetry, the opposite breast generally serves as the model for the reconstruction. When the opposite breast is attractive, the goal of reconstruction is to match it. Preoperative planning is an important factor in obtaining the best results (Bostwick, 1983). The timing of the reconstruction should be considered when planning the initial therapy because it can be done at the same time as the mastectomy (Georgiade and associates, 1981; Noone and associates, 1982). Consultation with the oncologic surgeon can determine whether the patient is best suited for immediate or for delayed reconstruction. Proper placement of the mastectomy incision and preservation of skin, often with the aid of a tissue expander, can facilitate reconstruction and enhance the final result. Preoperative consultation can identify the patient's specific expectations, which are the final determinant of the expected result.

Preoperative consultations should also include an assessment of the opposite breast, which can influence the type of reconstruction needed to achieve symmetry. The oncologic status of the opposite breast must also be considered by the reconstructive surgeon in planning the operation (Adami, Bergstrom, and Hansen, 1985; Sattin and associates, 1985).

Timing

The timing of the breast reconstruction is an important consideration. Because the foremost focus during the initial treatment is on the oncologic considerations, the timing of breast reconstruction has usually been delayed until primary treatment and adjuvant therapy have been carried out. Delayed reconstruction is most frequently recommended; however, immediate reconstruction, when carried out on selected patients by an experienced team, can be of considerable benefit (Stevens and associates, 1984; Georgiade and associates, 1985).

It is no longer considered necessary for the woman to live with the mastectomy defect to appreciate the reconstructed breast, even with all of its shortcomings. Some women find it difficult simultaneously to face the specter of breast cancer and also to lose the primary symbol of their femininity. The resulting anxiety may lead some women to delay or refuse mastectomy because of fear of mutilation as well as loss of the breast. Immediate reconstruction, however, can permit proper local treatment. The patient must understand that immediate breast reconstruction is the initial procedure after a total mastectomy. Other operations are required to further refine the appearance of the breast, to adjust the opposite breast, and to reconstruct the nipple areola.

The simplest approach is usually selected for reconstruction at the time of mastectomy. A submusculofascial implant or a tissue expander can be positioned after the mastectomy. Symmetry is difficult to achieve during one procedure, and although the reconstruction is begun at the time of the mastectomy, other procedures may be necessary to complete the reconstruction.

It is important that the reconstructive surgeon work closely with the oncologic surgeon in planning the immediate breast reconstruction. The incisions should properly incorporate the area of the breast biopsy as well as the nipple areola, but any other excess skin should not be sacrificed, because it will be useful for the breast reconstruction. The fascia, particularly over the lower chest, should be preserved if it is not in proximity to the tumor in order to provide a better submusculofascial cover.

Although there is a trend toward more immediate breast reconstructions, more patients undergo delayed reconstruction after the mastectomy and any other adjunctive treatments. Reconstruction, therefore, is usually initiated about three to nine months after the mastectomy, although it can be delayed indefinitely. Since most women cannot outgrow their sense of deformity, some patients request reconstruction up to 20 years after the mastectomy. Most of the currently popular procedures for breast reconstruction were also unavailable 20 years ago and patients were often told that reconstruction was not possible.

A delay in the reconstruction is helpful for most women who are considering the procedure. It allows them to be sure that they are suitable candidates for reconstructive surgery, and also to select a reconstructive surgeon and the type of procedure most likely to meet their expectations. It also permits an evaluation of the opposite breast and a decision concerning its management.

The delayed breast reconstruction is usually done in two stages. The breast and chest wall are reconstructed during the first stage (Fig. 79–1). Any correction of the opposite breast can be done at this time or at the second operation. During the second procedure the nipple areola is reconstructed and any other correction of the reconstructed breast is made to achieve optimal form and symmetry. When the tissue expansion technique is selected, an additional stage may be necessary to place the permanent implant prior to the reconstruction of the nipple areola (Radovan, 1982).

Breast reconstruction is sometimes done when the patient has systemic metastatic disease. This situation requires close consultation between the reconstructive surgeon and the oncologist. If the breast cancer is in remission and the patient is fully informed, breast reconstruction is done. Usually the simplest reconstructive technique is preferred in order to hasten the patient's recovery and create minimal operative trauma.

Method Selection

In selecting the method of breast reconstruction the primary considerations are the patient's expectations, the status of the op-

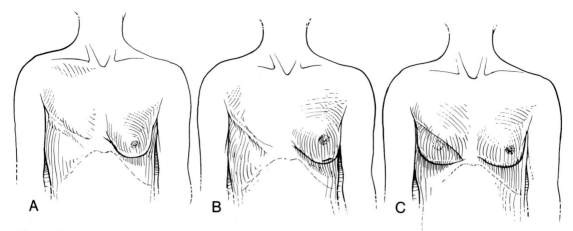

Figure 79–1. *A,* A patient with a right modified radical mastectomy and mild hypoplasia of the opposite breast. *B,* After submusculofascial augmentation of the left breast. This technique defines the opposite breast, which will be matched to obtain a symmetric breast reconstruction. *C,* After reconstruction of the right breast mound to match the augmented left breast.

posite breast, and breast symmetry. The appearance and oncologic status of the other breast are important determinants of symmetry. The plastic surgeon must first assess the other breast and determine whether the breast can be matched with breast reconstruction or whether it will need to be modified because of oncologic or esthetic considerations. Symmetry is very important because if the patient has undergone breast reconstruction and still has to wear an external prosthesis to achieve symmetry, she will usually be disappointed. The type of technique for breast reconstruction is occasionally determined by the patient's wishes regarding the opposite breast. Some patients prefer a flap type of breast reconstruction so that the opposite breast can be matched without the need for an operation or scarring.

Breast reconstruction with the local tissues available after mastectomy is the simplest and a frequently preferred method of breast reconstruction after total mastectomy and modified radical mastectomy (Fig. 79–2) (Woods, Irons, and Arnold, 1980; Gruber and associates, 1981). The introduction of tissue expansion (see Chap. 13) into the techniques of breast reconstruction has made it possible to reconstruct breasts with a silicone breast implant where in the past a flap was required. The overexpansion of the skin also improves the chances of ptosis and of a softer result with the silicone breast implant.

A basic decision must be made during the planning of the breast reconstruction whether the available local tissues are sufficient or whether the use of distant tissue will be necessary (Fig. 79–3). When additional skin or muscle is needed for the reconstruction, the latissimus dorsi flap is a most versatile and reliable source of tissue (Schneider, Hill, and Brown, 1977; Bostwick, Vasconez, and Jurkiewicz, 1978). The transverse rectus abdominis musculocutaneous (TRAM) flap is an even larger source (Hartrampf, Scheflan, and Black, 1982). It provides excess tissue from the lower abdomen and allows breast reconstruction without the need for implants. Breast reconstruction with microsurgical transfer of tissue from the buttocks region (the gluteus maximus musculocutaneous flap) is a highly refined type of procedure (Shaw, 1983). It is selected by an experienced surgeon when other methods are neither suitable nor available, and when the patient requires autologous tissue for the reconstruction. The method also permits reconstruction without the need for a breast implant.

RECONSTRUCTION WITH AVAILABLE TISSUE

This is a preferred method of breast reconstruction for many patients because it is technically the simplest and requires less surgical intervention than the other methods. It is also more predictable and should be selected only when there is a good chance of symmetry, even though a correction of the other breast will be necessary (Fig. 79–4). The silicone breast implant is placed beneath the

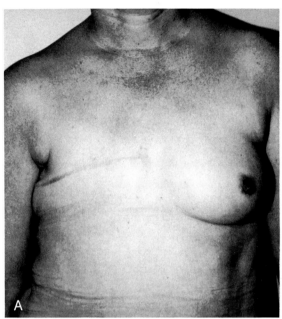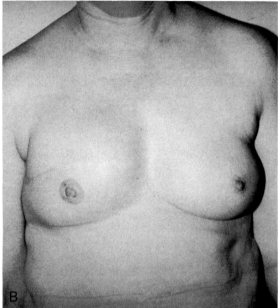

Figure 79–2. Breast reconstruction with available tissue. *A,* A 38 year old woman two years after undergoing a modified radical mastectomy for Stage I breast cancer. *B,* One year after breast reconstruction, with a silicone breast implant placed beneath the musculofascial layer, using the available tissues. (From Harris, J. R., Hellman, S., Henderson, I. C., and Kinne, D. K.: Breast Diseases. Philadelphia, J. B. Lippincott Company, 1987, p. 670.)

musculofascial layers of the chest wall. Usually at least a 250 to 350 ml silicone breast implant is placed during the initial procedure, and an even larger silicone breast implant can be placed if necessary during the

Figure 79–3. Breast reconstruction with available tissue. Preoperative mesurements are important in assessing the type of breast reconstruction. When the skin deficiency is greater than 6 cm in the vertical or horizontal dimensions, a flap is usually needed. When it is less, tissue expansion is possible. The mastectomy defect is illustrated on the patient's left side.

second operation, at the time of the reconstruction of the nipple areola (Dick and Brown, 1986).

The advantages of this method of breast reconstruction are its simplicity and predictability. Breast reconstruction can be done through the mastectomy scar by placement of the silicone breast implant beneath the submusculofascial layer without the need for another incision. The implant is situated behind the planes of the mastectomy, and does not camouflage any local recurrences of the tumor. The use of this method of breast reconstruction does not obviate the need for other techniques, and other methods can be used later if this one achieves a less than optimal result.

Breast reconstruction with available tissue is a satisfactory choice when the tissues after the total mastectomy or modified radical mastectomy are of good quantity and quality and the other breast can be matched with either one or two procedures. This method is contraindicated when the overlying skin is deficient or irradiated or when a radical mastectomy has been performed. These situations usually require the use of tissue expansion or musculocutaneous flaps to achieve an optimal breast reconstruction.

The planning of this method should cover

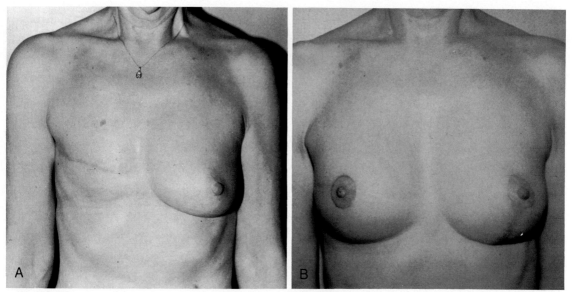

Figure 79–4. *A,* A 52 year old woman after a modified radical mastectomy. *B,* Appearance after breast reconstruction with a silicone breast implant inserted beneath the musculofascial layer and a mastopexy of the opposite breast. A second stage nipple-areola reconstruction was done with sharing of the nipple and application of a full-thickness upper inner thigh skin graft. (From Bostwick, J.: Breast reconstruction following mastectomy. Contemp. Surg., *30*:16, 1987.)

both the breast reconstruction and the management of the opposite breast. The final result must be clearly defined and conceptualized when the initial silicone breast implant is selected. The size of the implant may be determined by the estimated final size of the opposite breast. Another method for selecting the size is to place different-sized silicone breast implants in the brassiere and see which approximates in size the opposite breast. It is also helpful if the size and weight of the mastectomy specimen is available. It is generally preferable to select a silicone breast implant that is slightly larger rather than smaller than the other side. There usually is less projection of the reconstructed breast, and if the silicone breast implant must be changed, it is usually easier to reduce rather than enlarge the size. The ptosis and softness of the breast reconstruction are enhanced when the size is reduced.

The surgical approach begins with the preoperative markings, placed to define the limits of the submusculofascial pocket. The technique can be used when there is less than a 4 cm skin discrepancy with the opposite breast. When the discrepancy is greater, either the tissue expansion or a flap technique is usually necessary, especially if there is to be no surgical correction of the opposite breast. The pocket for the silicone breast

implant is usually marked 1.5 to 2.0 cm below the opposite inframammary crease. This is because there is a tendency for the implant to move upward in the postoperative period with the development of a fibrous capsule about it. The mastectomy scar is also noted and if it is wide or tight, it is excised and closed with a layered suture technique. The mastectomy scar is the most common site for local recurrence, and it must be examined for any nodularity. A fine needle aspirate can be helpful in the diagnosis. It is often helpful to use Z-plasties of the mastectomy scar in the area of the axilla to avoid a scar contracture.

The lateral mastectomy scar is excised and the dissection carried down to the pectoralis major muscle. The lateral fibers of the muscle are separated and the dissection is extended beneath the musculofascial layer. The dissection is done bluntly to minimize bleeding and to avoid dissection through the intercostal muscles (Fig. 79–5).

After the submusculofascial layer has been elevated, the patient is placed in the sitting position and the silicone breast implant is prepared for implantation. Preplaced sutures are situated in the margins of the pectoralis major muscle; the implant is selected and positioned and the sutures are tied. Any modification of the opposite breast is made during the same procedure so that the patient can

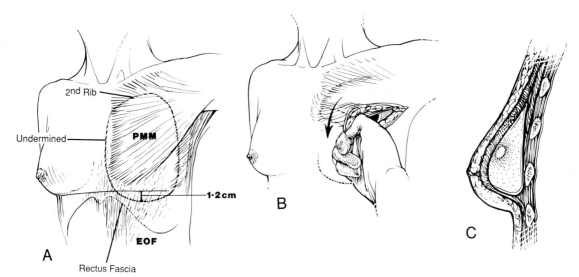

Figure 79–5. Breast reconstruction with available tissue. *A,* The reconstruction is begun by planning the reconstruction to match the opposite breast. The area to be undermined beneath the submusculofascial layer is defined. This pocket includes the pectoralis major muscle (PMM), the serratus anterior muscle, the external oblique fascia (EOF), and the rectus abdominis fascia. Note that the dissection is extended 1 to 2 cm below the opposite inframammary crease. *B,* The submusculofascial position is approached through the lateral mastectomy scar. The musculofascial layer is elevated primarily with blunt dissection. Sharp dissection is necessary to divide fascial bands. *C,* The implant is positioned appropriately to give position and size that are symmetric with the opposite breast.

finish the first operation with a symmetric result (Fig. 79–6). The nipple-areola surgery and any other operations on the breast mound are performed at the second stage, usually three months later.

There generally are fewer complications from this type of breast reconstruction than from the more complex operations. The most frequent problems, such as improper silicone breast implant size, cannot be regarded as true complications. The implant size and position can often be improved during the second operation. There is also development of a fibrous capsule about all silicone breast

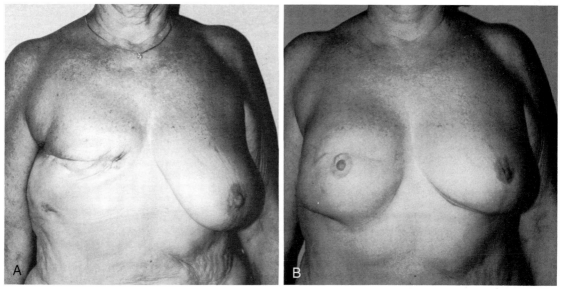

Figure 79–6. Breast reconstruction with available tissue. *A,* A 58 year old woman after a right modified radical mastectomy for Stage I breast cancer. She also had ptosis and hypertrophy of the opposite breast. *B,* Breast reconstruction was accomplished with a submusculofascial implant on the right and a left breast reduction. At a second operation two months later, nipple-areola reconstruction was performed with half of the opposite nipple and an upper medial thigh graft.

implants. This is usually acceptable to the patient if she is informed that it is a normal development. The tightness of the capsule can often be relieved by a capsulotomy at the second stage. If the capsular contracture persists, this may be an indication for replacement with a polyurethane-covered implant. This should be placed in contact with tissue without scar capsule, to achieve optimal softness. This condition may necessitate a capsulectomy at the time of the placement (Hester, 1988). If the patient has recurrent difficulties with the implants, they can be removed and replaced with autogenous tissue (flaps) from the abdomen or buttocks.

RECONSTRUCTION WITH TISSUE EXPANSION

Breast reconstruction with tissue expansion (Argenta, 1984) is a modification of the technique of using available tissue, as discussed above. Tissue expansion utilizes the principle of gradual stretching of the tissues of the chest wall that will be covering the silicone breast implant (see Chap. 13). In this manner the tissues available after the mastectomy can accommodate a larger implant than could be positioned during the first operation. The gradual stretching of the tissues also provides cover for the implant with a relative abundance of soft tissue, which simulates ptosis in the reconstructed breast. Spe-

cific suturing to the inframammary crease is often necessary to obtain optimal definition of this area. Reconstruction with tissue expansion extends the application of breast reconstruction utilizing available tissue and decreases the indications for the use of musculocutaneous flaps.

The tissue expander is an inflatable device made with an elastomer material similar to the covering of the silicone breast implant. There is usually a separate implantable fill valve (reservoir), or the fill valve can be located on the device. The tissue expander is placed in the submusculofascial position, like a silicone implant for breast reconstruction with available tissue, as previously described. The separate fill valve is usually placed subcutaneously, either lateral to or below the reconstructed breast (Fig. 79–7). A small amount of saline is inflated into the device through the fill valve to make sure that it is functioning properly. After several weeks when wound healing is progressing satisfactorily, the tissue expander is gradually inflated by instilling approximately 100 ml percutaneously into the fill valve, and this is repeated about every week. The fluid instillation must be done slowly under sterile conditions and the patient and the surgeon must both understand that this is a relatively slow method of breast reconstruction. For optimal results, the patient and surgeon must have patience. The tissue expander is overfilled approximately 200 ml over the estimated

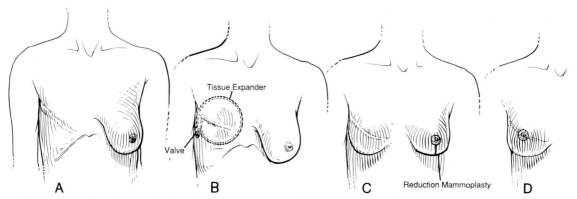

Figure 79–7. Breast reconstruction with tissue expansion. *A,* Breast reconstruction with tissue expansion is planned when there is a relative deficiency of tissue or when ptosis is necessary in the reconstructed breast to achieve symmetry with the opposite breast. *B,* A tissue expander is selected that has a wider base than the future breast. The tissue expander is placed in a submusculofascial position, as is the silicone breast implant for the available tissue type of reconstruction. The fill valve is placed laterally in the subcutaneous tissue. *C,* When necessary, a breast reduction or mastopexy is performed on the opposite breast for symmetry. If there is flattening in the upper pole of the opposite breast, a submusculofascial breast implant is positioned at the time of the mastopexy or reduction mammoplasty. *D,* After the tissue expander is overinflated and deflated, it is replaced with a permanent breast implant. The nipple-areola reconstruction is done at this time or as a separate procedure approximately three months later.

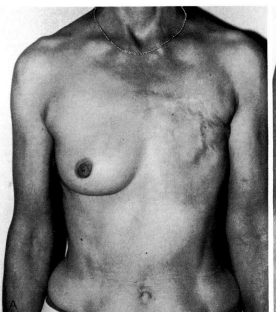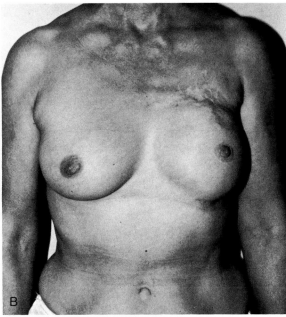

Figure 79–8. Breast reconstruction with tissue expansion. *A,* A woman after a modified radical mastectomy for Stage I breast cancer. The soft tissues were deficient and the opposite breast was flat. *B,* The breast reconstruction was done with tissue expansion, and a silicone breast implant was also placed beneath the opposite breast to give symmetry. (From Bostwick, J.: Breast reconstruction. Emory Univ. J. Med., *1*:297, 1987.)

volume of the opposite breast and is allowed to remain in position for several months so that the tissues can become accommodated to their expanded condition. At the time of the second operation, the tissue expander is removed and replaced by a permanent silicone breast implant of the proper size to achieve symmetry with the opposite breast. Nipple-areola reconstruction is usually accomplished several months later (Figs. 79–8, 79–9, 79–10).

An expander that can be converted to a permanent silicone breast implant has been developed, and offers some advantages over the traditional type of tissue expander. This device is a double-lumen implant with an outer implant containing silicone gel. There are two valves that lead to an expandable inner lumen. The device is inflated like other tissue expanders; however, when satisfactory size and position are determined, the fill valve can be removed and the device becomes a permanent double-lumen silicone breast implant (Becker, 1984).

The advantage of breast reconstruction with the technique of tissue expansion is that flaps are not required in most patients who have had a modified radical mastectomy or total mastectomy. The opposite breast can

usually be matched without the need for additional scars (Fig. 79–11). The technique permits reconstruction for some patients who might not otherwise have acceptable reconstruction with silicone breast implants alone. Breast reconstruction was done, however, for many years with serial insertion of progres-

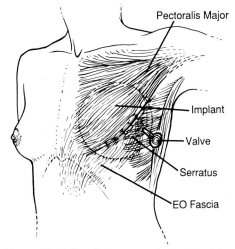

Figure 79–9. The tissue expander is placed in a sub-musculofascial position, generally through the lateral mastectomy scar. At a second procedure, the inframammary crease is defined by an internal capsulorrhaphy. EO = external oblique.

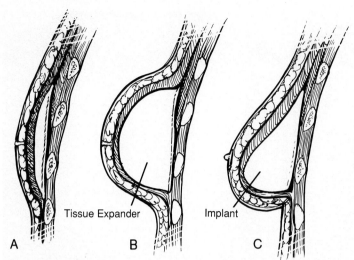

Tissue Expander   Implant

A   B   C

Figure 79–10. Breast reconstruction with tissue expansion. *A,* The tissue expander is placed in the submusculofascial position and is ready for expansion. *B,* Serial expansion is begun approximately two to three weeks after placement of the tissue expander. The breast is expanded by 100 to 150 ml in weekly increments until it is approximately 200 ml larger than the opposite breast. *C,* At a second operation, the tissue expander is exchanged for a permanent breast implant to match the opposite breast.

sively larger silicone implants, but the tissue expansion is certainly an improvement over this method. Tissue expansion also does not prevent the use of other methods of breast reconstruction. If there is a less than adequate or an unsatisfactory result with this method, the TRAM or the latissimus dorsi flap can be used. The expanded skin actually makes secondary breast reconstruction with these methods easier because often the skin has been sufficiently stretched.

A disadvantage of tissue expansion is the need for a silicone breast implant. The implant has the potential for the development of capsular contracture with resultant firmness and distortion of the breast. Tissue expansion can also add an extra operation to the breast reconstruction. In addition, the patient must come to the surgeon's office at weekly intervals for gradual fill of the device (Fig. 79–12). There have also been failures of the device with early deflation. When fill of the tissue expansion implant has been rapid, there has been exposure of the device through thin skin.

Skin expansion is a satisfactory method of breast reconstruction when the patient has had a modified radical or total mastectomy and when the opposite breast is full with some element of glandular ptosis. It is also a good choice when there is satisfactory skin cover and the breast reconstruction needs to be larger than can be achieved with a silicone breast implant in one operation (>400 ml). It is also indicated when ptosis is desirable in the reconstructed breast. It is unsatisfactory when the skin cover is thin or when there is evidence of advanced irradiation changes.

The patient must understand that the method is slow and includes several stages.

When a breast reconstruction with tissue expansion is planned, the management of the opposite breast must be considered also. The final size of the opposite breast influences the size of the tissue expander and is important in achieving symmetry. Because the diameter of the tissue expander should be sufficient to cover the base of the future breast, a potential volume of at least 600 to 700 ml is selected. Smaller tissue expanders have a base that is too narrow for the average woman's permanent silicone breast implant. The tissue expander size is also selected to give at least 200 ml of additional fill above the estimated volume of the final permanent implant. Overexpansion provides ptosis of the breast reconstruction and probably reduces the intensity and firmness of the capsular contraction.

The markings are similar to those for breast reconstruction with available tissue. Since the tissue expander tends to expand the tissue in the central part of the breast and since there is movement of the tissue expander in a superior direction, it is placed approximately 2 to 3 cm below the opposite inframammary crease. The markings for correction of the opposite breast can also be made at this time. It is helpful to have a model for reconstruction of the missing breast (Fig. 79–13). An alternative strategy is to correct the opposite breast at a later stage, if it is uncertain whether a correction will be needed, or if the patient has not decided that she wants a correction of the opposite breast. The position for placement of the separate fill valve for the tissue expander is also marked. The

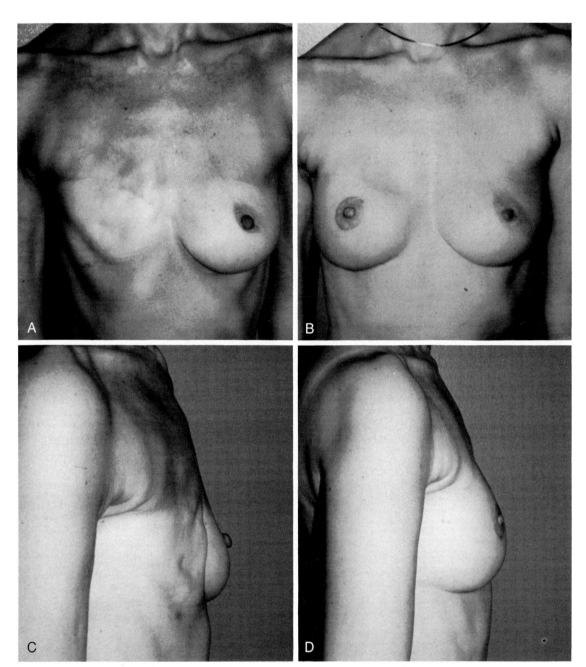

Figure 79–11. Breast reconstruction with tissue expansion. *A,* A 48 year old woman who had had a modified radical mastectomy for breast cancer. She wanted to match the opposite breast, which was somewhat hypoplastic and flattened in its upper pole. She underwent tissue expansion. *B,* After the initial placement of a silicone breast implant, approximately 100 ml larger than the anticipated final size at the second operation, a polyurethane-covered Meme implant (190 ml) was subsequently positioned to give symmetry with the opposite breast. A nipple-areola reconstruction was done at a later stage by sharing the opposite nipple and applying an upper medial thigh graft. *C,* Preoperative profile. *D,* Postoperative profile. (From Bostwick, J.: Breast reconstruction using modifed tissue expansion for matching a small opposite breast. Perspect. Plast. Surg. *1:*79, 1987.)

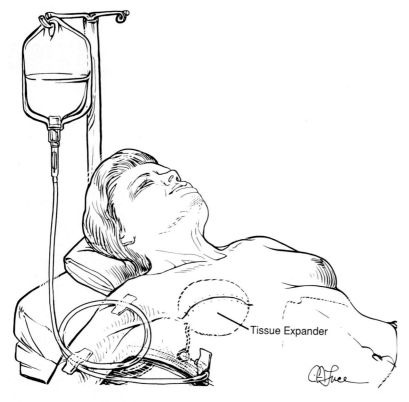

Figure 79–12. Tissue expansion with normal saline solution is done in the office under sterile conditions with antiseptic preparation of the injection site and sterile intravenous tubing.

Tissue Expander

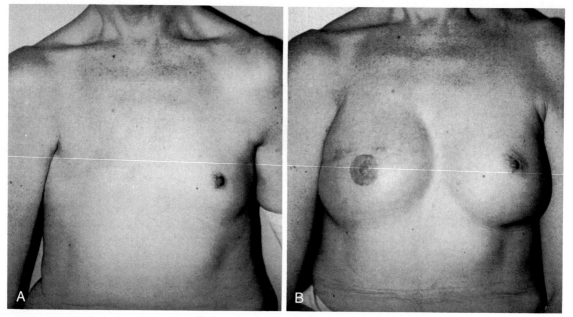

Figure 79–13. Breast reconstruction with tissue expansion. *A,* A woman who had had a modified radical mastectomy and also had hypoplasia of the opposite breast. She desired a breast augmentation and breast reconstruction. *B,* After breast reconstruction with tissue expansion, a silicone implant was placed in the submusculofascial position on the left. An implant approximately 100 ml larger in volume was placed in the opposite submusculofascial position. At the time of nipple-areola reconstruction, a 100 ml smaller implant was positioned to give symmetry.

fill valve should be placed in a subcutaneous position even though the tissue expander is placed in the submusculofascial position.

The submusculofascial layer is approached through the mastectomy scar. The dissection is extended through the pectoralis major muscle, and blunt dissection is made to create a pocket beneath the submusculofascial layer. The fibers of origin of the pectoralis major muscle are separated from the sternum and from the level of the third rib. This maneuver allows for better projection and expansion without contractions of the pectoralis major muscle. When this muscle is strong and tends to distort the breast reconstruction, selective denervation of the lateral fibers of the pectoralis major muscle is performed near the thoracoacromial pedicle between the pectoralis major and the pectoralis minor muscles. After the pocket has been dissected, the patient is placed in the sitting position and the tissue expander is positioned so that, when filled, it will give symmetry with the opposite breast. A small separate tunnel is created and the fill valve is positioned so that it can be easily identified for later fluid instillation in the office. Usually, only 100 to 200 ml of saline are instilled into the tissue expander at the time of insertion. The actual serial filling and expansion are begun in the office two to three weeks after the operation, when there is satisfactory wound healing.

After the tissue expander has been overfilled approximately 200 ml more than the volume of the other breast, the placement of the permanent silicone breast implant is scheduled for one to two months later. One method of determining the volume of the permanent silicone breast implant is to withdraw fluid from the tissue expander until the volume is the same as that of the opposite breast. The nipple-areola reconstruction is usually done at a third operation.

Breast reconstruction with tissue expansion has more complications than reconstruction with a silicone breast implant only. All the complications of silicone breast implant can occur in addition to problems unique to the tissue expander and its fill. Reconstruction with tissue expansion is also reserved for more challenging situations than those in which the insertion of a silicone breast implant alone would be sufficient. There seems to be a definite but low incidence of infection with the tissue expansion technique. This finding is attributed to the introduction of bacteria at the time of saline injection in the office, and sterile technique is necessary at the time of filling. The inflatable devices, as well as the valves, have failed and kinking has developed in the fill tubing.

RECONSTRUCTION WITH LATISSIMUS DORSI FLAP

Breast reconstruction with silicone breast implants and the use of the available tissues after modified radical mastectomy constitute the simplest and most reliable method of breast reconstruction. There are situations in which this type of reconstruction and the technique of tissue expansion do not give a satisfactory result for the patient. When an implant is not sufficient for a satisfactory reconstruction, additional tissue needs to be brought to the breast area with a flap. A flap reconstruction is also selected to preserve the appearance of the opposite breast. Many patients would prefer a donor scar on either the back or lower abdomen to one on the remaining breast. The two most commonly used musculocutaneous flaps are the latissimus dorsi and the TRAM flaps. Both provide additional tissue to supplement the breast reconstruction.

The latissimus dorsi musculocutaneous flap facilitates breast reconstruction by adding back skin to supplement the missing skin, and muscle to replace or supplement any muscle deficiency. The muscle can enhance the cover of a silicone breast implant, and contribute to the softness and natural appearance of the reconstruction. The latissimus dorsi flap is versatile and reliable and is a safe and predictable choice when additional tissue is required for the reconstruction. Breast reconstruction with the latissimus dorsi is more complex than with available tissues. After the flap is elevated from the back and transposed to the area of the reconstruction, the reconstruction proceeds as described with a silicone implant.

The latissimus dorsi flap is a particularly good choice when a flap is needed, when the patient is interested in axillary fill, or when she has had a radical mastectomy (Fig. 79–14). It is most useful for thin patients who are not good candidates for the TRAM flap. The latissimus dorsi is also indicated for patients with thin, tight or irradiated skin, and for those with imminent exposure of a

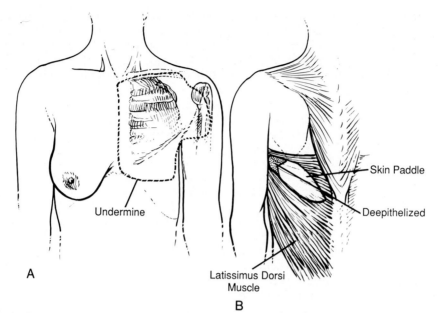

Figure 79–14. Breast reconstruction with the latissimus dorsi flap. *A,* Breast reconstruction after a radical mastectomy. To recreate the anterior axillary fold, the dissection pocket *(interrupted line)* must be extended to the arm in the area of insertion of the pectoralis major muscle. *B,* The latissimus dorsi musculocutaneous flap is designed on the back over the latissimus dorsi muscle. The skin paddle is designed below the bra line. The lateral aspect of the skin paddle is deepithelized *(dotted area)* for additional augmentation of the axillary area.

silicone breast implant through attenuated skin. The latissimus dorsi flap can provide additional fullness in the lower outer quadrant of a breast reconstruction and can contribute to ptosis in the final reconstruction (Figs. 79–15, 79–16) (Maxwell, 1981; Wolf and Biggs, 1982).

The anatomy of the latissimus dorsi contributes to its usefulness in breast reconstruction. It is a large, triangular muscle some-

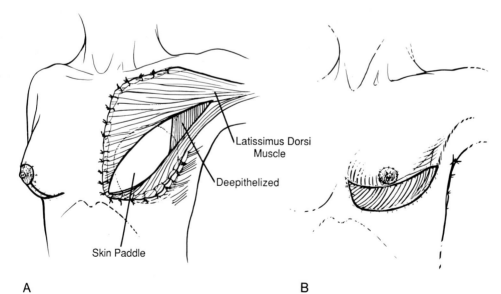

Figure 79–15. Breast reconstruction with the latissimus dorsi flap. *A,* The flap is transferred anteriorly, based on the thoracodorsal pedicle. The deepithelized area is used for anterior axillary fold fill. The latissimus dorsi muscle is sutured to the divided origins of the pectoralis major muscle. *B,* An alternative, preferred position for the latissimus dorsi skin island for the modified radical mastectomy patient is in the inframammary crease area.

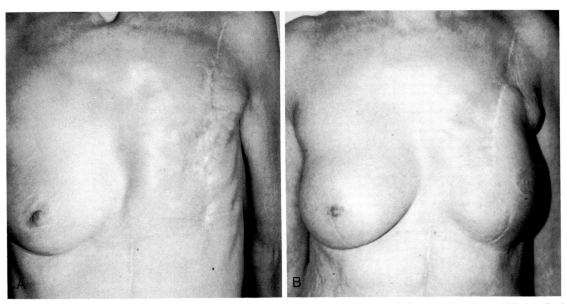

Figure 79–16. Breast reconstruction with the latissimus dorsi flap. *A,* A patient after an extended modified radical mastectomy. *B,* The latissimus dorsi muscle flap was positioned vertically to replace the deficit and to give soft tissue cover of the silicone breast implant. An augmentation mammoplasty was performed on the opposite breast.

what greater in area than the pectoralis major muscle. It is an outstanding example of a musculocutaneous flap. Its primary pedicle is the thoracodorsal vessel, which is about 10 cm long and is based on the axillary vessels (Fig. 79–17). There are many perforators over the entire surface of the muscle that can support overlying skin islands designed in many patterns. This attribute adds to the versatility of the flap. If the thoracodorsal pedicle has been injured, the flap can be elevated on the collateral vessels entering the latissimus dorsi from the outer surface of the serratus anterior muscle (Fisher, Bostwick, and Powell, 1983). The strongest set of

perforators supporting the flap are along the lateral margin of the muscle, under the primary intramuscular vessel. The design of the skin island and the muscle is prepared after the tissue requirements of the breast reconstruction have been determined.

Planning for breast reconstruction with the latissimus dorsi flap must take into account both skin and muscle requirements (Biggs and Cronin, 1981). The versatility of the latissimus dorsi flap allows custom flap designs to meet the specific requirements. When skin is needed in the lower portion of the breast reconstruction (Fig. 79–18), the skin island can be designed along the lateral mar-

Figure 79–17. The thoracodorsal artery, which is approximately 10 cm long, is the primary blood supply of the latissimus dorsi musculocutaneous island flap. There are significant branches, however, from the serratus anterior muscle that connect with the thoracodorsal artery as its pedicle enters the latissimus dorsi muscle.

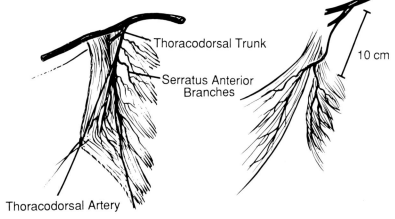

Thoracodorsal Trunk

Serratus Anterior Branches

10 cm

Thoracodorsal Artery

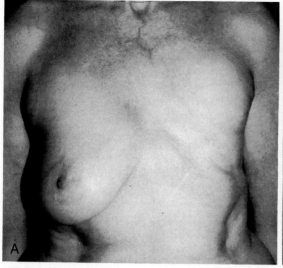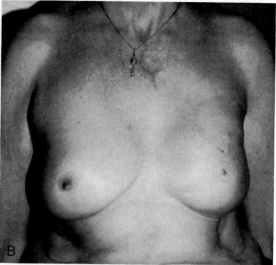

Figure 79–18. Breast reconstruction with the latissimus dorsi flap. *A,* A patient after a left-sided modified radical mastectomy. *B,* A latissimus dorsi muscle flap was positioned in the inframammary crease and a silicone breast implant was positioned under this to match the opposite breast, on which a small reduction was performed.

gin of the muscle or in the transverse lines of the back beneath the brassiere (Fig. 79–19). When there is need for breast reconstruction after radical mastectomy, the skin island is designed under the brassiere or along the lateral margin of the muscle. The insertion of the latissimus dorsi is divided, moved anteriorly, and reattached to the divided end of the pectoralis major muscle (Fig. 79–20).

The final result must be defined after consultation with the patient and committed firmly to memory before the specific planning of the flap. The tissue and silicone breast implant requirements are determined to give symmetry with the opposite breast, or with the opposite breast after it has been corrected. The amount of skin required can be estimated by measuring the skin of the opposite breast in the vertical and horizontal dimensions, and planning the size of the island to give symmetry. Preoperative markings should clearly define the skin island, the extent of the latissimus dorsi muscle to be harvested, the position of the latissimus dorsi flap on the back and in relationship to the underlying muscle, and the pocket for the implant. An estimate of the implant size should also be made.

The surgical approach to breast reconstruction with the latissimus dorsi flap begins after the preoperative markings have been made. The latissimus dorsi flap is harvested first with the patient in the lateral position. The skin island is circumscribed and the amount of muscle to be transferred is exposed. The

muscle is incised and the flap is elevated toward the axilla. The serratus anterior muscle is preserved. In addition, the serratus anterior collateral vessels going from the outer surface of the muscle to the entrance of the thoracodorsal pedicle are preserved, because there may have been injury to the pedicle at the time of the mastectomy. After the thoracodorsal pedicle is identified and seen to be intact, the insertion of the latissimus dorsi onto the humerus can be divided if this is needed to reconstruct the anterior axillary fold of the radical mastectomy defect. The mastectomy incision is opened and the mastectomy deformity is recreated. A tunnel is made high in the axilla, and the latissimus dorsi flap is transposed on its pedicle to the mastectomy defect. The high axillary tunnel allows the pedicle of the flap to fill the axillary defect, which is apparent after the axillary lymph node dissection. The back incision is closed and a suction drain is left in place because there is a tendency for serous fluid to accumulate.

For breast reconstruction after a radical mastectomy, the latissimus dorsi flap is positioned to provide augmentation to the axilla and the infraclavicular region. Usually a large portion or all of the flap is deepithelized to give satisfactory contour without an external scar. The silicone breast implant is positioned to give optimal contour of the breast mound in the interests of symmetry. When the correct-sized implant would result in ex-

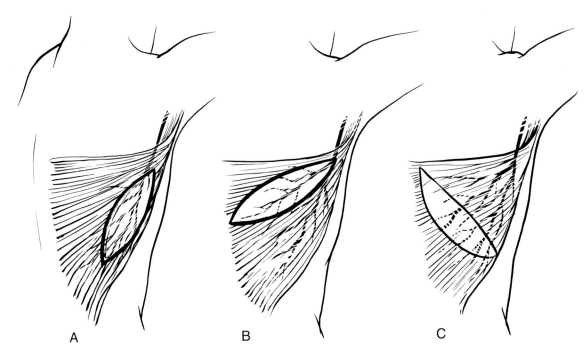

Figure 79–19. Breast reconstruction with the latissimus dorsi flap. *A,* The latissimus dorsi skin island can be designed in a variety of positions over the latissimus dorsi muscle. When it is oriented laterally, the transposed flap can reach the inframammary crease, and only a portion of the latissimus dorsi muscle is necessary. *B,* When the latissimus dorsi skin island is oriented beneath the brassiere strap in the back and is transposed anteriorly, the lower portion of the latissimus dorsi muscle can fill the infraclavicular area. *C,* When the latissimus dorsi skin island is oriented obliquely across the back, it is in the natural skin lines and gives the most inconspicuous donor scar. The design also provides a large portion of muscle for anterior transposition, and the skin island can be positioned at the inframammary crease of the breast reconstruction.

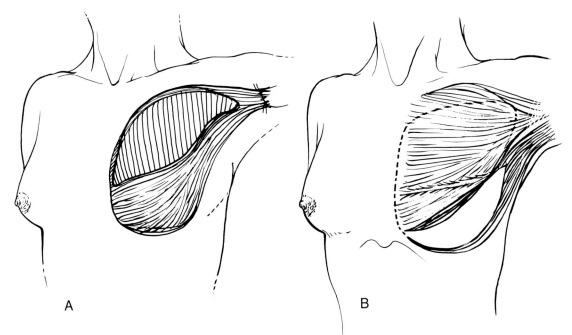

Figure 79–20. Breast reconstruction with the latissimus dorsi flap. *A,* When there is sufficient skin but a deficiency in the upper portion of the chest wall, the latissimus dorsi skin island can be deepithelized *(vertical lines)* to provide fill for the breast. The latissimus dorsi muscle insertion is divided posteriorly, transposed, and sutured to the cut end of the pectoralis major muscle tendon. *B,* After a modified radical mastectomy, the latissimus dorsi musculocutaneous island flap can be used to supplement skin in the lower outer portion of the breast, and the latissimus dorsi muscle can be sutured to the pectoralis major muscle above *(interrupted line)* to give complete muscle coverage of the implant.

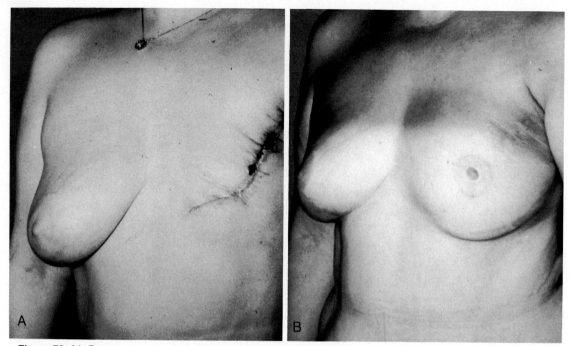

Figure 79–21. Breast reconstruction with the latissimus dorsi flap. *A,* A patient who had a tight skin closure after a left modified radical mastectomy. *B,* Breast reconstruction was done with a latissimus dorsi flap and insertion of a submusculofascial implant. A small reduction mammoplasty was performed on the opposite breast. (From Bostwick, J.: Breast reconstruction following mastectomy. Contemp. Surg., 27:19, 1985.)

cessive soft tissue stretching, a tissue expander can be inserted and filled later in the postoperative period.

After a modified radical mastectomy, the latissimus dorsi muscle is positioned to give satisfactory cover of the breast implant. It is usually sutured to the lower margin of the pectoralis major muscle and along a line above the inframammary crease. The skin island is positioned in the opened mastectomy scar when the scar is low and oblique (Fig. 79–21). It is not attractive to place the latissimus dorsi skin island in a high incision; it is better to place it in a separate oblique incision in the lower outer quadrant of the reconstructed breast. This maneuver enhances the symmetry and ptosis of the breast reconstruction. The silicone breast implant is appropriately selected to give symmetry with the opposite breast.

When the skin is thin but of adequate volume and there is imminent exposure of the silicone breast implant, the latissimus dorsi muscle alone is elevated through small incisions and transposed anteriorly into the reconstruction area to give implant soft tissue coverage and to enhance the security and appearance of the reconstruction.

Complications of breast reconstruction with the latissimus dorsi flap may be the same as those of any flap procedure, such as partial or total necrosis. The complication of total flap necrosis has been less than 1 per cent and of partial necrosis less than 5 per cent in the author's series. The most frequent complication has been the development of seroma of the back donor site; this is reduced by the use of the siliconized drain. The patient should avoid significant motion of the shoulder (and thereby the back skin) because the skin must become adherent to the base of the dissection to avoid a seroma. All the complications associated with use of a silicone breast implant in reconstruction with available tissues are possible because of the concomitant need for an implant (Lejour and associates, 1985).

RECONSTRUCTION WITH TRAM FLAP

Breast reconstruction with the lower abdominal skin and fat provides an abundant source of tissue for the patient who desires a reconstruction without a silicone breast implant and who also wants an abdominoplasty (Dinner, Dowden, and Scheflan, 1983). The TRAM flap is an ellipse of skin and fat harvested from the abdominal wall and based on the perforators from the underlying rectus abdominis muscle (Fig. 79–22). The flap is indicated for breast reconstruction when the patient needs flap tissue to permit a reconstruction that can satisfy her expectations of symmetry. For the selected patient, this flap is preferable to the latissimus dorsi because the reconstruction can be done without a silicone breast implant, because the abdominal excess is reduced, and because the donor scar is transverse in the lower abdomen rather than on the back or side. The TRAM flap is indicated when the latissimus dorsi muscle is denervated, divided, or atrophic. The flap is also useful for the patient who has had complications with a silicone breast implant, since the implant can be replaced with the patient's own tissues. The TRAM flap is also indicated to preserve the appearance of the opposite breast. The versatility of the flap and the large amounts of skin and fat that can be moved to the breast area are factors that permit the achievement of symmetry with a greater range of shapes of the opposite breast. The TRAM flap is also a good choice for the patient with a radical mastectomy who has a large tissue deficit in the axillary and infraclavicular region. The latissimus dorsi flap is often insufficient for heavy patients with a major tissue deficit. The TRAM flap is indicated for the patient with a large breast; reconstruction with the silicone implant is often disappointing in such patients.

There are definite limitations to the use of the TRAM flap, and patients must be selected carefully in order to avoid serious problems (Scheflan and Dinner, 1983). Previous irradiation to the base of the flap or to the

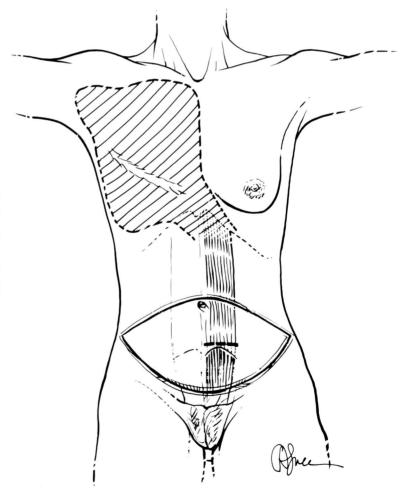

Figure 79–22. Breast reconstruction with the TRAM flap. The flap is designed as an abdominoplasty in the lower abdominal area and is transferred to the chest, pedicled on an upper rectus abdominis muscle containing the superior epigastric artery. The rectus abdominis muscle is divided at the level of the arcuate line.

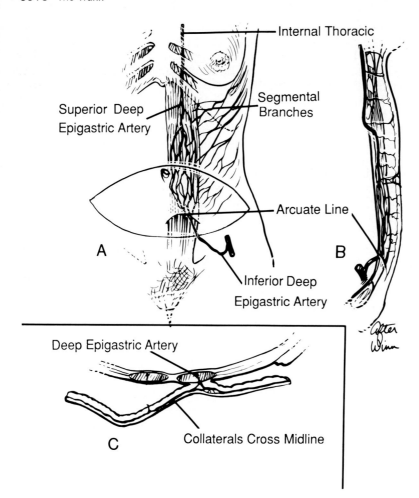

Internal Thoracic

Superior Deep
Epigastric Artery

Segmental
Branches

Arcuate Line

A

Inferior Deep
Epigastric Artery

B

Deep Epigastric Artery

C   Collaterals Cross Midline

Figure 79–23. The TRAM flap. *A,* The superior deep epigastric artery and the inferior deep epigastric artery collateralize just above the level of the umbilicus. These vessels send perforators to the subcutaneous tissue to supply the tissue of the flap. *B,* There are direct perforators from the rectus abdominis muscle into the subcutaneous tissue and skin, and a rich plexus is apparent in the subdermal area. The arterial perforators are concentrated around the umbilical region. *C,* The perforators from the rectus abdominis extend to the subdermal plexus, and the skin and subcutaneous tissue on the contralateral side are supplied by blood flowing through the subdermal plexus.

mediastinum, or surgical division of the pedicle, can seriously compromise the flap and even lead to flap necrosis. Patients older than 65 years, very obese patients, and those with microcirculation problems such as diabetes mellitus should usually undergo reconstruction with alternative methods. Long-term cigarette smoking (more than 20 pack/years) has an acute and chronic effect on the microcirculation, and the reliability of the flap is compromised in these patients. The operation is demanding physically and emotionally for the patient and should not be performed if she is not prepared for a major operation with significant pain and a long convalescence. It is also demanding for the surgeon, who should be experienced with the technique (Bunkis and associates, 1983).

The anatomy of the TRAM flap is complex and the predictability of the microcirculation to its random portions is variable (Taylor and Palmer, 1987). The TRAM flap depends on an intact system of vessels from the neck to the random tissue in the lateral lower abdomen (Fig. 79–23). The internal thoracic artery terminates in the superior epigastric artery just under the costal margin (Miller and associates, 1988). This vessel branches within the rectus abdominis muscle and sends perforators to supply the overlying fat and skin. There is a large concentration of perforators around the umbilicus and these are included in the TRAM flap to provide maximal reliability (see Chap. 10). The flap has direct perforators supplying it above the ipsilateral rectus abdominis muscle. There is a random portion of the flap across the midline and lateral to the muscle. The distal lateral portion of the flap on the contralateral side is often unreliable. The major random blood supply is across the midline in the subdermal plexus, and the flap should be thinned below Scarpa's fascia. When there is concern for the microcirculation of the flap in its random portions, the flap can be moved to the area for breast reconstruction with both rectus abdominis muscle pedicles. This strategy doubles the blood flow and venous drainage of the flap and reduces by half the tissue requirements (Ishii and associates, 1985). Another strategy for enhancing the blood flow to the flap is to preserve the deep inferior epigastric vessels and perform an anastomosis to the axillary vessels. This is particularly helpful when there has been surgical division of the upper pedicle.

When planning a breast reconstruction with the TRAM flap, the surgeon must first define the model for the reconstruction. If the opposite breast is attractive and the goal is to match it, the measurements of the vertical and horizontal skin deficits are made and this amount of skin is included in the flap. The flap must be planned in reverse to be certain that it will fit properly. The volume of the tissue deficit and the amount of tissue to be replaced must also be estimated. It is undesirable to have to add a silicone breast implant or tissue expander if the TRAM flap technique is selected.

The TRAM flap is usually designed as a transverse ellipse of excess tissue in the lower abdomen—the tissue usually discarded during an esthetic abdominoplasty. The donor site of the TRAM flap should be managed as an esthetic abdominoplasty with a flat abdominal wall and a low, thin scar (Fig. 79–24) (Hartrampf, 1984). The flap is versatile and can be used for breast augmentation only when the skin cover is satisfactory.

Planning must not be undertaken until there is a clear idea in the surgeon's mind of the expectations of the patient. Planning at the mastectomy site must define the position of the incisions and scars for the TRAM flap. There is usually an elliptic scar that crosses the original mastectomy scar, curves around, and courses along the inframammary crease.

The plan for the inframammary crease must not make it too inferiorly positioned

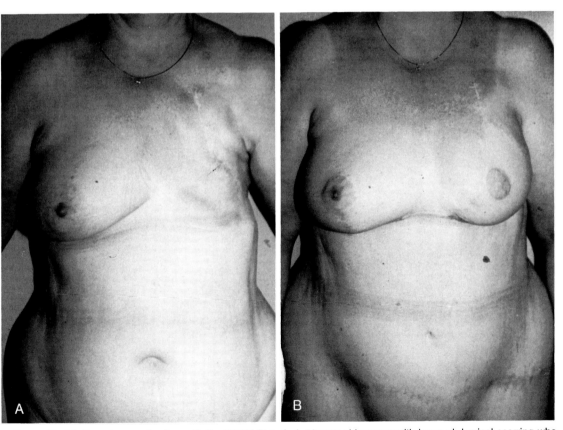

Figure 79–24. Breast reconstruction with the TRAM flap. *A*, A 56 year old woman with lower abdominal scarring who had a left modified radical mastectomy. *B*, Breast reconstruction was done with a contralateral TRAM flap, and a reduction mammoplasty was performed on the opposite breast. The nipple areola was reconstructed at a second operation approximately three months later. (From Berger, K., and Bostwick, J.: A Woman's Decision: Breast Care, Treatment and Reconstruction. St Louis, MO, Quality Medical Publishing, 1988.)

because it is usually displaced a few centimeters with the tighter abdominal closure. Correction of the opposite breast should also be included in the preoperative planning, and the reconstruction planned to match the corrected opposite breast.

During the surgical procedure it is important to maximize the microcirculation to the flap. Vasoconstriction should be avoided. The flap is also cold sensitive, and both the patient and the administered fluids should be warmed. The anesthesiologist should not administer nitrous oxide because it causes distention of the bowel, which can lead to difficulty with the abdominal closure.

After the definitive preoperative markings have been made, incisions are made around the TRAM flap and beveled upward to include more of the periumbilical perforators. The upper abdominal flap is elevated over the costal margin. The contralateral pedicle is used when the breast reconstruction requires skin and fat. The ipsilateral TRAM flap is used alone when the breast reconstruction

requires only filling. The TRAM flap is elevated until it is only over the direct strip of rectus abdominis muscle perforators in the periumbilical region, and just below it. The muscle is divided below, along with the deep inferior epigastric artery at the level of the arcuate line. The rectus abdominis muscle and the TRAM flap are elevated out of the rectus abdominis sheath. After the breast defect has been defined on the chest wall, the TRAM flap is passed through a generous tunnel into the breast area. It is positioned to give optimal appearance and symmetry with the opposite breast. Part of the flap is sometimes deepithelized and used for upper fill or lower projection (Figs. 79–25, 79–26, 79–27) (Elliott and Hartrampf, 1983).

The abdominal wall closure is done directly with large sutures. Prolene mesh is placed over the closure to provide additional security and to reduce the possibility of postoperative stretching of the abdominal wall. Suction drains are placed in all operative sites.

When two pedicles are necessary, such as

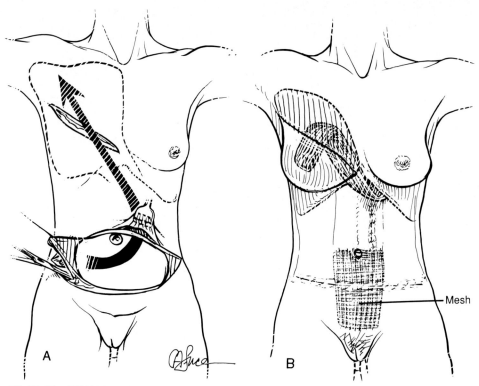

Figure 79–25. The TRAM flap. *A*, After the TRAM flap has been mobilized on the contralateral rectus abdominis muscle, the mastectomy site is opened to reestablish the mastectomy deformity. The TRAM flap is transposed through a generous tunnel into the breast area. It is fashioned into the shape of a breast to match the opposite side. *B*, The abdominal closure is accomplished by approximation of the fascia, and plication of the opposite side is done to ensure symmetry. Lower plication is done when necesary to enhance the tightness of the lower abdomen. Abdominal wall strength is increased by placing a sheet of prolene mesh over the repair.

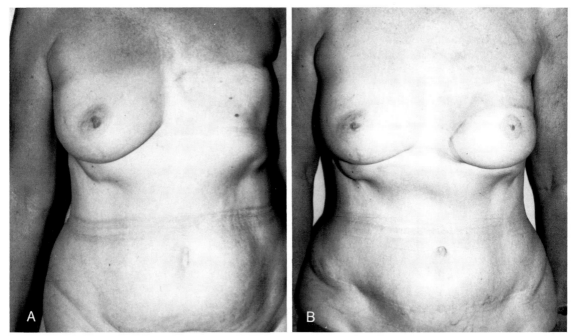

Figure 79–26. Breast reconstruction with the TRAM flap. *A,* A woman who requested breast reconstruction to match the opposite breast. She desired a flatter abdomen and did not want an operation on the opposite breast. *B,* The breast reconstruction was done with the TRAM flap technique. There was sufficient lower abdominal tissue for breast reconstruction without the need for a silicone breast implant. The nipple areola reconstruction was done on an outpatient basis three months later. (From Bostwick, J.: Breast reconstruction. Emory Univ. J. Med., *1*:300, 1987.)

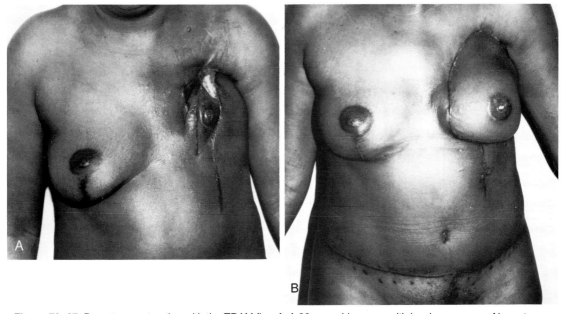

Figure 79–27. Breast reconstruction with the TRAM flap *A,* A 36 year old woman with local recurrence of breast cancer after a latissimus dorsi musculocutaneous flap breast reconstruction following a modified radical mastectomy. She underwent a radical mastectomy with postoperative radiation therapy for treatment of the recurrence. *B,* The mastectomy wound did not heal and developed radiation necrosis. The area of the radiation necrosis was excised and the breast reconstruction was done with a TRAM flap. (From Bostwick, J., Stevenson, T. R., Nahai, F., Hester, T. R., Coleman, J. J., and Jurkiewicz, M. J.: Radiation to the breast. Complications amenable to surgical treatment. Ann. Surg., *200*:543, 1984.)

for bilateral breast reconstruction or for enhancement of the TRAM flap, direct donor site closure is also possible. Some of the lateral fascia of the rectus abdominis muscle is preserved, and some of the lateral rectus abdominis muscle perforators are sacrificed.

Nipple-areola reconstruction is done several months later, not at the time of the TRAM flap, because the decreased flow in the flap usually does not support vascularization of the skin graft.

Complications from the TRAM flap are primarily related to decreased perfusion. These are best avoided by careful patient selection, avoidance of vasoconstriction of the flap in the intraoperative period, and administration of oxygen in the postoperative period (Georgiade and associates, 1984).

Abdominal wall complications are related to protrusion of the intra-abdominal contents against the weakened abdominal wall. A secure abdominal closure, reinforced with prolene mesh, usually avoids this problem. If protrusion occurs, the abdominal wall is plicated, and this closure is supported with prolene mesh.

RECONSTRUCTION WITH GLUTEUS MAXIMUS FLAP

When the other flap techniques are inappropriate or unavailable, or have been used in previous attempts, the breast can be reconstructed with the fat and skin from the buttocks, with the technique developed by Fujino, Harashina, and Enomoto (1976) and refined by Shaw (1983). The gluteus maximus musculocutaneous flap is taken from the superior gluteus maximus area and transferred to the chest. The flap vessels are connected to the internal mammary vessels by microsurgical technique. The donor site and reconstructive strategy are appealing for many patients because many women have an excess of tissue in this area. The technique uses autogenous tissue, and therefore can avoid the silicone breast implant. Sufficient tissue is provided to obtain an attractive result, and the donor scar is easily hidden on the buttocks beneath brief clothing.

The amount of tissue needed for the breast reconstruction is determined and planned for the buttocks region over the superior gluteal artery. The tissue, along with a segment of the gluteus maximus overlying the superior

gluteal artery, is elevated on the vascular pedicle (Figs. 79–28, 79–29). The buttocks tissue with the superior gluteal artery pedicle is transferred to the breast area. The internal mammary artery is prepared just under the fourth and fifth costal cartilages, and the superior gluteal artery is anastomosed to the internal mammary artery. The venous recipient vessel accompanying the internal mammary artery is often of inadequate size, and vein grafts from the axillary vessels or the external jugular vein are used for the anastomosis. There usually is better projection from the gluteus maximus musculocutaneous flap than from the TRAM flap, and there is not usually a need for insertion of a silicone breast implant.

Breast reconstruction with this microvascular technique is highly refined and technically demanding. The survival of the new breast mound depends on successful anastomosis of the vessels and maintenance of patency in the postoperative period. Failure can indicate the necessity to reoperate and revise the anastomoses.

PROPHYLACTIC MASTECTOMY

Some women have a high risk of developing breast cancer. Prophylactic mastectomy is an operation designed to reduce this risk by removing a high percentage of the breast tissue. This option has become more attractive for the woman at high risk since the development of satisfactory methods of immediate breast reconstruction (Jarrett, Cutler, and Teal, 1978; Woods, Irons, and Arnold, 1980). The operation is controversial, and even though the solution sounds appealing in terms of preventing the development of breast cancer and restoring the breast, serious esthetic, operative, and psychologic complications can arise (Goin and Goin, 1982).

There are several major high risk factors that increase a woman's chances of developing breast cancer. Although the cause of breast cancer is unknown, it appears to be affected by a number of genetic, pathologic (Dupont and Page, 1985), environmental, and sociobiologic factors. A family history of breast cancer in a first degree maternal relative (mother or sister), especially when the cancer develops bilaterally or premenopausally, increases the risks significantly. A previous cancer in one breast doubles the chances of it developing in the opposite breast. Younger patients are also at greater risk of developing a second breast cancer (Adami, Bergstrom, and Hansen, 1985). In addition, there are certain other pathologic indicators of increased risk such as multifocal areas of breast cancer, lobular carcinoma in situ, changes of epithelial hyperplasia and atypias, and multiple areas of in situ intra-ductal carcinoma. Fibrocystic disease does not indicate an increased risk, although certain pathologic changes that often coexist with this condition do increase the risk.

Women who are at high risk of developing breast cancer and are considering prophylac-tic mastectomy should weigh the pros and cons of the operation before making a deci-sion.

Prophylactic mastectomy should involve to-tal mastectomy to remove most of the breast tissue at risk. The incision is usually either in the inframammary crease or through a lateral incision that may extend around the areola. If there is no significant amount of breast ptosis, the nipple areola is not removed and is preserved with the breast skin. The ductal tissue is removed and checked by path-ologic frozen sections. When there is a major amount of ptosis, the excess skin is removed as in a reduction mammoplasty, and the nip-

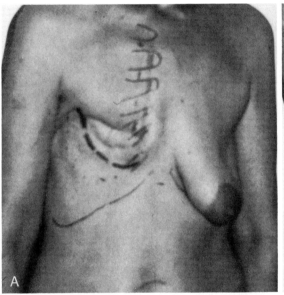
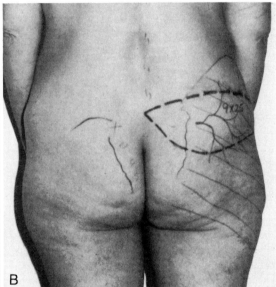
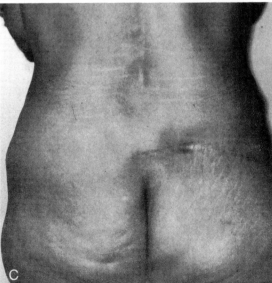

Figure 79–28. Gluteus maximus free flap reconstruc-tion. *A,* Recipient site. Note the incision at the location of the proposed inframammary fold. The internal mammary artery is also outlined. *B,* Donor site with skin island and muscle based on the superior gluteal vessels. *C,* Healed donor site. (Courtesy of Dr. William Shaw, Institute of Reconstructive Plastic Surgery, New York University Med-ical Center.)

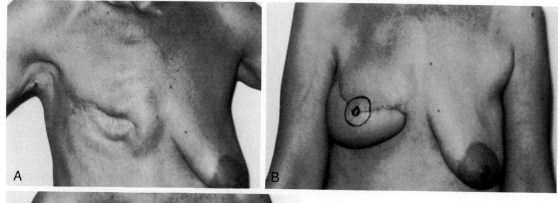

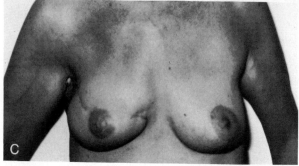

Figure 79–29. Gluteus maximus free flap. *A*, Preoperative view after a modified radical mastectomy and unsuccessful reconstruction. *B*, After reconstruction with the gluteus maximus free flap and before nipple-areola reconstruction and contralateral breast reduction. *C*, Final appearance. (Courtesy of Dr. William Shaw, Institute of Reconstructive Plastic Surgery, New York University Medical Center.)

ple areola is moved to its new position as a graft. Breast reconstruction is done at the time of the prophylactic mastectomy. The musculofascial layer is elevated and the silicone breast implant is placed in the proper position (Fig. 79–30). When the soft tissues are deficient or when there is concern for the viability of the skin, a tissue expander is placed beneath the musculofascial layer and inflated a few weeks later after the tissues have healed.

Prophylactic mastectomy is an operation subject to a number of complications. All the complications of mastectomy are also associated with the potential problems of immediate breast reconstruction, as well as those of any breast reconstruction with the silicone breast implant. In addition to the possibility of infection and hematoma, there can be loss of skin of the breast and of the nipple areola. If the silicone breast implant is not completely covered by the musculofascial layer, exposure of the silicone breast implant can result, and removal will be required. There seems to be a higher incidence of capsular contracture about the silicone breast implant with this operation. If this problem becomes intractable, it may be necessary to provide additional cover for the silicone breast implant with a latissimus dorsi flap, or the

implant can be replaced with the patient's own tissue in the form of a bilateral TRAM flap or a gluteus maximus flap.

MANAGEMENT OF THE OPPOSITE BREAST

The opposite breast is an important consideration in breast reconstruction. Symmetry is difficult to achieve because of the oncologic, reconstructive, and esthetic considerations involved. The oncologic management can range from careful monitoring of the opposite breast to a prophylactic mastectomy, as discussed above. The pathology of the original tumor as well as the risks related to the opposite breast are factors to be evaluated before the breast reconstruction is undertaken.

The patient's psychologic attitude toward the opposite breast influences the type of breast reconstruction. If she does not want anything done to the opposite breast, the indications are for a flap type of breast reconstruction to achieve symmetry. Some patients may rather have a flap reconstruction than change an opposite breast that they feel is attractive.

Esthetic considerations can also influence

the type of breast reconstruction and the modification of the opposite breast. When the latter is small and flat, it may not be possible to match it with a silicone breast implant. These patients may prefer to have an augmentation mammoplasty to enlarge the small breast, and the reconstruction must be planned to match the augmented breast. The augmentation mammoplasty is usually done via the inframammary approach. Any suspicious areas in the breast can be biopsied at this time. The silicone implant is placed in the submusculofascial position so that it does not interfere with future breast examination, imaging, and treatment.

When the opposite breast is hypoplastic and ptotic, it is difficult for the surgeon to match it without modification. The reconstruction is planned to match the opposite breast after it has been corrected with a submusculofascial silicone implant and a mastopexy. The latter is designed to elevate the nipple areola and remove the excess skin vertically beneath the nipple areola and, if necessary, horizontally in the inframammary crease.

When the opposite breast is hypertrophic and heavy, it is difficult to obtain symmetry without a reduction mammoplasty, which is usually done at the time of the breast recon-struction. By correcting both breasts at the same time, the surgeon is more likely to achieve symmetry. Occasionally, when there is a large volume of lower abdominal tissue, a heavy opposite breast can be matched with a lower TRAM flap. The most reliable strategy to obtain symmetry is to do a reduction of the opposite breast and to plan the reconstruction to match the reduced breast. It is important to understand the patient's expectations concerning the size and contour of the reduced breast. It is often necessary to use a flap for breast reconstruction in order to be sure that the expected size is achieved.

When a prophylactic mastectomy is done at the time of the reconstruction, the opposite breast may be either hypoplastic, ptotic, or hypertrophic. The adjustment of the opposite breast in these situations requires esthetic correction of the nipple-areola position, placement of the correct-sized silicone implant, and removal of any extra skin. This is one of the most complex corrections in breast reconstruction. When a TRAM flap procedure is being performed, the patient should know that it can be done only once. It is also possible to perform a total mastectomy and carry out the breast reconstruction on both sides with a bilateral TRAM flap.

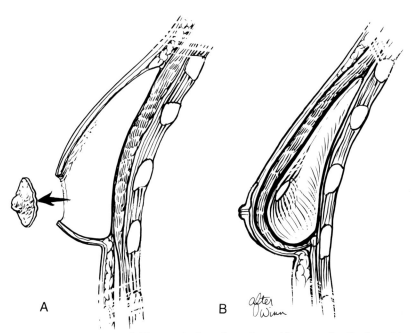

Figure 79–30. Prophylactic mastectomy. A, The mastectomy is performed by removing the breast in the superficial aspect of the superficial fascia but preserving the deep fascia. B, A total musculofascial cover is developed to protect the silicone breast implant. The nipple area is regrafted at the new position or is reconstructed at a second operation a few months later. Note the implant under the musculofascial layer.

RECONSTRUCTION OF NIPPLE AREOLA

Nipple-areola reconstruction should be done after breast symmetry has been achieved. Several years ago when breast reconstruction was developing and the results were not symmetric, nipple-areola reconstruction even detracted from the result and emphasized the asymmetry. Nipple-areola reconstruction is now an integral part of breast reconstruction, and the goal is to reconstruct a nipple areola similar in appearance to the opposite one.

Before nipple-areola reconstruction is done, the breast reconstruction should be stable and there should be breast symmetry. If the breast changes after the nipple-areola reconstruction, asymmetry will be apparent. If the areola is placed on skin that stretches in the postoperative period, the appearance of the areola could be distorted. The position, size, shape, and projection of the nipple-areola

reconstruction should be determined preoperatively with the patient standing, her arms at her side. The patient should participate in the determination of these variables of the breast reconstruction. The nipple-areola position should look correct when viewed directly as well as when seen by the patient in looking down.

Nipple-areola reconstruction is best done with donor material that most closely matches the opposite nipple areola (Fig. 79–31). When there is a reduction mammoplasty of the opposite breast, some of the extra peripheral areola can be used for the areola reconstruction. If this material is not available, a good choice is the pigmented skin of the upper inner (medial) thigh crease. The ellipse of skin is taken from the crease as a full-thickness graft, and any underlying hair roots are removed while the graft is being thinned. This donor site is painful, and patients usually prefer another site. A full-thickness skin graft removed from the area

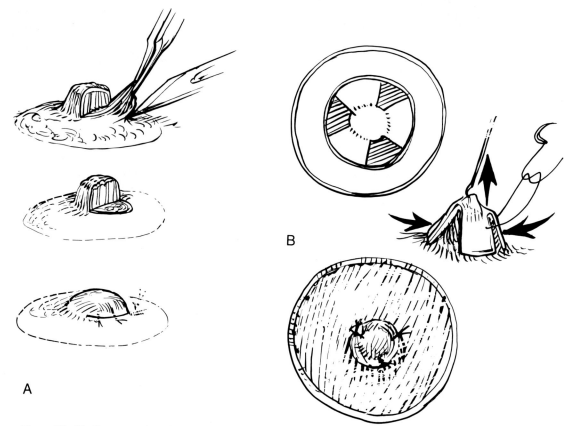

Figure 79–31. Reconstruction of the nipple areola. *A,* Nipple sharing is a satisfactory method of nipple reconstruction when the opposite nipple has adequate size and projection. The lower half of the nipple is excised and the donor site is closed primarily. The nipple is placed at the center of the future areola site. *B,* An alternative method of nipple-areola reconstruction is the quadrapod flap (Little). The flap is elevated, based on a central mound, and the lateral portions of the elevated tissue are used for lining the vertical portion of the nipple. A circumferential full-thickness skin graft is used for the areola reconstruction.

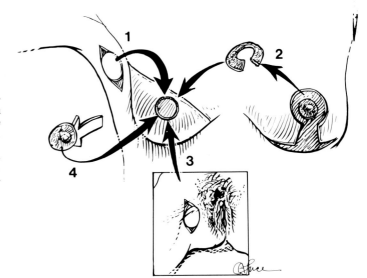

Figure 79–32. Reconstruction of the areola. Sources include (1) skin from the axilla or regions of the mastectomy scar, (2) the opposite areola, (3) the upper inner thigh, and (4) a skin graft from the resected areola, which is repositioned after appropriate frozen section examination. A tattoo is often necessary to provide the proper color after nipple-areola reconstruction.

of a mastectomy or abdominal scar can be used for the areola reconstruction; however, the color needs to be darkened later with a tattoo (Fig. 79–32).

The diameter of the areola graft should be the same as the recipient site so that the graft does not contract with healing.

Symmetry of the nipple is also important and half of the opposite nipple is a satisfactory choice, both for color match, texture, and symmetry, when it is large and possibly ptotic. When the opposite nipple is not available, as in bilateral reconstructions or when it is too small, nipple reconstruction can be done with local flaps of the chest skin centered over the proposed nipple site (Little and Spear, 1988). The "skate" flap procedure is a versatile and effective technique for nipple reconstruction. After defining the diameter of the areola, a third of the future areola surface area is deepithelized. The "wings" of the skate flap are elevated, going deeper into the dermis as the future diameter of the nipple is approached. The nipple is elevated with some fat on the flap centrally, and the wings of the flap are brought around and sutured to each other to give the proper projection of the nipple. There is some atrophy of the nipple in the first few postoperative months, so the nipple should be left about one-third larger than the desired final size. It is easy to reduce a slightly larger nipple but difficult to enlarge it. After the nipple is reconstructed, the areola graft is positioned over the recipient area and sutured circumferentially. A silicone stent for the areola with a plastic nipple protector immobilizes the nipple-areola reconstruction for one week.

Approximately two to three months later, the color of the reconstructed nipple areola is evaluated relative to the opposite side. The proper color is determined and the reconstructed nipple areola is tattooed to obtain that color.

REFERENCES

Adami, H., Bergstrom, R., and Hansen, J.: Age at first primary as a determinant of the incidence of bilateral breast cancer. Cumulative and relative risks in a population-based case-control study. Cancer, 55:643, 1985.

American Cancer Society: Cancer facts and figures, 1987. New York, American Cancer Society, 1987.

Anderson, D. E.: Breast cancer in families. Cancer, 40:1855, 1977.

Argenta, L. C.: Reconstruction of the breast by tissue expansion. Clin. Plast. Surg., 11:257, 1984.

Becker, H.: Breast reconstruction using an inflatable breast implant with detachable reservoir. Plast. Reconstr. Surg., 73:678, 1984.

Berger, K., and Bostwick, J.: A Woman's Decision: Breast Care, Treatment and Reconstruction. St. Louis, MO, C. V. Mosby Company, 1984.

Biggs, T. M., and Cronin, E. D.: Technical aspects of the latissimus dorsi flap in breast reconstruction. Ann. Plast. Surg., 6:381, 1981.

Bostwick, J.: Aesthetic and Reconstructive Breast Surgery. St. Louis, MO, C. V. Mosby Company, 1983.

Bostwick, J.: Breast reconstruction following mastectomy. Contemp. Surg., 27:19, 1985.

Bostwick, J.: Breast reconstruction following mastectomy. Contemp. Surg., 30:16, 1987.

Bostwick, J.: Breast reconstruction. Emory Univ. J. Med., 1:297, 300, 1987.

Bostwick, J.: Breast reconstruction using modified tissue expansion for matching a small opposite breast. Perspect. Plast. Surg., 1:79, 1987.

Bostwick, J., Stevenson, T. R., Nahai, F., Hester, T. R., Coleman, J. J., and Jurkiewicz, M. J.: Radiation to the breast. Complications amenable to surgical treatment. Ann. Surg., *200*:543, 1984.

Bostwick, J., III, Vasconez, L. O., and Jurkiewicz, M. J.: Breast reconstruction after a radical mastectomy. Plast. Reconstr. Surg., *61*:682, 1978.

Bunkis, J., Walton, R. L., Mathes, S. J., Krizek, T. J., and Vasconez, L. O.: Experience with the transverse lower rectus abdominis operation for breast reconstruction. Plast. Reconstr. Surg., *72*:819, 1983.

DeVita, V. T., Hellman, S., and Rosenberg, S. A. (Eds.): Cancer, Principles and Practice of Oncology. Philadelphia, J. B. Lippincott Company, 1985.

Dick, G. O., and Brown, S. A.: Breast reconstruction using modified tissue expansion. Plast. Reconstr. Surg., *77*:613, 1986.

Dinner, M. I., Dowden, R. V., and Scheflan, M.: Refinements in the use of the transverse abdominal island flap for postmastectomy reconstruction. Ann. Plast. Surg., *11*:362, 1983.

Dupont, W. D., and Page, D. L.: Risk factors for breast cancer in women with proliferative breast disease. N. Engl. J. Med., *312*:146, 1985.

Elliott, L. F., and Hartrampf, C. R., Jr.: Tailoring of the new breast using the transverse abdominal island flap. Plast. Reconstr. Surg., *72*:887, 1983.

Fisher, B., Bauer, M., Margolese, R., Poisson, R., Pilch, Y., et al.: Five-year results of a randomized clinical trial comparing total mastectomy and segmental mastectomy with or without radiation in the treatment of breast cancer. N. Engl. J. Med., *312*:665, 1985.

Fisher, J., Bostwick, J., III, and Powell, R. W.: Latissimus dorsi blood supply after thoracodorsal vessel division: the serratus collateral. Plast. Reconstr. Surg., *72*:502, 1983.

Fujino, T., Harashina, T., and Enomoto, K.: Primary breast reconstruction after a standard radical mastectomy by a free flap transfer. Plast. Reconstr. Surg., *58*:372, 1976.

Georgiade, G. S., Georgiade, N. G., McCarty, K. S., Jr., Ferguson, B. J., and Seigler, H. F.: Modified radical mastectomy with immediate reconstruction for carcinoma of the breast. Ann. Surg., *193*:565, 1981.

Georgiade, G. S., Riefkohl, R., Cox, E., McCarty, K. S., Seigler, H. F., et al.: Long-term clinical outcome of immediate reconstruction after mastectomy. Plast. Reconstr. Surg., *76*:415, 1985.

Georgiade, G. S., Voci, V. E., Riefkohl, R., and Scheflan, M.: Potential problems with transverse rectus abdominis myocutaneous flap in breast reconstruction and how to avoid them. Br. J. Plast. Surg., *37*:121, 1984.

Goin, M. K., and Goin, J. M.: Psychological reactions to prophylactic mastectomy synchronous with contralateral breast reconstruction. Plast. Reconstr. Surg., *70*:355, 1982.

Gruber, R. P., Kahn, R. A., Lash, H., Maser, M. R., Apfelberg, D., and Laub, D. R.: Breast reconstruction following mastectomy: a comparison of submuscular and subcutaneous techniques. Plast. Reconstr. Surg., *67*:312, 1981.

Haagensen, C. D.: Diseases of the Breast. 3rd Ed. Philadelphia, W. B. Saunders Company, 1986.

Halsted, W. S.: The results of operations for the cure of cancer of the breast performed at the Johns Hopkins Hospital from June 1889 to January 1894. Ann. Surg., *20*:497, 1894.

Harris, J. R., Hellman, S., Henderson, I. C., and Kinne, D. K.: Breast Diseases. Philadelphia, J. B. Lippincott Company, 1987.

Hartrampf, C. R., Jr.: Abdominal wall competence in transverse abdominal island flap operations. Ann. Plast. Surg., *12*:139, 1984.

Hartrampf, C. R., Scheflan, M., and Black, P. W.: Breast reconstruction following mastectomy with a transverse abdominal island flap. Anatomical and clinical observations. Plast. Reconstr. Surg., *69*:216, 1982.

Hester, T. R.: The polyurethane covered silicone breast implant. Perspect. Plast. Surg., *2*:135, 1988.

Holleb, A. I.: The American Cancer Society Cancer Book. New York, Doubleday & Company, 1986.

Ishii, C. H., Jr., Bostwick, J., III, Raine T. J., Coleman, J. J., III, and Hester, T. R.: Double-pedicle transverse rectus abdominis myocutaneous flap for unilateral breast and chest-wall reconstruction. Plast. Reconstr. Surg., *76*:901, 1985.

Jarrett, J. R., Cutler, R. G., and Teal, D. F.: Subcutaneous mastectomy in small, large, or ptotic breasts with immediate submuscular placement of the implants. Plast. Reconstr. Surg., *62*:702, 1978.

Lejour, M., Alemanno, P., De Mey, A., Gerard, T., Duchateau, J., et al.: Analysis of fifty-six breast reconstructions using the latissimus dorsi flap. Ann. Chir. Plast. Esthet., *30*:7, 1985.

Little, J. W., and Spear, S.: Nipple-areola reconstruction. Perspect. Plast. Surg., *2*:1, 1988.

Maxwell, G. P.: Latissimus dorsi breast reconstruction: an aesthetic assessment. Clin. Plast. Surg., *8*:373, 1981.

Miller, L. B., Bostwick, J., Hartrampf, C. R., et al.: The superiorly based rectus abdominis flap: predicting and enhancing its blood supply based on an anatomical and clinical study. Plast. Reconstr. Surg., *81*:713, 1988.

Noone, R. B., Frazier, T. G., Hayward, C. Z., and Skiles, M. S.: Patient acceptance of immediate reconstruction following mastectomy. Plast. Reconstr. Surg., *69*:632, 1982.

Radovan, C.: Breast reconstruction after mastectomy using the temporary expander. Plast. Reconstr. Surg., *69*:195, 1982.

Sando, W., and Jurkiewicz, M. J.: An approach to repair of radiation necrosis of the chest wall and mammary gland. World J. Surg., *10*:206, 1986.

Sattin, R. W., Rubin, G. L., Webster, L. A., Huezo, C. M., Wingo, P. A., et al.: Family history and the risk of breast cancer. J.A.M.A., *253*:1908, 1985.

Scheflan, M., and Dinner, M. I.: The transverse abdominal island flap: indications, contraindications, results, and complications. Ann. Plast. Surg., *10*:24, 1983.

Schneider, W. J., Hill, H. L., and Brown, R. G.: Latissimus dorsi myocutaneous flap for breast reconstruction. Br. J. Plast. Surg., *30*:277, 1977.

Shaw, W. W.: Breast reconstruction by superior gluteal microvascular free flaps without silicone implants. Plast. Reconstr. Surg., *72*:490, 1983.

Stevens, L. A., McGrath, M. H., Druss, R. G., Kister, S. J., Gump, F. E., and Forde, K. A.: The psychological impact of immediate breast reconstruction for women with early breast cancer. Plast. Reconstr. Surg., *73*:619, 1984.

Taylor, G. I., and Palmer, J. H.: The vascular territories (angiosomes) of the body: experimental study and clinical applications. Br. J. Plast. Surg., *40*:113, 1987.

Wolf, L. E., and Biggs, T. M.: Aesthetic refinements in the use of the latissimus dorsi flap in breast reconstruction. Plast. Reconstr. Surg., *69*:788, 1982.

Woods, J. E., Irons, G. B., Jr., and Arnold, P. G.: The case for submuscular implantation of prostheses in reconstructive breast surgery. Ann. Plast. Surg., *5*:115, 1980.

80

Frederick M. Grazer

Abdominoplasty

HISTORY

Body esthetics has its roots in antiquity, as far as 30,000 B.C. Before the modern surgical era beginning in the 1870's, limited resections were performed to contour the abdominal wall. Alterations to body contour had been made by such external methods as tattooing or scarification, the wearing of girdles, and alterations in clothing such as binding of the feet or head (Grazer and Klingbeil, 1980).

The first dermolipectomies of the abdominal wall were performed by surgeons who were repairing massive umbilical hernias. The dermolipectomy facilitated the herniorrhaphy and relieved the patient of a pendu-lous abdomen. In his thesis (1960), Voloir alluded to a case report of an abdominal wall lipectomy by Demars and Marx (1890) in France. Kelly (1899) called attention to the dermolipectomy in the United States. Case reports subsequently became more numerous in Europe, especially in France and Germany. At the French Congress of Surgery in 1905, Gaudet and Morestin reported transverse closure of the umbilicus in the repair of large hernias, in conjunction with resection of excess skin and fat and preservation of the umbilicus. Desjardins (1911) resected a composite of skin and fat weighing 22.4 kg through a vertical elliptic abdominal incision. In 1911 Amedée Morestin, the younger brother of Hippolyte Morestin, published five cases of dermolipectomy performed through transverse elliptic incisions. In Germany, Weinhold (1909) recommended a midline type of excision. Jolly (1911) favored a low transverse elliptic excision; Schepelmann (1918, 1924) preferred a vertical midline excision extending from the xyphoid to the pubis.

Subsequently, in the evolution of the technique of dermolipectomy of the abdominal wall, three methods have been advocated: (1) vertical midline resection, (2) transverse resection, and (3) a combination of the vertical and transverse methods.

The classic lipectomy incisions are shown in Figure 80–1. They include those of Kelly (1899, 1910), Weinhold (1909), Babcock (1916, 1939), Schepelmann (1918, 1924), Küster (1926), Flesch-Thebesius and Wheisheimer (1931), Thorek (1924), Pick (1949), Barsky (1950), Galtier (1955), and Gonzalez-Ulloa (1960). Castanares and Goethel (1967) published a modification of the classic techniques in which they combined the vertical and transverse excisions with little or no

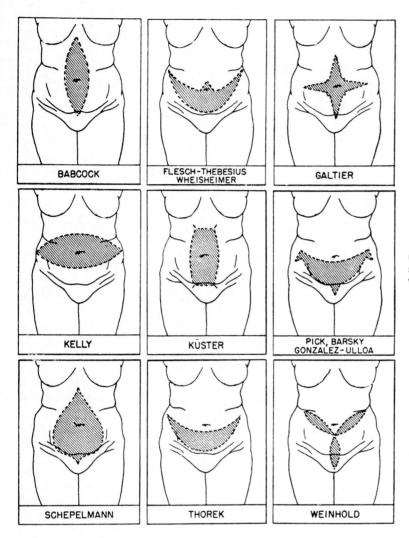

BABCOCK

FLESCH-THEBESIUS
WHEISHEIMER

GALTIER

KELLY

KÜSTER

PICK, BARSKY
GONZALEZ-ULLOA

SCHEPELMANN

THOREK

WEINHOLD

Figure 80–1. Classic incisions used for abdominoplasty and reconstruction of the anterior abdominal wall.

undermining, which greatly reduced the operating time. Grazer (1973) reviewed his technique in 44 abdominoplasties and recommended a low transverse incision with a vertical limb extending to the old umbilicus. Fischl (1973) considered that, in patients with excess skin and striae in the absence of an abdominal apron, a vertical abdominoplasty, which removes an ellipse of skin, is preferable. Schwartz (1974) advocated elevating the fat apron by suspension by towel clips to a rubber tube stretched between the metal posts used for gynecologic stirrups. Heavy interrupted sutures were then passed through the base of the suspended apron, and in this way excessive blood loss was prevented. Regnault (1975) reported a lower transverse incision in the shape of a "W."

The 1960's to the 1980's witnessed a period of contour refinement stimulated by the reports of Pitanguy and associates (1974), Baroudi (1975), Regnault (1975), and Psillakis (1984). During this period, it became obvious that the low transverse incision was the preferred choice for patients undergoing abdominoplasty. Surgery performed during this period is characterized by the low placement of the abdominal incision, emphasis on the small umbilicus, and the achievement of long-term contour results (Figs. 80–2, 80–3) (Grazer, Klingbeil, and Mattiello, 1980).

The introduction of suction assisted lipectomy (SAL) or liposuction in the 1980's, a technique popularized by Illouz (1983) and Kesselring (Kesselring and Meyer, 1978; Kesselring, 1982), provided another way to

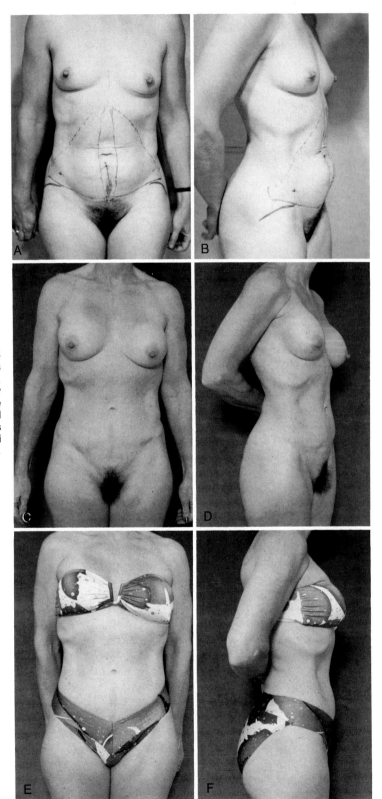

Figure 80–2. *A,B,* A 40 year old, 115 lb female had had three cesarean sections with diastasis recti and scar deformity. *C,D,* Sixteen years after abdominoplasty combined with breast augmentation. Note the near-disappearance of the vertical abdominal scar. The same patient is seen 16 years postoperatively in a bikini bathing suit *(E)* frontal and *(F)* side view.

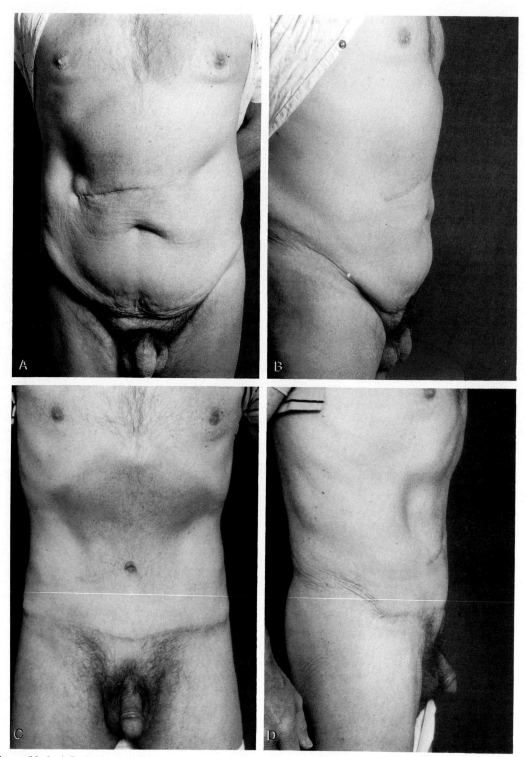

Figure 80–3. *A,B,* A 50 year old male had weighed 300 lb and had lost 105 lb following ileojejunal bypass surgery. *C,D,* Seven years after abdominoplasty. His weight has remained unchanged. Note the transposed subcostal scar at the level of the umbilicus.

improve the results in body contouring patients, especially in the abdomen (see Chap. 81).

The internal sculpturing produced by plication and suctioning combines the precepts of refinement and technique. This chapter discusses the procedures and techniques of the abdominoplasty and mini-abdominoplasty with reference to the reverse abdominoplasty and the suctioning techniques that furnish the overall refinements so essential for a satisfactory result.

EQUIPMENT

Liposuction or "sculpture from within" requires proper equipment. The ability to suction fat is achieved with a vacuum pump, noncollapsible silicone tubing, and cannulas of various sizes (see Chap. 81).

Pump. The vacuum pump must achieve vaporization pressure of the tissues, which is approximately 743 mm Hg at sea level. The pressure adequately vaporizes the fat, especially when the smaller cannulas are used. Lower vacuum pressures can be used but only if one employs large-aperture cannulas (Kesselring and Meyer, 1978).

Silicone Tubing. Noncollapsible silicone tubing, approximately 6 feet in length, is used to attach the cannula to the vacuum pump.

Cannulas. The author prefers to use smaller cannulas for all suctioning procedures. The average cannula size for the abdomen is 5 mm or less. The most versatile is the 3.7 mm cannula with multiple apertures (Mercedes 3 hole) (Fig. 80–4).

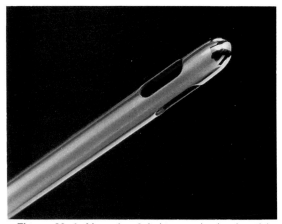

Figure 80–4. Mercedes 3 hole cannula developed by Grams and Grazer.

PATIENT SELECTION AND PREOPERATIVE PLANNING

With the introduction of suction techniques, better results can often be achieved by less surgery. For example, before suction assisted lipectomy, many localized abdominal deformities could be corrected only with a standard abdominoplasty or a mini-abdominoplasty. Therefore, a greater variety of therapeutic options has evolved for two reasons: the recognized value of the mini-abdominoplasty and the advances in suctioning techniques. Many patients who were not suitable candidates for abdominoplasty can now be treated with suction, and measurable results obtained.

Although the parameters for the abdominoplasty have been broadened, patient selection remains the foremost decision before any surgery is entertained.

As with any elective procedure, good health is the primary consideration in patient selection. The decision whether to perform suction alone, a traditional abdominoplasty, or a mini-abdominoplasty obviously depends on the integrity of the skin and subcutaneous tissues. The patients illustrated in Figures 80–5, 80–6, and 80–7 represent typical candidates in each category. Figure 80–5 demonstrates the typical candidate for suction assisted lipectomy alone: localized deformity, satisfactory skin turgor, and the potential for the skin to contract after suctioning. In Figure 80–6 the typical candidate for traditional abdominoplasty is presented: deformity existing both above and below the umbilicus. The typical candidate for the mini-abdominoplasty has the deformity located primarily below the umbilicus (Fig. 80–7).

Age is of very little consideration. The old rule of thumb ("any patient over the age of 45 is not a good candidate") is no longer valid. The true test is skin turgor and contractibility, not age. Suctioning has been successfully accomplished in selected individuals in their 70's and 80's.

The informed consent, individualized by each surgeon, should include a discussion of the most frequent complications such as wound infection, wound separation, hematoma, seroma, and nerve damage as well as some of the rare problems: pulmonary fat embolism syndrome and thromboembolic phenomena with the remote possibility of death (Grazer and Goldwyn, 1977). Costs

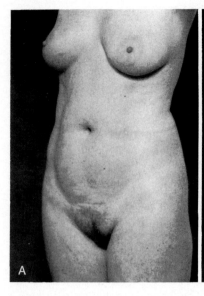
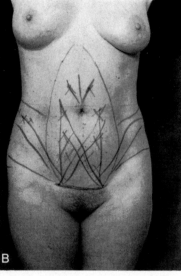

Figure 80–5. A candidate for suctioning alone. The patient is 39 years of age and has satisfactory skin turgor with localized adipose tissue of the anterior abdominal wall that is amenable to suction assisted lipectomy (SAL). *A,* Preoperative appearance. *B,* Outline of the incisions and the areas to be suctioned.

should be completely covered including all the hidden costs at the hospital, surgery center, or office. The consent procedure should also include a discussion of the possibility of secondary procedures. In the author's experience with suctioning alone, 20 to 30 per cent of the patients require secondary therapy.

Since body contour surgery is elective, no detail can be left to chance. Assuming that the selected patient has a completely normal preoperative history and physical examination, the surgeon should next evaluate the medication and dietary histories.

Many drugs have an influence on platelet activity, especially aspirin and other anti-inflammatory agents such as naproxen (Naprosyn). It is imperative that such medications be discontinued two weeks before surgery in order to prevent excessive bleeding. With a history of other sophisticated medications such as antihypertensives, it is recommended that the anesthesiologist be consulted ahead of time.

A detailed dietary history is important. Patients on starvation diets do not heal well. Some of the fish oil concentrates used in some diets may influence platelet activity and result in excessive bleeding (Peterson, 1987).

Patients should also be warned about preoperative sunburn and the importance of the complete absence of any open skin defect that could be a potential site of infection.

It is recognized that smoking has a profound influence on the potential for skin slough, particularly in extensive undermining (Forrest, Pang, and Lindsay, 1985). All patients must be cautioned to stop smoking for *at least two weeks* before surgery.

Inpatient vs. Outpatient Surgery. Most patients undergoing suction alone and mini-

Figure 80–6. A candidate for abdominoplasty with generalized abdominal wall weakness, diastasis recti, and striae gravidarum.

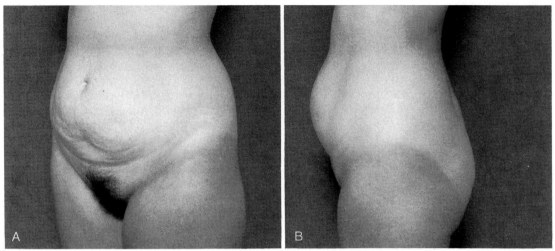

Figure 80–7. A candidate for mini-abdominoplasty: A 39 year old female who demonstrates that the deformity is restricted to the area below the umbilicus with loss of elasticity, while the upper abdomen is firm and flat. *A,* Three-quarter view. *B,* Profile.

abdominoplasty can be handled on an outpatient basis. It is advisable that major combined procedures with the potential for moderate blood loss should be performed on an inpatient basis.

Autologous Blood. The author has been using autologous blood for over ten years and recommends it as a routine in combined procedures or in procedures in which suction volumes exceed 2500 ml. Two or more units should be donated by the patient one or two months before surgery, and the patient is also started on oral iron therapy.

PREVENTION OF COMPLICATIONS

The major potential complications that may occur with abdominoplasty, as with other related body contour procedures, are those one might expect when large amounts of soft tissue are undermined or traumatized. These include infection, wound separation, hematoma, seroma, nerve damage, skin and subcutaneous tissue necrosis, hypovolemic shock, deep venous thrombosis, and pulmonary problems (atelectasis, pulmonary emboli, or fat embolism syndrome).

Prevention of infection begins with proper skin preparation. Most surgeons use one of the iodine-containing compounds. The patient should shower with one of the iodine solutions the night before surgery. In view of the possibility of contamination with extensive undermining of flaps and the use of suctioning, intravenous antibiotics are given during the surgical procedure.

Wound separation usually parallels wound infection but may also be caused by overresection, which results in an excessively tight closure.

Since hematoma and seroma are one of the inevitable consequences of surgery, meticulous hemostasis is essential. Drains are used only with surgical undermining, not with suction alone.

Some degree of nerve damage is inevitable and its extent must be ascertained. It is mostly transitory and primarily sensory. In full abdominoplasty, small areas of permanent anesthesia usually exist around and below the umbilicus. Preoperative discussion with the patient is essential.

Skin and subcutaneous tissue necrosis is a multifactorial problem related to infections, skin tension, smoking, and the state of hydration of the patient.

Volume Loading

Patients undergoing abdominoplasty surgery are usually placed on fluid restriction for at least six to seven hours. Consequently, there is a fluid deficit volume of at least 1500 to 2000 ml. If there is sudden blood loss and tissue trauma due to surgery, the microcirculation suffers at the expense of maintaining the homeostasis of the organism. Fluids are shifted out of the tissues into the major circulation. To prevent this fluid shift, volume loading is recommended. Volume loading (10–12 ml per kg of body weight) of a crystalloid such as Ringer's lactate in the holding room or operating room before the induction of anesthesia is most beneficial and modifies the detrimental fluid shifts.

Pulmonary Thrombosis, Pulmonary Fat Embolism Syndrome

Before 1975, the author had experienced four nonfatal pulmonary emboli in the space of two years while performing approximately 100 abdominoplasties per year. A subsequent publication by Grazer and Goldwyn (1977) indicated that approximately one in 100 patients undergoing abdominoplasty would develop a serious thromboembolic episode, and approximately one in 1000 patients would die. These statistics still prevail. After investigation into the etiology of pulmonary embolism and pulmonary fat embolism syndrome, it was concluded that surgical trauma to fat resulted in a series of complicated changes in the circulation, and in rare cases gave rise to pulmonary fat embolism syndrome or pulmonary emboli. As part of an ongoing study of abdominoplasty patients, fat globules have been found in the blood in randomly selected cases.

Beginning in 1975, because of the work of Evarts and associates (1976) and Peltier (Peltier, 1965, 1971; Peltier and associates, 1974), the author began administering a standard 5 per cent dextrose and 5 per cent alcohol intravenous solution in all abdominoplasty patients at the start of the procedure. The solution contains a total of 50 gm of alcohol, which can be administered in a period extending from 30 minutes up to three hours. This amount of alcohol presents an average blood level of approximately 80 mg per cent, which is below the intoxication level and is the equivalent of approximately three cocktails. Because alcohol is an anesthetic, the anesthesiologist must reduce the regular amount of anesthetic administered (Kettunen and associates, 1983; Mathews, 1983; Grazer and Klingbeil, 1983).

The above alcohol regimen was originally developed by correlating orthopedic clinical studies. These demonstrated that, in long bone fractures, tissue trauma resulted in the release of fat, which was broken down to free fatty acids that lodged in the lungs and produced the fat embolism syndrome (Fig. 80–8) (Sladen, 1980). The trauma and/or the movement of large amounts of fatty tissue associated with the abdominoplasty procedure or the suctioning of large volumes of fat is capable of producing the same pulmonary fat embolism syndrome and the more potentially lethal pulmonary emboli. It has now been clearly demonstrated in the laboratory that alcohol prevents the breakdown of free fat to fatty acids. It also stimulates the formation of tissue plasminogen activator and the production of prostacyclin (Levin and associates, 1981; Laug, 1983; Goldhaber and associates, 1986). Both have aggregate antiplatelet activity and antithromboembolic activity, and also act as vasodilators.

TECHNIQUE FOR SUCTIONING OF ABDOMEN ONLY

In patients who have satisfactory skin turgor with the deformity localized primarily in the lower abdomen, suctioning (SAL) alone may give the desired result (see Fig. 80–5). Small volumes of under 750 ml can be suctioned under local anesthesia. The author prefers a solution of 0.3 per cent lidocaine (Xylocaine) with 1:320,000 epinephrine, which (1) tends to reduce blood loss and (2) provides the patient with some degree of pain relief during the immediate postoperative period. For volumes exceeding 750 ml, it is preferable to use either an epidural anesthesia or a general anesthesia in addition to the lidocaine-epinephrine solution.

When large volumes of fatty tissue are removed, blood loss estimation is valuable in determining the point at which a patient may require blood replacement. The use of a "lipocrit" (Grazer, 1986b) is helpful. This is done by determining the amount of blood in the aspirate following centrifugation of a 10 ml aliquot. The following formula can be used. If there are 10 per cent packed cells per 1000 ml aspirate, this equals 100 ml packed cells per 1000 ml aspirate. Therefore, if the patient has a hematocrit of 40, to convert this number to whole blood one multiplies 2.5 × 100 ml,

PATHOPHYSIOLOGY OF PULMONARY DESTRUCTION
(Mechanical/Chemical Theory of Fat Embolism Syndrome)

Figure 80–8.

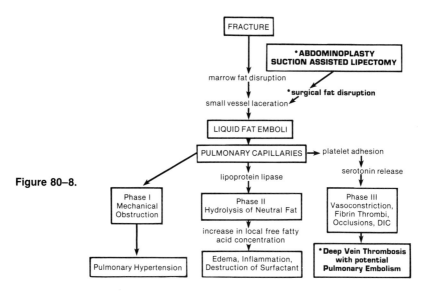

The three overlapping phases of pulmonary fat embolism syndrome: (1) mechanical obstruction; (2) hydrolysis of neutral fat resulting in free fatty acids that are toxic to the lungs; (3) activation of the coagulation system resulting in the release of vasoconstrictive mediators and localized disseminated intravascular coagulation (DIC). (Original: Stoltenberg, J.J. and Gustilo, R.B.: The use of methylprednisolone and hypertonic glucose in the Prophylaxis of fat embolism syndrome. Clin. Orthop. 143:211, 1979. First modification: Goldhaber, Samuel Z., Pulmonary Embolism and Deep Venous Thrombosis. W.B. Saunders Company, Philadelphia, 1985, p. 228, Figure 11-5.)

* **Grazer-Mathews modifications:**
   Note: phases I, II, III usually occur within the first 72 hours, while pulmonary thromboemboli usually occur after 5 days.

which represents 250 ml whole blood per 1000 ml aspirate or 25 per cent blood loss in the aspirate. If the patient has a hematocrit of 30, simply multiply by 3.3 to obtain a figure of 330 ml. A figure of 10 per cent packed cells gives an approximate 33 per cent blood loss in the aspirate. In the last 100 "lipocrits" performed by the author, the values have been running at 12.5 to 15 per cent, with the average packed cell sediment in the range of 5 to 6 mm.

Surgical access to the subcutaneous fat of the abdomen and flanks can be approached through stab incisions in the groin, the inguinal crease, or the periumbilical area. The use of three hole cannulas below a 5 mm diameter is preferred (see Fig. 80–4). By keeping the cannula between the fingers of the operator's free hand with the cannula pointing away from the fascia and deeper structures, abdominal cavity penetration can be prevented (Fig. 80–9). Figures 80–10 to 80–13 demonstrate the use and results of suction alone.

FULL ABDOMINOPLASTY

There are nine major points to consider in the technique of abdominoplasty: (1) selection of the incision; (2) elevation of the panniculus and the decision as to whether suction is indicated, and if so, before or after elevation; (3) plication of the diastasis recti, if indicated; (4) closure; (5) tailoring of the umbilicus; (6) suctioning of the upper abdomen, if indicated; (7) suctioning of adjacent deformities such as the hips, flanks, and trochanteric areas, when indicated; (8) trimming of the flaps and suctioning of the dog-ears, if present; and (9) drains and dressings.

Selection of Incision. Incision selection depends on the patient body type and the choice of bathing apparel, if this is important to the patient. It is recommended that the patient provide the type of preferred bathing suit style for marking (Fig. 80–14). The author favors the modified W-plasty for the high French cut bathing suits, the incision lines coming up within the iliac crest (Figs. 80–15

SAL ALONE

STAB INCISION SITES

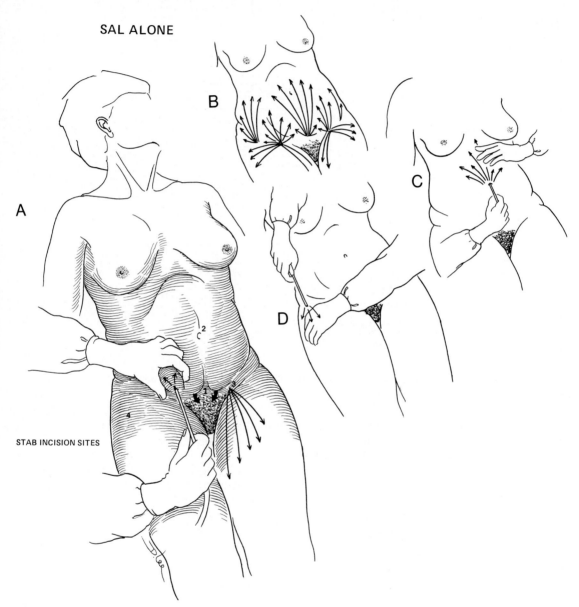

Figure 80–9. Technique of suctioning the abdomen. The multiple sites for approaching the abdomen for suctioning are indicated: note the numbered sites. *A*, *B*, and *D* demonstrate approaches to the anterior thigh, which is frequently suctioned in conjunction with primary abdominal suctioning or with abdominoplasty.

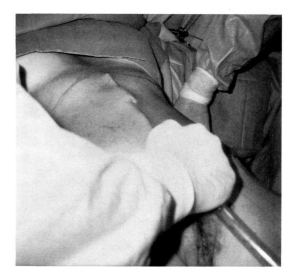

Figure 80–10. Demonstration of the development of the median raphé by superficial suctioning of the midline (see also Fig. 80–25).

to 80–17). The skinline incision is preferred for obese patients and for males. In many long-waisted patients it is not possible to eliminate the umbilical site, and the inverted T incision is employed (Fig. 80–18).

Before surgery, the patient is marked in the bathing suit in the standing position. At the time of surgery, careful confirmation of the markings is made with the string compass technique, using the xiphoid process as the apex of the triangle to ensure symmetric incisions (Grazer and Klingbeil, 1980). The patient is carefully positioned on the operating table with the table break at the level of the trochanters so that, when the patient is brought into flexion, maximal flexion is achieved.

Elevation of Panniculus. Depending on the amount of subcutaneous fatty tissue and the amount of redundancy in the abdominal panniculus, the surgeon may prefer to suction some of the adjacent areas of the flank as well as thin out the mons pubis and the panniculus before surgical dissection (Fig. 80–19). The surgeon may alternatively elect to elevate the panniculus and do the suctioning after the panniculus is elevated. In either case, the abdominal panniculus should be elevated with electrodissection, which minimizes the blood loss and allows a small amount of subcutaneous fat to remain on the fascia (Fig. 80–20). Circumscription of the umbilicus is aided by elevation with skin hooks (Fig. 80–21).

Plication of Diastasis Recti. After the panniculus has been elevated to the xiphoid and costal margins, with the umbilicus circumscribed in the form of a small vertical ellipse (Fig. 80–21), the plication of the rectus sheath is accomplished (Figs. 80–22, 80–23).

A nonabsorbable suture is used for the first layer of closure, followed by a running layer of absorbable suture. This technique allows the nonabsorbable sutures to be buried and the superficial sutures to be absorbed, thereby preventing the formation of palpable knots through the subcutaneous tissue in thinner patients. In patients in whom the plication of the rectus sheath does not correct the contour deformities of the anterior abdominal wall, the first alternative choice is the waistline suture of Jackson (see Fig. 80–20) in which the same plicating sutures are used across the midportion of the abdomen and occasionally the lower portion of the abdomen, midway between the pubis and the umbilicus. Another possible technique is the transposition of the external oblique fascia as described by Psillakis (1984) (Fig. 80–24).

Closure. After the appropriate plication techniques have been carried out, a rubber button is sutured to the umbilicus for purposes of identifying it through the skin by palpation. The patient is placed in the flexed position and vertical cuts are made for fitting the panniculus; all the excess tissue is resected. The panniculus is pulled in an inferior direction and tacked into position. The wounds are approximated with buried Vicryl sutures and interrupted nylon sutures, with final closure by Proximate skin staples and Steri-strip tapes. In three to four days, the

Text continued on page 3948

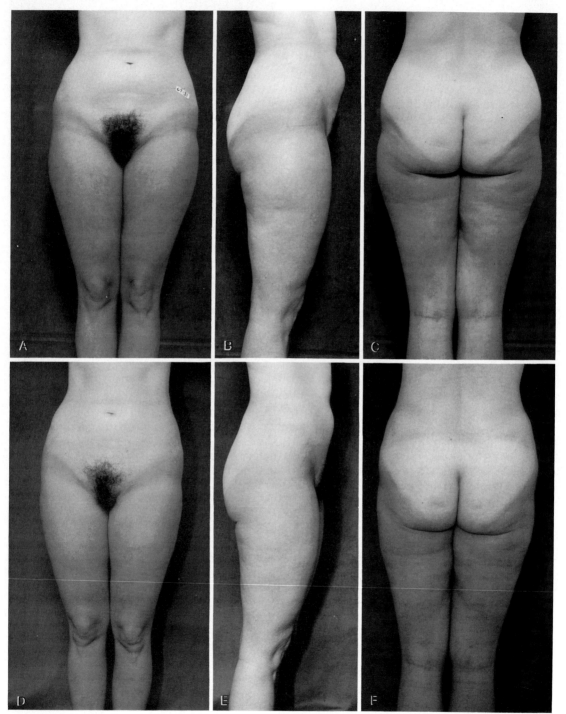

Figure 80–11. Abdominal suctioning alone. *A to C,* A 30 year old nulliparous female with Type III trochanteric deformity and anterior abdominal wall deformity. *D to F,* One year after approximately 1300 ml aspiration of fatty tissue from the hips, thighs, and abdomen.

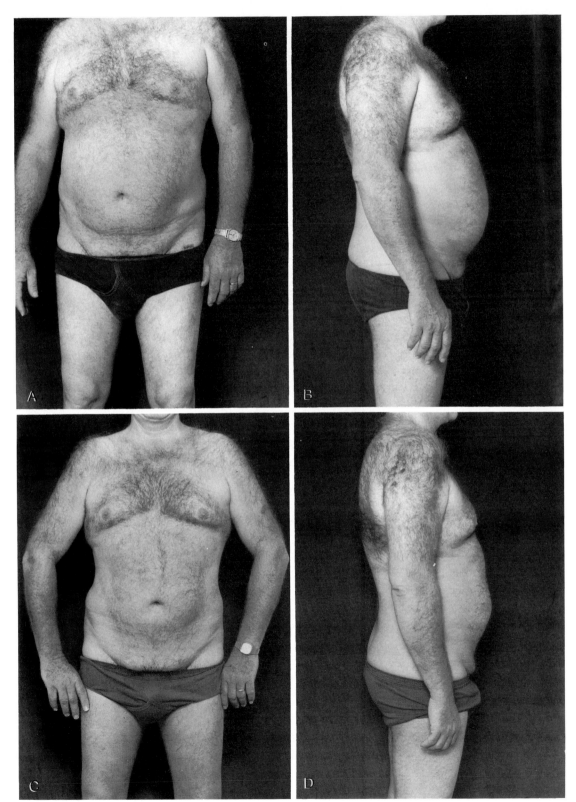

Figure 80–12. Abdominal suctioning alone. *A, B,* A 54 year old diabetic male. *C, D,* One year after approximately 1100 ml aspiration of fatty tissue. Following suction surgery, the patient's tolazamide requirements were reduced by half.

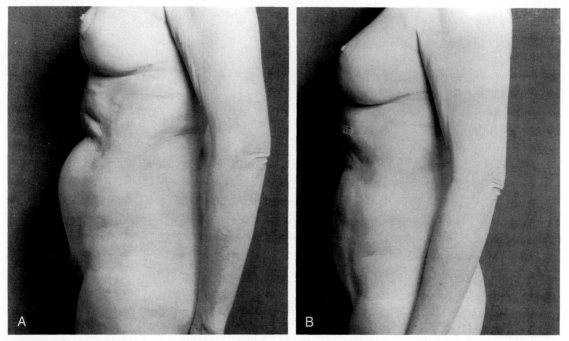

Figure 80–13. Abdominal suctioning alone. *A,* Preoperative view of a 53 year old female who had a previous mastectomy followed by reconstruction. *B,* One year after suctioning of the abdomen.

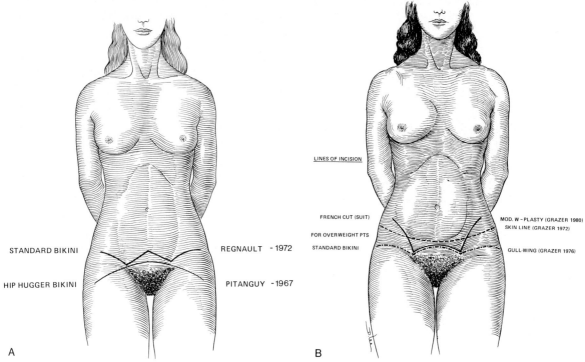

Figure 80–14. Abdominoplasty incisions. *A,* Earlier low placement of incision lines. *B,* The author's preferred incision lines.

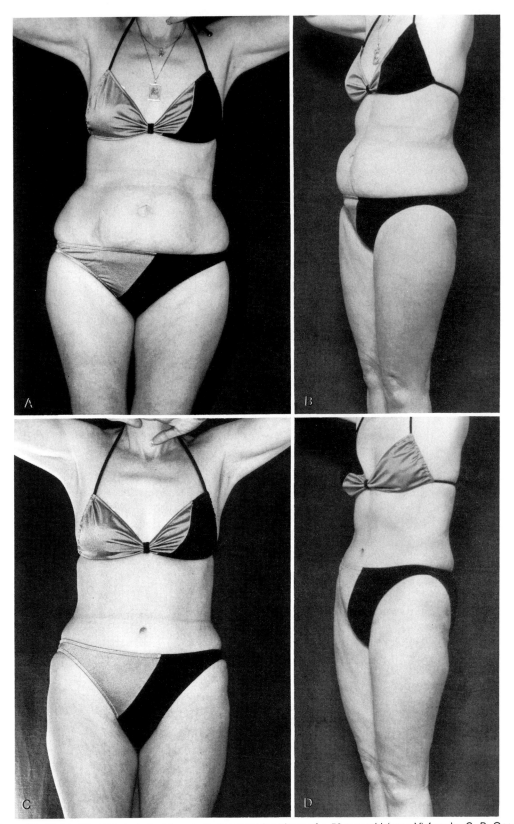

Figure 80–15. Modified W-plasty incision. *A, B,* Preoperative views of a 50 year old (para V) female. *C, D,* One year after abdominoplasty demonstrating the incision for a high cut swimsuit line.

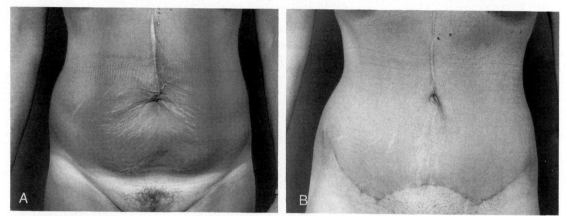

Figure 80–16. Modified W-plasty incision. *A,* Preoperative view of a 49 year old (para II) female. *B,* Six months postoperatively demonstrating the incision.

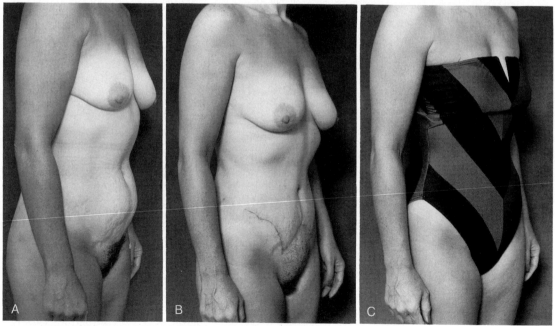

Figure 80–17. Modified W-plasty incision. *A,* Preoperative view of a 40 year old multiparous female. *B,* One month postoperatively. *C,* Demonstrating the need for the incision design for a French cut swimsuit.

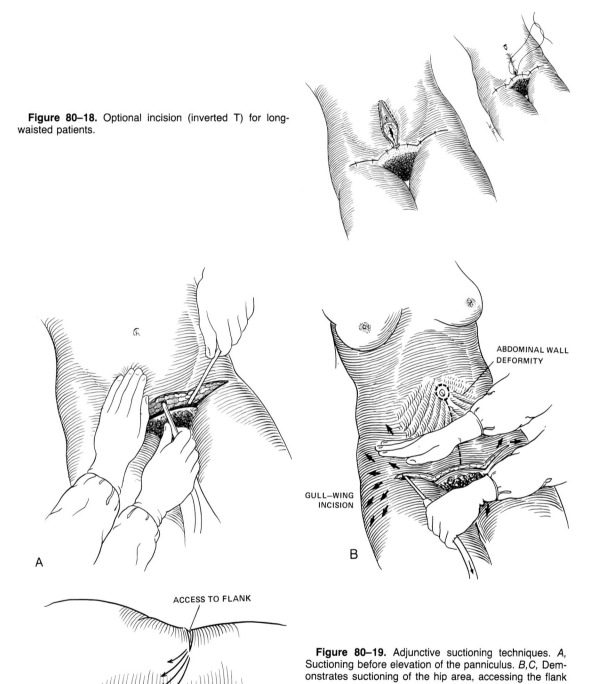

Figure 80–18. Optional incision (inverted T) for long-waisted patients.

ABDOMINAL WALL DEFORMITY

GULL—WING INCISION

B

A

ACCESS TO FLANK

C

Figure 80–19. Adjunctive suctioning techniques. *A,* Suctioning before elevation of the panniculus. *B,C,* Demonstrates suctioning of the hip area, accessing the flank area.

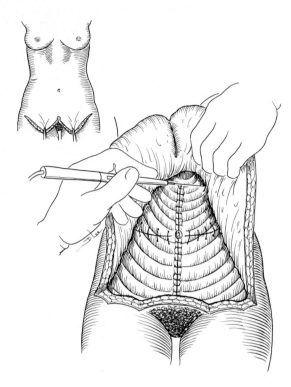

Figure 80–20. The Jackson waistline sutures across the midportion of the abdomen. Note the use of electrocautery. Inset shows downward displacement of the flap before resection.

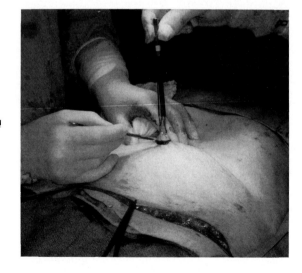

Figure 80–21. The umbilicus is circumscribed in a small vertical ellipse and is everted with skin hooks.

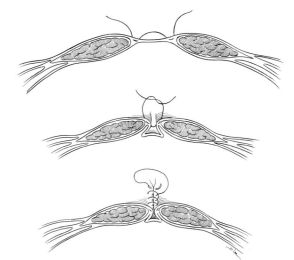

Figure 80–22. Plication of the diastasis recti with a two-layer imbrication.

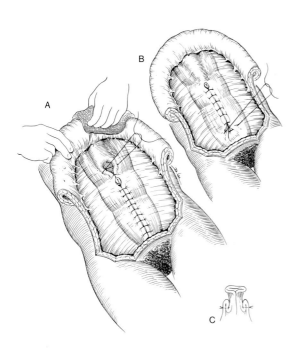

Figure 80–23. *A,B,* Plication technique. *C,* Shortening of umbilical stalk.

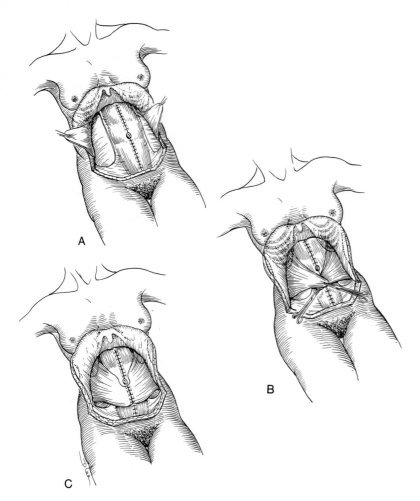

A

B

C

Figure 80-24. Psillakis plication technique of correcting lower abdominal fullness. *A,* Elevation of external oblique fascial flaps. *B,* Transposition of flaps. *C,* Flaps sutured over the rectus abdominis.

skin staples are removed leaving no permanent marks and the Steri-strip tapes are reapplied.

Tailoring the Umbilicus. Before the rubber button is pulled through the abdominal flap, deepening of the median raphé is accomplished through suctioning (Fig. 80–25). This procedure produces a more youthful contoured look to the abdomen. After the rubber button is palpated, a vertical incision is made through the subcutaneous tissues to provide an opening for the umbilicus and for the entry of cannulas. It is important that this incision should not be more than 1 to 1.5 cm in length. With two small Senn retractors, the skin is retracted and the rubber button again identified. At this point, the surgeon may prefer to suction the flanks of the patient and contour the upper portion of the abdomen, inserting the cannula through the new umbilical site stab wound or through the newly closed incision sites.

When this maneuver is completed, and depending on the thickness of the abdominal panniculus, additional suctioning of the abdomen may be desired with smaller cannulas; 2.4 mm to 3.7 mm diameter cannulas work best. After the umbilical stalk is brought through the flap, the rubber button is cut free and the umbilicus exteriorized with two small single skin hooks. Without resecting any skin, and after defatting around the umbilical stalk (Fig. 80–26), the abdominal skin is sutured to the rectus fascia at the base of the umbilical stalk. This maneuver is done in the 3, 6, and 9 o'clock positions (Fig. 80–26) (Baroudi, 1975). This method of suturing prevents the umbilicus from being pulled back into the depths of the wound. By not placing the 12 o'clock suture, the small hooding characteristic of the youthful umbilicus is developed (Fig. 80–27). If the umbilical stalk is somewhat elongated, imbrication must be done at the time of plication; a suture through

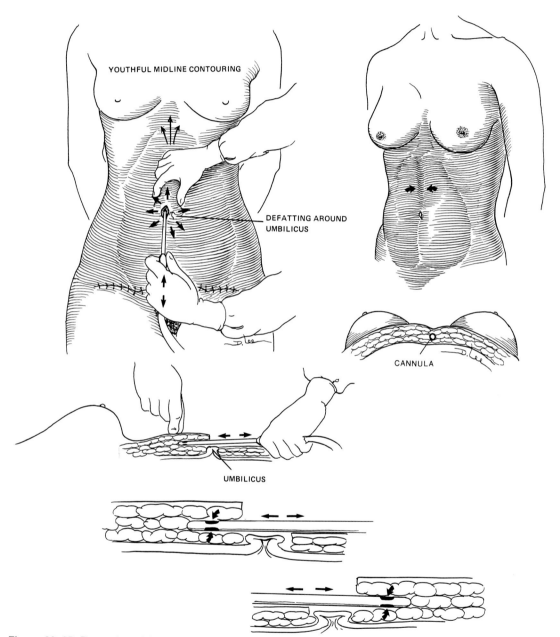

Figure 80–25. Deepening of the median raphé is accomplished through suctioning of the midline (see also Fig. 80–10).

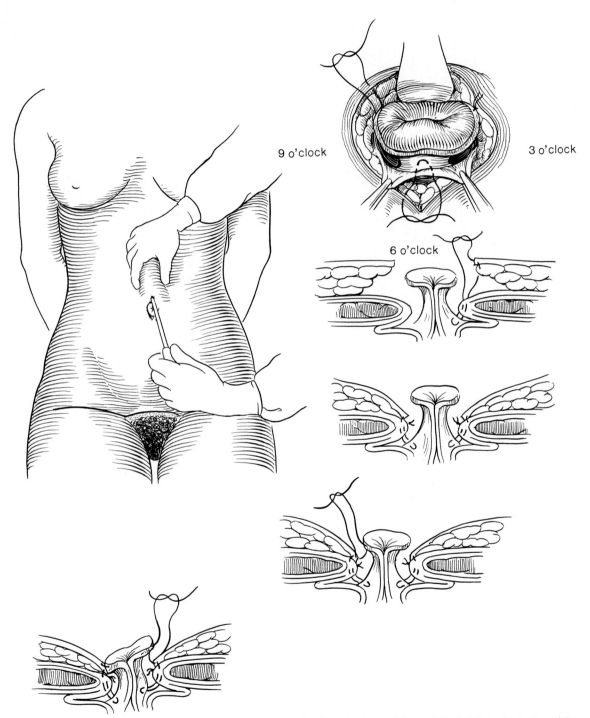

Figure 80–26. Suturing of the abdominal skin to the rectus fascia at the base of the umbilical stalk in the 3, 6, and 9 o'clock positions. A second layer sutures the umbilical skin to the abdominal skin.

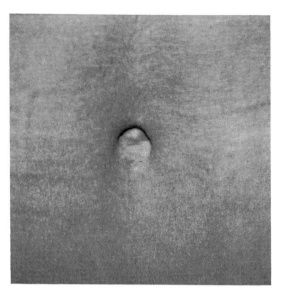

Figure 80–27. A youthful, hooded effect of the umbilicus accomplished by suturing at the 3, 6, and 9 o'clock positions (see Fig. 80–26).

the umbilical stalk reduces its length (see Fig. 80–23C). After the abdominal skin has been sutured to the base of the umbilical stalk in the 3, 6, and 9 o'clock positions, the mushroom portion or the skin of the umbilicus is sutured deeply into the interstices of the wound by burying the cicatrix deeply within the recesses of the umbilicus. This technique provides a normal-appearing umbilicus and places the small scar in a less conspicuous site.

Suctioning of Upper Abdomen. Suctioning of the upper abdomen has been a controversial issue among plastic surgeons, since it is possible that the suctioning could compromise the circulation to the flap. With the use of small cannulas, this risk is significantly reduced since the smaller cannula limits the amount of disturbance, and only a limited amount of fat is extracted. Light suctioning of the upper abdomen provides a more pleasing contour and result in abdominoplasty.

Suctioning of Adjacent Deformities. During abdominoplasty, suction of adjacent deformities can easily be included in the procedure, especially contouring of the hips and flanks (see Figs. 80–9, 80–19C). By extending the cannula in an inferior direction, the medial thigh area may also be suctioned.

Trimming of Flaps and Suctioning of Dog-ears. Final tailoring of the abdominal panniculus includes trimming of the flaps and

suctioning of any dog-ears. Care with the final tailoring of the panniculus results in a smoother, more refined incision line (Fig. 80–28).

Drains and Dressings. Two 7 mm or 10 mm Jackson-Pratt drains are let out either through stab incisions in the mons pubis or through the incision itself. The patient is placed in a supportive garment; either a Velcro abdominal binder (Fig. 80–29) or, if extensive suctioning has been performed on the hips and thighs, a girdle of the Caromed or foundation type is used (Fig. 80–30). A molded plaster of Paris splint is a useful adjunct for patients who have some element of nausea, vomiting, and coughing; when laid on top of the other dressing, it has been helpful during the first 24 hours. It appears to minimize seroma formation by providing pressure on the flap. However, when the plaster strips are molded to the body over the binder, the heat generated by crystallization makes the splint hot and it must be removed until it is cooler.

MINI-ABDOMINOPLASTY

The mini-abdominoplasty is a less extensive operation than the full abdominoplasty (Fig. 80–31). It is indicated when the deformity is limited primarily below the umbilicus (Fig. 80–32).

The choice of the incision is essentially the same as that for the full abdominoplasty; however, the lateral extent of the incision is not as long.

It is recommended that before the lower abdominal segment is elevated, the entire abdominal wall be suctioned, when indicated, either through the incision line or through stab incisions made before the full incision. After the elevation has been accomplished up to the umbilicus, the surgeon can determine if the lower rectus sheath requires plication, a maneuver carried out with the same suturing technique as for the full abdominoplasty.

If there is fullness above the umbilicus, the umbilical stalk can be skeletonized without detaching it. Dissection can extend 3 or 4 cm above the umbilical stalk for the purposes of putting plication sutures above the umbilicus. The final closure is made with the same suture described for a regular abdominoplasty.

The use of a drain is recommended, either

WITH SAL

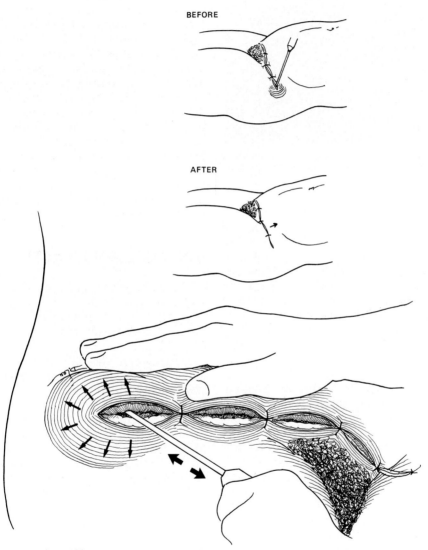

BEFORE

AFTER

Figure 80–28. Final tailoring of the abdominal panniculus with suctioning of the dog-ears.

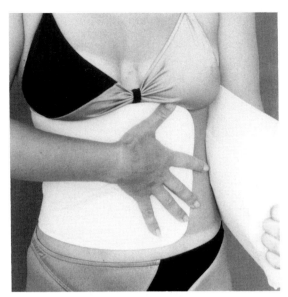

Figure 80–29. Velcro abdominal binder—a choice for support after abdominoplasty. Its use is dependent on the extent of the suctioning.

abdominoplasty had been performed one and one-half years previously.

COMBINED PROCEDURES

Combined procedures with abdominoplasty have not resulted in an increased morbidity provided that the selected patient has been appropriate and autologous blood, which may be essential, is available. Figure 80–35 illustrates breast augmentation through the abdominal approach with a Dingman breast dissector. Figure 80–36 demonstrates breast augmentation and abdominoplasty. Figure 80–37 shows a patient with breast mastopexy and augmentation and abdominoplasty who later underwent a belt lipectomy and suctioning. Figure 80–38 demonstrates breast reduction and abdominoplasty with subsequent suctioning after weight gain.

a Jackson-Pratt 7 mm drain or the minidrain, which is a 19 gauge butterfly attached to a Vacutainer tube. In general, the combination of suction and flap elevation leads to greater seroma formation. The usual abdominal Velcro binder (see Fig. 80–29) is all that is required unless the hips and thighs are suctioned. In these cases the additional use of a form-fitting girdle such as the Caromed or foundation garment is helpful (see Fig. 80–30).

REVERSE ABDOMINOPLASTY

In certain selected individuals the use of the reverse abdominoplasty is indicated. In these patients the deformity, which may include surgical scars, is confined to the upper abdomen. The incision for the reverse abdominoplasty is made in the upper abdominal region under the inframammary fold (Fig. 80–33). The reverse abdominoplasty can be considered in conjunction with a breast reduction as a combined procedure, although it is not recommended as a combined procedure with breast augmentation. Figure 80–34 illustrates a 58 year old female who had a 156 lb weight loss and subsequent reverse abdominoplasty with breast reduction after a full

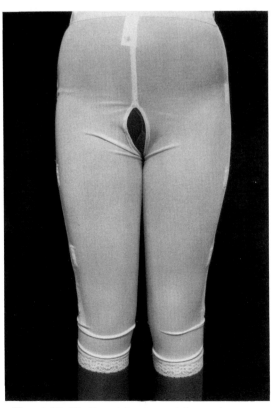

Figure 80–30. Foundation-type girdle used when the hips and thighs are suctioned in conjunction with an abdominoplasty.

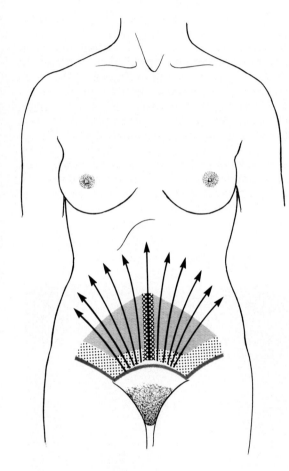

Figure 80–31. The mini-abdominoplasty procedure.

suctioning
undermining
resection
plication
mini-abdominoplasty

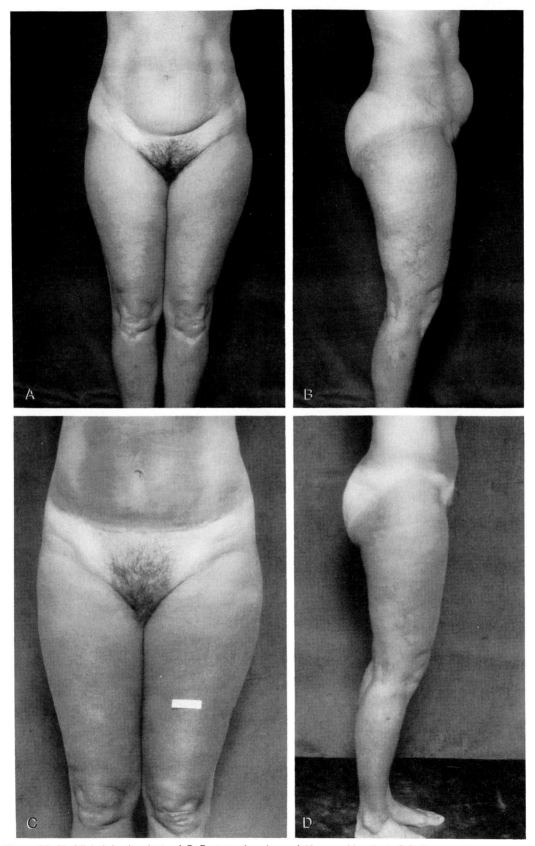

Figure 80–32. Mini-abdominoplasty. *A,B,* Preoperative views of 40 year old patient. *C,D,* Five months postoperatively with associated suctioning of the hips and thighs.

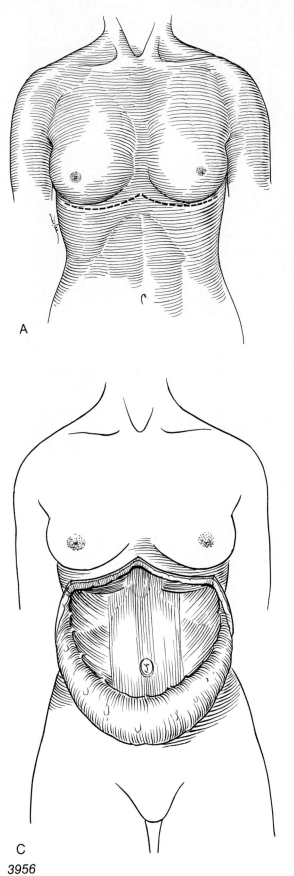
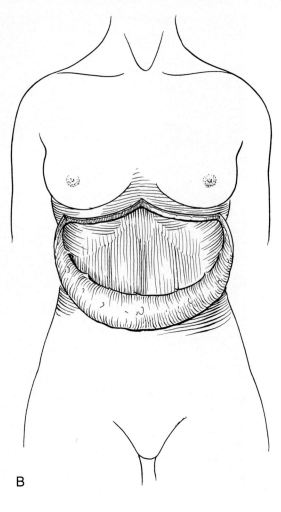

Figure 80–33. *A,* Incision for reverse abdominoplasty in the inframammary fold. *B,* Partial upper abdominoplasty. *C,* Full reverse abdominoplasty with transposition of the umbilicus.

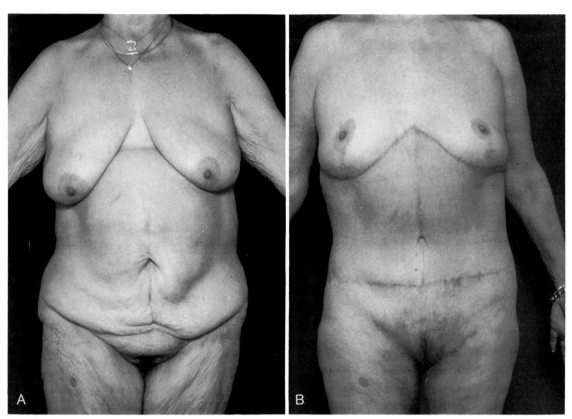

Figure 80–34. Reverse abdominoplasty. *A,* A 58 year old (para III) female who weighed 300 lb but lost 156 lb. *B,* After maintaining her weight at 144 lb, she underwent a partial reverse abdominoplasty with breast reduction after a preliminary abdominoplasty.

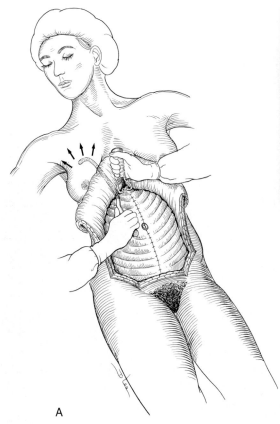

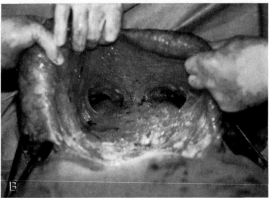

Figure 80–35. Combined breast augmentation and abdominoplasty. *A,* Technique of breast implantation through the abdominoplasty incision. Dissection can be done with a Dingman breast dissector. *B,* Demonstrates the pockets for placement of the breast implants.

A

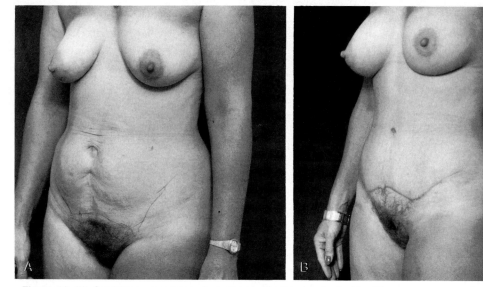

Figure 80–36. Combined procedures. *A,* A 42 year old female who had had three cesarean sections. She underwent abdominoplasty and breast augmentation with implantation through the abdominoplasty incision. *B,* Five months postoperatively.

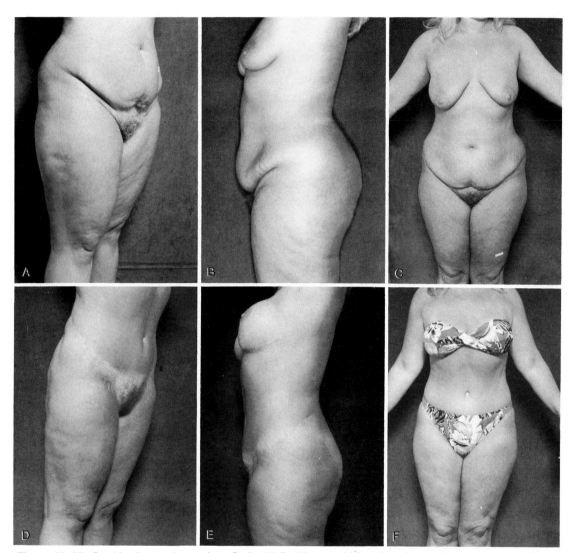

Figure 80–37. Combined procedures. *A* to *C,* A 186 lb, 33 year old female before abdominoplasty and bilateral mastopexy with breast augmentation. *D* to *F,* Results one year postoperatively with additional suctioning and belt lipectomy.

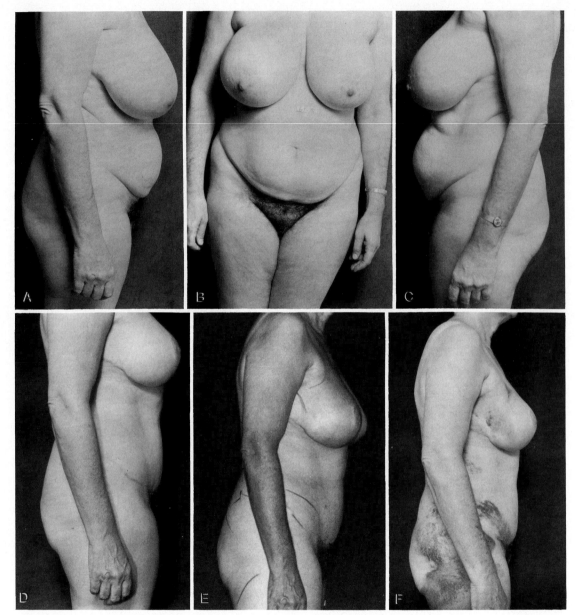

Figure 80–38. Combined breast reduction, abdominoplasty, and suctioning. *A,* to *C,* A 53 year old female weighing 155 lb. *D,* One year after abdominoplasty and breast reduction. *E,* The patient had weight gain after surgery and has been marked for suctioning. *F,* Extent of suctioning.

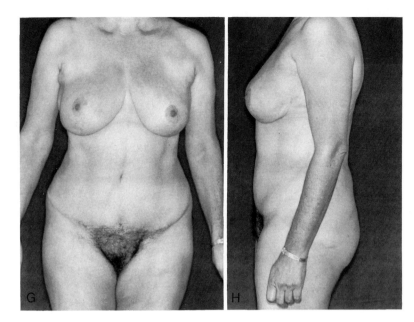

Figure 80–38 *Continued G, H,* Final result after both procedures.

POSTOPERATIVE MANAGEMENT

An abdominoplasty patient is maintained in a flexed position on the day of surgery and is ambulated within 24 hours following surgery. People handled on an outpatient basis are encouraged to maintain a semiflexed position for 24 hours. In suctioned patients there is no required position. Removal of the drain is almost always possible within 24 to 48 hours. The Velcro binder is worn for two or three weeks after surgery.

The author administers oral cephalosporin for three to four days postsurgically.

The use of ultrasound helps to resolve any ecchymosis and small irregularities such as lumps. In patients undergoing suction alone, ultrasound is utilized as soon as the patient is pain free; in combined procedures, it is given a few days postsurgically according to the patient's pain comfort level. Ultrasound is applied at 2 watts per second squared for a ten minute period over the areas in question. This usually continues twice a week for two or three weeks.

For patients undergoing suctioning alone, normal activity can be resumed as soon as all the ecchymosis and edema has subsided, usually two to three weeks. For an abdominoplasty patient, the rule of thumb for normal activity is three to four weeks. For strenuous activities such as aerobics a period of four to six weeks is recommended.

SECONDARY/REVISION PROCEDURES

In secondary/revision procedures, suction techniques are recommended no earlier than four months postoperatively. Following an abdominoplasty, it is preferable to wait six months to one year. Revisions usually consist of scar revision; suctioning of irregular areas of the abdomen, as well as the hips and thighs; and deepening of the abdominal median raphé.

Unsatisfactory postoperative scarring is not unusual. Scar revisions may be done six months to one year after surgery. Steroids can be injected into the hypertrophic scars.

REFERENCES

Babcock, W. W.: The correction of the obese and relaxed abdominal wall with especial reference to the use of buried silver chain. Am. J. Obstet. Gynecol., *74*:596, 1916.

Babcock, W. W.: Plastic reconstruction of the female breasts and abdomen. Am. J. Surg., *43*:269, 1939.

Baroudi, R.: Umbilicaplasty. Clin. Plast. Surg., *2*:431, 1975.

Barsky, A. J.: Principles and Practice of Plastic Surgery. Baltimore, Williams & Wilkins Company, 1950.

Castanares, S., and Goethel, J. A.: Abdominal lipectomy: a modification in technique. Plast. Reconstr. Surg., 40:379, 1967.

Desjardins, P.: Résection de la couche adi d'obesité extrème (lipectomie). Rapport par Dartigues. Paris Chirurg., 3:466, 1911.

Evarts, C. M., Hoaglund, F. T., Jacobs, R., and Peltier, L. F.: Symposium: fat embolism syndrome. Contemp. Surg., 9:49, 1976.

Fischl, R. A.: Vertical abdominoplasty. Plast. Reconstr. Surg., 51:139, 1973.

Flesch-Thebesius, M., and Wheisheimer, K.: Die Operation des Hängebauches. Chirurg., 3:841, 1931.

Forrest, C. K., Pang, C. Y., and Lindsay, W. K.: Detrimental effect of nicotine on skin flap viability and blood flow in random skin flap operations on rats and pigs. Surg. Forum, 36:611, 1985.

Galtier, M.: Traitement chirurgical des obesités de la paroi abdominale avec ptose. Mém. Acad. Chir., 81:12, 341, 1955.

Goldhaber, S. Z., Vaughan, D. E., Markis, J. E., Selwyn, A. P., Meyerovitz, M. F., et al.: Acute pulmonary embolism treated with tissue plasminogen activator. Lancet, 2:886, 1986.

Gonzalez-Ulloa, M.: Belt lipectomy. Br. J. Plast. Surg., 13:179, 1960.

Grazer, F. M.: Abdominoplasty. Plast. Reconstr. Surg., 51:617, 1973.

Grazer, F. M.: Suction-assisted lipectomy, suction lipectomy, lipolysis, and lipexeresis (discussion). Plast. Reconstr. Surg., 72:620, 1983.

Grazer, F. M.: Unfavorable results in body contouring operations including psychological aspects. *In* Goldwyn, R. M. (Ed.): The Unfavorable Result in Plastic Surgery, Avoidance and Treatment. 2nd Ed. Boston, Little, Brown & Company, 1984.

Grazer, F. M.: Lipexhairesis versus lipexeresis (letter). Plast. Reconstr. Surg., 77:857, 1986a.

Grazer, F. M.: Quantitative analysis of blood and fat in suction lipectomy aspirates (discussion). Plast. Reconstr. Surg., 78:770, 1986b.

Grazer, F. M., and Goldwyn, R. M.: Abdominoplasty assessed by survey, with emphasis on complications. Plast. Reconstr. Surg., 59:513, 1977.

Grazer, F. M., and Klingbeil, J. R.: Abdominoplasty. *In* Courtiss, E. (Ed.): Aesthetic Surgery. Trouble: How to Avoid it and How to Treat It. St. Louis, C. V. Mosby Company, 1978, pp. 204–222.

Grazer, F. M., and Klingbeil, J. R.: Body Image: A Surgical Perspective. St. Louis, C. V. Mosby Company, 1980.

Grazer, F. M., and Klingbeil, J. R.: Pulmonary complications following abdominal lipectomy (discussion). Plast. Reconstr. Surg., 71:814, 1983.

Grazer, F. M., Klingbeil, J. R., and Mattiello, M.: Abdominoplasty. *In* Goldwyn, R. M. (Ed.): Long Term Results in Plastic and Reconstructive Surgery. Boston, Little, Brown & Company, 1980.

Grazer, F. M., and Mathews, W. A.: Fat embolism (correspondence). Plast. Reconstr. Surg., 79:671, 1987.

Hinderer, U. T.: The dermolipectomy approach for augmentation mammaplasty. Clin. Plast. Surg., 2:359, 1975.

Illouz, Y. G.: Body contouring by lipolysis: a 5 year experience with over 3000 cases. Plast. Reconstr. Surg., 72:591, 1983.

Jolly, R.: Die Operation des Fettbauches. Berl. Klin. Wochenschr., 29:1317, 1911.

Kelly, H. A.: Report of gynecological cases. Johns Hopkins Med. J., 10:197, 1899.

Kelly, H. A.: Excision of the fat of the abdominal wall—lipectomy. Surg. Gynecol. Obstet., 10:229, 1910.

Kesselring, U. K.: Suction curette for removal of subcutaneous fat (letter to the Editor). Plast. Reconstr. Surg., 63:560, 1979.

Kesselring, U. K.: Suction curettage to remove excess fat for body contouring (letter to the Editor). Plast. Reconstr. Surg., 69:572, 1982.

Kesselring, U. K., and Meyer, R.: A suction curette for removal of excessive local deposits of subcutaneous fat. Plast. Reconstr. Surg., 62:305, 1978.

Kettunen, R., Timisjärvi, J., Saukko, P., and Koskela, M.: Influence of ethanol on systemic and pulmonary hemodynamics in anesthetized dogs. Acta Physiol. Scand., 118:209, 1983.

Küster, H.: Operation bei Hängebrust und Hängeleib. Monatsschr. Geburtsh. Gynäk., 73:316, 1926.

Laug, W. E.: Ethyl alcohol enhances plasminogen activator secretion by endothelial cells. J.A.M.A., 250:772, 1983.

Levin, R. I., Jaffe, E. A., Weksler, B. B., and Tack-Goldman, K.: Nitroglycerin stimulates synthesis of prostacyclin by cultured human endothelial cells. J. Clin. Invest., 67:762, 1981.

Mathews, W. A.: Pulmonary complications following abdominal lipectomy (discussion). Plast. Reconstr. Surg., 71:816, 1983.

Morestin, A.: La restauration de la paroi abdominale par résection etendue des téguments et de la graisse souscutanée et le plissement des aponévroses superficielles envisagé comme complément de la cure radicale des hernies ombilicales. Thèse, Paris, 1911.

Ogburn, P. L., Jr., and Brenner, W. E.: The physiologic actions and effects of prostaglandins. Current Concepts. Kalamazoo, MI, Upjohn Company, 1983, p. 19.

Peltier, L. F.: The diagnosis of fat embolism. Surg. Gynecol. Obstet., 121:371, 1965.

Peltier, L. F.: The diagnosis and treatment of fat embolism. J. Trauma, 11:661, 1971.

Peltier, L. F., Collins, J. A., Evarts, C. M., and Sevitt, S.: A panel by correspondence. Fat embolism. Arch. Surg., 190:12, 1974.

Peterson, R.: Letter to the Editor. Cal. Soc. Plast. Surg. Newsletter, 11:3, 1987.

Pick, J. F.: Surgery of Repair: Principles, Problems, Procedures. Abdomen (Abdereplasty). Vol. 2. Philadelphia, J. B. Lippincott Company, 1949, p. 435.

Pitanguy, I., Yobar, A. A., Pires, C. E., and Matta, S. R.: Aspectos atuais das lipectomias abdominais. Bol. Cir. Plast. Rev. Bras. Cirurgia, 19:149, 1974.

Psillakis, J. M.: Plastic surgery of the abdomen with improvement in the body contour: physiopathology and treatment of the aponeurotic musculature. Clin. Plast. Surg., 11:465, 1984.

Regnault, P.: Abdominoplasty by the W technique. Plast. Reconstr. Surg., 55:265, 1975.

Schepelmann, E.: Ueber Bauchdeckenplastik mit besonderes Berucksichtigung des Hängebauches. Beitr. Klin. Chir., 111:372, 1918; Zentralbl. Gynäk., 48:2289, 1924.

Schwartz, A. W.: A technique for excision of abdominal fat. Br. J. Plast. Surg., 27:44, 1974.

Sladen, A.: Pulmonary fat embolism. Surg. Rounds, 3:46, 1980.

Stoltenberg, J. J., and Gustilo, R. B.: The use of methylprednisolone and hypertonic glucose in the prophylaxis of fat embolism syndrome. Clin. Orthop., *143*:211, 1979.

Teimourian, B., Adham, M. N., Gulin, S., and Shapiro, C.: Suction lipectomy—a review of 200 patients over a six-year period and a study of the technique in cadavers. Ann. Plast. Surg., *11*:93, 1983.

Teimourian, B., and Fisher, J. B.: Suction curettage to remove excess fat for body contouring. Plast. Reconstr. Surg., *68*:50, 1981.

Thorek, M.: Plastic Surgery of the Breast and Abdominal Wall. Springfield, IL, Charles C Thomas, 1924.

Voloir, P.: Opérations plastiques sus-aponévrotiques sur la paroi abdominale antérieure. Thèse, Paris, 1960.

Weinhold, S.: Bauchdeckenplastik. Zentralbl. Gynäk., *38*:1332, 1909.

81

Frederick M. Grazer

Body Contouring

It is human nature to strive for the ideal. The perception of "ideal proportions" has varied with the passage of time from antiquity to the present (Grazer and Klingbeil, 1980).

The melding of the two disciplines, traditional body contour (soft tissue) surgery and suction assisted lipectomy (SAL), did not occur until the early 1980's (see Chap. 80). At its inception, suction was confined to the trochanteric "saddlebags," the arms and abdomen, but the technique has evolved to include treatment of deformities of the whole body. The advances made with SAL of the face, arms, trunk, breasts, buttocks, thighs,

knees, and ankles parallel those of SAL of the abdomen. In the current philosophy of body contouring, SAL can be applied to all body contouring procedures, depending on specific indications. There is virtually no part of the body featuring unwanted fatty tissue that cannot be altered by either surgical excision or suction, or both (Grazer and Davis, 1987).

All surgical body contouring procedures involve one of the following approaches: (1) surgical reduction/alteration alone, (2) suction alone, or (3) surgical reduction and suctioning (Grazer, 1983; Grazer, 1984c; Ersek and associates, 1986).

BODY FAT AND DISTRIBUTION

There are three major categories of fat distribution that impact body contouring: (1) the effects of genetic predisposition, (2) the effects of environment, and (3) the natural process of aging.

Genetic Predisposition

The genetic predisposition of the individual is the most distinctive since certain localized deformities cannot be corrected without surgery. An example is the "saddlebag" deformity, which no amount of dieting or exercise will correct; it persists even in a nonobese state (Fig. 81–1). Siblings of genetically obese parents generally tend to be obese.

Environmental Effects

The environmental features of body shape that are determined by diet and exercise are

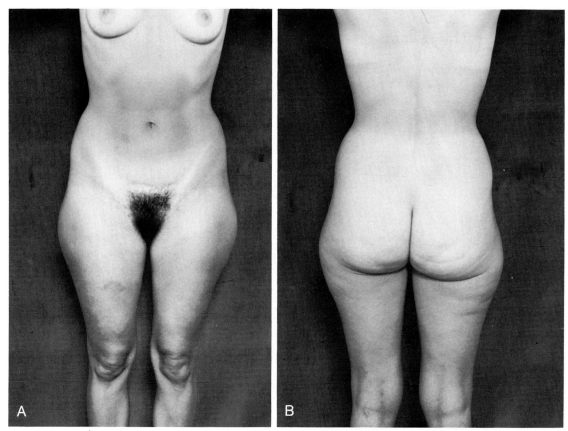

Figure 81–1. *A, B,* A 39 year old female whose weight generally does not exceed 115 lb and whose localized deformities continue to exist even after dieting (below 100 lb) and an exercise regimen.

the controllable aspects of an individual's figure proportion within the genetic template. In most non–Third World countries, obesity has become a major disease entity. Diet and exercise have given new emphasis to the techniques of body contouring through the reduction of skin volume and/or subcutaneous tissue. Bray (1976) postulated, in relation to the changing body composition initiated at gestation and continuing through adult life, that at approximately 1 year of age there is a peak of total body fat followed by a drop until puberty, with a steady rise thereafter (Fig. 81–2).

Natural Effects of Aging

The natural effects of aging, in conjunction with genetic predisposition, dictate changes in localized fat volume and excess skin in several ways: (1) redistribution of fat; (2) loss of body muscle mass, which is replaced in

some individuals with fatty tissue; and (3) loss of tissue elasticity. Each of these categories has a direct and distinct relationship to the amount of adipose tissue and the square area making up the human integument. Obesity is defined as an excess of body fat. On an anatomic basis, obesity is divided into two types: (1) hypertrophic obesity, in which the body has a normal number of fat cells but the size of the cell is enlarged; and (2) hyperplastic obesity, characterized both by the enlargement of the fat cells and by an increased number of fat cells (Sjöström, 1980).

Popular theory maintains that, beginning in infancy, adipose tissue develops mainly by an increase in the number of fat cells. At some predetermined time, generally around puberty, the *number* of fat cells becomes fixed, and from this point the increase in adipose tissue occurs solely by means of an increase in the *size* of the individual fat cells (Fig. 81–3). Evidence (Sjöström, 1980) derived from a small sample of middle-aged women contra-

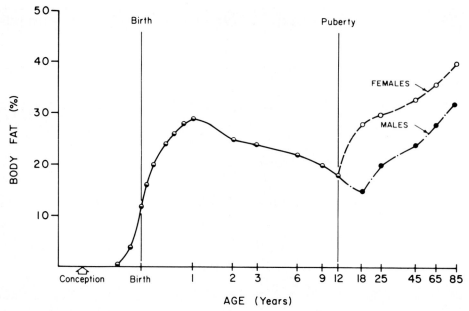

Figure 81–2. Changing body composition from gestation through adult life. (From Friis-Hansen: *In* Brozek, J. (Ed.): Human Body Composition. Oxford, Pergamon Press, 1965, pp. 191–209. Reprinted with permission from Pergamon Journals, Ltd., Copyright 1965.)

dicts this theory and indicates that there may be an increase in the number of fat cells as well as in the size of the cell.

What impact does either theory have on the patient with localized fat deformities? Can we safely tell a patient that, after the fat cells have been removed, they will not return to that site? The photo in Figure 81–4 depicts a patient who had 1700 ml of fatty tissue removed from the trochanteric region. Subsequently she had a 17 lb weight gain with no reappearance of the primary deformity. From the author's perspective, whether or not there may be an increased number of cells with weight gain, the primary deformity does not reappear. Removal of these cells early in life before they become hypertrophic may prevent the genetic predisposition of

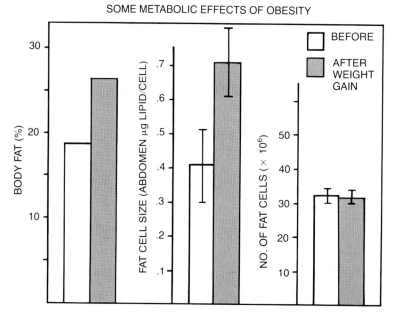

Figure 81–3. Effect of weight gain on the size and number of fat cells. In normal weight men the storage of fat occurred entirely by increasing the size of fat cells. (Adapted from Salans, L. B., Horton, E. S., and Sims, E. A.: Experimental obesity in man: cellular character of the adipose tissue. J. Clin. Invest., *50*:1005, 1971. Reproduced by copyright permission of the American Society for Clinical Investigation.)

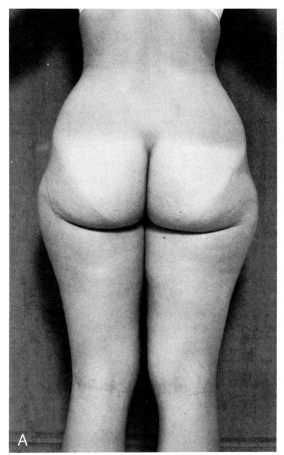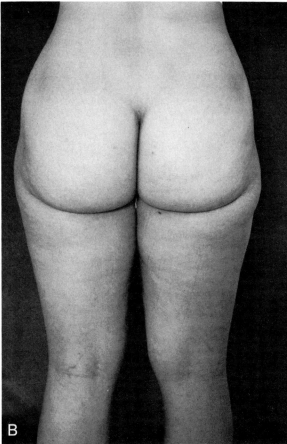

Figure 81–4. A 28 year old female, weighing 165 lb preoperatively *(A)*, underwent suctioning of the hips and thighs. 1700 ml of fatty tissue was aspirated and at three months postoperatively she weighed 158 lb. One year postoperatively *(B)*, the patient had experienced a 17 lb weight gain, reaching 175 lb *without* the reappearance of the primary trochanteric deformity.

such anomalies as the double chin, saddle-bags, or maldistribution of body weight. For example, in infants and children who are overweight, there is an increase in the number of fat cells (Fig. 81–5). This finding may represent genetic or environmental influences (such as overfeeding or consumption of a diet high in fat or refined sugars).

MORBID OBESITY

One of the leading causes of death in this century consists of the problems associated with the grossly overweight and the morbidly obese; morbid obesity is defined as the condition of being "overweight 100 lb or more" (Davis, 1984).

There are differences in the approach to surgical intervention in the process of the morbidly obese and the patient who has lost significant weight by undergoing any form of short circuiting (bypass) of the gastrointestinal tract such as ileojejunal bypass, gastric stapling, and the gastric balloon (see Chap. 80, Fig. 80–34A). The malabsorption that accompanies surgical bypass can produce significant changes in the body's wound healing mechanism. Another is the marked excess of redundant skin, which is often a trap for the neophyte surgeon who tends to overestimate what can be accomplished.

An important fact, often overlooked, is that patients who have been morbidly obese and reduce by 100 to 150 lb retain the increased vascular bed, and consequently bleeding at the time of surgery is always more than one usually expects. Autologous blood is especially vital in these cases.

With the elimination of large amounts of fat either by diet or by surgical/suction reduction, there is evidence of significant phys-

CELL NUMBER OBESE

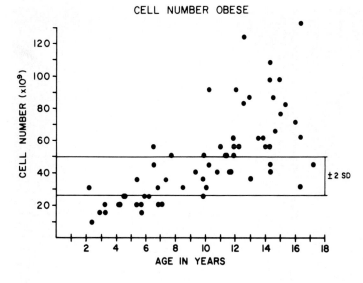

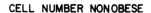

CELL NUMBER NONOBESE

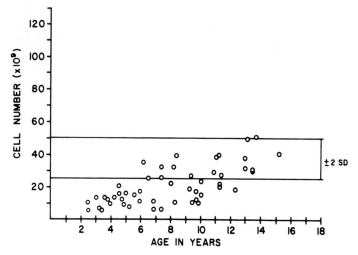

Figure 81–5. Number of fat cells in obese and nonobese children, respectively. Although an overlap is obvious, the progressive rise in number of fat cells in the obese children between the ages of 4 and 12 years indicates the importance of the multiplication of fat cells. (From Knittle, J. L.: Obesity and the cellularity of the adipose depot. Triangle, *13*:57, 1974.)

iological and chemical changes (Figs. 81–6 and 81–7), particularly in respect to diabetes.

In addition to the cardiovascular problems associated with the morbid obesity disease process, there is the prevalence of diabetes in relation to body weight (Fig. 81–8). Although not all obese patients develop diabetes, there is a definite relationship between insulin production and ideal body weight since it is known that obesity increases the demand on the pancreas to produce insulin (Fig. 81–9).

In the author's patients over the past three years, a parallel between obesity and serum insulin production has been demonstrated

(Fig. 81–10). Suctioning of the patients has produced an improvement in the prediabetic and diabetic conditions (see Chap. 80, Fig. 80–12). Often when an obese diabetic patient diets, the serum insulin level is modified. Suctioning creates the same modification of serum insulin levels. If suction techniques could be applied at strategic times in the life of the obese, it might be possible to modify the severity of the diabetic process. When more is learned about fat metabolism, there will no doubt be a place for SAL in altering body fat levels to influence and improve the physiologic parameters governing lipid chemistry.

Text continued on page 3973

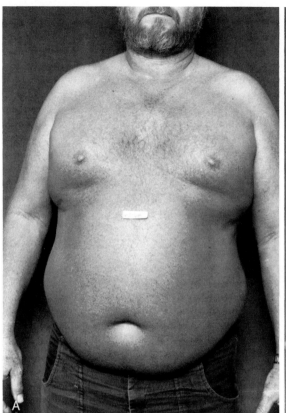

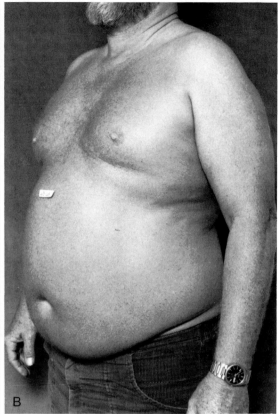

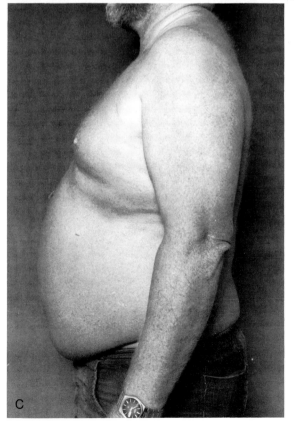

Figure 81–6. A 47 year old male weighing 245 lb approaching the morbidly obese classification underwent SAL of the flanks, back, abdomen, and breasts. A total of 5000 ml of fatty tissue was aspirated. Two units of autologous blood were administered. After surgery there was continual weight loss along with a reduction of fasting serum insulin levels (see also Fig. 81–7). *A* to *C,* Preoperative appearance.

Illustration continued on following page

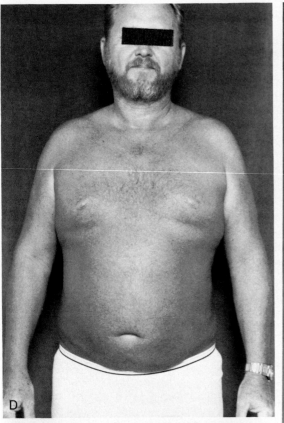

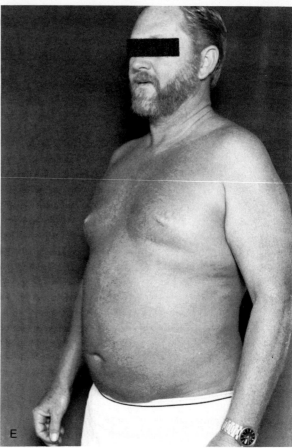

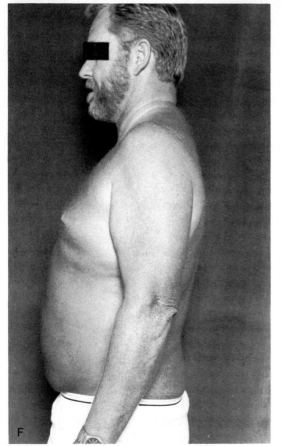

Figure 81–6 *Continued D* to *F,* Postoperative appearance at one year.

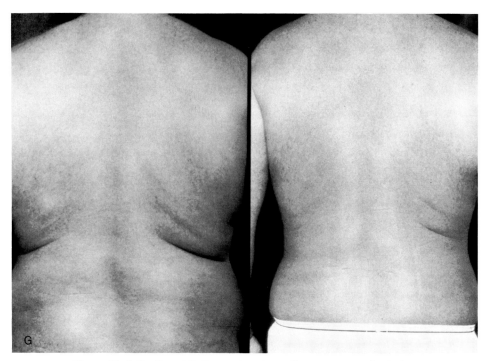

Figure 81–6 *Continued G,* Pre- and postoperative appearance, back view.

	PRE-OP	5000 cc ASPIRATED (11 lbs.)	1 MONTH POST-OP	9 MONTHS POST-OP
WEIGHT	245 lbs.		229.5 lbs	211.5 lbs
CHEST	48"		44.5"	44.5"
HIPS	48"		43.5"	41.5"
INSULIN LEVEL	43 Micro U/ml		Less than 5.0 Micro U/ml	5.0 Micro U/ml

Figure 81–7. Data on the patient illustrated in Figure 81–6: weight, measurements, and serum insulin level. Changes occurred without a change in life style. The patient was a nondiabetic.

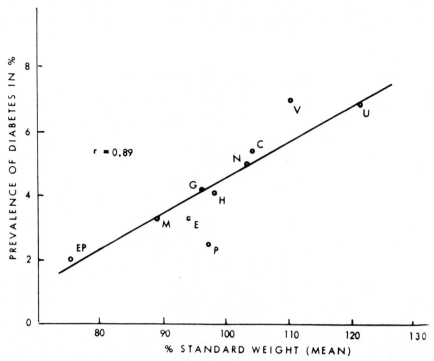

Figure 81–8. Prevalence of diabetes mellitus in relation to body weight. Standard weights for samples from ten countries were compared with the prevalence of diabetes mellitus in the same groups. The population with the higher standard weight showed a higher prevalence of diabetes. U = Uruguay; V = Venezuela; C = Costa Rica; N = Nicaragua; G = Guatemala; H = Honduras; E = El Salvador; P = Panama; M = Malaya; EP = East Pakistan. (From West, K. M., and Kalbfleisch, J. M.: Influence of nutritional factors on prevalence of diabetes. Diabetes, *20*:99, 1971. Reproduced with permission from the American Diabetes Association, Inc.)

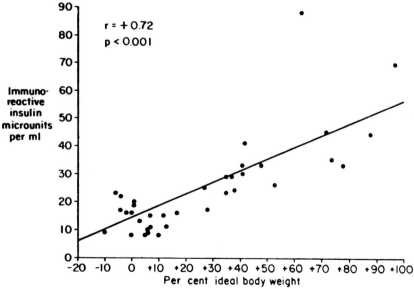

Figure 81–9. Relation of insulin and ideal body weight. As the percentage of ideal body weight increased, immunoreactive insulin levels also rose. (From Bagdade, J. D., Bierman, E. L., and Porte, D., Jr.: The significance of basal insulin levels in the evaluation of the insulin response to glucose in diabetic and nondiabetic subjects. J. Clin. Invest., *46*:1549, 1967. Reproduced by copyright permission of the American Society for Clinical Investigation.)

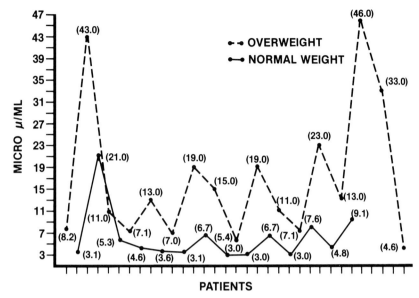

Figure 81–10. Correlation between an increased insulin level and overweight patients before surgery.

EQUIPMENT

The following equipment is necessary for body contouring: (1) a vacuum pump, (2) approximately 6 feet of silicone or vinyl tubing, and (3) several sizes of cannulas (Figs. 81–11 to 81–13).

Physics of Suctioning and Cannulas. Suction devices have been utilized in surgery since the Venturi principle of creating vacuum was proposed. The use of vacuum to aspirate blood, other body fluids, and tissue scrapings is common in surgery.

Kesselring (Kesselring and Meyer, 1978) developed a wide-mouth cannula attached to a low vacuum suction for aspirating fatty tissue (Fig. 81–13B). He designed his cannula with a large aperture, which is used facing the skin surface. After separating the fat from the underlying fascia, he shaves the fat under low vacuum suction using approximately ½ atmosphere of vacuum.

In 1977, Illouz (1983) began to use smaller blunt cannulas with smaller apertures that required a higher vacuum (Fig. 81–14). To grasp the concept of the use of vacuum in suctioning cannulas, it is helpful to understand the physics of vacuum.

Physics of the Vacuum.* A perfect vacuum is 1 atmosphere, which equals 30 inches

*Provided by Grams Medical.

Hg, which equals 760 mm Hg, which equals 1033 gm per sq cm, which equals 14.7 lb per square inch. Vacuum is defined as the absence of air. Even though air is light, the total weight from sea level to outer space is equivalent to 14.7 lb per square inch, or 1033 gm per sq cm in metric, which is called 1 atmosphere. This varies slightly, depending on the atmospheric condition. The column of mercury that can be raised in a glass tube at maximal vacuum is 760 mm or 29.92 inches, and it is this measurement that is most commonly used in identifying vacuum on mechanical gauges.

In the presence of water at 20°C, it is not possible to obtain a vacuum higher than 743 mm Hg or 29.25 inches Hg, because at this vacuum water vaporizes. This also applies to tissue fluid and it can be easily observed as a bubbling action in the collecting bottle. This physical change is known as vapor pressure. At higher elevation, vapor pressure can be obtained, but the reading on the gauge will be less, depending on the altitude.

Near-complete vacuum as high as a fraction of a millimeter of mercury can be obtained by mechanical pumps. Positive-displacement pumps fall into two categories, reciprocating and rotary. Reciprocating pumps can be either piston or diaphragm type and generally are not capable of producing vapor pressure vacuum. Rotary pumps have

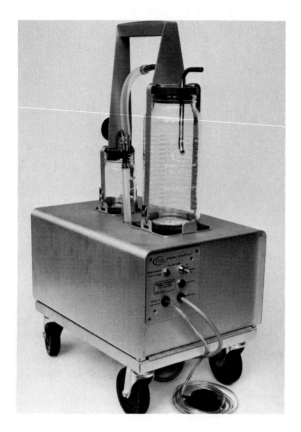

Figure 81–11. Typical vacuum pump with graduated collecting bottle. A one-third horsepower, two-stage mechanical rotary pump achieves vapor pressure vacuum in 15 seconds in a 2.5 liter bottle.

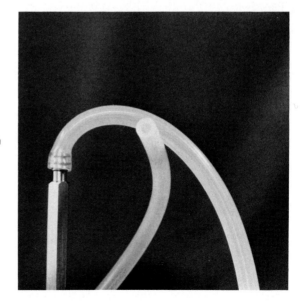

Figure 81–12. Thick wall tubing does not collapse with 743 mm of vacuum pressure.

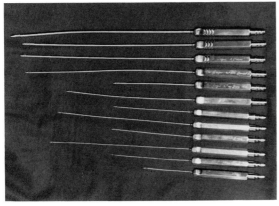

A

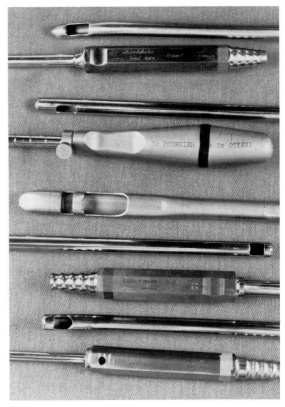

B

Figure 81–13. *A,* The author's preferred set of cannulas. All are three-aperture style and range from 6 mm to 1.5 mm outside diameter. The shaft length ranges from 32 cm to 8 cm exclusive of the handle. The cannulas below 3.7 mm diameter are easily bent to any configuration. *B,* Original cannulas. *Two bottom,* Illouz blunt type. *Middle,* Wide-mouth Kesselring type. Above the Kesselring type is the Fournier-Otteni type, which has a less blunt tip than the Illouz. *Top,* Grazer-Grams with the bullet-shaped tip. (Courtesy of Takehiro Shirakabe, M.D., Osaka, Japan.)

the fewest moving parts and are best suited for deep vacuum application. A high vacuum pump has precision fitting parts with minimal clearances. The precision parts inside a high vacuum require oil for lubrication. Since evacuated air has to pass through the pump, the exhausted air may be contaminated. In vacuum application, only a small amount of air is exhausted. A properly designed and maintained exhaust filter can clear the air to conform to standards required in the operating room.

Free air displacement of a pump is determined by its internal dimensions. The higher the free air displacement, the more horsepower it takes to drive it and the faster the jar is evacuated. It is desirable to have instant high vacuum, but this is determined by the size of the vacuum jar and the available power in the operating room. A one-third horsepower motor and pump with a free air displacement of 3 cubic feet per minute should produce body fluid vapor pressure in less than 15 seconds in a 2.5 liter jar (see Fig. 81–11).

Vacuum hose dimensions have no effect on maximal vacuum at the cannula tip. However, for practical reasons, internal dimen-sions should not be smaller than the inside dimensions of the cannula.

Tubing. Tubing should be manufactured from silicone or vinyl. It must not collapse with full vacuum (see Fig. 81–12).

Cannulas. Cannulas come in a variety of sizes and shapes (see Fig. 81–13). One has to be a pragmatist when it comes to selecting the type for each procedure. After multiple prototypes, the author has found that the smaller-sized three-aperture tip (equally spaced around the tip) cannula produces less trauma to the soft tissue, and removes as much fat as a large one-aperture cannula (see Chap. 80, Fig. 80–4).

Since cannula size is directly related to the amount of trauma, the smallest cannula possible per body area size should be used. Usual sizes range from 1.5 to 6 mm. The 8 to 10 mm cannulas are used only on the largest suction volumes.

PATIENT SELECTION AND PREOPERATIVE PLANNING

Patient selection requires that the surgeon have an esthetic eye as well as a knowledge of the effects of soft tissue trauma, a knowledge of physiology, and clinical judgment to determine the elasticity and retractibility of skin and soft tissue. Age is not a deterrent (Fig. 81–14). The quality of tissue elasticity and tissue turgor actually determines whether the patient is a good candidate. Appropriate amounts of tissue can be suctioned at any age provided that the turgor and elasticity of the overlying skin envelope is adequate.

Preoperative assessment should include the state of the patient's health, diet, medications, and medical and family history.

The informed consent forms should include both general and specific information regarding complications. General information should touch upon what the patient can realistically expect and what the surgeon can realistically produce. Specific information should include all possible complications. The use of visual information such as videos and photos of results, including scars and complications, is also important. Specific complications are discussed later.

Body contouring procedures can be done on an outpatient basis except for patients (1) who have health problems or (2) in whom the amount of surgical resection required or suction volumes in excess of 2500 ml mandate their being an inpatient. Most extended combined procedures should be done on an inpatient basis.

There is considerable variation among surgeons in decisions regarding general versus local anesthesia. Several criteria must be considered:

1. Patient desires and fears.
2. Volume aspirated.
3. Amount of surgical resection.
4. Length of surgical procedures.
5. Volume of local anesthesia required.
6. Associated medical problems.

The following procedures are amenable to local anesthesia:

1. Face and neck suctioning.
2. Face lift with suctioning.
3. Brachioplasty with or without suctioning.
4. Removal of axillary breasts, mastopexy.
5. Mini-abdominoplasty (with or without suctioning).
6. Suctioning of the abdomen (volume under 750 ml).
7. Suctioning of the hips and thighs (volume under 750 ml).

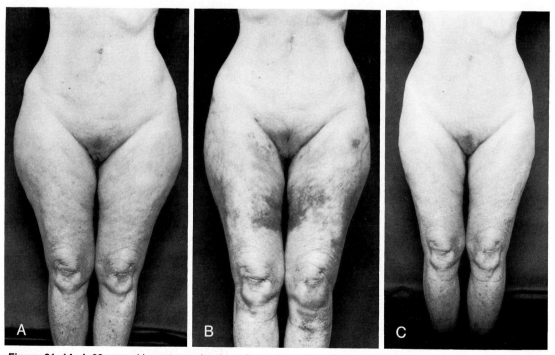

Figure 81–14. A 62 year old great grandmother who underwent suctioning of the hips and thighs. 2000 ml of fatty tissue were aspirated. *A*, Preoperative appearance. *B*, Ecchymosis 48 hours postoperatively. *C*, Postoperative appearance at one year, showing adequate contraction of the skin envelope.

8. Small thigh reductions.

9. Suctioning of the calves and ankles.

The use of autologous blood is strongly advocated. In addition to volume loading (see Chap. 80, p. 3935), autologous blood is recommended in suction volumes exceeding 2500 ml or surgical resections resulting in more than 1 unit of blood loss. The rule of thumb is usually 1 to 2 units of blood replacement for every 2500 ml of fat aspirated.

It must be recognized that for every milliliter of blood lost in the suction aspirate, approximately 0.5 to 1 ml extravasates into the tissues. In elective surgery, the use of bank blood is not advocated owing to the increasing high risk of hepatitis and acquired immune deficiency syndrome (AIDS). Family or other designated donors have become an alternative. Depending on the estimated blood replacement needed, an average patient in good health can donate 2 or 3 units of whole blood within one month of surgery without the blood being frozen. For more than 3 units of blood, the patient should start several months before the anticipated surgery and have the blood bank freeze the cells and plasma. It is possible to donate blood at one center and have it transferred by courier or air express, if distance requires it, to the hospital where the surgery is to be performed.

In order to estimate blood loss for a given case when the only procedure is SAL, a lipocrit is most helpful (see Chap. 80, p. 3936).

After centrifugation, there is a separation of the aspirate into four components: the oil rises to the top, fat cells comprise the second layer, serum components comprise the third layer, and the packed red cell button is evident in the fourth layer (Fig. 81–15). The packed cell button at the bottom can be converted to the amount of whole blood lost when the patient's hematocrit is known. In a combined suction and traditional contouring procedure, the lipocrit determination should be added to the usual blood loss estimates including blood-soaked sponges.

It is important that *all* patients be marked in the standing position prior to any body contour surgery including suctioning. Marks are frequently washed off during the preparation process, but a green Pentel felt-tip pen is a superior product that can help to prevent this.

COMPLICATIONS

Many of the abdominal complications discussed in Chapter 80 have also occurred with

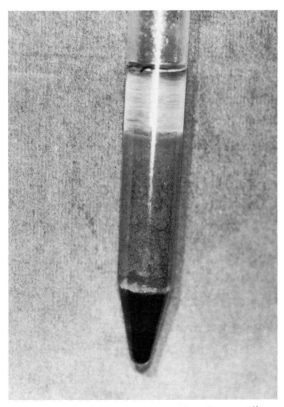

Figure 81–15. 10 ml aliquot spun down in a centrifuge. Note the four components: 1, Top—clear pure triglycerides; 2, Central component—fat cells and connective tissue; 3, 4, Bottom has two components: (a) cell button on the immediate bottom, and (b) the supernatant above the cell button, containing plasma serum, local anesthetic, and broken-down hemoglobin. The blood and serum components represent approximately 10 per cent of the entire volume in this sample.

all other forms of body contouring. They include the usual complications for any surgical procedure of the same magnitude, i.e., infection, hematoma, wound separation, tissue necrosis, pulmonary problems (e.g., atelectasis, pulmonary fat embolism syndrome, pulmonary emboli), neurologic injuries, pigment changes, and contour irregularities. The most frequent complication is that of oversuctioning. Correction includes resuctioning adjacent areas, skin reduction to tighten the skin envelope, and autologous fat grafting (Fig. 81–16).

Arms, Breasts, and Thorax. Most commonly, the arms are treated in conjunction with other body contouring procedures. The author is unaware of any major fat embolism or pulmonary emboli related to surgery in the areas containing the arms, breasts, and thorax. The circulation to the arm and hand may be compromised by excessively tight

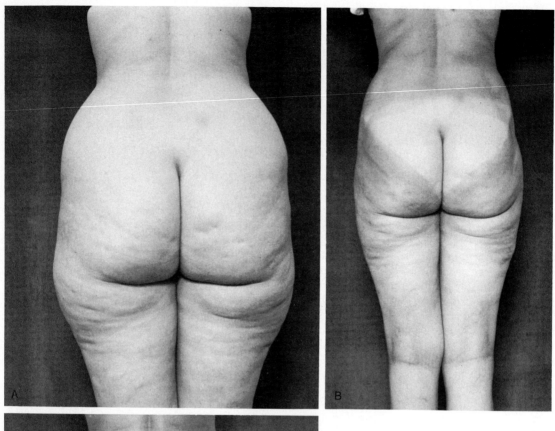

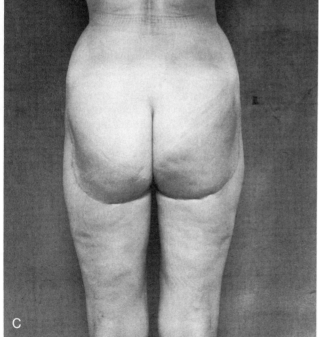

Figure 81–16. *A,* A 39 year old female before 1500 ml buttock-trochanteric aspiration. *B,* Secondary touch-up of the SAL did not correct the loose infragluteal roll. *C,* After skin and subcutaneous tissue reduction.

wound closure or by the formation of a hematoma necessitating release of sutures or aspiration of the hematoma. Hypertrophic scarring occurs in 10 to 20 per cent of brachioplasty patients and is the most frequent complaint arising from this surgery. Secondary scar revision improves approximately 50 per cent of patients in whom hypertrophic scarring occurs.

Hip and Thigh Reduction. Major potential complications are wound separation, wound infection, necrotizing fasciitis/septicemia, hematoma, hypovolemic shock, pulmonary emboli, and pulmonary fat embolism syndrome. Minor complications include contour irregularities, hypertrophic scarring, skin loss, sensory damage, and hyperpigmentation.

Knees, Calves, and Ankles. A greater risk of circulatory problems involving hematoma and seroma is encountered in the suctioning of the lower extremities. Persistent lymphedema, lymphorrhea, pain, pigment changes, infection, hematoma, and seroma may be experienced by the patient. Skin loss is a rare complication in these areas (Pfulg, 1982).

PREVENTION OF COMPLICATIONS

Suggested steps in the reduction of complications peculiar to each anatomic area provide a specific agenda:

1. Proper patient selection.
2. Preoperative work-up of the patient (including the goals of both patient and surgeon, preoperative assessment, general information, and informed consent).
3. How much surgery is contemplated?
4. Autologous blood/adequate blood bank availability.
5. Volume loading.
6. Antibiotics.
7. Patient position on the operating table.
8. Monitoring devices for the patient in an outpatient setting, i.e., pulse oxymeters, disconnect alarms, continuous cardiac monitoring devices.
9. Duration of surgery.
10. Meticulous hemostasis.
11. Indwelling catheter when necessary for inpatients or a temporary catheter for outpatients.
12. Use of drains when required (in patients undergoing suction alone, no drains are needed).

13. Adequate patient surveillance.
14. Postoperative visit (on the day after surgery).
15. Alcohol protocol (see Chap. 80) in all abdominal cases, in patients in whom the volume of fat aspirate in other body areas exceeds 250 ml, and/or in large subcutaneous reductions. (Note: Pulmonary fat embolism syndrome has occurred in a patient in whom only 180 ml was aspirated from the abdomen.)
16. Steroids: Solu-Medrol or its generic equivalent (methylprednisolone) with similar criteria as for the alcohol protocol, using 500 mg intravenously in all suction volumes exceeding 250 ml.
17. Adequate postoperative compression.

TECHNIQUE

Face, Chin, and Neck

After the early success of the SAL technique applied to other parts of the body, it became apparent that the technique would naturally lend itself to the face, chin, and neck. Teimourian (1983) and Courtiss (1985) popularized the use of the plastic abortion cannula for suctioning the face and neck. Grazer (1984b) and others discussed suctioning with smaller stainless steel cannulas as shown in Figure 81–13. Shirakabe (1987) has popularized the flexible cannula.

As described at the start of this chapter, controversy still exists concerning the possibility of an increase in the number of fat cells after adult life is reached. It is the author's contention that, if the fat cell bed in the face, chin, and neck is removed early in life, there is no matrix for more primordial fat cells to be laid down in the future.

Since genetics is so important in determining body type, early recognition of some family traits such as the "double chin" allows the early implementation of suctioning to contour and reduce unwanted fat deposits early in life in order to prevent their occurrence in adulthood (Fig. 81–17).

Suctioning Alone. There are four recommended sites for inserting the cannula in a patient with excessive face, chin, or neck fat in whom a face lift is not necessary but only suction is required: (1) the temple hair-bearing area, (2) immediately below the earlobe in the retroauricular sulcus, (3) in the vestibule of the nose, and (4) the submental area (Fig. 81–18).

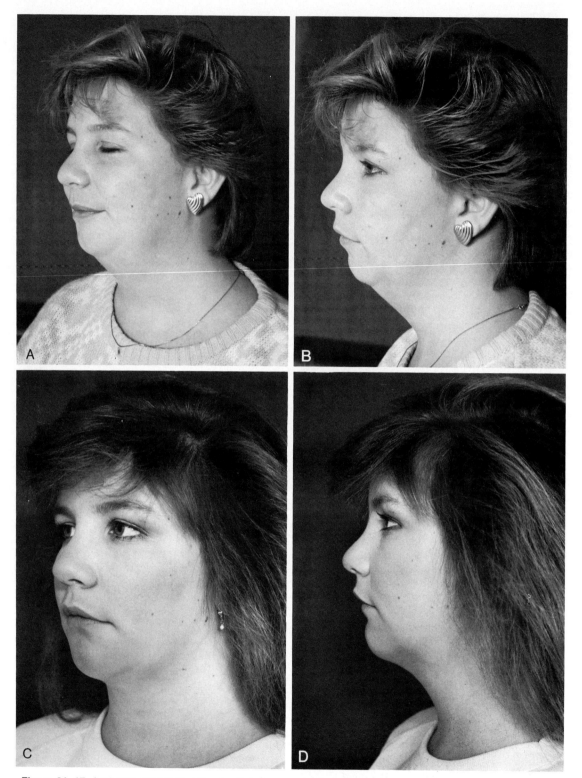

Figure 81–17. A 16 year old female with a familial obese neck who underwent three procedures within an eight month period to achieve the final result. The total volume aspirated was 200 ml. The patient had a chin implant placed in the initial surgery. She has gained 17 lb since her first surgery, none of which has appeared in her face. *A, B,* Preoperative appearance. *C, D,* Postoperative appearance at eight months.

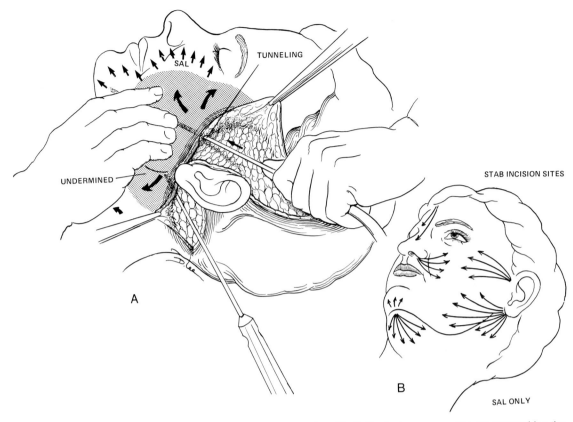

TUNNELING

SAL

UNDERMINED

STAB INCISION SITES

A

B

SAL ONLY

Figure 81–18. The face lift. *A,* Suctioning in conjunction with a face lift. *B,* Suctioning access sites for approaching the face and neck when skin resection is not necessary.

It is not necessary to use drains, and the wound can be closed with a single suture. When the surgery is performed as an isolated procedure, the author has noted no nerve injuries or areas of necrosis (Grazer, 1984b).

In addition to the genetic predisposition, there are congenital fatty abnormalities in children that are also amenable to suctioning (Fig. 81–19). Facial suctioning also lends itself well to the "fat face," "chipmunk cheeks," "moon face," "double chin" or to patients with problem areas who wish to defer a face lift procedure.

Suctioning (SAL) to reduce steroid-induced facial deformities in conjunction with the "buffalo hump" may return the patient to the pre–steroid therapy appearance (Fig. 81–20).

SAL in Conjunction with Face Lift. Suctioning of the face in conjunction with a face lift (see Fig. 81–18) is done both before and after the SMAS flap (see also Chap. 43) has been elevated (Figs. 81–21, 81–22).

With all facial suctioning the 1.5, 1.8, and 2.4 mm, three-holed (Mercedes) cannulas are utilized. Most of the face, cheek, chin, and neck areas can be reached through the four separate stab incision sites previously noted. Insertion of the cannula with the aperture side toward the skin edge does not, in itself, cause irregularities. The question always arises as to whether the holes face up or down with the three-hole cannula. With this cannula, one aperture is always facing the skin surface and no problems have resulted. In the beginning, some evidence of early contour depression was experienced owing to overaspiration only. Correction was made by a face lift.

Arms and Thorax

One of the signs of the aging process is the "hanging" of the triceps, which is usually associated with muscle mass loss as well as the accumulation of subcutaneous fat. The classic corrective procedure has been the reduction of skin and subcutaneous fat.

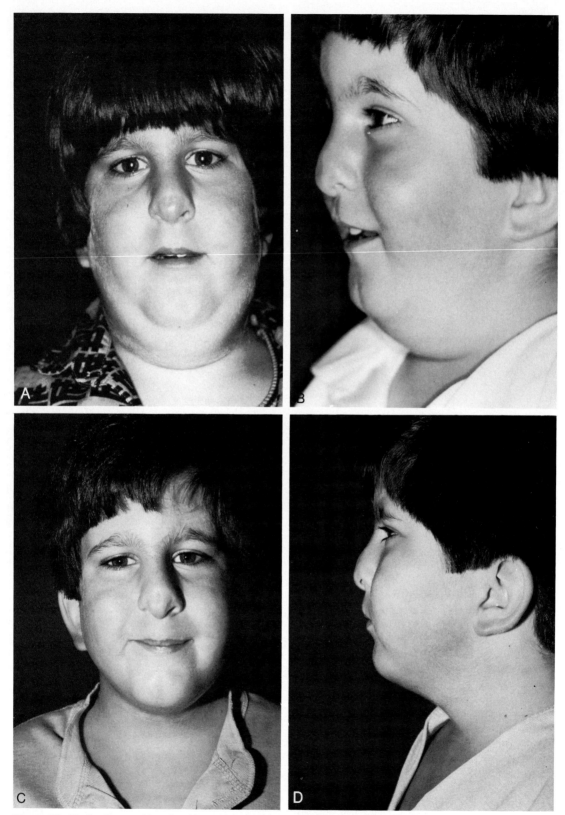

Figure 81–19. An 8 year old male with multiple anomalies: bilateral clubfeet, nasal tip deformity, and abnormal fat distribution of the face and neck. 125 ml was suctioned. *A, B,* Preoperative appearance. *C, D,* Postoperative appearance at six months.

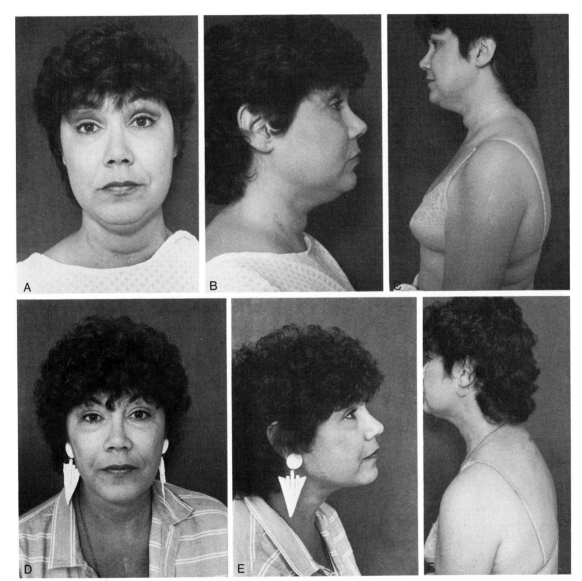

Figure 81–20. A 42 year old female patient who successfully underwent heart-lung transplantation for pulmonary hypertension. She had several years of steroid therapy resulting in facial changes and a "buffalo hump" deformity. *A* to *C,* Preoperative appearance. *D, E,* Postoperative appearance at four months after aspiration of 1400 ml of fat from the face and neck areas. *F,* Postoperative appearance at four months with absence of the buffalo hump. 200 ml was aspirated from the posterior neck.

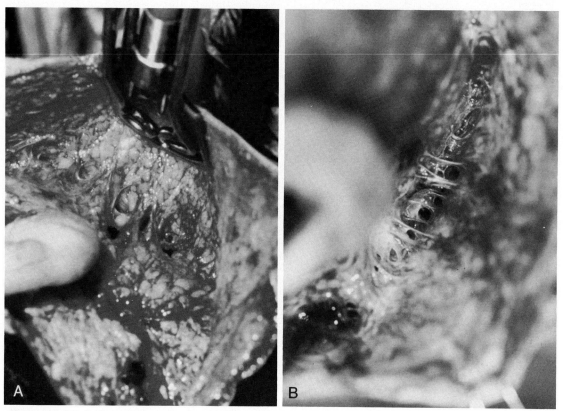

Figure 81–21. *A,* The multiple aspiration sites during a face lift. *B,* Close-up appearance of the fibrous septa, each of which contains small vessels.

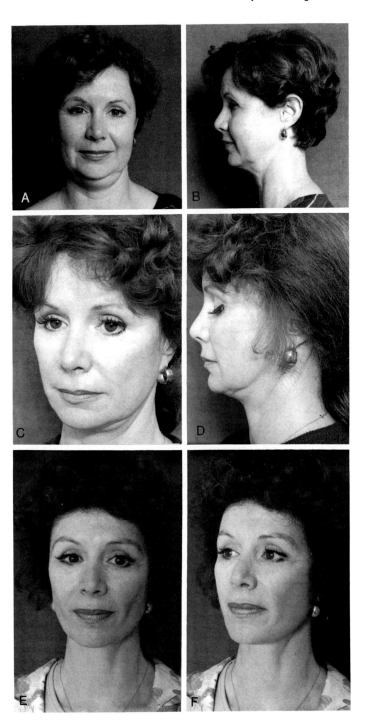

Figure 81–22. Combined face lift and SAL. *A, B,* Preoperative appearance before the face lift. The patient had previously undergone blepharoplasty. *C, D,* Postoperative face lift, but before SAL. *E, F,* Appearance one year after face and neck SAL.

Suction alone can reduce the fatty tissue from the arms; however, to provide the best esthetic result, most patients also require reduction of the skin envelope.

Brachioplasty Without Suctioning. Before the advent of SAL, arm circumference was reduced by excising a longitudinal portion of the skin and subcutaneous tissue (Figs. 81–23, 81–24) (Grazer and Klingbeil, 1980). This is still a highly effective and acceptable technique. The objective is to reduce the skin envelope and the subcutaneous fat while placing the resulting scar in the most inconspicuous location in the medial aspect of the arm. The landmarks for the incision line lie in the brachial sulcus located from the midpoint of the axilla to the medial epicondyle. To determine how much to re-

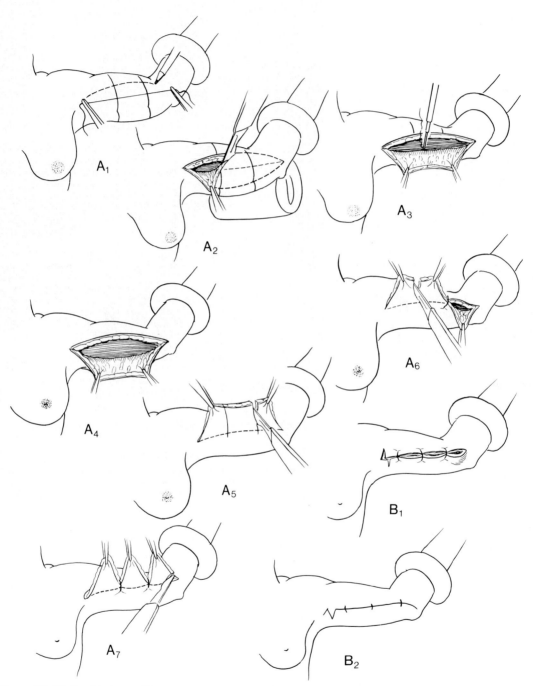

Figure 81–23. Brachioplasty without suctioning. A_1 to A_7, The essentials of the technique. A string is drawn from the medial epicondyle to the center of the axilla for positioning of the final scar. B_1, B_2, Note the important crossmarkings. Z-plasty is not always necessary.

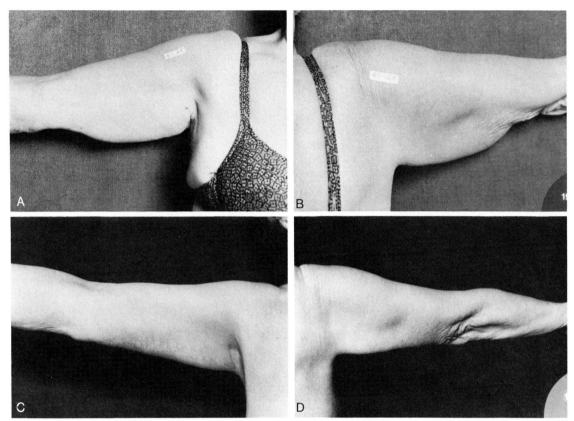

Figure 81–24. A 64 year old female who underwent a classical brachioplasty. *A, B,* Preoperative appearance. *C, D,* Postoperative appearance at seven years. Note the optimal scar position.

move, the surgeon must use the pinch test. The end result of the removal leaves NO undermining, thereby eliminating the potential for seroma collection. To monitor the patient, a blood pressure cuff is usually placed on one of the lower extremities. Subcutaneous wound closure is with buried absorbable sutures such as 4-0 Vicryl. Skin closure is with fine prolene and/or skin staples and Steri-Strip tapes. Drains are not usually indicated. The preferred dressing is a 4 inch Kerlix wrap. Postoperatively the patient should keep the arms elevated on two pillows for 24 to 48 hours.

Postoperative monitoring of the patient for the first 24 hours is essential to detect circulation or nerve embarrassment from such conditions as hematoma, seroma, or excessively tight wound closure. If any of these occur, corrective measures must be undertaken, i.e., evacuation of the hematoma or seroma, or release of the sutures to allow the tissue to recover. Sutures are removed on day 4 or 5. Steri-Strip tape or paper tape is worn across the seam for approximately one month after surgery.

Occasionally a Z-plasty in the axilla may be necessary if a contracture develops postoperatively. This development can usually be predetermined by hyperextending the axilla. If there is evidence of a tight band, a Z-plasty should be done at the time of surgery.

Suctioning Alone. In patients in whom there is an increase in girth but adequate turgor and elasticity of the skin, suction alone suffices. The arm should have no triceps hang since SAL alone only accentuates the condition without skin reduction. The prime preoperative concern is whether the skin will shrink sufficiently to give a cosmetically acceptable result.

Technique. Most suction of the arm can be done under local anesthesia. General anesthesia is usually necessary when surgery is performed in combination with other body contouring operations such as on the thighs or abdomen.

The patient is placed in the supine position

with arms extended on rests or boards. After the instillation of the local anesthetic solution, the approach to the arm is through the medial epicondyle and occasionally through the lateral epicondyle. The author prefers the smaller cannulas—3.7 mm and smaller, and long enough to reach the axilla (approximately 30 cm in length). Suctioning can be accomplished circumferentially through the epicondyle site. The intravenous line, when indicated for sedation or general anesthesia, can be draped out of the field with a stockinette. Suctioning is begun in the triceps area with gradual movement around the circumference of the arm as indicated (Fig. 81–25).

A stab incision in the axilla may occasionally be necessary to suction the axilla and adjacent upper arm. Stab incisions are closed with nonabsorbable prolene or nylon sutures. Usual volumes removed are in the 100 to 200 ml range. Compression of the arm is provided by a Jobst elastic stocking or a 4 inch Ace wrap. It is recommended that the patient wear the compressive dressing until all edema and ecchymosis have subsided, which usually takes ten days to three weeks (Fig. 81–26).

Thoracobrachioplasty and Thoracobrachiobreastplasty Without Suctioning. These procedures may be performed via the traditional surgical approach (see Fig. 81–23) or by the newer combination of suction and skin reduction (see Fig. 81–25). Figure 81–27 illustrates the results from the traditional reduction technique.

Thoracobrachioplasty and Thoracobrachiobreastplasty With Suctioning. The technique of skin reduction with SAL (see Fig. 81–25) differs from the classic reduction in that after the SAL (Fig. 81–28) the skin is tailor tacked to determine the amount to deepithelize. The deepithelized dermis is invaginated (Grazer, 1984b). After final closure, additional suctioning is advised to reduce wound tension if the wound appears too tight (Fig. 81–28C). This technique may also be extended to include the thorax and forearm (Fig. 81–29, and see Fig. 81–25).

Breasts

Axillary Breasts and Breast Reduction. One of the sequelae of breast reduction is the lack of correction of the axillary breast or axillary fullness. Suctioning of this area, using a 2.4 or 3 mm cannula, improves the esthetic appearance of the breasts.

Using any of the standard techniques for breast reduction, the surgeon can improve the results with SAL. At the time of the operation, SAL may be employed to reduce tension on the suture line and correct any minor asymmetry without taking the wound down (Figs. 81–30, 81–31) (see also Chap. 80, Fig. 80–38). When the amount of reduction falls short of the patient's or surgeon's goal, secondary suction may be considered. However, if this is done, suction samples should be sent for tissue evaluation as a random breast biopsy. SAL of the breast should not be done as a primary procedure but only as an adjunct. The 2.4 or 3.7 mm cannula is most commonly used.

Breast Reconstruction. In breast reconstruction, the tailoring of the latissimus myocutaneous flap or the transverse abdominal myocutaneous (TRAM) flap (see Chap. 79) with suctioning has been beneficial to reduce bulk and provide a better contour for the newly constructed breast (Fig. 81–32). The usual cannula sizes are 2.4 to 3.7 mm for this type of refinement (Bostwick, Hester, and Nahai, 1985).

Gynecomastia. There are three forms of gynecomastia: the glandular, the fatty glandular, and the simple fatty type. The classic technique has consisted of the circumareolar subcutaneous mastectomy for all three forms of gynecomastia, with the exception of those in which there is ptosis and excess of skin.

Glandular. Patients with a glandular component require surgical removal of the gland, which frequently results in a deep depression where the gland existed with fatty fullness in all directions. With the combination of SAL and glandular reduction, a more symmetric result is obtained (Fig. 81–33).

Nonglandular. Cases that are primarily fatty in nature and generally exhibited in the middle-aged male respond to SAL alone (Fig. 81–34).

Gynecomastia with Ptosis. Patients who have significant breast enlargement and ptosis do not respond to suction alone and require skin reduction (Fig. 81–35).

Complications of surgery for gynecomastia include asymmetry, hematoma, seroma, nipple slough, and infection.

Hips and Upper Thighs

In properly selected patients, SAL has significantly broadened the field of body contour

Text continued on page 4000

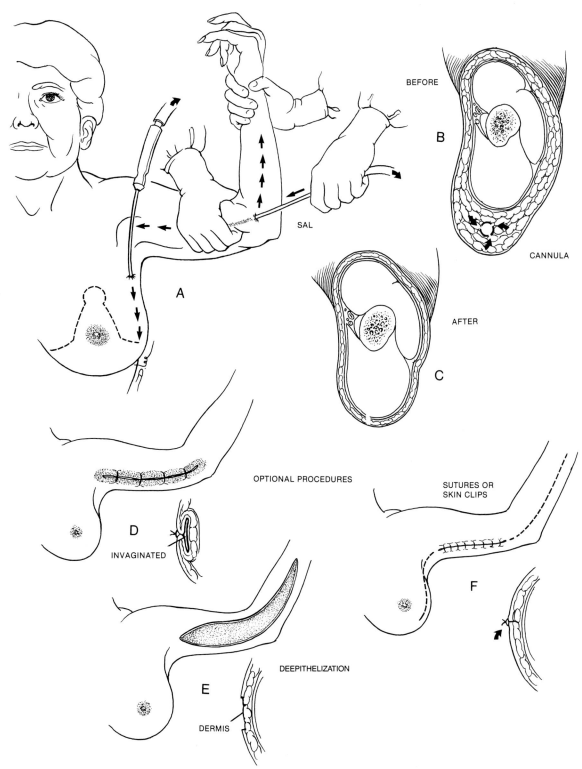

Figure 81–25. Combination approaches to the arm, thorax, and breast. *A,* Suction alone or the first step before skin reduction. *B,* Cannula position in the subcutaneous tissue. *C,* Expected postoperative result. *D,* After suctioning tailor tacking to determine the amount of deepithelization. *E,* Deepithelization. *F,* Final closure.

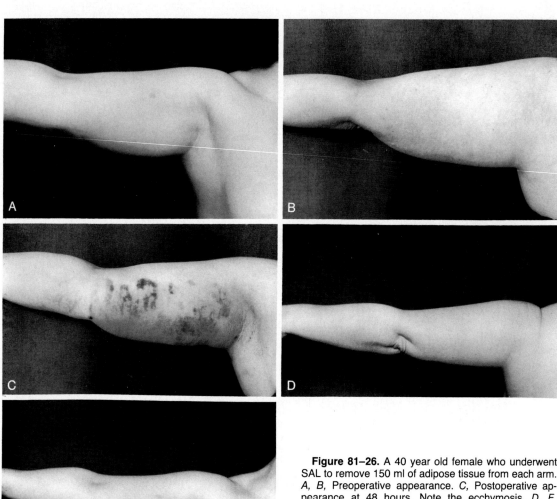

Figure 81–26. A 40 year old female who underwent SAL to remove 150 ml of adipose tissue from each arm. *A, B,* Preoperative appearance. *C,* Postoperative appearance at 48 hours. Note the ecchymosis. *D, E,* Postoperative appearance at one year.

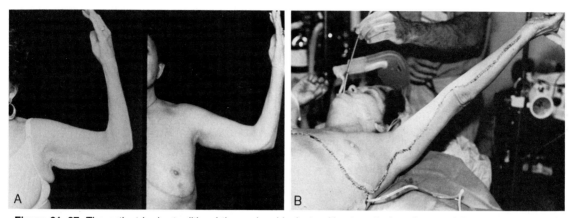

Figure 81–27. The patient had a traditional thoracobrachioplasty without suctioning after a weight loss from a morbid obese state of 300 lb. *A,* Pre- and postoperative appearance with arm extended. *B,* Intraoperative view of extent of resection.

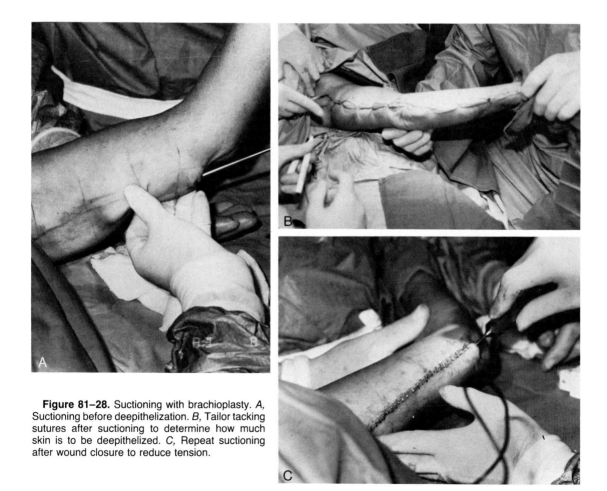

Figure 81–28. Suctioning with brachioplasty. *A,* Suctioning before deepithelization. *B,* Tailor tacking sutures after suctioning to determine how much skin is to be deepithelized. *C,* Repeat suctioning after wound closure to reduce tension.

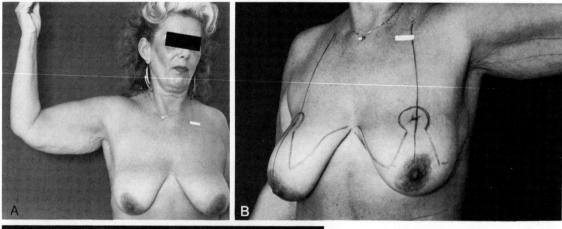

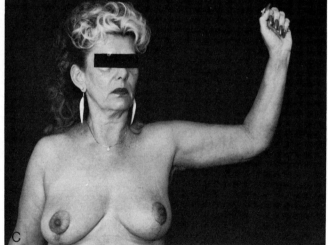

Figure 81–29. A 58 year old female who underwent thoracobrachiobreastplasty. *A,* Preoperative appearance. *B,* Preoperative view with breast markings for the McKissock technique. *C,* Early postoperative result. 100 ml was aspirated from each arm.

MCKISSOCK BREAST REDUCTION

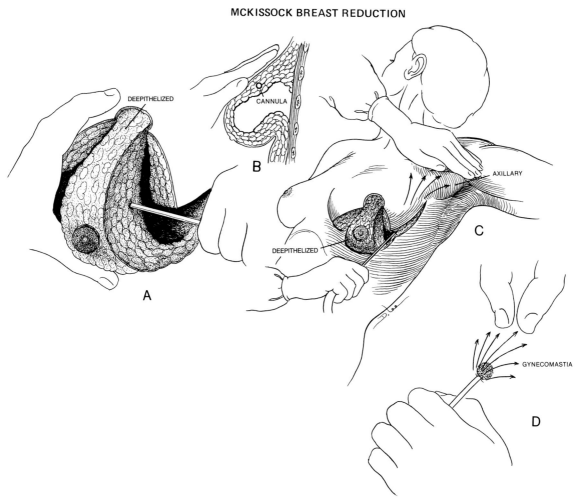

Figure 81–30. Ancillary suction techniques to aid in breast reduction. *A, B,* The bulk of the vertical pedicle can be reduced without affecting the blood supply. *C,* Suctioning of the axillary breast. *D,* Periareolar site for suctioning areas of gynecomastia. The optional site is through the axilla. (McKissock, 1972.)

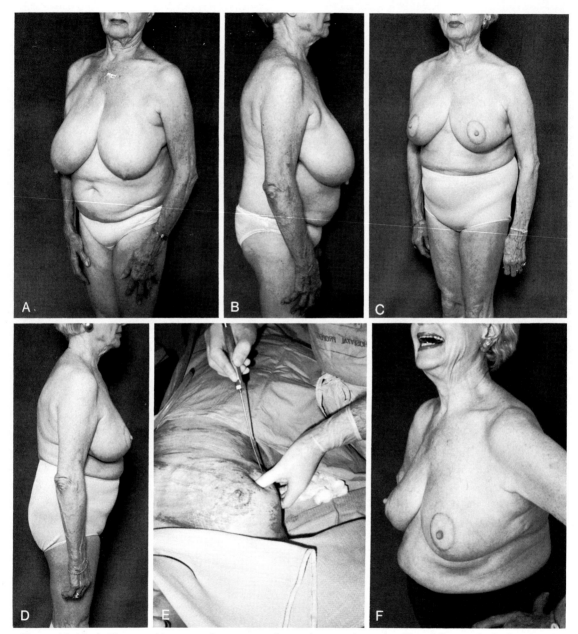

Figure 81–31. A 70 year old woman demonstrates breast hypertrophy and axillary fullness. *A, B,* Preoperative appearance. *C, D,* Postoperative appearance: note the absence of axillary fullness. The patient was happy with the postoperative results after removal of 250 gm from each breast, even though she had insisted that the surgeon not reduce the breast tissue as much as he preferred. At a later date the patient returned, feeling that added reduction would be desirable. *E,* An additional 100 ml was removed by suctioning of the breasts after primary breast reduction. *F,* Final result. Sample biopsies were taken from the aspirated fat.

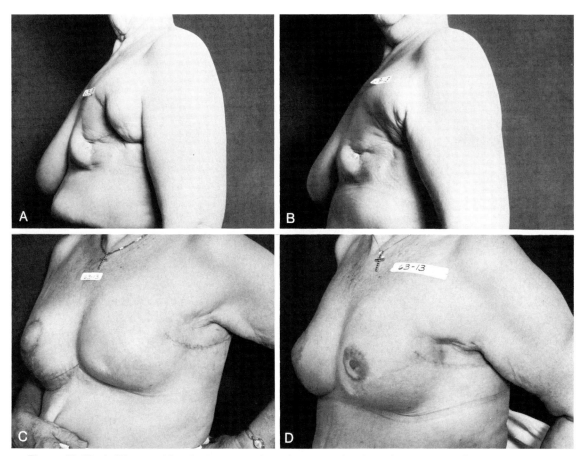

Figure 81–32. A 67 year old patient was on chemotherapy at the time of consultation. She could not undergo reconstruction because of the chemotherapy, nor could she wear an external prosthesis because of the axillary deformity. The deformity was suctioned, after which the patient was able to tolerate a prosthesis. Reconstruction was completed after the chemotherapy regimen ended. *A,* Preoperative appearance. Note the extensive depression and the bulk of the axillary fullness. *B,* Postoperative appearance after axillary suctioning. The patient was able to tolerate the prosthesis with the axillary fullness reduced. *C,* First-stage breast reconstruction with additional suctioning to refine the contour. *D,* Final result showing right breast reduction and suction tailoring to achieve better contour (one year postoperatively).

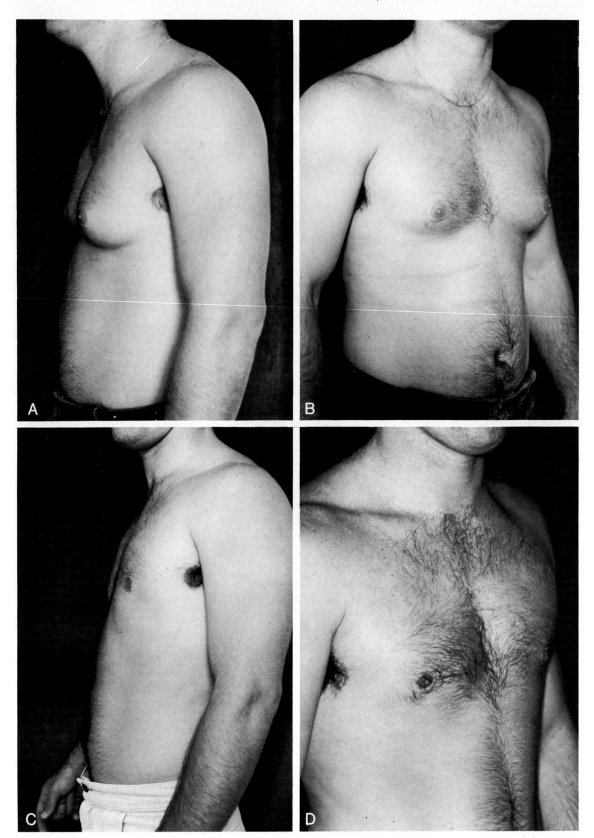

Figure 81–33. A 25 year old male who underwent a combination glandular resection with suctioning (SAL) through the periareolar area. *A, B*, Preoperative views showing a typical glandular gynecomastia. *C, D*, Postoperative appearance one year later. Note the absence of the postoperative depression deformity.

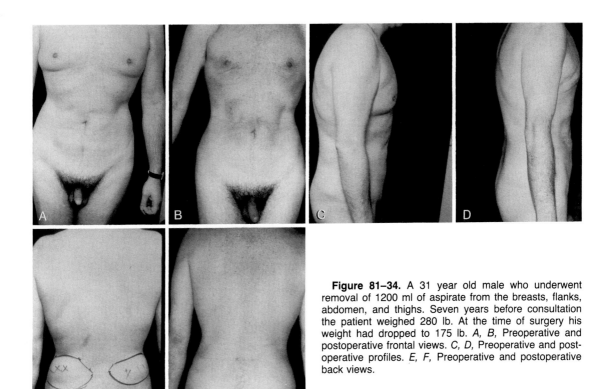

Figure 81–34. A 31 year old male who underwent removal of 1200 ml of aspirate from the breasts, flanks, abdomen, and thighs. Seven years before consultation the patient weighed 280 lb. At the time of surgery his weight had dropped to 175 lb. *A, B,* Preoperative and postoperative frontal views. *C, D,* Preoperative and postoperative profiles. *E, F,* Preoperative and postoperative back views.

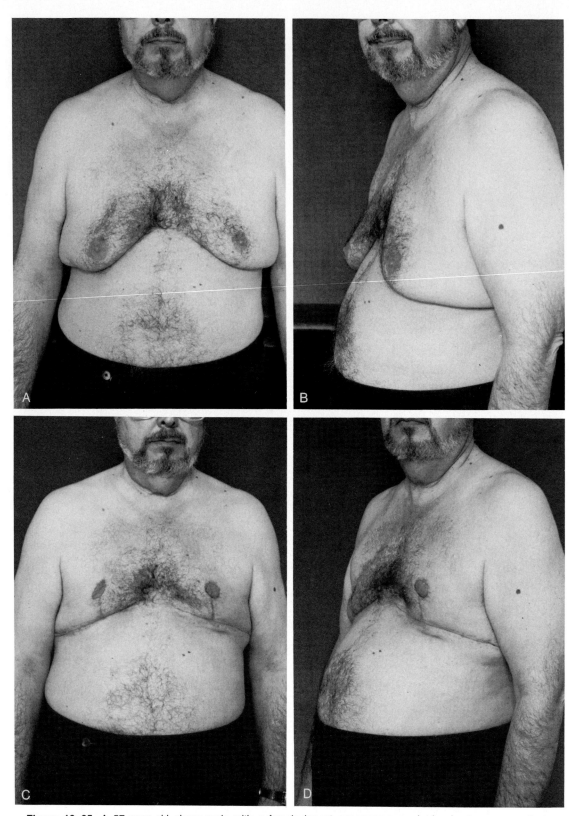

Figure 18–35. A 57 year old obese male with a female breast appearance required subcutaneous mastectomy, mastopexy, and suctioning. *A, B,* Preoperative views showing pendulous, female-like breasts. *C, D,* Postoperative appearance at four months after mastectomy, mastopexy, and suctioning (SAL). An abdominoplasty is planned for the future.

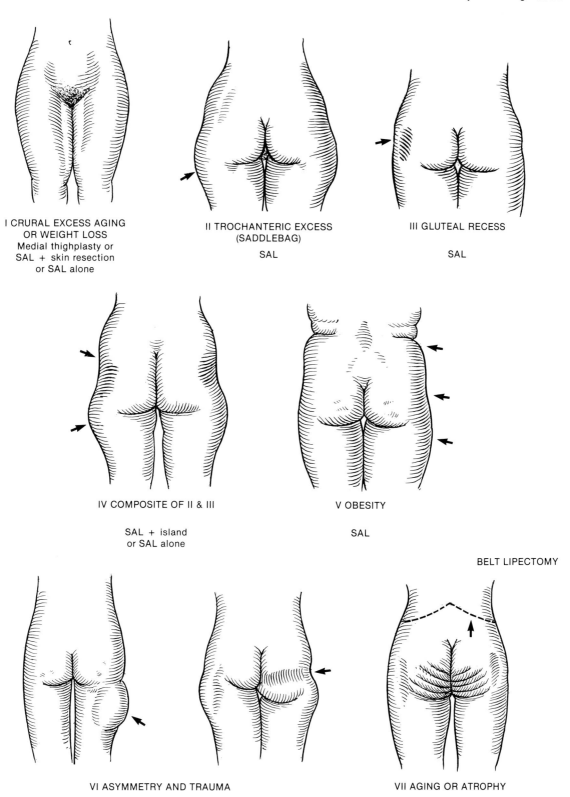

Figure 81–36. Classification of hip/thigh deformity.

surgery by allowing corrections of hip and thigh defects with essentially no scarring. However, some patients also require skin envelope reduction to achieve a satisfactory result. Grazer and Klingbeil (1980) developed a classification based on the anatomic deviations of the spectrum of hips and thigh defects. It was updated in 1984 to reflect the addition of SAL as a therapeutic modality (Grazer, 1984b, Shaer, 1984).

There are seven classifications that cover hip and thigh deformities (Fig. 81–36). For those patients with adequate skin turgor, suction alone usually suffices. Types I, IV, VI, and VII usually require skin reduction (Grazer and Klingbeil, 1980; Grazer, 1984b). The classifications are based on variations of the anatomy from the normal, including skin, subcutaneous fat, and muscle and bone structure that reflect the genetic template, environmental status, aging, or occasionally congenital deformities.

Type I Deformity. These deformities may occur as an isolated fullness of the medial thigh or in combination with any of the other six classified deformities (Figs. 81–37, 81–38).

SAL of Medial Thighs Alone. *Primary suctioning* may be performed in patients with adequate skin turgor who need only medial thigh improvement. However, most patients have other associated hip and/or thigh defects.

The patient is prepared and draped in the supine position. After injections of local anesthetic solution, stab incisions are made in the hair-bearing mons pubis or the inguinal crease, or both (see Fig. 81–40A, B). A 3.7 mm cannula or one of comparable size suffices. Care must be taken not to overaspirate this area (Fig. 81–39).

Complications. These include (1) irregularities, (2) hyperpigmentation, and (3) use of too long or too large a cannula, resulting in overaspiration.

In the Type I deformity, which exhibits loose skin in the medial thigh, skin reduction is frequently necessary. This may be accomplished by an en bloc resection (Fig. 81–40) or by suctioning the deformity, deepithelizing the skin, and invaginating the deepithelized segment in the manner described previously for the arms. Care must be taken to place the final incision line sufficiently high in the

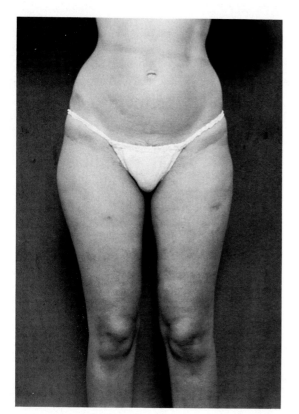

Figure 81–37. A 35 year old female demonstrating the typical appearance of Type I deformity with fullness of the medial thighs.

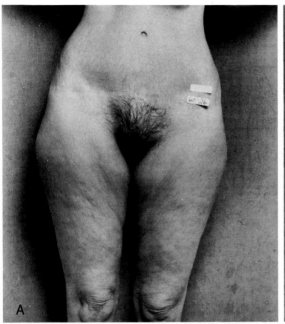

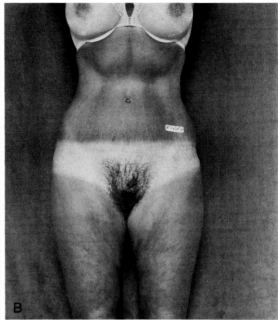

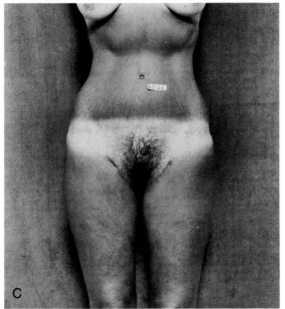

Figure 81–38. A 46 year old female who had undergone a previous abdominoplasty after losing 70 lb. *A,* Before suction (SAL) of hips and medial thighs. *B,* Postoperative appearance with persistent Type I deformity. *C,* Postoperative appearance after medial thighplasty. Note the correction and absence of the medial thighs touching each other.

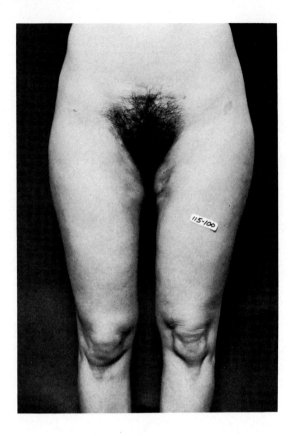

Figure 81–39. A 35 year old patient illustrating all types of complications: oversuctioning, skin redundancy, and hyperpigmentation. Note the irregularities and hyperpigmentation as a result of oversuctioning with too large a cannula.

inguinal crease so that it is not exposed below the bathing suit line (Fig. 81–41).

The combination of SAL and deepithelization has less potential for hematoma formation. Isolated Type I deformities can be surgically corrected under local anesthesia in the supine or frog-leg position.

Type II Deformity. This type of deformity is characterized by the "saddlebag" or "riding breeches" appearance. Suctioning is sufficient to reduce and refine these abnormalities (Fig. 81–42). Few patients with this type of deformity require more than suctioning (Fig. 81–43). For small deformities requiring less than 750 ml aspiration, local anesthesia suffices.

Type III Deformity. This type of deformity is characterized by the medial gluteal depression in addition to the trochanteric deformity. This deformity can be corrected by SAL alone usually requiring general anesthesia (Fig. 81–44).

Type IV Deformity. This deformity has also been known as the "viola" or "violin" deformity (Illouz, 1983). Type IV is a combination of the "saddlebag" and upper hip fullness.

Correction may require either suctioning alone or a combination of SAL with skin reduction under general anesthesia. The patient in Figure 81–45 underwent a medial thighplasty in 1980 *without suction*, employing the island technique (Fig. 81–46). This correction could have been made with *suction only* if the SAL procedure had been available at that time. However, in patients with more redundant tissue, the procedure of choice is suction with skin reduction by means of the "island technique." Figure 81–47 demonstrates the result of *suction and skin reduction*.

Type V Deformity (Obesity). Many patients with the endomorphic body type fall into this category. Frequently there is a significant body disproportion, e.g., a small thorax in comparison to a large lower trunk. These patients, who are generally obese, can respond to SAL alone as long as there is satisfactory skin tone (Fig. 81–48, and see Fig. 81–42). This 32 year old female underwent three separate SAL procedures: 5400 ml was removed during the first procedure, 3500 ml during the second procedure, and 3100 ml

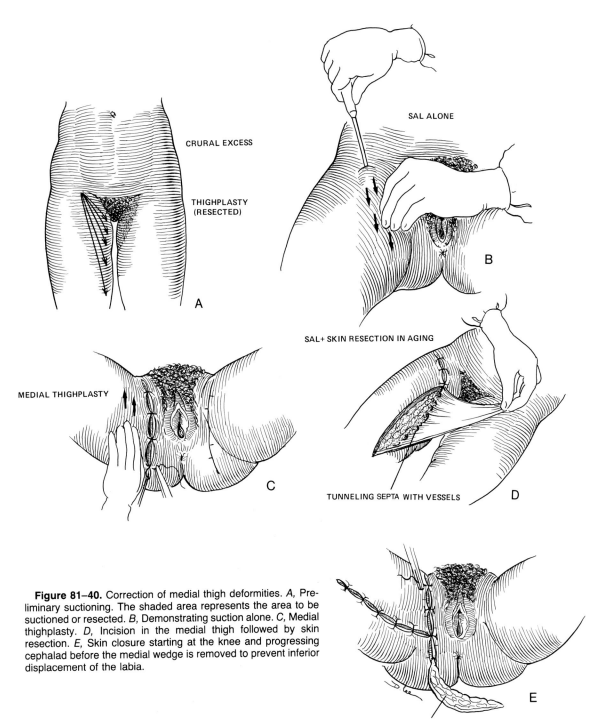

CRURAL EXCESS

THIGHPLASTY
(RESECTED)

A

SAL ALONE

B

MEDIAL THIGHPLASTY

C

SAL+ SKIN RESECTION IN AGING

TUNNELING SEPTA WITH VESSELS

D

WEDGE FROM MEDIAL THIGHPLASTY

E

Figure 81–40. Correction of medial thigh deformities. A, Preliminary suctioning. The shaded area represents the area to be suctioned or resected. B, Demonstrating suction alone. C, Medial thighplasty. D, Incision in the medial thigh followed by skin resection. E, Skin closure starting at the knee and progressing cephalad before the medial wedge is removed to prevent inferior displacement of the labia.

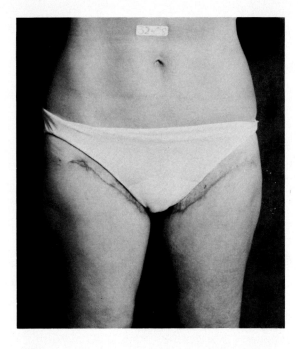

Figure 81–41. Improper placement of medial thigh reduction incisions.

during the third procedure. Over a two year period, a total of 12,000 ml of fatty tissue was aspirated from the hips and thighs. The patient donated two units of autologous blood for each procedure. The surgeries were performed under general anesthesia with an average 48 hour hospital stay.

Type VI Deformity. The Type VI deformity is characterized by asymmetry—congenital and/or post-traumatic deformities. The latter can frequently be improved by SAL alone (Fig. 81–49). Others require combined procedures utilizing the SAL and island techniques already depicted. This category also includes the oversuctioned or unevenly suctioned patient (see Fig. 81–16). General anesthesia is usually required because of the extent of the procedure.

Type VII Deformity. The type VII deformity is characterized by aging, atrophy, and/or weight loss. Morbid obesity, treated by one of the short-circuiting gastrointestinal surgical procedures, results in massive skin redundancy. This type primarily requires skin reduction with SAL used for refinement as needed. The deformities can involve the abdomen, buttocks, thigh, hip, and belt area (Fig. 81–50) (see also Chap. 80, Fig. 80–34).

SUCTIONING TECHNIQUES FOR HIPS AND THIGHS

For procedures involving SAL alone, the author prefers to begin with the patient in the prone position. With volumes approximating 750 ml or less of total aspirate, local anesthesia may be considered, but the author prefers general or epidural anesthesia. In most cases, in addition to general anesthesia, a local anesthetic solution (0.3 per cent lidocaine with 1:320,000 epinephrine) is infiltrated. This technique is a variant of the "wet technique" that Illouz (1983) described when he injected a hypotonic saline solution to "aid in the rupture of the adipocytes," a maneuver that he theorized would make SAL easier.

Fournier and Otteni (1983) proved that there was no difference between the "wet" and "dry" techniques. However, the author noted significant reduction in blood loss because of the vasoconstrictive properties provided by the epinephrine (Grazer, 1984b; Hetter, 1984a). The mixture is made as follows: three 50 ml bottles of 0.5 per cent lidocaine with 1:200,000 epinephrine diluted with 90 ml of injectable saline, giving a concentration of 0.3 per cent lidocaine with 1:320,000 epinephrine. It should be noted that the mixture totals 750 mg of lidocaine, which exceeds the manufacturer's recommended package dose. In a clinical study (Grazer, 1984b), it was noted that, when the entire 750 mg dose was injected into the patient and suctioning was begun within ten minutes of injection time, serum lidocaine levels did not exceed 1 μg per ml. Blood samples were taken 10, 20, and 40 minutes after the injection. The blood samples confirmed that subcutaneous absorp-

Text continued on page 4015

SAL ALONE

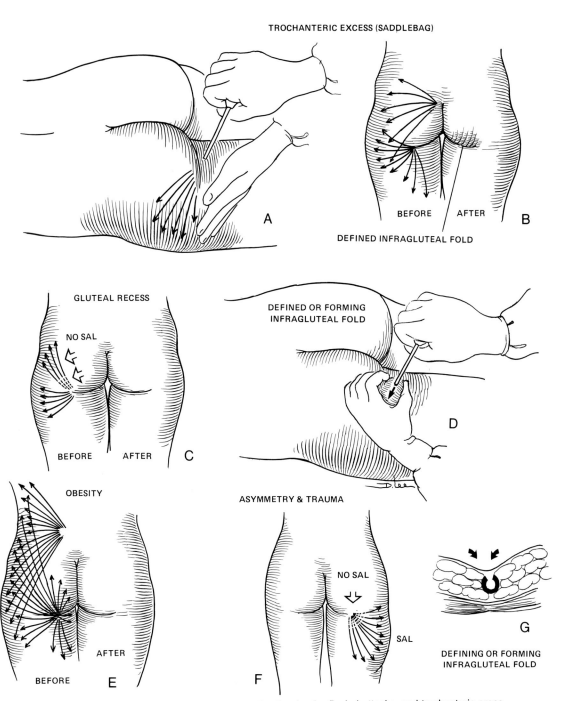

Figure 81–42. The various cannula sites for the flank, buttocks, and trochanteric areas.

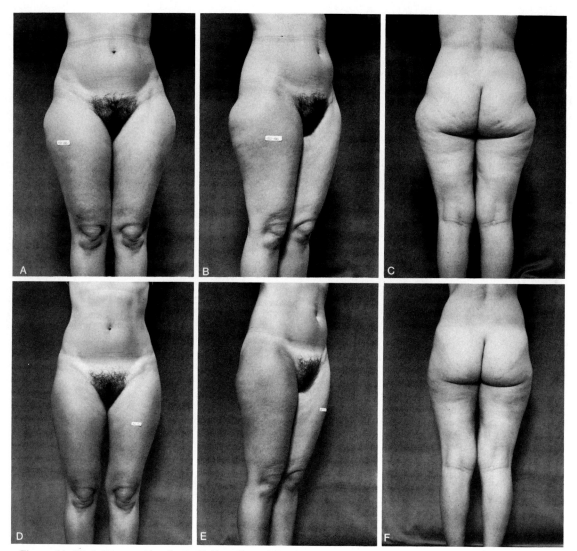

Figure 81–43. A 35 year old patient with Type II or "riding breeches" deformity. A total of 1300 ml of fatty tissue was aspirated. *A* to *C,* Preoperative views. *D* to *F,* Postoperative views.

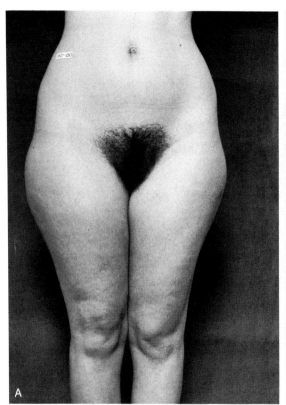 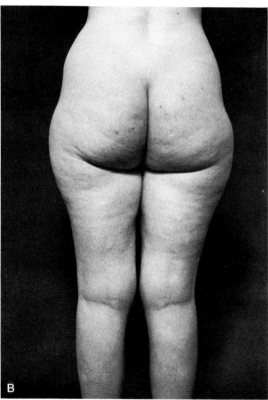

Figure 81–44. A 31 year old female with medial gluteal depression in addition to the "saddlebag" deformity. The postoperative views show the result of removal of 1400 ml of fatty aspirate. The measurements were as follows:

		Preoperative	Postoperative
Hips		43″	36″
Thighs	(r)	25″	20¼″
	(l)	25″	20½″

A, Preoperative frontal view showing Type III deformity.
B, Preoperative back view.

Illustration continued on following page

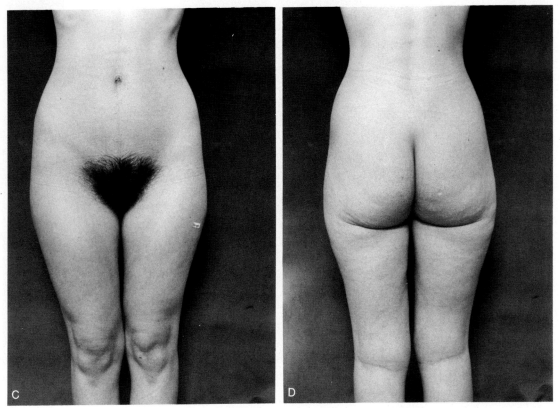

Figure 81–44 *Continued C,* Postoperative frontal view. *D,* Postoperative back view.

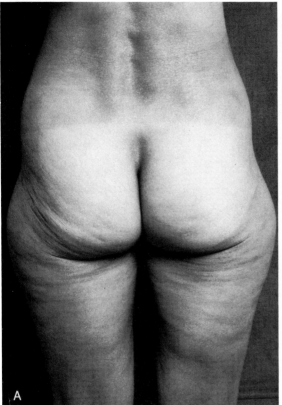

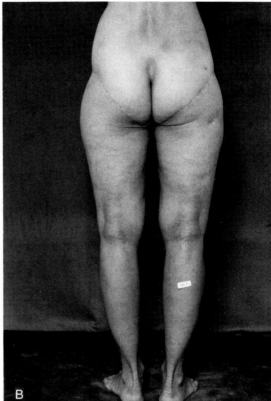

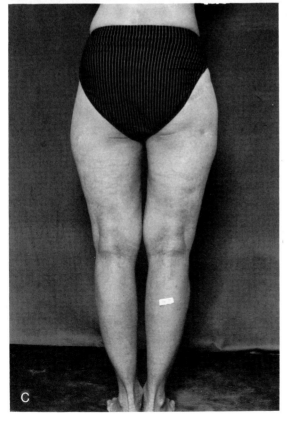

Figure 81–45. A 37 year old patient had a traditional medial and posterior thighplasty before the advent of surgery using the "island technique." Note the potential deformity in the upper hip area. The scars are well hidden in a bathing suit. *A,* Preoperative appearance showing a form of Type IV deformity. *B,* Postoperative appearance at seven years. *C,* Postoperative appearance showing the result in a bathing suit.

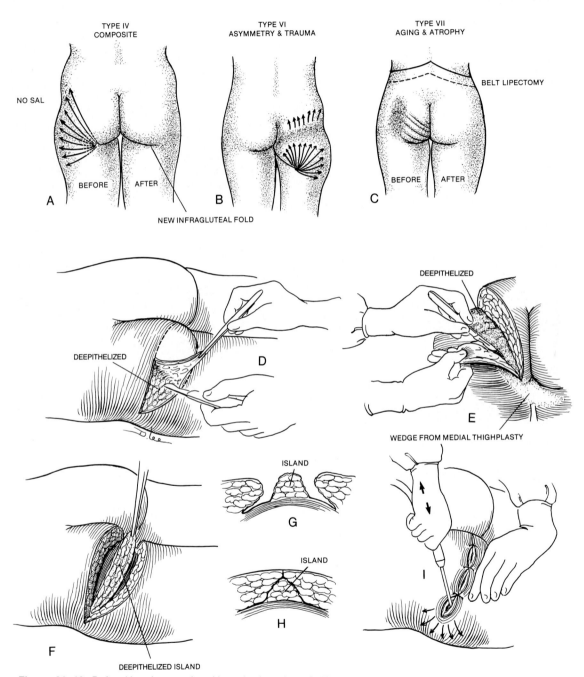

Figure 81–46. Deformities that require skin reduction. *A* to *C,* Three such deformities. *A* and *B* will require skin reduction as well as suctioning. *C,* Skin reduction alone may be all that is necessary. *D* to *H,* The technique for reducing the skin envelope and leaving the island to diminish the gluteal recess. *I,* Additional suctioning for final contour improvement.

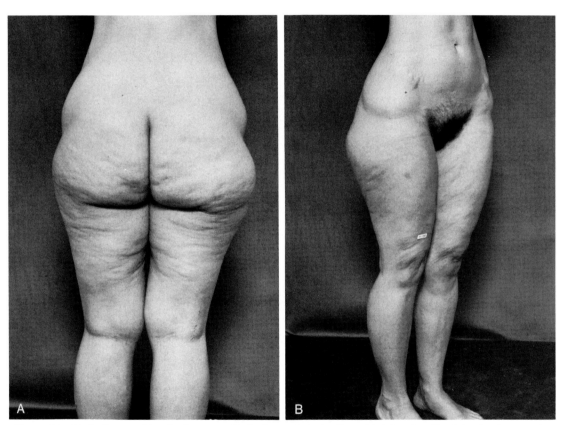

Figure 81–47. A 43 year old patient preoperatively demonstrated a Type IV deformity with slight obesity as well as severe relaxation of the skin envelope. Bilateral thighplasty using the "island technique" with suction assisted lipectomy brought her conformation to more acceptable standards. The Type IV and V deformity caused a severe disproportion of the lower trunk. Five inches of skin were removed from the medial thighs followed by a skin reduction of 6 inches through the trochanteric and upper gluteal areas. Approximately 1400 ml of fatty aspirate was removed. A, B, Preoperative appearance showing Type IV "viola/violin" truncal deformity in association with Type V obesity.

Illustration continued on following page

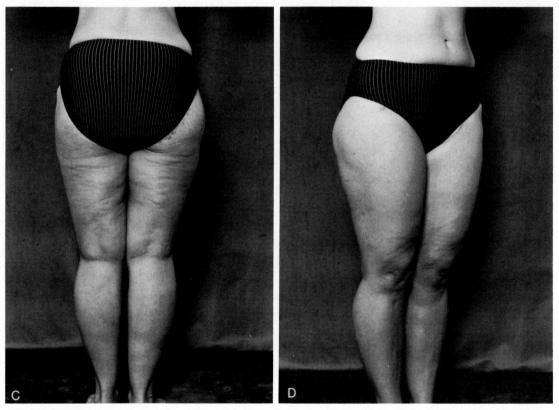

Figure 81–47 *Continued C, D* Postoperative appearance showing result after bilateral thighplasty. *D,* Note the adequate coverage of the scars by the bathing suit.

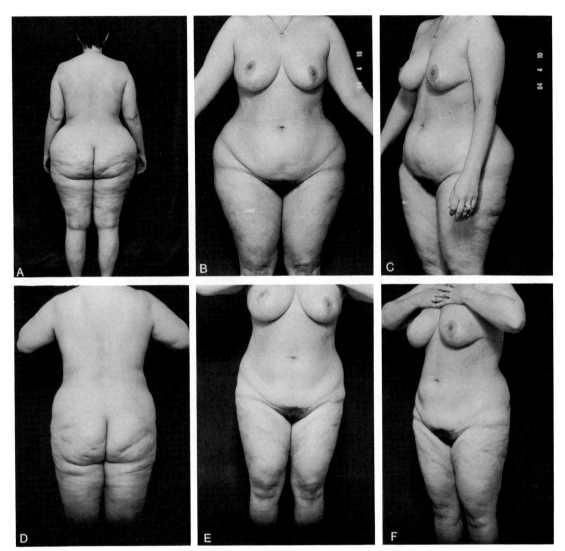

Figure 81–48. A 32 year old patient who typifies the Type V (obesity) configuration and truncal deformity. She underwent three procedures in which a total of 12,000 ml of fatty tissue was removed. Ten years previously, the patient had had a breast reduction. Measurements were as follows:

		Preoperative		Postoperative (two years later)
Weight		186 lb	Height 5'2''	181 lb
Hips		52½"		45"
Waist		34½"		31¾"
Thighs	(r)	30¼"		25½"
	(l)	30"		25½"
Knees	(r)	17¼"		15½"
	(l)	16½"		16"

A to *C,* Preoperative views. *D* to *F,* Postoperative views.

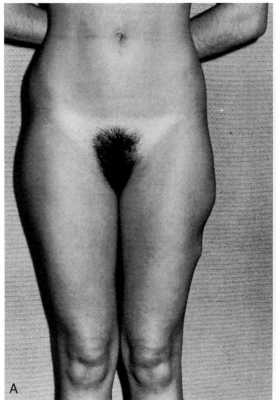

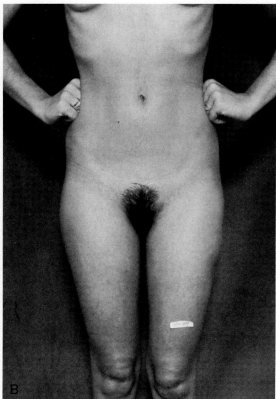

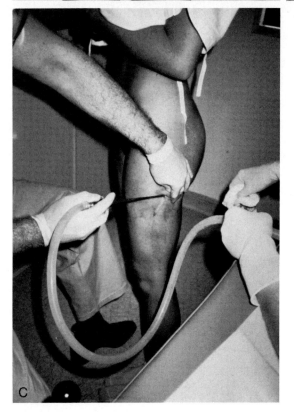

Figure 81–49. A 27 year old female who exhibits a post-traumatic deformity aggravated by excision. *A,* Preoperative appearance. *B,* Postoperative appearance. Acceptable correction was achieved by suctioning above and below the deformity. *C,* Technique: suctioning performed under local anesthesia with the patient in the standing position.

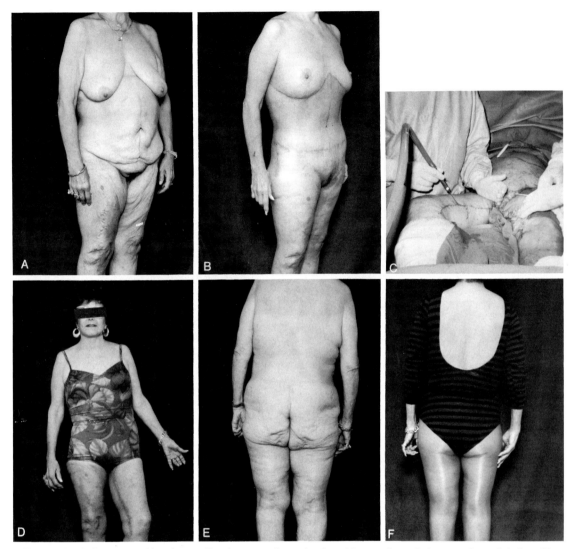

Figure 81–50. A 58 year old patient typifies the excessive redundant skin experienced after massive weight loss (Type VII deformity). The morbid obesity was treated by employing an ileojejunal bypass, which resulted in a weight loss of 150 lb. The patient underwent multiple body contour procedures: breast reduction/mastopexy, brachioplasty, abdominoplasty, thighplasty, buttocks lift, and belt skin reduction. *A,* Preoperative appearance. *B,* Appearance three years after the first procedures began. *C,* Suction after wound closure to reduce tension on the suture line and to obtain final contour refinement. *D,* Medial thigh scars. *E,* Preoperative appearance. *F,* Postoperative appearance in tights.

tion did not reach its maximal limit in the bloodstream for at least 30 to 40 minutes. However, with suctioning beginning 30 minutes before maximal absorption is attained, much of the lidocaine is aspirated. In order to increase the safety margin, one-half of the volume is injected at a time and the aspiration is performed on first one side of the body and then the other. No adverse reactions were noted in a personal series exceeding 1500 cases in which this formula and protocol were used.

After the local solution is injected, the deformity is approached through four sites—two stab incision sites in the infragluteal fold and two high in the buttocks near the perianal area (see Fig. 81–42). For large patients and for individuals with large deformities, a 6, 8, or 10 mm cannula is used; for average-sized patients a 3.7 mm cannula is preferred.

The use of small caliber cannulas obviates the necessity for *pretunneling.* After closure of the stab incision sites, the patient is frequently reprepped and redraped in the supine position for SAL of the medial thighs or the

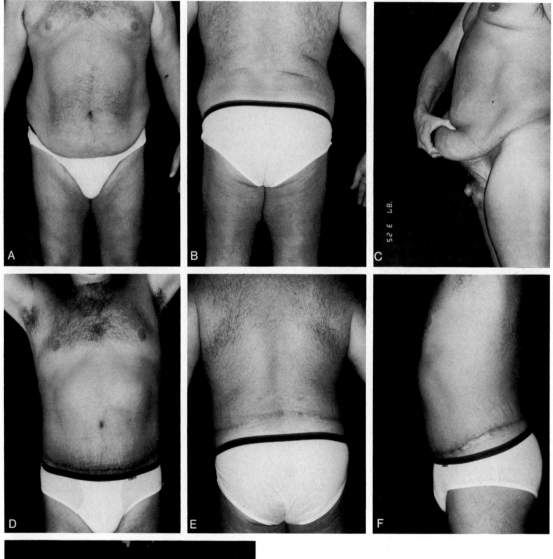

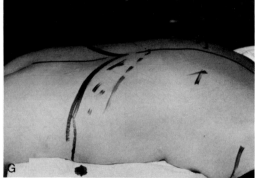

Figure 81–51. A 41 year old male who weighed 290 lb preoperatively but was unable to lose more than 50 lb before surgery. He underwent an abdominoplasty and belt lipectomy with suctioning. *A* to *C,* Preoperative appearance. *D* to *F,* Postoperative appearance. Note the continuation of the belt lipectomy. *G,* Posterior marking. The "X" designates the areas to be suctioned.

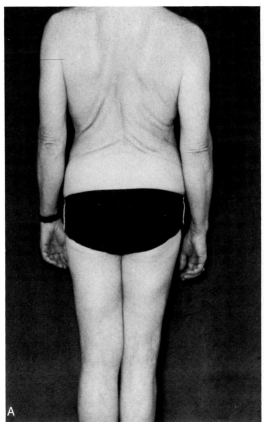 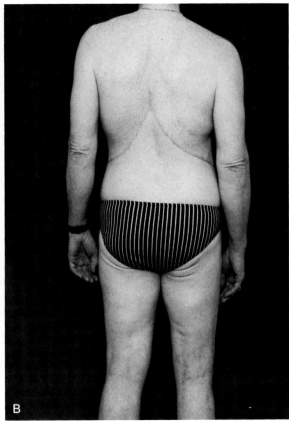

Figure 81–52. A 55 year old male had complained of redundant skin of the middle and lower back. Belt lipectomy was modified to conform to the defect area. *A*, Preoperative view. Note the pyramid of redundant skin. *B*, Postoperative view.

anterior trochanteric deformity (see Fig. 81–40).

After the wounds are closed but before the patient is placed in the postoperative garment, the surgeon must ascertain whether the bladder is distended. Volume loading frequently makes voiding difficult in the immediate postoperative period. If indicated, the patient is catheterized on the operating table. This maneuver accomplishes two objectives: (1) it makes the patient more comfortable and (2) the volume obtained is an indication of the patient's hydration. For example, in a one-hour operation, if the volume obtained is less than 300 ml, the patient may require additional fluid replacement in the immediate postoperative period.

After catheterization, the patient is placed in a girdle (see Fig. 81–62).

BELT LIPECTOMY

The belt lipectomy is useful in reducing some of the sag of the upper buttocks area and/or reducing the flank and back folds, each of which may be noted with weight reduction or the aging process (see Fig. 81–36).

At the time of surgery, the patient in Figure 81–51 weighed 290 lb after an approximate 50 lb weight loss. A belt lipectomy was performed in conjunction with an abdominoplasty and SAL. After reduction of the skin envelope, SAL was employed to give the torso a uniform appearance. The procedures involved the resection of 1200 gm of tissue from the flanks, 3700 gm removed from the abdominal panniculus, 2000 ml of aspirate suctioned from the flanks and abdomen, and approximately 300 ml suctioned from the breasts to reduce the pseudogynecomastia. These procedures required three units of autologous blood.

The patient in Figure 81–52 was concerned by the folds along the flanks and lower back. These were improved by a modification of the belt lipectomy, placing the incision close to the primary defect.

The belt lipectomy is a helpful adjunct in

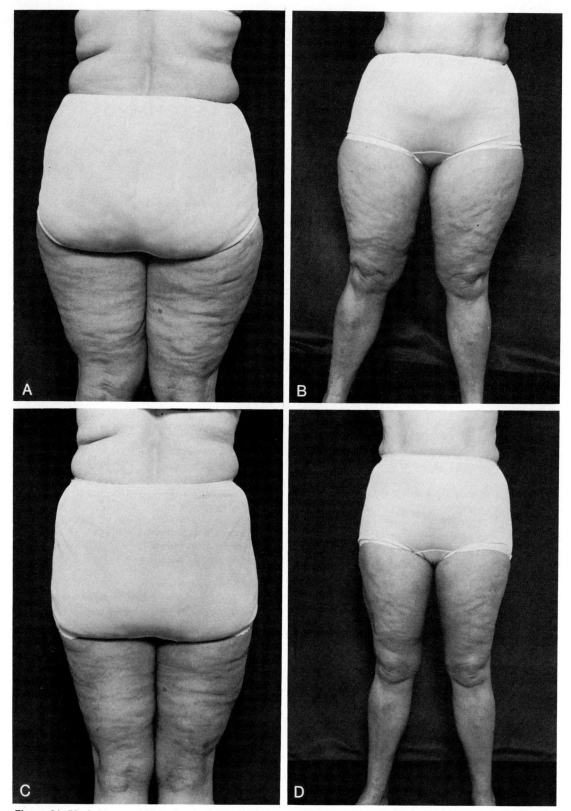

Figure 81–53. A 60 year old female who had a medial thigh reduction and 4200 ml of fatty tissue aspirated from the flanks, buttocks, and medial, lateral, and anterior thighs. *A, B,* Preoperative appearance. *C, D,* Postoperative appearance. Note that the scars are not evident in these positions.

skin envelope reduction for the morbidly obese patient after massive weight loss (see Fig. 81–50).

MEDIAL THIGHPLASTY

Patients who are candidates for medial thighplasty usually demonstrate a combination of the Type V and Type VII deformities (see Fig. 81–50). In patients requiring extensive suctioning of heavy thighs or sagging of the skin envelope, skin reduction is also essential. The technique employs suctioning and skin reduction in the vertical axis with only a *minimal amount* of skin reduction in the inguinal and infragluteal areas. General anesthesia is required.

For example, the 60 year old patient in Figure 81–53 required skin reduction as well as suctioning, since the skin turgor and elasticity were lax. A total of 4200 ml of fatty tissue was aspirated from the flanks, buttocks, and thighs (medial, lateral, and anterior) in addition to a medial thigh reduction. Estimated blood loss was approximately 1100 ml; 1½ units of autologous blood, one unit of packed cells, and two units of Hespan were administered as volume replacement. Immediate postoperative measurements indicated a reduction of 2 inches at the thigh and 1¾ inches at the knee levels (see Fig. 81–40).

REDUCTION OF ANTERIOR THIGHS

Ten years after a lateral and anterior thighplasty, the patient in Figure 81–54 had concerns of persistent thickness of the thighs and the obviously low placement of the groin incisions. Suctioning of 1200 ml of fatty tissue allowed the skin to be advanced so that the scars could be placed more superiorly in the groin area.

Knees, Calves, and Ankles

Recontouring of the knees is usually done in combination with other related deformities. In medial thigh reductions it is common to extend the scar to the knees to reduce the bulk of the knee fat pads. Lipomatous deform-

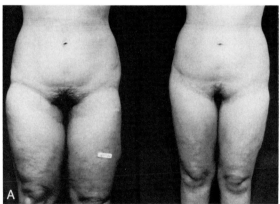
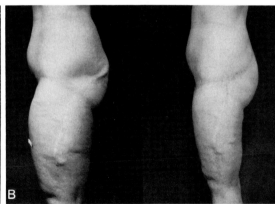
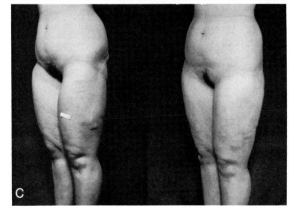

Figure 81–54. A patient who at the age of 25 years had undergone anterior and lateral thighplasties, the inguinal incisions being placed 3 inches below the inguinal crease. Suctioning the thighs circumferentially made possible advancement of the scars to a less conspicuous inguinal site. The patient also underwent buttocks-thighplasty. Pre- and postoperative views: *A,* frontal; *B,* lateral; *C,* oblique.

KNEE CALF & ANKLE

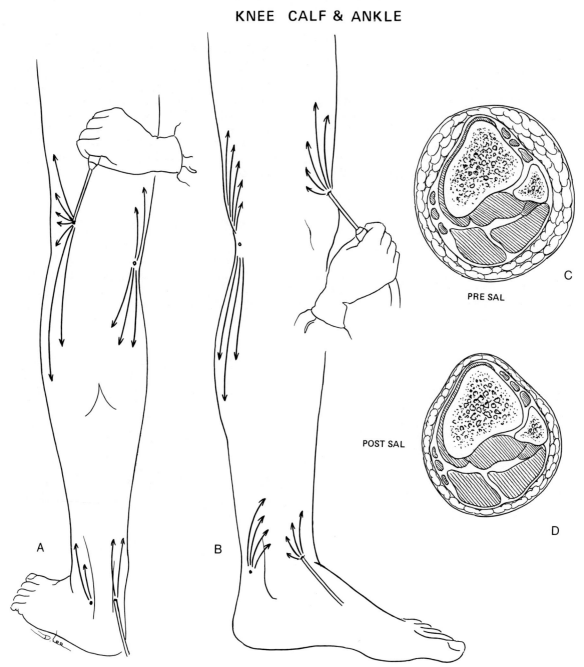

PRE SAL

POST SAL

Figure 81–55. Stab incision sites for suctioning of the knee, calf, and ankle regions.

ities in the knee area can easily be addressed (Figs. 81–55, 81–56).

Only in rare cases is skin reduction of the calves indicated. Therefore, only suctioning of the calves and ankles is recommended (Figs. 81–57, 81–58). Suctioning is accomplished with the patient in the supine and/or prone position, and can be performed under local anesthesia using a long 2.4 or 3.7 mm cannula.

COMBINED PROCEDURES

Many of the patients illustrated in this chapter had combined procedures. The most important consideration in electing combined procedures is the safety of the patient, which involves the following considerations:

1. Patient selection.
2. Preoperative patient assessment.
3. Informed consent.
4. Length of surgery.
5. Autologous blood.
6. Estimated blood loss.
7. Prevention of complications.
8. Volume loading.
9. Antibiotics.
10. Postoperative management.

SEQUENCE OF PERFORMING COMBINED PROCEDURES

Suctioning Alone. The procedures may include the face, neck, chin, arms, abdomen, hips, thighs, flanks, and extremities. With suction alone to multiple areas, the author prefers to begin with the patient in the prone position, and complete the procedure with the patient in the supine position.

Suction Plus Skin Reduction. These procedures include face lift, brachioplasty, breast reduction, abdominoplasty, and thighplasty. A major thigh reduction with abdominoplasty is not recommended because of the risk of possible lymphatic obstruction.

The sequence of combined procedures is dependent on the safety of the patient along with the logistics to determine which order is most efficient. Many combinations are possible, such as the following:

1. Abdominoplasty	1. Brachioplasty
2. Face lift	2. Face lift
or	*or*
1. Abdominoplasty	1. Brachioplasty
2. Brachioplasty	2. Thighplasty

The preferred sequence, when applicable, is a breast reduction or mastopexy followed by abdominoplasty and/or face lift. Face lifting is reserved as the last procedure when done in combination, since the movement of the anesthesiologist is required only once.

Any combined procedure that would exceed five to six hours of actual operating time should not be undertaken, otherwise the safety of the patient might be compromised.

AUTOLOGOUS FAT INJECTION

Recent advances include the injection of autologous fat to fill in facial lines and small body defects. In the past, dermis-fat grafts (see Chap. 14) have had limited success (Peer, 1950, 1956, 1977). The use of autologous fat is beginning to supplant that of collagen without any of the apparent drawbacks and complications sometimes encountered with collagen (see Chap. 22). At the present time, autologous fat grafting is so popular that its extensive use has outstripped basic research.

Many laboratories are intensely searching for evidence that autologous fat cells survive and persist. Although this evidence is still lacking, the value of the procedure lies in its safety. Autologous fat grafting is a simple procedure because of the ease of harvesting and subsequent injection into selected sites. As a technique, it *awaits the test of time*.

Some authors have theorized that there may be privileged donor sites (Davis, 1984). At this time, however, the preferred donor site is the abdomen since the fat cells in that area are easiest to retrieve and there is less likelihood of creating a donor site defect.

Autologous fat grafting has proved useful as an adjunct in the face lift procedure to plump out glabellar frown lines (Fig. 81–59), crow's feet in the eye area, the nasolabial folds, and the creases of the aging upper lip. It has also been used successfully to correct contour deformities associated with depressions resulting from oversuctioning. The use of the autologous fat injection for breast augmentation, as advocated by Bircoll (1987), is deplored. The monthly hormonal changes that take place in the breast can cause the formation of cystlike lesions; some patients can also develop calcifications. The esthetic results are marginal, especially if large volumes are required.

Text continued on page 4026

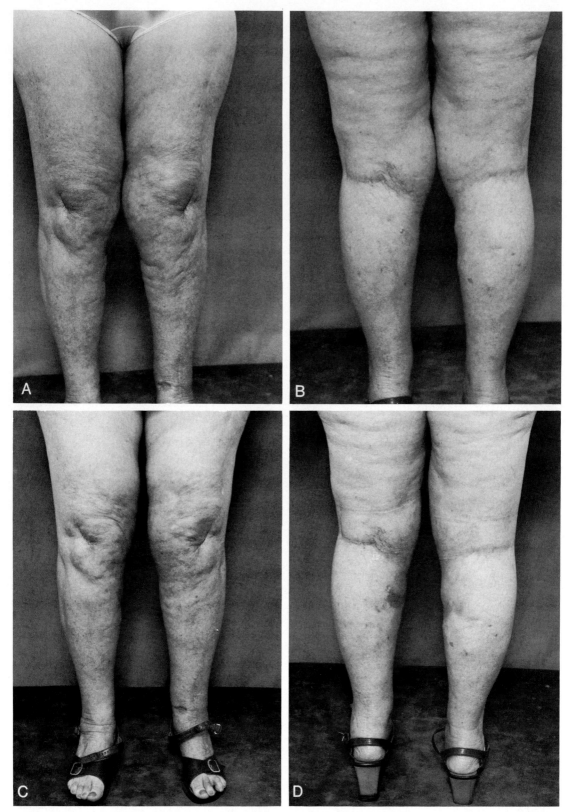

Figure 81–56. A 65 year old patient had an unstable gait due to arthritis, which was exacerbated by the increasing size of the giant lipomas situated bilaterally at the medial knee. 500 ml of fatty tissue was aspirated from the left knee, 500 ml from the right knee, and an additional 250 ml from the immediate adjacent areas of both knees. *A, B,* Preoperative appearance. *C, D,* Postoperative appearance.

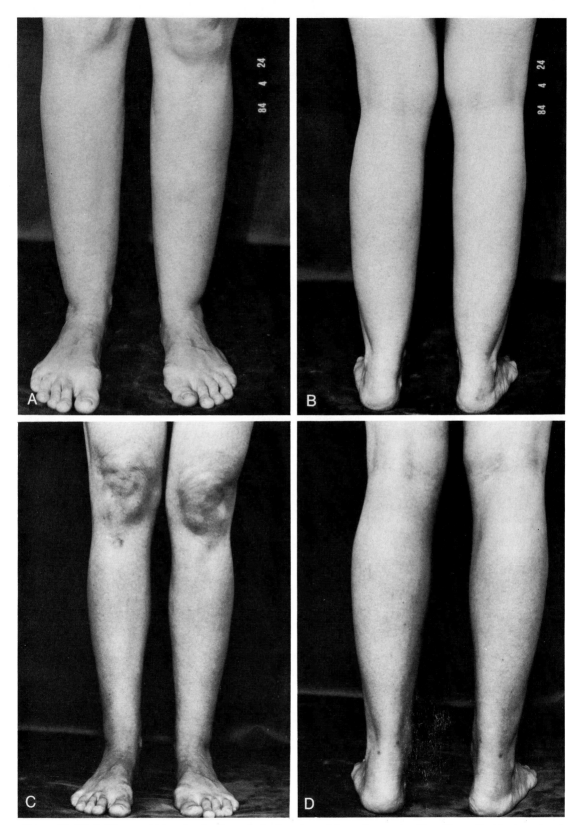

Figure 81–57. A 33 year old female showing a lack of contour of the calves and ankles. The patient had previously undergone SAL for a contour deformity in the trochanteric areas of the thighs and knees. *A, B,* Preoperative appearance. Note the contour deformity caused by the pseudolipodystrophy in the ankle area. *C, D,* Postoperative appearance at one year.

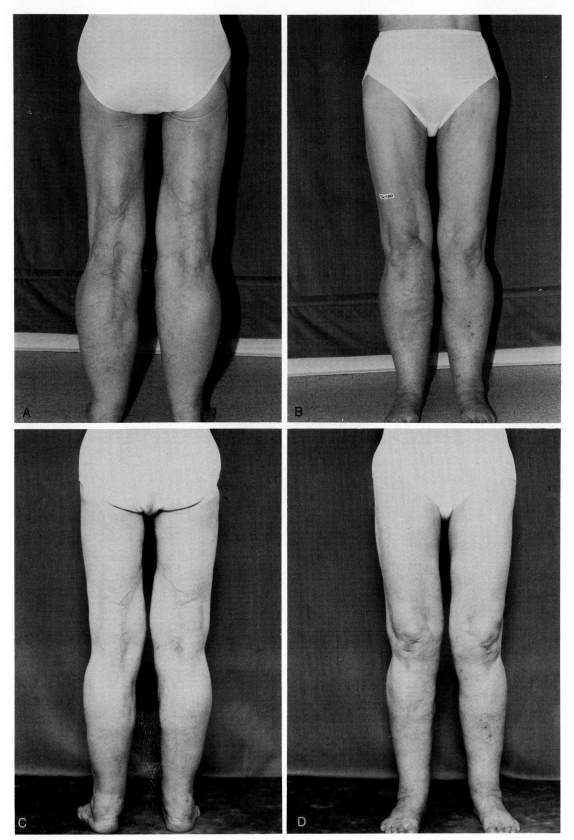

Figure 81–58. A 60 year old female showing lipodystrophy of the extremities below the knees. There is no subcutaneous fat above the knees. In three SAL procedures, a total of 1800 ml of fatty tissue was aspirated. *A, B,* Preoperative views. *C, D,* Postoperative views.

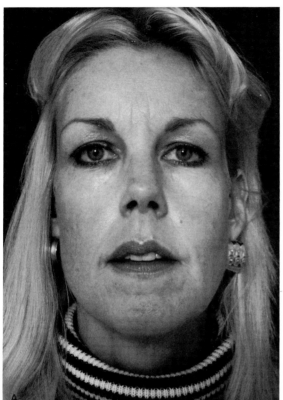

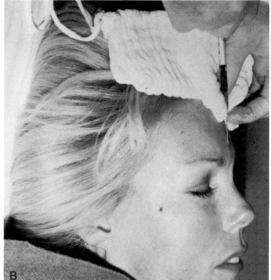

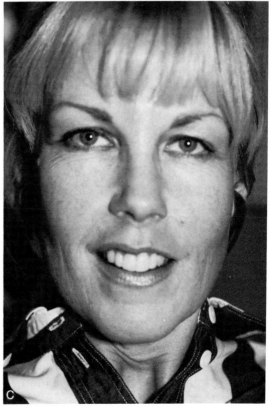

Figure 81–59. A 39 year old patient with deep glabellar frown lines aggravating her otherwise youthful appearance. *A,* Preoperative appearance. *B,* Injection of the harvested fat cells in the glabellar frown lines with a 21 gauge needle. *C,* Postoperative appearance six months after the injections.

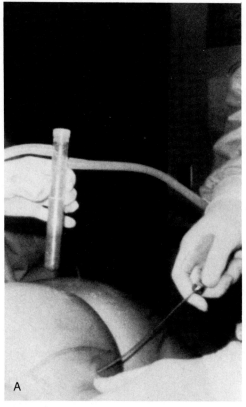
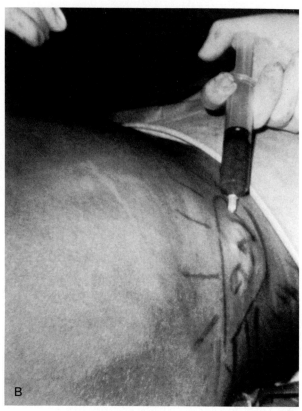

Figure 81–60. Harvesting fat cells from the buttocks with a Luki branchoscopy tube. *A,* The Luki tube interposed between two segments of silicone tubing. *B,* Injection of fat cells into a flank defect.

INSTRUMENTATION AND TECHNIQUE

Clinically, there are elaborate techniques for harvesting fat cells, including methods of sedimentation plus the addition of such agents as insulin to "preserve" the cells (Ellenbogen, 1986; Ersek and associates, 1987).

The 1.5 mm cannula may be used to collect fatty tissue. For large volumes (20 to 200 ml), the sterile Luki bronchoscopy collection tube, which is interposed in the system between the vacuum and the cannula, is preferred (Fig. 81–60). This tube is available in every operating room.

An alternative technique for harvesting smaller volumes, usually employed in the face, is to aspirate fatty tissue with a syringe and an 18 gauge needle (Fig. 81–61). Harvesting the fatty tissue by this method is accelerated, after a vacuum is created in the syringe by drawing back the plunger, moving the syringe back and forth rapidly.

It is common to overfill a defect by 50 per cent primarily to account for the resorption rate as well as to compensate for the imme-

diate swelling of the injection sites. Although data on long-term results are lacking, soft tissue augmentation with autologous fat cells shows considerable promise.

ADJUNCTS FOR FAT SUCTIONING

Garments. These include a Poli foundation or the Caromed type girdle, Velcro binders, TED stockings, a chin strap, and a Reston sponge (Fig. 81–62).

Antibiotics. Antibiotics are used in all major cases, given by the intravenous route at the time of surgery (1 gm of cephalosporin) and by oral intake for the next three to five days (250 mg four times a day). With this regimen, postoperative infection has been rare.

Ultrasound. The use of ultrasound has had mixed reactions from plastic surgeons. Beginning as early as the patient can tolerate the pressure of the ultrasound head, the usual treatment is 1.5 to 2 watts per second squared

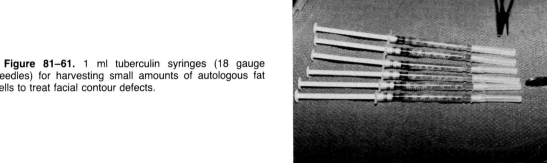

Figure 81–61. 1 ml tuberculin syringes (18 gauge needles) for harvesting small amounts of autologous fat cells to treat facial contour defects.

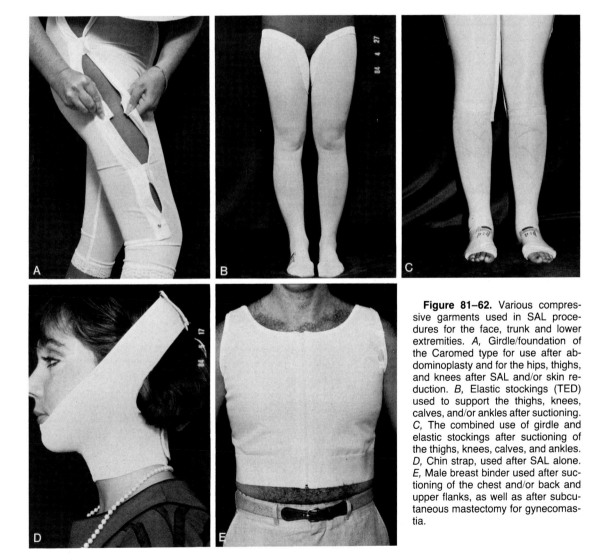

Figure 81–62. Various compressive garments used in SAL procedures for the face, trunk and lower extremities. *A,* Girdle/foundation of the Caromed type for use after abdominoplasty and for the hips, thighs, and knees after SAL and/or skin reduction. *B,* Elastic stockings (TED) used to support the thighs, knees, calves, and/or ankles after suctioning. *C,* The combined use of girdle and elastic stockings after suctioning of the thighs, knees, calves, and ankles. *D,* Chin strap, used after SAL alone. *E,* Male breast binder used after suctioning of the chest and/or back and upper flanks, as well as after subcutaneous mastectomy for gynecomastia.

for a ten minute period over each ecchymotic area, two to three times a week until the ecchymosis has disappeared. It helps to smooth out small irregularities as well as accelerate the dissolution of the ecchymotic areas. It is recommended that ultrasound treatment be administered by a physical therapist or knowledgeable health professional.

Normal Activity. Normal activity can usually be resumed two to three weeks after SAL. In skin reduction, full activity is usually permitted after six weeks.

Secondary/Revision Procedures. Approximately 20 to 30 per cent of all SAL patients require secondary procedures. Revisions are usually done under local anesthesia, when less than 200 ml of fat is aspirated. A revision is not recommended earlier than four months after surgery. For revisions requiring skin reduction, a minimum of six months is suggested.

REFERENCES

Bircoll, M.: Cosmetic breast augmentation utilizing autologous fat and liposuction techniques. Plast. Reconstr. Surg., *79*:267, 1987.

Bostwick, J., Hester, T. R., and Nahai, F.: Microvascular and musculocutaneous flaps: aesthetic contour enhancement with suction assisted lipectomy. 18th Annual Meeting, American Society of Aesthetic Plastic Surgeons, Boston, MA, 1985.

Bray, G. A.: The Obese Patient. Philadelphia, W. B. Saunders Company, 1976.

Courtiss, E. H.: Suction lipectomy of the neck. Plast. Reconstr. Surg., *76*:882, 1985.

Davis, T. S.: Morbid obesity. Clin. Plast. Surg., *11*:517, 1984.

Ellenbogen, R.: Free autogenous pearl fat grafts in the face—a preliminary report of a rediscovered technique. Ann. Plast. Surg., *16*:179, 1986.

Ersek, R. A., Bircoll, M., Aiache, A., Chagchir, A., and Weber, J.: Panel: Autologous fat injection. 20th Annual Meeting, American Society of Aesthetic Plastic Surgeons, Los Angeles, 1987.

Ersek, R. A., Zambrano, J., Surak, G. S., and Denton, D. R.: Suction-assisted lipectomy for correction of 202 figure faults in 101 patients: indications, limitations, and applications. Plast. Reconstr. Surg., *78*:615, 1986.

Fournier, P. F., and Otteni, F. M.: Lipodissection in body sculpturing: the dry procedure. Plast. Reconstr. Surg., *72*:598, 1983.

Grazer, F. M.: Suction-assisted lipectomy, suction lipectomy, lipolysis, and lipexeresis. Plast. Reconstr. Surg., *72*:620, 1983.

Grazer, F. M.: Unfavorable results in body contouring operations including psychological aspects. *In* Goldwyn, R. M. (Ed.): The Unfavorable Result in Plastic Surgery, Avoidance and Treatment. 2nd Ed. Boston, Little, Brown & Company, 1984a.

Grazer, F. M.: Suction assisted lipectomy—its indications, contraindications, and complications. *In* Habal, M. B. (Ed.): Advances in Plastic and Reconstructive Surgery. Vol. 1. Chicago, Year Book Medical Publishers, 1984b.

Grazer, F. M. (Ed.): Body contouring surgery. Clin. Plast. Surg., *11*:3, 1984c.

Grazer, F. M.: Reflections on Body Imagery. Commercial video, 1984d.

Grazer, F. M.: Quantitative analysis of blood and fat in suction lipectomy aspirates (discussion). Plast. Reconstr. Surg., *78*:770, 1986.

Grazer, F. M., and Davis, T. S.: Body contouring and abdominal lipectomy. *In* Sohn, S. A. (Ed.): Fundamentals of Aesthetic Plastic Surgery. Baltimore, Williams & Wilkins Company, 1987.

Grazer, F. M., and Klingbeil, J. R.: Body Image: A Surgical Perspective. St. Louis, C. V. Mosby Company, 1980.

Hetter, G. P.: The effect of low-dose epinephrine on the hematocrit drop following lipolysis. Aesth. Plast. Surg., *8*:19, 1984a.

Hetter, G. P.: Optimum vacuum pressures for lipolysis. Aesthetic Plast. Surg., *8*:23, 1984b.

Illouz, Y. G.: Body contouring by lipolysis: a 5-year experience with over 3000 cases. Plast. Reconstr. Surg., *72*:591, 1983.

Illouz, Y. G.: Surgical remodeling of the silhouette by aspiration lipolysis or selective lipectomy. Aesthetic Plast. Surg., *9*:7, 1985.

Kesselring, U. K.: Regional fat aspiration for body contouring. Plast. Reconstr. Surg., *72*:610, 1983.

Kesselring, U. K.: Facial liposuction. *In* Kesselring, U. K. (Ed.): Facial Plastic Surgery. International Quarterly Monographs, *4*:1, Fall, 1986.

Kesselring, U. K., and Meyer, R.: A suction curette for removal of excessive local deposits of subcutaneous fat. Plast. Reconstr. Surg., *62*:305, 1978.

McKissock, P. K.: Reduction mammaplasty with a vertical dermal flap. Plast. Reconstr. Surg., *49*:245, 1972.

Peer, L. A.: Loss of weight and volume in human fat grafts. Plast. Reconstr. Surg., *5*:217, 1950.

Peer, L. A.: The neglected free fat graft. Plast. Reconstr. Surg., *18*:233, 1956.

Peer, L. A.: Transplantation of fat. *In* Converse, J. M. (Ed.): Reconstructive Plastic Surgery. 2nd Ed. Philadelphia, W. B. Saunders Company, 1977, pp. 251–261.

Pfulg, M. E.: Complications of suction for lipectomy (correspondence). Plast. Reconstr. Surg., *69*:562, 1982.

Shaer, W. D.: Gluteal and thigh reduction: reclassification, critical review, and improved technique for primary correction. Aesthetic Plast. Surg., *8*:165, 1984.

Shirakabe, T.: A new device for suction-assisted lipectomy: a flexible cannula. Ann. Plast. Surg., *18*:257, 1987.

Sjöström, L.: Fat cells and body weight. *In* Stunkard, A. J. (Ed.): Obesity. Philadelphia, W. B. Saunders Company, 1980, pp. 72–100.

Stunkard, A. J. (Ed.): Obesity. Philadelphia, W. B. Saunders Company, 1980.

Teimourian, B.: Face and neck suction-assisted lipectomy associated with rhytidectomy. Plast. Reconstr. Surg., *72*:627, 1983.

Teimourian, B.: Suction Lipectomy and Body Sculpturing. St. Louis, C. V. Mosby Company, 1987.

Teimourian, B., and Fisher, J. B.: Suction curettage to remove excess fat for body contouring. Plast. Reconstr. Surg., *68*:50, 1981.

82

Charles H. M. Thorne
John W. Siebert
James C. Grotting
Luis O. Vasconez
William W. Shaw
Paul F. Sauer

Reconstructive Surgery of the Lower Extremity

HISTORY

Centuries ahead of his time Celsus (25 B.C.–50 A.D.) introduced the axioms of wound closure: removal of all foreign bodies, absolute hemostasis, and careful placing and spacing of sutures (Kirk, 1944; Mettler, 1947; Vitali, 1971; Aldea and Shaw, 1986). Unfortunately, after the fall of the Roman Empire the precocious tenets of Greek medicine were largely forgotten, and Galen's theory that suppuration was essential to healing characterized the treatment of lower extremity wounds. One thousand years later, Ambroise Paré (1509–1590) almost singlehandedly led medicine out of the Middle Ages (Fig. 82–1).

Paré recommended amputation through viable tissue, described phantom pain, became the first surgeon to perform a surgical revision of an amputation for a better prosthetic fitting, and introduced the modern concept of choosing an amputation site according to the plans for a prosthesis (Paré, 1575; Garrison, 1929; Aldea and Shaw, 1986).

The concepts of debridement and immobilization were introduced in the eighteenth and nineteenth centuries, respectively. Pierre-Joseph Desault (1744–1795), the chief surgeon at the Hotel Dieu in Paris, coined the term "debridement." The concept of immobilization was introduced by Ollier (1825–1900), who developed the plaster cast (Brown, 1965).

Toward the end of World War I, Orr from Nebraska treated open fractures of the lower extremity by incising the wound to ensure drainage, and then placing the leg in a plaster cast. This "closed plaster treatment" influenced Trueta, who treated open fractures during the Spanish Civil War (1935–1938). He took the idea one step farther, performing a true surgical debridement before placement of the cast. Trueta observed that infection could be avoided if all devitalized tissue was excised (Trueta, 1940, 1944; Byrd, 1988).

In World War II, no revolutionary concepts were developed but refinements were made in the treatment of lower extremity injuries, employing the principles of debridement and immobilization that had been set forth earlier. Improved transportation, the introduction of antibiotics, resuscitative measures including blood banking, and aseptic techniques resulted in a decrease in wound mortality from 8 per cent in World War I to 4.5 per cent in World War II (Lange and associates, 1985; Aldea and Shaw, 1986). In addi-

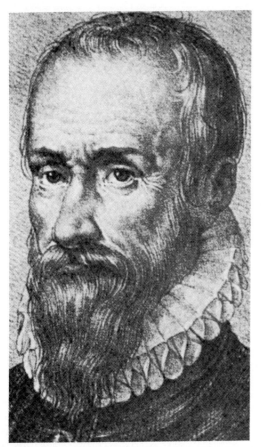

Figure 82–1. Ambroise Paré, 1509–1590. (From Spector, B.: One Hour of Medical History. Boston, Beacon Press, 1931.)

tion, the incidence of postfracture osteomyelitis decreased from approximately 80 per cent in World War I to about 25 per cent at the end of World War II.

Because of limitations in the ability to reconstruct large soft tissue and bone defects, entrance into the modern era of fracture treatment awaited the development of microsurgery. It was only after microsurgical techniques provided unlimited amounts of tissue for reconstruction of even massive defects that truly adequate debridement of lower extremity injuries could be performed with confidence.

The techniques of lower extremity reconstruction are sufficiently well developed that care must be taken to avoid the "salvage" of nonfunctional, insensate, or chronically painful extremities. Complex reconstructive efforts must be restricted to those patients in whom the reconstruction is likely to yield a result superior to that which can be provided by amputation.

The history of lower extremity surgery is predominantly that of lower extremity trauma, particularly trauma inflicted during wartime. However, modern concepts of immediate coverage and the emphasis on ultimate function have recently been applied to other aspects of lower extremity surgery, including surgery for congenital problems, tumors, chronic osteomyelitis, and diabetic peripheral vascular disease.

Modern understanding of muscular anatomy, cutaneous blood supply, and microsurgery has made such a contribution to lower extremity reconstruction that plastic surgeons now interact with general surgeons, vascular surgeons, oncologic surgeons, pediatric surgeons, and trauma surgeons in the care of virtually all types of lower extremity problems.

PRINCIPLES

Evaluation of any lower extremity wound begins with an analysis of what is missing and what vital structures are exposed. Any local or systemic factors that may alter the approach to a particular patient are assessed. For example, the presence of infection, a history of radiation therapy, or the presence of widely metastatic cancer obviously affect decision making. Having assessed the defect in the context of the individual patient, the surgeon must project what the ultimate function of that extremity will be and plan the sequence of therapeutic steps to yield that result. If such planning does not begin at the initial evaluation, multiple, poorly organized procedures may result in an amputation that could have been performed swiftly after the patient was first seen, sparing the patient (and the physician) considerable frustration.

The classic reconstructive ladder (primary closure, skin graft, local flap) is helpful but is not the sole criterion used for planning a reconstructive procedure. One is no longer forced to close the wound with the simplest available technique. In other words, one need not start at the bottom of the reconstructive ladder and work through failures, and then plan a microvascular transfer that was indicated at the outset.

Reconstruction of the lower extremity has traditionally been planned by dividing the lower leg into thirds. The flaps available in

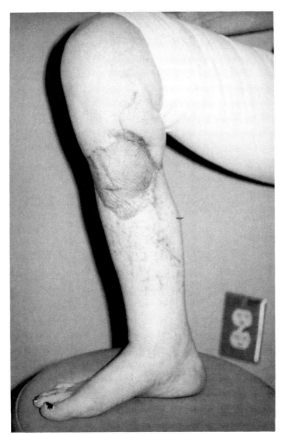

Figure 82–2. After transfer of a medial gastrocnemius musculocutaneous flap. Note the donor site scarring. A meshed skin graft was also employed for coverage purposes. The normal contour of the calf has been sacrificed.

each third are then enumerated (gastrocnemius flap for proximal third, soleus flap for middle third), free tissue transfer being reserved for the lower third of the leg. Although this traditional method (like the reconstructive ladder) can be helpful, the surgeon must decide what is the optimal technique for the particular defect, not necessarily the most expeditious. Frequently, free tissue transfer yields a more esthetic result without expenditure of local muscle, and provides primary wound healing more quickly than any alternative technique (Fig. 82–2).

ANATOMY

Unique Features

Lower extremity surgery requires an understanding of the ways in which such reconstruction differs from that for the upper extremity.

First, the weight-bearing requirements of the lower extremity provide the most obvious difference. Paradoxically, the weight-bearing function makes reconstruction of the lower extremity simpler than that of the upper extremity; to restore the more complex capabilities of the upper extremity is often beyond the scope of current surgical techniques. Adequate function can frequently be restored to the lower extremity, however, if only a stable post with adequate soft tissue coverage and protective sensation is provided. For the same reasons, lower extremity prostheses are more successful than their upper extremity counterparts.

Second, the lower extremity is almost always in a dependent position, and therefore deep vein thrombosis, venous stasis problems, and chronic edema are more common than in the upper extremity. As a result, free tissue transfer to the lower extremity is more likely to be compromised by venous drainage problems than are similar operations in the upper extremity.

The third unique feature of the lower extremity is the increased incidence of atherosclerosis in the arterial system. Any reconstructive procedure requires assessment of the arterial circulation, and in the lower extremity the operation occasionally demands augmentation of arterial inflow in addition to free tissue transfer.

Fourth, the greater length over which nerve regeneration must occur after injury or nerve grafting is relevant. It is this fact that makes replantation of an above knee amputation contraindicated in some circumstances.

Finally, the subcutaneous location of the tibia, the main weight-bearing bone of the leg, poses unique problems in fracture healing. Unlike the femur, which for the most part is buried in muscle, the tibia has a poorly vascularized environment. In open fractures of the tibia, therefore, sufficient muscle does not exist to restore the periosteal blood supply to the fractured bone, so that there is a predisposition to nonunion and infection.

Bones and Joints

LaMont (1986) reviewed the functional anatomy of the lower limb, and his insights have been used in compiling the following section.

The most mobile joint in the lower extremity is the hip. Unlike the shoulder, which is also a "ball and socket" joint, the hip joint is stable under large loads. Whereas the glenoid fossa in the shoulder is shallow and the surrounding ligaments are relatively weak, the acetabular socket in the hip joint is deep and the capsular ligaments are extremely strong, thus allowing the hip joint to withstand the application of large forces over a wide range of motion.

The blood supply to the femoral head is dual: the major component is the retinacular plexus entering the neck; the minor component is the vessel within the ligamentus teres. Avascular necrosis secondary to hip dislocation is primarily a result, therefore, of disruption of the retinacular vessels in the femoral neck.

The knee is the largest joint in the body. Injuries to the knee ligaments are frequently overlooked in major lower extremity injuries, especially when attention is focused on re-vascularizing the limb and providing soft tissue coverage. Unrepaired ligamentous injuries, however, lead inexorably to long-term disability. Two sets of ligaments stabilize the knee. The collateral ligaments prevent excessive valgus or varus deformities, while the cruciate ligaments prevent motion in the anterior and posterior directions.

The medial and lateral menisci, "C-shaped" fibrocartilagenous discs seated on the tibial plateau, help to distribute and cushion the loads imposed on the knee joint. If possible, these structures should also be preserved or repaired.

It is important to consider the minimal range of knee motion that is associated with everyday activities. Average activity requires from near-full extension to approximately 120 degrees of flexion. Walking on a flat surface requires 70 degrees of flexion, descending stairs 90 degrees of knee flexion, and normal sitting 100 degrees of flexion. Consequently, near-*normal* motion of the knee joint is essential for comfortable function. A complex surgical reconstruction that successfully revascularizes and provides soft tissue coverage to a mutilated lower extremity, but which fails to address an unstable knee joint, is therefore doomed to failure.

The ankle is a hinge joint allowing little side to side motion. The distal tibia and fibula form a mortise over the body of the talus. The tibia bears most of the weight, with the fibula bearing only one-sixth of the load placed on the leg. As long as the distal fibula is present so that the ankle joint is intact, the shaft of the fibula can be removed without causing disability.

Stability of the ankle joint is also dependent on the syndesmosis between the tibia and fibula, consisting of the anterior and posterior tibiofibular ligaments and the interosseus membrane. Disruption of the tibiofibular syndesmosis allows widening of the ankle mortise and subsequent degenerative changes. The subtalar joint also absorbs forces that would otherwise be transmitted directly to the ankle joint.

In order to appreciate the importance of stable joints, it is instructive to review the forces borne by the various lower extremity joints during normal function. Walking, for example, imposes forces on the hip joint as high as 1.5 times the body weight. During running the forces on each hip joint equal five times the body weight. The knee joint bears loads up to three times the body weight during normal ambulation, which is increased to five times the body weight during stair climbing. Forces are further amplified at the ankle joint, where loads up to five times the body weight are imposed during normal gait (LaMont, 1986).

Compartments

The fascial compartmentalization of the lower extremity provides a convenient framework for studying the anatomy and it is also of clinical relevance. The muscles of the thigh are enclosed by the deep fascia; fascial septa divide them into three compartments, each compartment hvaing its own motor nerve. The *anterior muscle group (compartment)* muscles flex the thigh and extend the leg and are innervated by the femoral nerve. The *medial muscle group (compartment)* provides thigh adduction and is innervated by the obturator nerve. The *posterior muscle group (compartment)* is responsible for thigh extension and leg flexion and receives motor innervation from the sciatic nerve.

Compartment syndromes, although rare in the thigh, are common in the lower leg where fascial septa divide the muscles into four compartments (Fig. 82–3). The muscles in the *anterior compartment* arise from the tibia, fibula, and interosseous membrane and are innervated by the deep peroneal nerve. The *lateral compartment* muscles that evert the

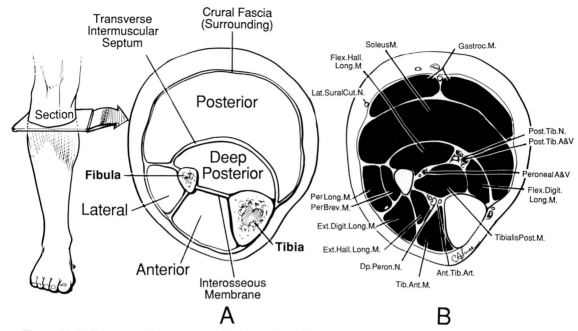

Figure 82–3. Compartmental anatomy of the leg. *A,* Fascial septa separate the calf into four compartments. *B,* The peroneal and posterior tibial arteries are located in the deep posterior compartment, which must be included in any fasciotomy.

foot are innervated by the superficial peroneal nerve. In the posterior leg there are two compartments: the *superficial posterior compartment* consisting of the gastrocnemius and soleus muscles, and the *deep posterior compartment* enclosing the plantar flexors of the foot innervated by the tibial nerve.

Arterial Anatomy

In the inguinal region, the external iliac and common femoral arteries are the source of numerous arterial branches that radiate in all directions like the spokes of a wheel (Fig. 82–4). The deep inferior epigastric artery (DIEA) and the deep circumflex iliac artery (DCIA) are branches of the external iliac artery located just proximal to the inguinal ligament. The DIEA provides blood supply to the rectus abdominis muscle, while the DCIA is the pedicle for the iliac bone microvascular free flap described by Taylor (1982). Distal to the inguinal ligament the superficial inferior epigastric artery (SIEA) and the superficial circumflex iliac artery (SCIA) arise from the common femoral artery. The SIEA is the pedicle that supplies the inferior epigastric skin flap described by Shaw and Payne (1946). The vessel runs

obliquely cephalad in the direction of the axilla, supplying a territory that extends to the costal margin, where it intersects the territory of the lateral thoracic artery. The SCIA courses laterally across the inguinal region to supply the territory of the groin flap, as originally described by McGregor and Jackson (1972).

Approximately 4 cm distal to the inguinal ligament, the common femoral artery bifurcates into the superficial femoral artery and the profunda femoris artery. The latter represents the predominant source of blood supply to the thigh. The lateral femoral circumflex artery, a branch of the profunda femoris, supplies the rectus femoris and vastus lateralis muscle through its transverse branch, the tensor fascia lata. The medial femoral circumflex artery arises at approximately the same level and provides blood supply to the gracilis muscle. In addition, there are four perforators of the profunda femoris artery that supply the thigh muscles and skin. The first profunda perforator forms an anastomosis with the superior and inferior gluteal arteries on the posterior thigh, forming the so-called cruciate anastomosis. The third profunda perforator is the largest and supplies the skin on the lateral aspect of the thigh.

The main trunk of the femoral artery con-

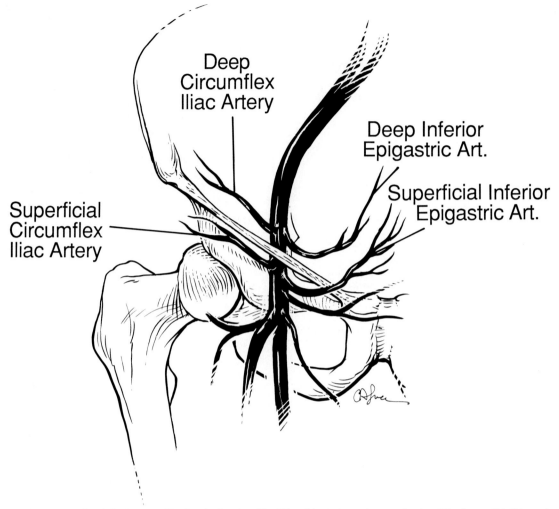

Figure 82–4. Arterial anatomy of the inguinal region. The "deep" branches arise proximal and the "superficial" branches arise distal to the inguinal ligament. Arterial branches are numerous in this region and are oriented in all directions like the spokes of a wheel. Fasciocutaneous flaps need not be designed according to classically described flaps (such as the groin flap), but rather can be based over the femoral vessels and oriented in any direction.

tinues distally as the superficial femoral artery (SFA). The SFA passes through the adductor hiatus to reach the posterior aspect of the thigh, where it becomes the popliteal artery. Proximal to the adductor hiatus the descending geniculate artery arises from the SFA. This vessel runs along the medial aspect of the knee and in turn gives off the saphenous artery, which accompanies the saphenous nerve and supplies the territory of the saphenous flap, as described by Acland and associates (1981). Superior and inferior geniculate branches above and below the knee provide an anastomotic network that serves as collateral circulation around the knee.

The popliteal artery provides paired sural branches to the medial and lateral gastrocne-

mius muscles and medial and lateral inferior geniculate arteries, as described above; it then bifurcates into the tibioperoneal trunk and the anterior tibial artery. The anterior tibial artery enters the anterior compartment of the leg, passing above the upper end of the interosseous membrane, descending on the anterior surface of the interosseous membrane, and providing branches to the muscles of the anterior compartment. The anterior tibial artery becomes the dorsalis pedis artery on the dorsum of the foot.

The tibioperoneal trunk in turn bifurcates into the peroneal artery and posterior tibial artery. The posterior tibial artery provides the nutrient artery to the tibia as well as branches to adjacent muscles in the deep posterior compartment. The peroneal artery descends adjacent to the fibula, posterior to the interosseous membrane, providing the nutrient artery to that bone. An important communicating branch to the posterior tibial artery arises in the distal aspect of the leg.

The dorsalis pedis artery may be absent or present only as a rudimentary structure in as many as 15 per cent of the population (Fig. 82–5) (Hidalgo and Shaw, 1986b). In most patients the dorsalis pedis artery bifurcates into the first dorsal metatarsal artery and the deep plantar artery, which dives between the first and second metacarpals to form the deep plantar arch. The first dorsal metatarsal artery, the most important structure in the dissection of toe free flaps or the dorsalis pedis flap, may run above, within, or deep to the first dorsal interosseous muscle. According to Huber (1941) the first dorsal metatarsal artery arises from the dorsalis pedis in only 76 per cent of individuals.

On the plantar surface of the foot, the arterial circulation is provided by the medial and lateral plantar branches from the posterior tibial artery (Fig. 82–6). The lateral plantar artery is significantly larger than the medial plantar vessel in 80 per cent of cases (Edwards, 1960). In the distal foot, the deep plantar branch from the dorsalis pedis artery and the terminal branch of the lateral plantar artery unite to form the plantar arch (Vann, 1943; Reiffel and McCarthy, 1980).

Nerves

The motor fibers to the lower extremity musculature are carried in the femoral, obturator, and sciatic nerves. The femoral and obturator nerves are derived from the lumbar plexus and represent the L2, L3, and L4 nerve roots. The femoral nerve exits the pelvis on the anterior surface of the iliopsoas muscle, passing beneath the inguinal ligament lateral to the femoral artery, and innervates the quadriceps muscles and the sartorius. The obturator nerve accompanies the obturator artery through the bony obturator canal and provides motor innervation to the adductor muscles. The sciatic nerve, the largest nerve of the body, is derived from the nerve roots L4, L5, S1, S2, and S3; it exits the pelvis through the sciatic foramen below the piriform muscle and lateral to the ischial tuberosity. At this level the tibial and common

peroneal divisions are together as a single nerve trunk but are anatomically separate within that nerve. The hamstring muscles are innervated by the tibial division of the nerve. Just proximal to the popliteal space the sciatic nerve divides into two, the tibial and common peroneal neves, which provide all motor input to the leg and foot.

The tibial nerve courses with the posterior tibial vessels in the deep posterior compartment of the leg, providing innervation to the muscles in both the superficial and deep posterior compartments. In the distal leg the nerve follows the posterior tibial artery behind the medial malleolus, where the medial calcaneal branch supplies the heel skin, and the tibial nerve divides into its terminal branches, the medial and lateral plantar nerves. The common peroneal nerve runs across the popliteal fossa around the fibular head and bifurcates into the superficial and deep peroneal nerves. The deep peroneal nerve is in the anterior compartment of the leg, where it accompanies the anterior tibial artery and provides motor innervation to the four muscles in the anterior compartment. The superficial peroneal nerve provides motor innervation to the peroneus muscles before piercing the fascia at approximately the junction of the middle and distal thirds of the leg. It subsequently courses subcutaneously to provide sensory innervation to the lateral aspect of the leg and the dorsum of the foot.

The sensory nerves of the lower extremity are generally more superficial than the motor nerves (Fig. 82–7). Although not essential to normal functioning (with the exception of plantar sensation), the sensory nerves when injured can be the source of significant morbidity. The anterior thigh skin is innervated by the anterior femoral cutaneous nerves (L2 and L3), which are branches of the femoral nerve. The lateral thigh skin is innervated by the lateral femoral cutaneous nerve (L2 and L3), a branch of the lumbar plexus. Sensibility to the proximal medial thigh is provided by the ilioinguinal nerve, and sensibility to the distal medial thigh by a cutaneous branch of the obturator nerve, the medial cutaneous nerve of the thigh. Posteriorly a direct branch of the sacral plexus, the posterior femoral cutaneous nerve (S1–S3) provides sensory innervation.

On the medial half of the lower leg (anterior and posterior) the saphenous nerve carries the sensory input. The lateral leg and

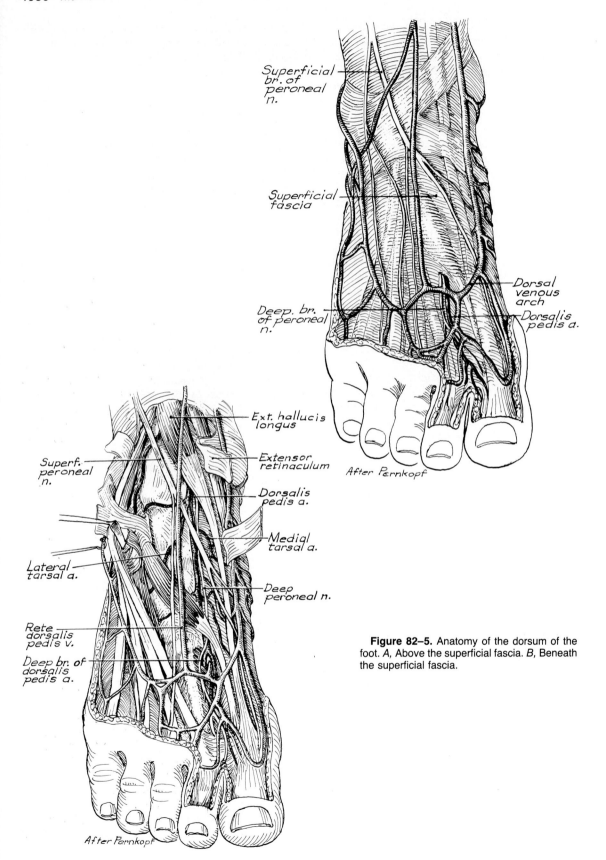

Superficial
br. of
peroneal
n.

Superficial
fascia

Deep. br.
of peroneal
n.

Dorsal
venous
arch

Dorsalis
pedis a.

After Pernkopf

Ext. hallucis
longus

Extensor
retinaculum

Superf.
peroneal
n.

Dorsalis
pedis a.

Medial
tarsal a.

Lateral
tarsal a.

Deep
peroneal n.

Rete
dorsalis
pedis v.

Deep br. of
dorsalis
pedis a.

After Pernkopf

Figure 82–5. Anatomy of the dorsum of the foot. *A,* Above the superficial fascia. *B,* Beneath the superficial fascia.

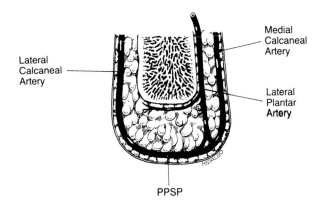

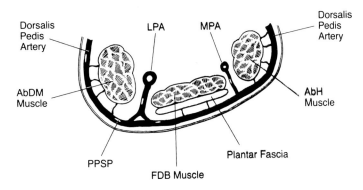

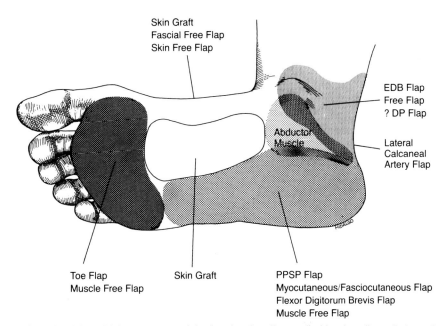

Figure 82–6. The skin of the midplantar aspect of the foot is primarily supplied by dorsalis pedis branches that course around the sides of the foot, and large lateral plantar artery branches that descend vertically to reach the proximal plantar subcutaneous plexus (PPSP). There are musculocutaneous vessels that contribute to the cutaneous blood supply from the abductor muscles (AbDM, abductor digiti minimi; AbH, abductor hallucis). (From Hidalgo, D. A., and Shaw, W. W.: Reconstruction of foot injuries. Clin. Plast. Surg., *13*:663, 1986.)

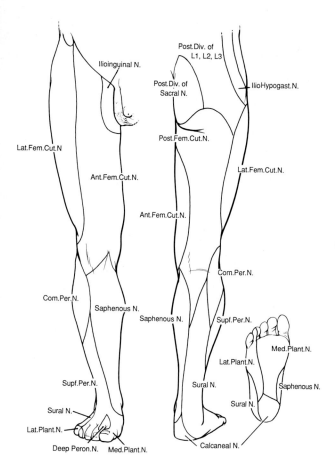

Figure 82–7. Sensory innervation of the lower extremity.

the dorsum of the foot are innervated by the superficial peroneal nerve, while the dorsal first web space is the only cutaneous territory served by the deep peroneal nerve. The posterior aspect of the leg and lateral foot sensory information is carried by the sural nerve, which runs behind the lateral malleolus, up the posterior calf, and between the two heads of the gastrocnemius to join the tibial nerve in the popliteal fossa.

On the sole of the foot, sensibility is provided by the three terminal branches of the tibial nerve. The medial calcaneal branch (S1 and S2) provides sensibility to the skin over the heel, while the medial and lateral plantar nerves provide sensibility to the skin on the sole of the foot. The medial plantar nerve is larger and provides sensibility to most of the plantar skin and the medial 3½ toes. The lateral plantar nerve innervates only the most lateral aspect of the foot and lateral 1½ toes. It is important to recall that the calcaneal nerve is superficial, lying only a few millimeters beneath the skin throughout its medial to lateral course (Shaw and Hidalgo, 1987). The medial and lateral plantar nerves,

which course in a deeper plane and provide sensory fibers to the skin, emerge between the flexor digitorum brevis muscle and the abductor hallucis on the medial side, and between the flexor digitorum brevis and the abductor digiti minimi on the lateral side. The plantar fascia is not penetrated by major sensory branches, making the plantar fascia a safe plane for dissection (Shaw and Hidalgo, 1987).

MUSCLE AND MUSCULOCUTANEOUS FLAPS

The lower extremity muscles described below are useful as muscle and musculocutaneous flaps (see also Chap. 11).

Gluteus Maximus

Origin and Insertion. The large, flat, quadrilateral gluteus maximus arises from the posterior gluteal line of the ilium, the

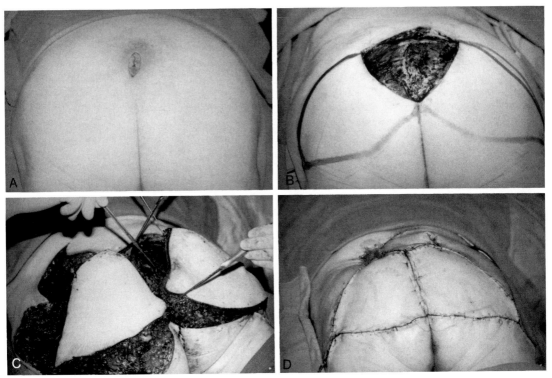

Figure 82–8. Gluteus maximus V-Y advancement flap. *A,* Radiation ulcer of the sacrum. *B,* After wound debridement and outline of flaps. *C,* Advancement of flaps. *D,* Wound closure.

posterior iliac crest, the lateral margin of the sacrum, and the coccyx and inserts into the iliotibial tract.

Vascular Supply. The gluteus maximus is a Type III muscle (Mathes and Nahai, 1982), receiving blood supply from two branches of the internal iliac artery, the superior and the inferior gluteal arteries. The superior gluteal artery exits the pelvis above the piriform muscle and the inferior gluteal artery, accompanied by the sciatic nerve, below the piriform muscle.

Motor Innervation. The inferior gluteal nerve (L5, S1, and S2) accompanies the inferior gluteal artery, passing caudal to the piriform muscle and innervating the gluteus maximus.

Applications. The gluteus maximus muscle is most commonly used as a musculocutaneous flap for the coverage of pressure sores (see Chap. 77). It is useful either as a musculocutaneous rotation flap or as a V-Y advancement flap to cover lesions of the sacrum (Fig. 82–8). In paraplegics, in whom there is no functional impairment related to rotating the insertion of the muscle, the gluteous maximus musculocutaneous flaps are excellent option for covering ischial pressure sores.

Shaw popularized microvascular transfer of a myocutaneous unit based on the superior gluteal artery for breast reconstruction (see Chap. 79).

Tensor Fascia Lata (TFL)

Origin and Insertion. The muscle takes origin from the anterior superior iliac spine and anterior aspect of the lateral iliac crest, and inserts on the iliotibial tract. The muscle is small with a long fascial extension.

Vascular Supply. The TFL is a Type I muscle (Mathes and Nahai, 1982). The pedicle is the transverse branch of the lateral femoral circumflex artery, which arises from the profunda femoris artery approximately 10 cm below the anterior superior iliac spine. The cutaneous portion of the TFL musculocutaneous flap extends distally over the fascial component. The skin territory is supplied proximally by musculocutaneous perforators and distally by the perforating branches from the profunda femoris artery.

Motor Innervation. The TFL is innervated by the superior gluteal nerve.

Applications. The muscle can be rotated

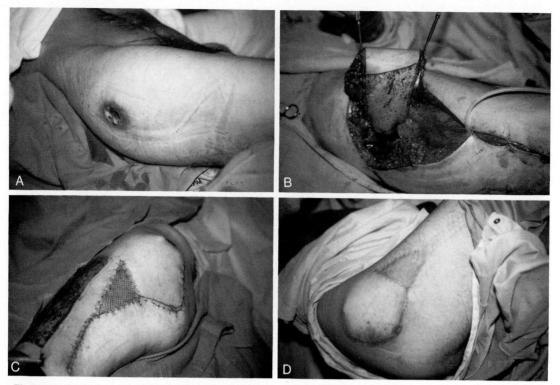

Figure 82–9. Tensor fascia lata musculocutaneous flap. *A,* Trochanteric pressure sore in a quadriplegic patient. *B,* Elevation of flap. Note the deepithelized distal portion that will provide filling of the depths of the defect. *C,* Closure after flap transfer. A skin graft is used to close part of the donor defect. *D,* Long-term result.

in an anterior direction as a musculocutaneous flap with a fasciocutaneous extension to reconstruct defects in the abdominal wall, suprapubic area, and adjacent groin and perineum. Alternatively, the flap can be rotated posteriorly to cover trochanteric defects (Fig. 82–9) (see Chap. 77). The flap is designed along the anterolateral thigh posterior to a line drawn from the anterior superior iliac spine to the lateral femoral condyle. The flap can be extended to within 8 to 10 cm of the knee joint, or further if a delay procedure is employed. It can be used as a microvascular free flap, but the donor defect is significant and it offers no advantage over other free flap donor sites. It can be transferred as a sensory flap, having a twofold cutaneous nerve supply: the cutaneous branch of T12 and the lateral femoral cutaneous nerve (L2–L3). In addition, the anterior 5 to 10 cm of the iliac crest can be transferred with the flap as a composite osteomusculocutaneous flap.

The distal one-third of the flap is not reliable without a delay procedure. In addition, transfer in an athletic patient may lead to lateral knee instability. Because the working portion of the flap is primarily fasciocuta-

neous, it is not an ideal flap for many defects. When covering pressure sores of the trochanter, for example, the fascia does not conform to an irregular bed as does a large muscle flap. The same is true for osteoradionecrosis of the pubis, a situation in which a muscle flap may be more efficacious (Mathes, Alpert, and Chang, 1982) by providing more complete filling of the defect.

Rectus Femoris

Origin and Insertion. The rectus femoris takes origin from the anterior inferior iliac spine and inserts into the patellar tendon.

Vascular Supply. The primary pedicle is the lateral femoral circumflex artery, and the distal muscle receives segmental blood supply (Type II).

Motor Innervation. The muscle is innervated by the femoral nerve (L2–L4).

Applications. The rectus femoris is clinically the most useful muscle in the thigh. Some of the indications for its use are similar to those of the TFL, but it provides more muscle bulk than the TFL flap. The rectus

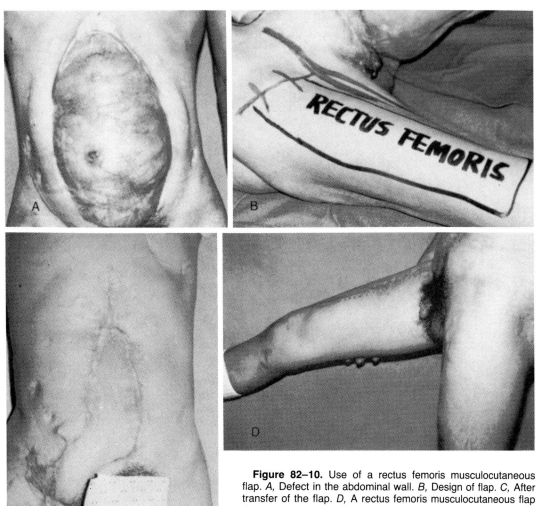

Figure 82–10. Use of a rectus femoris musculocutaneous flap. *A*, Defect in the abdominal wall. *B*, Design of flap. *C*, After transfer of the flap. *D*, A rectus femoris musculocutaneous flap donor area without loss of knee extension. (From Grotting, J. C., and Vasconez, L. O.: Regional blood supply and the selection of flaps for reconstruction. Clin. Plast. Surg., *13*:581, 1986.)

femoris can be transferred as superiorly as the upper abdomen (Fig. 82–10) with or without the overlying skin. One must ensure that the quadriceps tendon is reconstructed after transfer of the muscle by suturing together the tendons of the vastus lateralis and medialis.

Vastus Lateralis

Origin and Insertion. The origin of the vastus lateralis is the greater trochanter of the femur, the intertrochanteric line, and the intermuscular septum posteriorly. The tendinous portion of the muscles inserts into the patellar tendon.

Vascular Supply. The main pedicle is the lateral femoral circumflex artery. Multiple minor pedicles enter the distal muscle in a segmental pattern (Type II).

Motor Innervation. The muscle is innervated by the femoral nerve (L2–L4).

Applications. The primary use of the vastus lateralis is in the coverage of trochanteric defects. It is particularly useful after resection of the femoral head, which leaves a deep cavity requiring coverage with a bulky muscle.

Gracilis

Origin and Insertion. The gracilis muscle arises from the pubic tubercle and inserts

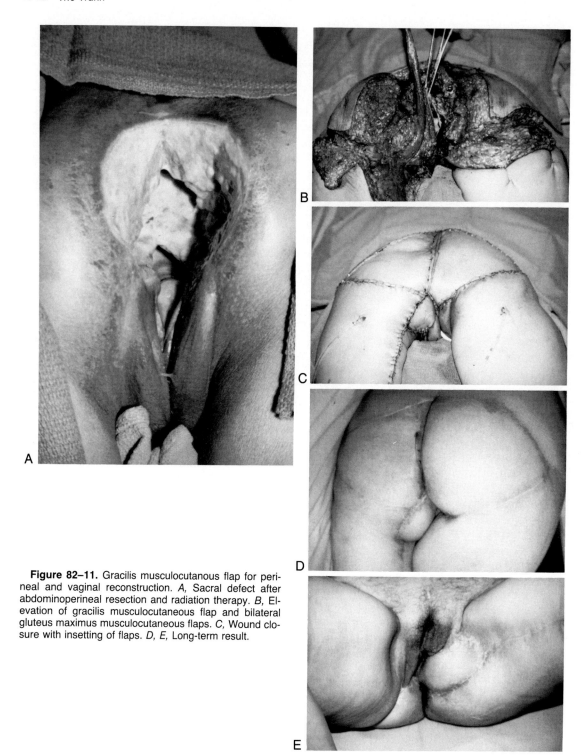

Figure 82–11. Gracilis musculocutanous flap for perineal and vaginal reconstruction. *A*, Sacral defect after abdominoperineal resection and radiation therapy. *B*, Elevation of gracilis musculocutaneous flap and bilateral gluteus maximus musculocutaneous flaps. *C*, Wound closure with insetting of flaps. *D, E*, Long-term result.

into the pes anserinus on the medial aspect of the proximal tibia.

Vascular Supply. The gracilis is a Type II muscle, the main pedicle being the medial femoral circumflex branch of the profunda femoris artery. Several minor pedicles from the superficial femoral artery enter the muscle distally.

Motor Innervation. The gracilis is innervated by a branch of the obturator nerve (L3 and L4).

Applications. As a muscle flap or as a

musculocutaneous flap, the gracilis is extremely useful for regional coverage of the perineum or vagina (Fig. 82–11). It has been used in penile and vaginal reconstruction, and coverage of ischial pressure sores. Because the cutaneous territory in obese or older individuals tends to hang posteriorly when they are in the supine position, one must verify that any skin paddle that is included is that which is perfused by the gracilis musculocutaneous perforators. The muscle is also a popular free flap donor site, particularly for small defects in the lower extremity. In addition, the gracilis can be transferred as a microneurovascular free flap for functional forearm muscle replacement and for facial reanimation.

Gastrocnemius

Origin and Insertion. The gastrocnemius has two heads, one arising from the medial femoral condyle and the other from the lateral femoral condyle. The two heads fuse in the midline and insert with the soleus to form the Achilles tendon.

Vascular Supply. The medial and lateral heads of the gastrocnemius muscle can be transferred separately as Type I muscles. The medial and lateral sural arteries, paired branches of the popliteal artery, provide the blood supply to the respective gastrocnemius muscle on each side.

Motor Innervation. The two heads are innervated separately by branches of the tibial nerve as it passes through the popliteal space.

Applications. The medial and lateral gastrocnemius flaps can be elevated as either muscle flaps or musculocutaneous flaps. The medial gastrocnemius is slightly larger and is more frequently used to cover defects over the knee and proximal third of the tibia (Fig. 82–12). When used as a musculocutaneous flap, a fasciocutaneous extension can be elevated to within 5 cm of the medial malleolus. Musculocutaneous flaps taken from this region, however, cause unsightly donor sites. It is generally preferable to transfer the flap as a muscle flap and cover it with a skin graft.

Soleus

Origin and Insertion. The soleus muscle takes origin from the tibia, the fibula, and the interosseus membrane. The insertion is with the gastrocnemius into the Achilles tendon, which in turn inserts on the calcaneus.

Vascular Supply. The soleus is a Type II muscle. The dominant pedicle enters the muscle proximally, and there are segmental perforators from the posterior tibial and peroneal artery that enter the medial and lateral halves of the muscle, respectively.

Motor Innervation. The muscle is innervated by a branch of the tibial nerve.

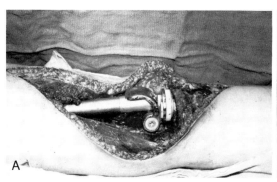
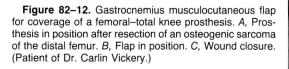
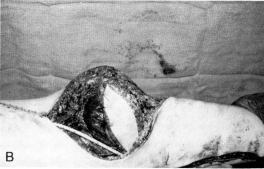
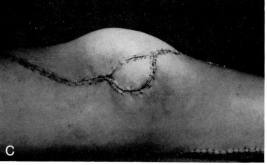

Figure 82–12. Gastrocnemius musculocutaneous flap for coverage of a femoral–total knee prosthesis. *A,* Prosthesis in position after resection of an osteogenic sarcoma of the distal femur. *B,* Flap in position. *C,* Wound closure. (Patient of Dr. Carlin Vickery.)

Applications. The soleus muscle is described as the muscle flap of choice for defects over the middle third of the tibia. While the muscle can cover defects in this region, it is frequently easier and more esthetically acceptable to use a microvascular free muscle flap from a distant location. In certain patients, however, the soleus offers a satisfactory solution for the midtibial defect. Because the posterior tibial artery provides perforators medially, and the peroneal artery provides segmental perforators to the lateral half of the muscle, either half of the muscle can be transferred individually, leaving the other half intact. Distally based soleus flaps are not recommended.

FASCIOCUTANEOUS FLAPS

The concept that a given cutaneous territory is supplied either by direct cutaneous vessels or by musculocutaneous perforators is a useful one but is an oversimplification. It is important to realize that most cutaneous territories have multiple sources of blood supply and do not necessarily conform to one of the traditional vascular patterns. In addition, the concept of fasciocutaneous flaps must be integrated into an understanding of cutaneous blood supply (Ponten, 1981). The skin of the lower extremity, for example, is supplied in a variety of patterns, depending on the location, and this is precisely why the same cutaneous territory can often be transferred as a musculocutaneous flap or a fasciocutaneous flap, depending on the reconstructive needs.

In 1981 Ponten reported the use of fasciocutaneous flaps in the lower leg in 22 patients. Barclay and associates (1982) confirmed Ponten's experience with fasciocutaneous flaps in the lower leg, reporting 16 clinical cases as well as anatomic dissections. Although fasciocutaneous flaps were originally described for use in the lower leg, the principle is also applicable to the thigh.

The skin of the anterior thigh receives blood supply from both musculocutaneous perforators from the rectus femoris muscle, as well as from multiple vessels in the inguinal region that contribute to the suprafascial plexus. Fasciocutaneous flaps on the anterior thigh, which extend from the inguinal region to the suprapatellar area, can safely be raised. The flap can be as wide as 15 cm; however, it is advisable to limit the width to one that can be closed primarily. When the perforators from the rectus femoris are divided in order to raise this cutaneous territory as a fasciocutaneous flap, the flap remains viable because it is based on the plethora of blood vessels in the inguinal region. In addition, according to Grotting and Vasconez (1986), a direct unnamed branch from the superficial femoral artery provides blood supply to the anterior thigh skin.

The skin on the medial thigh also receives blood supply from both musculocutaneous perforators through the gracilis muscle and from the numerous cutaneous vessels in the inguinal region. Fasciocutaneous flaps are therefore a viable option, but frequently provide advantage over the gracilis musculocutaneous flap. Baek (1983) described a medial thigh fasciocutaneous free flap based on an unnamed branch from the superficial femoral artery and its accompanying vein (Fig. 82–13). The pedicle arises proximal to the adductor canal; it is 5 cm in length and 2 to 4 mm in diameter. The distal aspect of the medial thigh receives blood supply from the saphenous branch of the descending geniculate artery. Above the knee the artery travels with the medial femoral cutaneous nerve, and below the knee with the saphenous nerve, where the saphenous artery supplies the skin calf.

The lateral thigh skin is perfused by perforators from the tensor muscle as well as by the second and third perforators from the profunda femoris artery. Whether flaps on the lateral thigh should be considered musculocutaneous flaps based on the perforators from the small tensor muscle or fasciocutaneous flaps based on the suprafascial plexus distally is a matter of semantics; in fact, flaps can be raised at the subfascial level over the lateral thigh. Baek (1983) described a free fasciocutaneous flap from the lateral thigh based on the third perforating branch from the profunda femoris artery and its venae comitantes (Fig. 82–14). In addition, this area

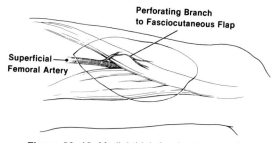

Perforating Branch
to Fasciocutaneous Flap

Superficial
Femoral Artery

Figure 82–13. Medial thigh fasciocutaneous flap.

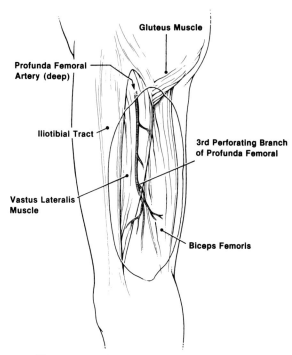

Figure 82–14. Lateral thigh fasciocutaneous flap.

has a constant cutaneous nerve supply based on the lateral femoral cutaneous nerve, and therefore is potentially usable as a sensate free flap. The fact that the pedicle enters the

flap at approximately its midpoint can make insetting of the flap difficult.

The posterior cutaneous blood supply of the thigh is derived from the hamstring muscle perforators as well as from cutaneous vessels. The inferior gluteal artery flap (Fig. 82–15) described by Hurwitz, Swartz, and Mathes (1981) is a robust fasciocutaneous flap based on the descending branch of the inferior gluteal artery, which enters the thigh midway between the greater trochanter and the ischial tuberosity, and runs with the posterior cutaneous nerve of the thigh. Even when the descending branch from the inferior gluteal artery is absent, the cruciate anastomosis involving the superior and inferior gluteal arteries and the first perforator from the profunda femoris artery provide a rich suprafascial plexus on which to base the flap.

The cutaneous blood vessels, therefore, form an anastomosing network in the suprafascial and subdermal planes. The musculocutaneous perforators tend to be concentrated in the proximal third of the thigh. The various territories overlap considerably, and when one source of blood supply to any particular cutaneous territory is altered by surgery, injury, or disease, other sources become the dominant blood supply to that region.

The skin over the anterior compartment of

Figure 82–15. Posterior thigh fasciocutaneous flap.

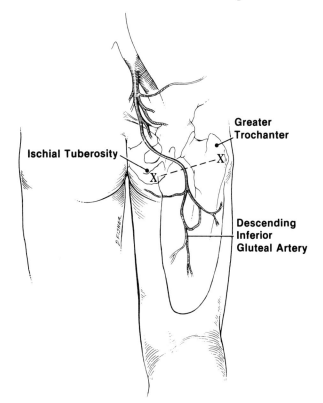

the leg is supplied by vessels originating from the anterior tibial artery, which run in the intermuscular septa and contribute to the plexus above the fascia. The lateral leg skin is supplied in a similar fashion, the origin of the septocutaneous vessels being the peroneal artery (Fig. 8–16, 82–17). The skin over the posterior leg can be carried on the musculocutaneous perforators from the gastrocnemius muscle, or rotated as a fasciocutaneous flap based on contributions from the geniculate anastomosis around the knee and perforators of the posterior tibial and peroneal arteries. In addition, according to Barclay and associates (1982), a constant cutaneous branch from the popliteal artery supplies the posterior leg skin. On the medial aspect, the cutaneous circulation is derived from the gastrocnemius perforators as well as from the saphenous artery originating above the knee (Fig. 82–18). On the lower leg, therefore, fasciocutaneous flaps can be raised medially, laterally, or posteriorly (Fig. 82–19).

On the plantar surface of the foot, the lateral plantar artery provides the major source of blood supply by a series of vertical cutaneous branches. As shown by Shaw and Hidalgo (1986), branches of the dorsalis pedis and lateral plantar arteries form a suprafascial, subcutaneous plexus in the proximal aspect of the sole of the foot. The plexus extends from the posterior heel to a point halfway between the heel and the metatarsal heads. This study also showed that no significant direct perforating vessels penetrate the plantar fascia, and therefore the skin over the flexor digitorum brevis muscle is not supplied in a significant way by musculocutaneous perforators. More laterally the skin over the abductor hallucis and abductor digiti minimi muscles has a more typical musculocutaneous blood supply. The subcutaneous

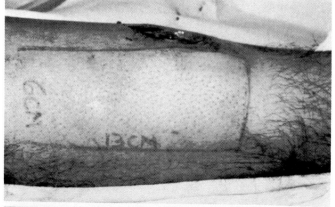
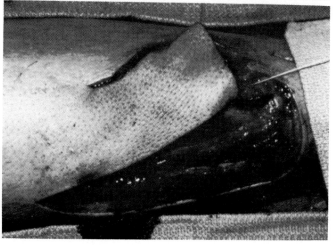

Figure 82–16. Use of a fasciocutaneous flap to close a defect in the anterior tibial region. Such a flap can be designed overlying the anterior tibial artery on the anterolateral leg based on septocutaneous vessels. Note the unsightly donor defect. (From Grotting, J. C., and Vasconez, L. O.: Regional blood supply and the selection of flaps for reconstruction. Clin. Plast. Surg., *13*:581, 1986.)

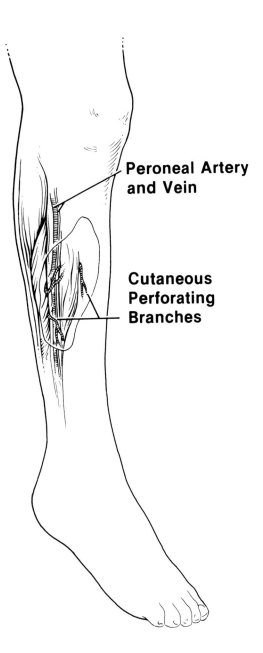

Peroneal Artery and Vein

Cutaneous Perforating Branches

Figure 82–17. Peroneal fasciocutaneous flap.

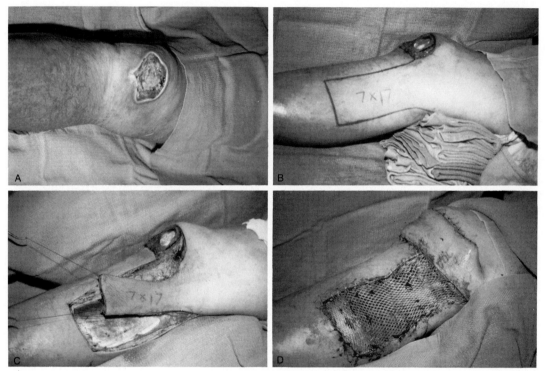

Figure 82–18. Medial calf fasciocutaneous flap. *A*, Post-traumatic knee defect. *B*, Outline of flap. *C*, Flap elevation. *D*, Flap in position with skin grafting of the donor site. The esthetic disadvantages of the flap are obvious.

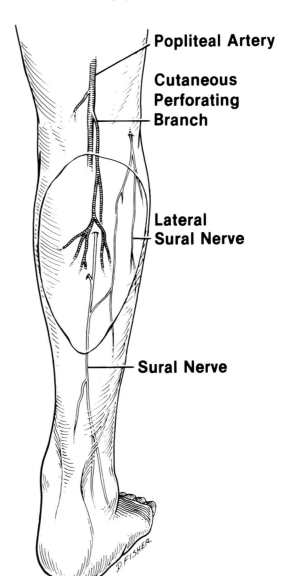

Popliteal Artery

Cutaneous Perforating Branch

Lateral Sural Nerve

Sural Nerve

Figure 82–19. Posterior calf fasciocutaneous flap.

vascular plexus over the heel allows local flaps to be raised in a suprafascial plane.

FREE FLAPS

Groin Flap

In 1973 Daniel and Taylor reported the free transfer of the groin skin and subcutaneous fat by use of microvascular anastomoses. Despite initial enthusiasm about the groin flap as a donor site, it has been almost completely replaced by other flaps recently described.

The artery to the groin flap (Fig. 82–20),

the superficial circumflex iliac artery (SCIA), demonstrates variable anatomy. Usually the SCIA and the superficial inferior epigastric artery (SIEA) arise separately from the femoral artery just distal to the inguinal ligament. Occasionally one of the two arteries is very small and the other is correspondingly large; occasionally both arteries arise from a common trunk (Hidalgo and Shaw, 1987; Harii and associates, 1975; Ohmori and Harii, 1975; Taylor and Daniel, 1975). The SCIA runs just above the deep fascia of the anterior thigh until it reaches the lateral border of the sartorius muscle, where it courses more superficially. The vein accompanies the SCIA

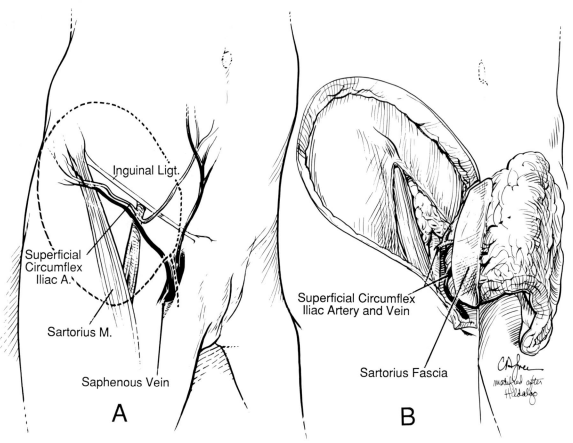

Figure 82–20. The groin free flap. *A,* The flap is centered on the arterial pedicle, which is parallel and caudal to the inguinal ligament. *B,* The flap is dissected from lateral to medial. When the lateral border of the sartorius is reached, the dissection is carried deep to the sartorius fascia so as not to injure the arterial pedicle.

from the flap, but as the femoral vessels are approached the vein diverges to run in a slightly more superficial plane to its termination in the saphenous vein before its entry into the femoral vein.

Ideally, the flap is designed by centering the skin ellipse on a line drawn parallel to and 2 cm below the inguinal ligament (Fig. 82–20).

The groin microvascular free flap has been relegated to "last resort" status because of the difficulty in dissection, the variable size and anatomy of the vessels, and the short pedicle length.

The authors rarely use the free groin flap for lower extremity reconstruction, reserving it for young female patients with contour defects of the thigh or calf. Shaw and Hidalgo (1987) recommended starting the dissection by identifying the saphenous vein. Following the saphenus vein toward the fossa ovalis, the surgeon exposes the venous pedicle. In-

cising the upper border of the flap and elevating it directly off the aponeurosis of the external oblique exposes the femoral artery as it emerges from beneath the inguinal ligament. At this point the arterial pedicle can be identified. Dissection is then begun laterally, taking the flap off the deep fascia until the lateral border of the sartorius is reached, and including the fascia over the sartorius with the flap so as not to injure the vessel that lies superficial to it.

Dorsalis Pedis Flap

The dorsum of the foot is a source of thin, pliable skin that would be more useful as a free flap donor site if it were not for the morbidity associated with its use.

The artery to the flap (Fig. 82–21) is the dorsalis pedis, which emerges on the dorsum of the foot beneath the extensor retinaculum

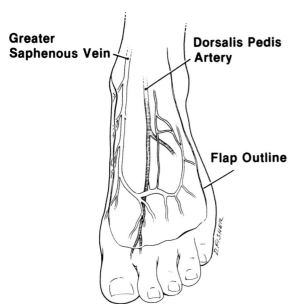

Greater Saphenous Vein

Dorsalis Pedis Artery

Flap Outline

Figure 82–21. Dorsalis pedis flap.

accompanied by the deep peroneal nerve on its medial side. The extensor hallucis brevis muscle and tendon pass over the dorsalis pedis artery distal to the extensor retinaculum. The more superficial dorsal venous arch of the foot provides venous drainage of the flap via the greater saphenous vein medially and the small saphenous vein laterally. Providing sensory innervation to the flap is the superficial peroneal nerve, the branches of which pass either superficial or deep to the venous arch.

The cutaneous blood supply on the dorsum of the foot is provided by vertical branches of the dorsalis pedis artery, which average 3.8 in number distal to the extensor retinaculum (Gilbert, 1976). The dorsalis pedis artery bifurcates into the first dorsal metatarsal artery and the deep plantar artery, which contributes to the deep plantar arch. The first dorsal metatarsal artery continues into the first web space, where it in turn bifurcates.

The arterial anatomy of the dorsalis pedis artery and its distal branches is variable and has been studied by several authors (McCraw and Furlow, 1975; May and associates, 1977; Man and Ackland, 1980). The deep peroneal nerve accompanies the dorsalis pedis artery and subsequently the first dorsal metatarsal artery to supply the skin of the first web space. It is therefore irrelevant to the innervation of the dorsalis pedis flap, which has

sensory innervation from the superficial peroneal artery.

Because the dorsalis pedis artery is absent or rudimentary in up to 15 per cent of the population, some authors have recommended that angiography be performed before elevation of a free flap on the dorsum of the foot. In fact, if a strong dorsalis pedis pulse is palpated, there is no reason to perform further examinations and a dorsalis pedis flap can be harvested. If no pulse is palpable, Doppler examination and possibly angiography are necessary prior to flap elevation.

Dissection is easiest when initiated distally, incising the skin at the bases of the toes. The first dorsal metatarsal artery is identified and ligated. It is important to remember that it may pass subcutaneously, within the interosseus muscle or deep to the muscle. As the flap is elevated, care is taken to raise the first dorsal metatarsal artery with the flap and at the same time leave the paratenon on the extensor tendons so that the donor site can be skin grafted. The flap is raised in a plane deep to the first dorsal metatarsal artery. Following the first dorsal metatarsal artery retrograde exposes the bifurcation of the dorsalis pedis artery and allows ligation of the deep plantar branch. Exposure is facilitated by distracting the first and second metacarpals. As mentioned, the cutaneous branches of the dorsalis pedis are relatively few in number and can easily be injured during the dissection if excessive traction is applied to the flap. Because the extensor hallucis brevis passes over the artery, it is necessary to divide the tendon medial to the artery and the muscle belly lateral to the artery in order to elevate the artery with the flap.

After raising the flap, defects in the paratenon are repaired and a skin graft is applied. A meticulous dressing followed by a plaster cast is applied and the leg is elevated for one week. The cast is removed, and graduated dangling is allowed until ambulation is begun approximately two weeks postoperatively.

The donor site morbidity of the dorsalis pedis free flap is its main disadvantage. Even if a skin graft successfully closes the wound, compulsive long-term care is required. Unstable coverage over the tendons is the rule even with satisfactory graft vascularization. In addition, the wound is often tender, an obvious disadvantage for the wearing of shoes.

"Foot Fillet" Flap

The skin of an unreplantable foot can be harvested circumferentially based on both the dorsalis pedis and posterior tibial arteries, or as the plantar skin alone (fillet of sole) based on the posterior tibial artery (Fig. 82–22). In the setting of a leg amputation where free flap transfer is required to salvage a below knee amputation, the foot fillet flap is an ideal choice. The tibial nerve provides the potential for sensory innervation.

If the flap includes the dorsal and plantar skin, both the dorsalis pedis artery and the posterior tibial artery must be included despite the connection between the two systems via the deep plantar branch. To facilitate dissection and to provide additional padding over the amputation stump, the flap is raised at a deeper plane than the standard dorsalis pedis flap, including the extensor tendons with the flap. On the plantar surface of the foot the plane of dissection is most conveniently performed on the surface of the bony architecture. In this way, the vascular pedicle is protected by a thick layer of tissue and dissection is expeditious.

Dissection is initiated by making an incision along the lateral foot and a circumferential incision at the base of the toes. The dorsal foot skin is raised from lateral to medial, raising the extensor tendons with the flap. The anterior tibial artery is located proximally at the level of the amputation and traced distally into the foot in order to verify that the artery is included in the flap. The most difficult part of the dissection, as with any free flap involving the dorsum of the foot or first web space, is the identification and preservation of the first dorsal metatarsal artery and the deep plantar artery. The plantar skin is then elevated at the level of the tarsal and metatarsal bones. Once again, as the pedicle is approached, it is safest to identify the posterior tibial artery proximally in the region of the stump, to trace it into the flap, and to make sure that the dissection is including the pedicle in flap elevation. The first metatarsal bone is transected at its base, a maneuver that allows preservation of the deep plantar branch. As mentioned above, if both the plantar and dorsal skin are harvested, anastomoses of both the dorsalis pedis and the posterior tibial arteries should be performed to the recipient vessels. Even though care has been taken to preserve the deep plantar branch of the dorsalis pedis artery, it has been the authors' experience that restoring circulation through either the dorsalis pedis or the posterior tibial artery results in inadequate perfusion of the other skin territory. Often the dorsal skin is not needed to close the amputation and the dissection can be confined to the plantar surface of the foot, which provides a sturdier form of coverage and necessitates anastomosis of only the posterior tibial artery. The theoretical advantage of restoring sensation to the stump by anastomosis of the tibial nerve has not been determined.

Gracilis Muscle Flap

The anatomy of the gracilis muscle has been discussed in the section on Muscle and Musculocutaneous Flaps (Fig. 82–23). Because the muscle is expendable, the donor site is inconspicuous, and since the pedicle is of satisfactory size and consistent location, the gracilis muscle is an excellent donor site. It is appropriate for small coverage problems in the lower extremity; however, it is usually inadequate to cover most major open fractures and cases of chronic osteomyelitis. The gracilis muscle has proved useful as a microneurovascular flap for facial reanimation as well as for functional replacement of the forearm musculature. In general, the skin over the proximal muscle is consistently perfused; however, the skin over the distal muscle is not reliable when the gracilis is used as a free flap.

The medial femoral circumflex vessel and its two venae comitantes run between the adductor longus and adductor brevis to reach the deep surface of the gracilis muscle approximately 10 cm below the pubic tubercle. The motor nerve, a branch of the obturator nerve, innervates the muscle adjacent to the vascular pedicle.

If a free muscle flap is required, an incision is made over the muscle, which lies posterior and parallel to a line extending from the pubic tubercle to the medial tibial condyle. If a musculocutaneous free flap is needed, a distal incision is made first to identify the gracilis tendon. Location of the tendon allows more precise design of the skin paddle to ensure its location over the gracilis muscle.

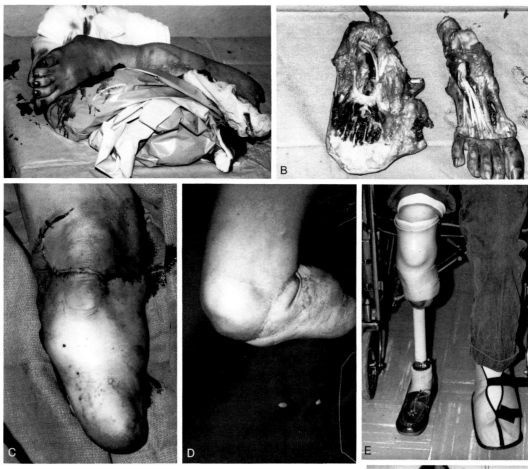

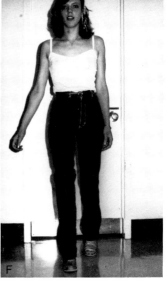

Figure 82–22. Foot fillet flap. *A,* An unreplantable below knee amputation. *B,* The foot fillet flap has been dissected from the amputated part. *C,* Inset of flap. *D,* Long-term result with evidence of a functioning knee joint. *E,* Patient wearing the prosthesis. *F,* Patient ambulating.

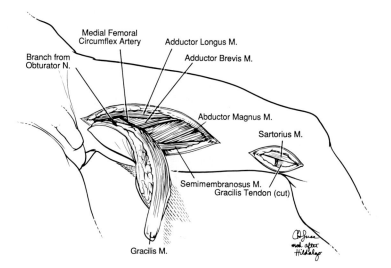

Figure 82–23. Gracilis free flap. The arterial pedicle and the motor nerve enter the muscle in close proximity to each other. A small distal incision allows identification of the gracilis tendon. The tendon is put on traction, permitting identification of the skin, which lies over the gastrocnemius belly.

Tensor Fascia Lata Flap

The TFL donor site provides abundant skin and subcutaneous tissue. The potential for sensory reinnervation exists because of the lateral femoral cutaneous nerve, which can be included with the flap. Because the pedicle enters the flap in its central portion, the flap is thick proximally and thin distally. Since the donor site morbidity can be formidable, the flap has largely been replaced by other donor sites. It should not be forgotten, however, as an abundant source of tissue to fill large defects.

The transverse branch of the lateral femoral circumflex artery is the pedicle that supplies the tensor muscle (Fig. 82–24). The lateral femoral circumflex artery also provides blood supply to the quadriceps muscles. The pedicle to a tensor muscle free flap can be made long, approximately 10 cm, by interrupting the branches to the other anterior thigh muscles. The motor innervation is provided by the inferior branch of the superior gluteal nerve (L4–L4, S1), which does not run with the vascular pedicle but reaches the tensor muscle from the posterior direction. The lateral femoral cutaneous nerve (L2–L3)

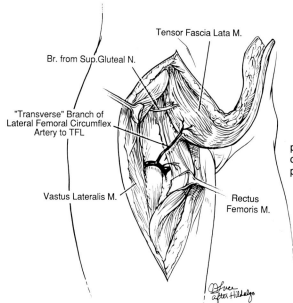

Figure 82–24. Tensor fascia lata free flap. The arterial pedicle and the motor nerve enter the muscle from different directions. The muscle itself is small and comprises a small portion of the overall flap area.

demonstrates consistent anatomy, running 1 cm medial and caudal to the anterior superior iliac spine. The upper part of the skin territory of the TFL is innervated by the cutaneous branches of T12.

The anterior border of TFL muscle lies on a line between the anterior superior iliac spine and the lateral aspect of the patella. Shaw and Hidalgo (1987) recommended identifying the pedicle as the initial maneuver by developing the space between the rectus femoris and vastus lateralis muscles. The vessel is on the surface of the vastus intermedius muscle and can be traced in a distal and a superior direction to identify the transverse branch to the tensor muscle. The flap can then be raised from distal to proximal in an expeditious fashion until the caudalmost aspect of the tensor muscle is identified. At this point the tensor muscle is separated from the rectus femoris to expose the vascular pedicle. The nerve can be identified as it enters the posterior surface of the muscle between the gluteus medius and minimus muscles, at a location above the greater trochanter.

Fibula Flap

Several characteristics of the fibula donor site make it an ideal source of vascularized bone for contralateral lower extremity problems. The flap (see Fig. 82–30) is raised on the peroneal artery, which is of adequate size and length for most clinical situations (Taylor, Miller and Ham, 1975). Segments of bone up to 25 cm in length are available. The periosteal blood supply is such that multiple osteotomies can be made in the bone, hinging it on the periosteum without compromising the vascularity of the flap. The proximal epiphysis can be included for long bone replacement in children. In addition, the fibula can be used as a double-barreled strut for defects in large bones such as the femur by leaving the periosteum intact. Donor site morbidity is generally minimal if care is taken not to injure the common peroneal nerve proximally and if sufficient fibula is left distally to avoid ankle instability.

The peroneal artery provides the nutrient branch to the fibula, entering at approximately the midportion of the bone. The peroneal artery also provides a network of periosteal blood vessels that allow osteotomy of the bone without interfering with the blood supply. The skin over the lateral aspect of the leg is supplied in part by perforating vessels from the peroneal artery that run with the septum between the lateral and posterior compartments.

Shaw and Hidalgo (1987) recommended preoperative angiography to assess the vascular anatomy of the leg from which the fibula is to be harvested. Because the vessels that supply the skin island run with the septum between the lateral and posterior compartments, it is important to design the skin island over a line posterior to the fibula, not directly over it.

Although the fibula flap can be dissected from either a lateral or a posterior approach, most operative situations favor supine positioning and therefore make the lateral approach more convenient. The leg is exsanguinated and the pneumatic tourniquet is inflated. If no skin island is to be included, a linear skin incision extending from the fibula head to the lateral malleolus is employed. If a skin island is desired, the boundaries of the flap are incised circumferentially to the level of the deep fascia. Care is taken not to injure the superficial peroneal nerve in the lower third of the leg. The flap is elevated off the lateral compartment muscles in a plane deep to the fascia. When the septum between the lateral and posterior muscle groups is identified, the occasional septocutaneous vessels can be seen running within the septum to supply the overlying skin. Similar dissection is performed from the posterior aspect of the incision, elevating the flap with the deep fascia off the posterior compartment muscles. Having now isolated the skin island on the septum, the surgeon continues the dissection down the anterior surface of the septum to the fibula and anteriorly around the fibula. The dissection is entirely extraperiosteal. Although there is no need to leave muscle on the periosteum per se, it is safer to leave a few muscle fibers rather than injure the periosteum by dissecting too close to it. The septum between the lateral and anterior compartments is incised to reveal the anterior compartment muscles. As the extensor digitorum longus, tibialis anterior, and extensor hallucis longus are elevated, the interosseus membrane is visualized. The interosseus membrane is divided, taking care not to injure the vessels deep to it. The fibula osteotomies are planned, depending on how much bone is needed to fill the defect. The osteotomies are performed, allowing distraction of the fibula from its bed and easier visualization of the remainder of the dissection. The tourniquet is deflated and the pulse from the peroneal vessel is palpated. These manuevers provide excellent visualization both anteriorly and posteriorly to the pedicle so that the final dissection of the vessels can be performed.

TRAUMA

Assessment

The initial assessment and treatment of patients with lower extremity trauma should be in accordance with the Advanced Trauma Life Support (ATLS) guidelines for multiple systems trauma dictated by the American College of Surgeons.

Underestimation of blood loss is the most common error in the early management of lower extremity injuries. In patients with a traumatic above knee amputation, open femur fractures, or open tibia-fibia fractures, there is the potential for life-threatening blood loss. Control and prompt replacement of blood loss in the emergency room prevents patients from entering the cycle of multiple transfusions, hypothermia, coagulopathy, or ARDS (adult respiratory distress syndrome). Hypotensive patients with lower extremity trauma whose blood pressure is not normalized with two liters of Ringer's lactate should receive uncrossmatched blood in the emergency room; transfusions should not be delayed until arrival in the operating room when frantic "catch-up" efforts must be made.

If examination of the lower extremity injury is performed in the emergency room, it should be done at a time when all consultants are present. Multiple examinations by numerous representatives of the various subspecialties lead inevitably to unnecessary blood loss, pain, and delay in transferring patients to the operating room. The critical components of the initial extremity assessment involve the neurovascular status. The remainder of the examination can be made more carefully, under more sterile conditions, and with less blood loss in the operating room.

The neurologic examination covers both motor and sensory components. A fixed neurologic deficit is probably related to the primary injury, whereas an evolving deterioration in the neurologic status is more likely related to ischemia or a compartment syndrome. A rapid assessment of the distal pulses and vascular status of the foot is made. A sterile dressing is applied to the wound and appropriate radiographs are taken. Tetanus prophylaxis is administered according to standard guidelines and intravenous antibiotics are given (Benson and associates, 1983; Yaremchuk, 1986).

As the experience with lower extremity trauma has increased, it has been found that prolonged examinations in the emergency room not only are unnecessary but are detrimental. A rapid neurologic and vascular examination can often be performed on an exposed foot without taking the dressing off when the patient is asleep in the operating room. At the very least, delays in the emergency room lead to significant blood loss and increased contamination of an open wound.

The second phase of management begins when the patient arrives in the operating room. The debridement is a fundamental step in the management of these injuries and is *not* relegated to the judgment of an inexperienced member of the team. Debridement is initiated with the pneumatic tourniquet inflated, and precise examination of the wound is undertaken. The surgeon must know exactly which structures are being debrided and which are being salvaged. All degloved skin is removed. Split-thickness skin grafts can be harvested from the degloved tissue by using the Reese dermatome. Crushed or devitalized muscle is methodically excised. Depending on the nature of the muscle injury, it may be better to remove the entire muscle than to simply cut across it, causing more bleeding. If the proximal, vascularized portion of a divided muscle is to be used for coverage of an underlying vital structure, only the distal muscle is removed. All major neurovascular structures in the vicinity of the injury are explored. Large bone fragments with significant soft tissue attachments are maintained, and small, free fragments are removed. If there is vascular compromise of the extremity, debridement is preceded by femoral arteriography on the operating room table. In addition, in the setting of ischemia, fasciotomies are immediately performed on the lower leg, releasing all four compartments. A two-incision approach (medial and lateral) is preferred.

After the primary debridement, the tourniquet is deflated and hemostasis obtained. A second debridement is performed with the tourniquet deflated. Upon completion of the secondary debridement, the tourniquet is reinflated and the wound is irrigated with a pulsatile jet lavage system.

Unless the leg has been devascularized (in which case revascularization may precede bone fixation), the next step is the application of appropriate fixation. Close cooperation with the orthopedic surgeons is essential. On the lower leg, an external fixator is usually applied. Above the knee, where there is more soft tissue coverage, an external or internal fixation system can be used.

The final step is the provision of soft tissue coverage. If the defect calls for a free flap, there is some controversy over the appropriate timing. Godina (1986) favored immediate coverage, whereas other surgeons (Yaremchuk, 1986) advocated serial debridement procedures, allowing marginal tissues to declare their viability and subsequently providing microvascular free flap coverage. It is the authors' recommendation that immediate coverage, or coverage within 72 hours, is preferable to repeat debridements over a longer period. It is true that repeated examinations of the wound reveal nonviable tissues, but the marginal tissues that have desiccated with the passing of time might have been salvaged if immediate coverage had occurred.

Definitive closure within 72 hours is also advantageous in terms of bone healing. If repeated debridements are performed over several days, the bone fragments desiccate or become excessively contaminated, necessitating removal of all free fragments of bone, including the large fragments. If immediate coverage is applied, however, the large fragments with soft tissue attachments can be salvaged, eliminating the need for a secondary bone grafting procedure or at least reducing the size of the bone defect. The advantages of acute coverage include a shorter hospital stay, less pain associated with dressing changes, decreased infection rate, and a superior long-term result.

It is equally important to determine which injuries are not appropriate for limb salvage. If the knee and the ankle are damaged with significant intervening soft tissue trauma, it is unlikely that any reconstruction will provide adequate function to justify salvage of the extremity. In addition, the presence of sensibility on the sole of the foot must be considered. An above knee injury with a wide zone of injury to the tibial component of the sciatic nerve has a poor prognosis. The indications for limb salvage are also discussed in the section on Replantation.

Open Fractures and Bone Healing

An understanding of the three sources of tibial blood supply provides a framework in which to assess the vascularity and potential healing ability of any tibial fracture. The posterior tibial artery provides the *nutrient artery* to the tibia, entering the bone posteriorly at the junction of the proximal and middle thirds of the bone (Fig. 82–25) (Rhinelander, 1974; Macnab and De Haas, 1974). The nutrient artery occupies an oblique groove in the tibial cortex, approximately 5 cm in length. Once inside the medullary cavity, the nutrient artery gives off proximal and distal branches that supply the cortex from its endosteal surface. The second source of blood supply is the *metaphyseal branches.* Neighboring arteries provide branches to the metaphysis of the tibia that anastomose within the medullary cavity with branches from the nutrient artery in the most proximal

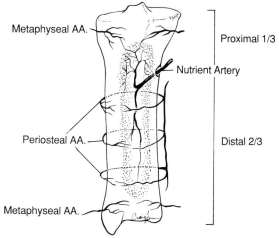

Figure 82–25. Blood supply of the tibia. The nutrient artery enters the cortex at the junction of the proximal and middle thirds of the tibia. Fractures through the diaphysis, therefore, necessarily injure the endosteal circulation, leaving the segmental periosteal arteries as the only source of blood supply to the fracture site. Because of the superficial location of the tibia, however, open fractures frequently also injure the periosteum, thereby rendering the fracture ischemic and prone to infection and nonunion.

and distal aspects of the bone. The *periosteal vessels* provide the third source of tibial blood supply. Unlike the endosteal blood vessels, which run longitudinally, the periosteal vessels are oriented perpendicular to the long axis of the bone. The periosteal circulation provides circulation to the outer one-third of the tibial cortex, while the endosteal circulation supplies the inner two-thirds.

If the tibia is fractured and displaced, the longitudinally oriented branches of the nutrient artery are of necessity disrupted. The bone distal to the fracture therefore is supplied by the transversely oriented periosteal blood supply, and the distal metaphysis by the metaphyseal arteries. As demonstrated by Rhinelander (1974), the normal dominance of the endosteal circulation is interrupted when a displaced fracture occurs, and the periosteal circulation becomes the chief source of blood supply to the healing fracture site. Any interruption in the periosteal blood supply therefore compromises the healing fracture and necessitates coverage of the bone by healthy tissue that can provide neovascularization to the periosteal structures.

A nondisplaced fracture that is rigidly stabilized demonstrates direct osseous healing by blood supply from the medullary cavity. This situation provides the most rapid type of bone healing. If either the blood supply to the fracture is compromised or the stabilization is not perfect, direct osseous healing does not occur and wound repair must be accomplished via a periosteal callus. Periosteal callus normally appears on approximately the third day with blood supply from the surrounding soft tissues and periosteum. The callus contains a zone of fibrocartilage that provides stabilization for the healing fracture, but leads to a much slower bony union than does direct osseous healing. Although it has not been definitively proved (Holden, 1972; Macnab and De Haas, 1974; Gothman, 1960), it appears that in the setting of damaged periosteum the surrounding soft tissue becomes the source of blood supply to the healing fracture. Delayed healing of displaced tibial fractures therefore is related to the subcutaneous location of the tibia and the resultant paucity of surrounding soft tissue.

Open fractures of the tibia have been classified by Gustillo and Anderson (1976) according to the degree of severity. A *Type I fracture* is an open fracture with a cutaneous wound less than 1 cm in length; a *Type II*

fracture involves extensive soft tissue damage; and a *Type III fracture* represents an open fracture or segmental fractures with extensive soft tissue damage that may require vascular repair. Byrd, Spicer, and Cierny (1985) enlarged the classification of open tibial fractures into four types in order of increasing energy of injury (Fig. 82–26). A *Type I fracture* represents low energy forces causing an oblique fracture of the tibia with a relatively clean cutaneous wound less than 2 cm in length. A *Type II fracture* indicates moderate energy forces causing either a displaced fracture or a comminuted tibia fracture with a skin wound greater than 2 cm in length, and accompanying moderate skin and muscle contusion without devitalized muscle. A *Type III fracture* results from high energy forces causing a significantly displaced or severely comminuted fracture or segmental fractures with extensive associated skin loss and devitalized muscle. A *Type IV fracture* pattern indicates extreme energy forces, a history of crush or degloving injury, or associated vascular injury requiring repair.

It is critical that both plastic surgeon and orthopedic surgeon evaluate the injury concomitantly at the time of the debridement. After the debridement has been accomplished, bone fixation can be provided by one of several techniques. For tibial fractures with significant associated soft tissue injury, the external fixator is almost always used. However, there have been no studies of internal fixation and the placement of *immediate* microvascular free muscle transfers. It seems likely that the success of external pin fixation over internal fixation is related to the extent of contamination at the time at which bone fixation is achieved. Since the wounds are frequently associated with severe soft tissue injury, successful placement of internal fixation would require a perfect debridement and placement of immediate soft tissue coverage for wound closure. In injuries of the femur, where abundant muscle is available for coverage, internal fixation is more often indicated.

As mentioned in the section on assessment of trauma, there is some disagreement regarding comminuted fractures as to whether all bone fragments should be debrided. The disagreement can be resolved if the timing of wound closure is considered. If an immediate closure of the wound is to be accomplished, either by local muscle tissue or by free tissue

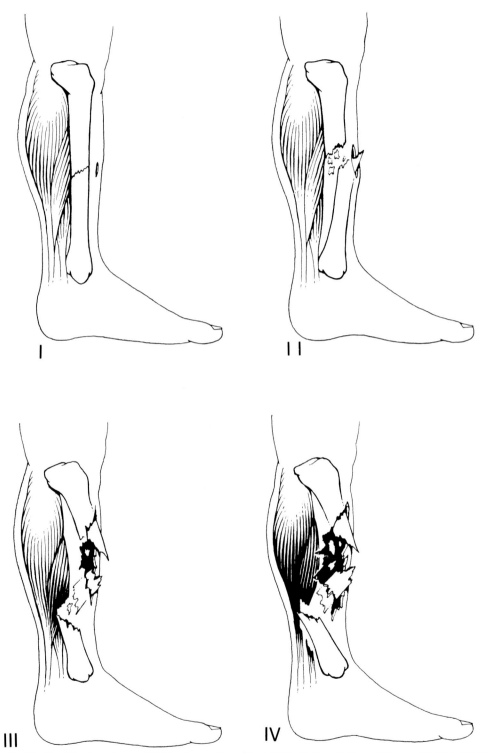

Figure 82–26. Classification of open tibial fractures. (From Byrd, H. S., Spicer, R. E., and Cierny, G.: The management of open tibial fractures. Plast. Reconstr. Surg., 76:719, 1985.)

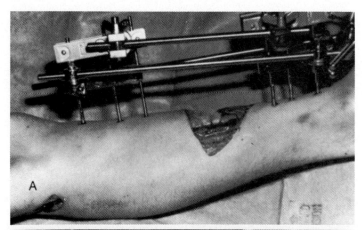

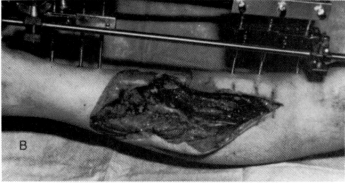

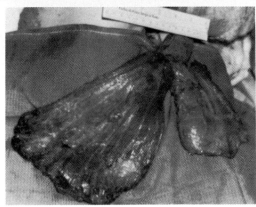

Figure 82–27. High energy–induced open tibial fracture. *A,* Medial view after stabilization in an anterior half-frame external fixator device. The construction of the frame allows easy access to the posterior tibial and popliteal vasculature for possible microsurgical anastomoses during free tissue transfer, as well as access to the gastrocnemius and soleus muscles when local muscle transfer is indicated. *B,* Lateral view showing access for bedside wound care. Note the pretibial skin demarcation in this wound five days after injury and after two formal operative debridements. *C,* The latissimus dorsi and serratus muscles harvested on a common thoracodorsal pedicle. This arrangement allows the transfer of a large amount of soft tissue for wound closure as well as the possibility of various flap orientations.

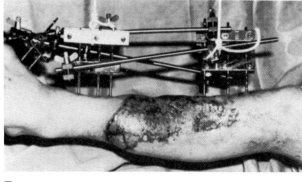

E

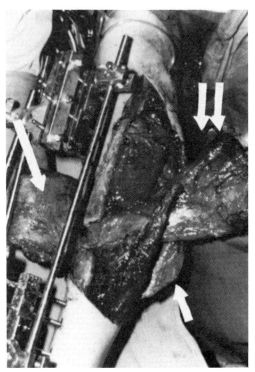

D

Figure 82–27 *Continued D,* The patient's knee is at the top of the photo. The thoracodorsal artery was anastomosed to the popliteal artery (via a vein graft) by a medial approach. The latissimus dorsi was placed under the tibial fracture site and the fibular remnant, and then split. The larger portion *(double arrows)* was directed proximally and draped over the tibia. The smaller portion of the split latissimus dorsi *(single short arrow)* was directed distally and draped over the fibular remnant. The serratus *(single long arrow)* was placed over the tibial fracture site. This arrangement effectively obliterated all dead space. *E,* After bone grafting, and six weeks after soft tissue closure using the combined serratus and split latissimus dorsi free muscle transfer. The bone graft was placed from a posterior "stocking seam" approach. (From Yaremchuk, M. J.: Acute management of severe soft-tissue damage accompanying open fractures. Clin. Plast. Surg., *13*:621, 1986.)

transfer, large pieces of bone that still have some soft tissue attachment can be salvaged. If, however, the wound is to be debrided serially over the course of several days or weeks, it is safer to remove all fragments of bone prior to soft tissue closure.

Soft Tissue Coverage After Trauma

The importance of obtaining early definitive wound healing after lower extremity trauma cannot be overemphasized. In the words of Cannon and Constable (1977), "The restoration of an intact cutaneous covering is the primary surgical requisite following trauma of the lower extremity because deep healing can be no better than the surface covering."

The time-honored concept of dividing the lower leg into thirds and discussing coverage in each third on the basis of the proximity of local muscle flaps remains useful, but must be subordinated to a more functional and esthetic evaluation of the wound. The surgeon should decide what form of coverage, given the individual circumstances, will provide the most functional and esthetic result, rather than perform necessarily the simplest procedure that will do the job. In other words, an open wound in the vicinity of the knee traditionally calls for a gastrocnemius muscle flap. The latter may indeed be the procedure of choice in that circumstance, but one must consider (1) that trauma to the posterior knee may have disrupted the blood supply to that muscle; (2) that the function of the lower extremity will undoubtedly be affected, albeit slightly, by sacrificing that component of plantar flexion; and (3) that it is necessary to compare the gastrocnemius flap to a microvascular free muscle flap, which, statistically, is at least as likely to be successful. The last consideration is an esthetic one: a gastrocnemius muscle flap effaces the normal contour of the posterior calf. A free muscle flap, however, allows more freedom in designing the exact flap for that particular wound, and at the same time does not have the undesirable esthetic impact of some lower extremity muscle flaps. Nonetheless, local muscle flaps have a definite place in lower extremity reconstruction, and are much more expeditious than free tissue transfer. The overall condition of the patient and the specific anatomy of the wound determine which technique is ideal in each circumstance.

The importance of debridement and the controversy over the timing of coverage have been discussed. The authors' preference is for immediate or acute coverage of all lower extremity injuries within 72 hours, barring other injuries or systemic problems that may preclude such intervention. Free tissue transfer to the lower extremity for trauma has been shown to reduce the number of operative procedures required as compared with traditional muscle flap techniques.

In an otherwise healthy young patient with isolated trauma to the lower extremity, immediate microvascular free tissue coverage of a lower extremity wound without preoperative angiography is a reasonable alternative. In an older patient with atherosclerosis, it is recommended that a formal arteriogram be obtained prior to free tissue transfer. In this circumstance, thorough debridement at the time of injury, followed by an arteriogram and free flap coverage of the wound, should be accomplished within 72 hours of the injury.

Acute injuries as well as some chronic conditions in the lower extremity frequently result in venous hypertension. It is preferable to use deep veins in the lower extremity for microvascular anastomosis unless examination of the deep veins and attempted irrigation of these structures reveal obvious venous hypertension. In that case, anastomoses should be performed to both the deep system and a superficial vein such as the greater saphenous. The propensity for spasm in the saphenous vein makes the superficial veins of the lower extremity a definite second choice for microvascular anastomosis. In acute injuries, intraoperative assessment of the venous systems suffices. However, in the setting of a chronic lower extremity condition such as osteomyelitis with swelling and pigmentation suggesting venous disease, it is reasonable to perform venography as well as arteriography before planning microvascular free flap coverage.

A free flap to the lower extremity, like any reconstructive procedure, is only as good as the preoperative plan (Fig. 82–27). Both the recipient vessels and the donor site anatomy are marked on the patient preoperatively. Estimates of pedicle lengths and tissue requirements are made so that intraoperative surprises are minimized. The need for vein grafts can usually be anticipated before the operation, so that harvesting of the vein graft can be incorporated into the operative plan.

Free flap coverage of the lower extremity is best performed with two operative teams. If there is any question about the quality of the recipient vessels, however, the recipient site should be dissected first; otherwise, the two teams can initiate the dissection simultaneously. After the recipient site has been prepared, any incisions in the area are temporarily closed to minimize both contamination and the swelling that accompany several hours of retraction.

After the recipient and donor site dissections are complete, the flap is transferred to the recipient defect. The flap is inset, at least preliminarily, before the vascular anastomoses are performed. It is theoretically preferable to perform the venous anastomosis first; in practice, however, whichever anastomosis allows easiest access to the second anastomosis is done first. Venous anastomoses are generally performed end to end, and arterial anastomoses end to side.

Postoperative management of lower extremity microvascular free flaps includes continuous elevation and monitoring of the flap. If thrombosis of a microvascular anastomosis can be detected early, reexploration often allows salvage of the free flap. In the NYU-Bellevue experience of 304 consecutive free flaps to the lower extremity, reexploration of failing lower extremity free flaps resulted in salvage of 50 per cent (Khouri and Shaw, 1987).

Because of the high energy nature of lower extremity injuries and the consequent magnitude of soft tissue deficits, the most common free flaps used to cover the lower extremity wounds are the latissimus dorsi, the rectus abdominis, and the scapular flaps.

In the NYU-Bellevue experience, the free flap failure rate after lower extremity trauma was 8 per cent, compared with 3 per cent for free flaps to other parts of the body and 0 per cent for free flaps to the lower extremity in nontraumatic cases (Khouri and Shaw, 1987). The increased failure rate in lower extremity trauma was related to the extent of the trauma; the larger wounds with the largest bone gaps and the highest rate of vascular compromise had the highest rate of free flap failure. In addition, there was a fivefold incidence of anastomotic thrombosis when vein grafts were required. The increased complication rate therefore is not inherent to the lower extremity, but rather secondary to the extent or magnitude of the trauma.

Vascular Injuries

Recognition of a vascular injury begins with the examination in the emergency room. Lack of distal pulses in the injured extremity or a reduction in the pulses on the injured side, compared with the noninjured extremity, necessitates a percutaneous transfemoral arteriogram in the operating room. This is a rapid procedure that provides radiographs of adequate quality to determine whether vascular repair is necessary.

The presence of distal pulses does not rule out significant vascular injury. It is well known that posterior knee dislocation and fractures of the distal femur can cause popliteal artery injury. The presence of an injury of this type is an indication for arteriography even if distal pulses are present, in order to rule out an intimal injury that may lead to vascular compromise. A patient presenting with a devascularized lower extremity requires four-compartment fasciotomy of the lower leg. At the conclusion of the arterial repair, repeat transfemoral arteriography is recommended to verify the patency of the anastomosis and the adequacy of distal runoff. The amount of contrast material used for the completion arteriogram is kept to a minimum to avoid nephrotoxicity in these patients, who inevitably have myoglobinemia and have already undergone one arteriogram.

Figure 82–28 shows the arteriogram from a 10 year old girl who fell down an elevator shaft and presented with a fracture of the distal femur and a devascularized lower leg. Transfemoral arteriography confirmed complete occlusion of the popliteal artery above the knee. The patient underwent four-compartment fasciotomy, reversed contralateral saphenous vein bypass from the superficial femoral artery at the adductor hiatus to the distal popliteal artery, and a completion arteriogram to confirm the patency of the bypass graft and three-vessel runoff to the foot.

Open Joint Injuries

Open joint injuries are a frequent component of lower extremity trauma. Patzakis and

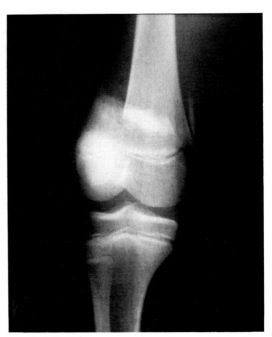

Figure 82–28. Popliteal artery occlusion. The patient is a 10 year old girl who fell down an elevator shaft, sustaining an open fracture of the distal femur. Arteriography demonstrated complete occlusion of the popliteal artery at the fracture site. She underwent four-compartment fasciotomy and a reversed contralateral saphenous vein bypass graft from the superficial femoral artery at the adductor hiatus to the distal popliteal artery.

associates (1975) studied 140 patients with open joint injuries in a prospective fashion. The authors recommended irrigation of the joint surface and primary wound closure without drains. Barford and Pers (1970) reported closure of five open knee joints with immediate gastrocnemius muscle flaps; there were no infections. Open interarticular injuries that are reduced and have sufficient soft tissue for closure do not generally present a problem. In injuries for which there is insufficient tissue for primary closure, immediate muscle flap closure is generally successful. In patients with open joint injuries who have delayed wound closure but in whom definite coverage is provided within 72 hours, the authors have not seen infectious complications.

Chronically open joints are a more difficult problem. However, aggressive debridement of granulation tissue, irrigation, and definitive muscle flap closure are worth the attempt. Drains should always be used in this circumstance. In addition to providing tissue for wound closure, it is essential that range of motion exercises be begun as soon as possible. In fact, such exercises can be initiated prior to definitive treatment of the wound in an attempt to combat scar contracture, which inevitably limits ultimate joint function. In summary, open joint injuries, like exposure of any vital structure, should be definitively covered, whether by primary closure, a local muscle flap, or a microvascular free flap, as soon as possible. Some authors recommend that drains not be used in the acute situation, but the authors have not found a problem with drains. In the setting of chronically contaminated open joints, the incidence of infection associated with joint coverage is much higher. Treatment consists of physical therapy, debridement of the joint, and definitive flap closure.

Nerve Injuries

Nerve injuries in the lower extremity are associated with a poorer prognosis than those in the upper extremity. While upper extremity injuries are frequently the result of industrial accidents, lower extremity injuries are generally related to high speed vehicular trauma. As a result, lower extremity nerve injuries are associated with more extensive damage to both the nerve and the surrounding soft tissue. In addition, injuries in the lower extremity tend to occur more proximally than in the upper extremity, a finding that makes nerve regeneration more problematic. Because of the difficulties associated with lower extremity nerve injuries, as with brachial plexus injuries, there is a tendency to procrastinate in the hope of spontaneous nerve regeneration. It is true that nerve repair in the lower extremity is often not completely successful, but whatever potential for success there may be is lost if surgery is delayed. The most common mistake in treating nerve injuries of the lower extremity is therefore the decision not to explore a nerve injury.

Assessing the potential for spontaneous nerve regeneration, or analyzing the need for nerve repair or grafting, requires detailed knowledge of the level and extent of nerve injury, the condition of the surrounding tissue, and the integrity of end organs that the nerve innervates. If a complete motor and sensory deficit exists when the patient is first examined in the emergency room, the nerve most likely has been divided or undergone irreversible injury related to traction. Progressive neurologic deterioration while a patient is in the emergency room, however, is more likely the result of ischemia related to arterial injury or to a compartment syndrome. If any doubt exists concerning the integrity of a lower extremity nerve, it should be explored. When there is a partial deficit in the setting of blunt trauma, indicating that the nerve is still in anatomic continuity, a delayed exploration can be justified. Even partial deficits require exploration after penetrating trauma.

The surgeon decides at the time of the injury how long to wait for spontaneous recovery, so that exploration is not repeatedly delayed beyond the time when improvement might be expected. If exploration of a nerve injury reveals complete transection, the timing of nerve repair depends on the mechanism of injury and the condition of the associated wound. For an uncontaminated, sharp transection of a major lower extremity nerve, the results occur when repair is accomplished within 72 hours.

A nerve repair, however, should not be performed in a highly contaminated wound when the integrity of the surrounding soft tissue is in question. In such a wound, meticulous debridement and delayed repair are in order. In crush or traction injuries in which long nerve gaps exist in the setting of comparable soft tissue deficits, the use of vascularized nerve grafts and reconstruction of the soft tissue with microvascular free flaps may be the optimal choice (Briedenbach and Terzis, 1984; Shaw and Hidalgo, 1987).

When a nerve has been injured in close proximity to the muscle it innervates, and when the distal stump cannot be located, neurotization of the muscle by direct implantation of the proximal motor nerve stump or a nerve graft from that stump into the muscle is a reasonable alternative (Wigand and associates, 1976).

Although nerve repairs in the lower extremity do not boast excellent results, the results are not as dismal as commonly believed. Protective sensibility returns more reliably than motor function, but if the sensibility is on the sole of the foot, it can make the difference between a functional and a nonfunctional extremity. Kline (1989, 1982) reported an improvement in 15 of 24 patients with complete sciatic nerve injuries. He found uniform return of useful tibial motor and sensory functions in four patients and partial recovery of footdrop in two patients whose sciatic nerve transections were explored and repaired primarily. In Seddon's (1972) series of 47 tibial nerve repairs, 62 per cent of patients had sensory recovery and 79 per cent functional motor recovery. It should be noted, however, that repair of the tibial nerve was also associated with hyperesthesia of the sole, which may be more incapacitating than the initial lesion.

Reconstruction of Bone Gaps and Chronic Non-Union

Osseous defects after lower extremity trauma can be reconstructed either at the same time as the soft tissue reconstruction or at a second stage. When designing the operative approach to an osseous defect, one must consider the presence or absence of infection, the size of the defect, the soft tissue requirements, the availability of various bone donor sites, and finally the time that it will take to restore the patient to full weight-bearing status. Small bone defects up to 6 cm in length, in the presence of adequate soft tissue, can be adequately restored with nonvascularized cancellous bone grafts (see Fig. 82–27), usually from the iliac crest. When such short osseous defects are associated with a large soft tissue defect, the options are to restore the soft tissue by free flap coverage with simultaneous bone grafting, or by a two-stage procedure consisting of free flap coverage with simultaneous bone grafting, or by a two-stage procedure consisting of free flap coverage and delayed cancellous bone grafting. If a simultaneous reconstruction of soft tissue and bone is performed, Swartz and Mears (1986) recommend the use of free osteocutaneous flaps (Fig. 82–29). A more conservative approach that provides a healthy soft tissue environment at the first stage and nonvascularized cancellous bone grafts at the second stage is more universally accepted at the present time (Shaffer and associates, 1985; Bieber and Wood, 1986). It must be recognized that a two-stage procedure requires a minimum of six weeks between operations, an interval that contributes significantly to the overall time needed to restore weight-bearing status.

For high energy injuries resulting in longer bone deficits associated with soft tissue requirements, it is generally agreed that a two-stage procedure is indicated. The zone of injury in such high velocity injuries makes immediate one-stage reconstruction with an osteocutaneous free flap somewhat risky. There is not general agreement, however, as to the method of reconstructing long bone defects in the lower extremity. If the soft tissue environment has been restored, long bone defects can be successfully bridged with nonvascularized bone grafts (Enneking, Eady, and Burchardt, 1980). Another alternative, if the fibula is intact, is to create a synostosis (Fig. 82–30) between the tibia and fibula by using cancellous bone graft above and below the defect, thereby bypassing the tibial defect (Harmon, 1945; Gregory, Chapman, and Hansen, 1984). This relatively simple technique provides an adequate alternative to a complex bone reconstruction.

The alternative, which has been embraced by microsurgeons to bridge long bone defects, is the vascularized bone flap. An ipsilateral pedicled fibula transfer is discouraged because the supplementary mechanical support of an intact fibula is destroyed. A free vascularized fibula flap from the contralateral extremity, however, is a potential solution (Fig. 82–31). Although it has not been shown that patients with free fibula flaps are able to ambulate in a shorter time than those receiving more conventional bone grafts, vascularized bone flaps heal in a fashion similar to fresh fractures, have a higher and faster rate of union than conventional grafts, and demonstrate more rapid remodeling and hypertrophy (Lau and Leung, 1982; Cutting and McCarthy, 1983; Tessier, Bonnel, and Allieu, 1985). The fibula is largely cortical, allowing secure fixation with cortical-cancellous screws. The bone flaps may be step cut or dowled to fit the bone on either end of the defects. In the femur, the fibula may be employed as a double-barreled flap by preserving a periosteal hinge, increasing the diameter of the bone flap to provide a better size match with the femur. Other donor sites such as the iliac crest and the scapula also provide vascularized bone flaps for smaller effects.

Two other techniques for treating osseous defects deserve mention. The Papineau technique (Mears and associates, 1983; Cierny and Mader, 1983) is a method of closing open bone defects. The bone defect is debrided and moistened with saline-soaked dressings until

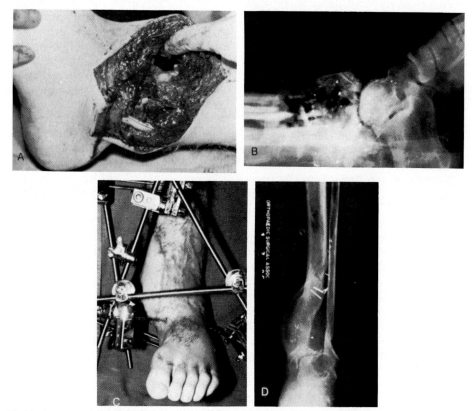

Figure 82–29. A 25 year old man sustained a gunshot wound of the distal tibia resulting in a through and through defect that spared the posterior tibial neurovascular bundle. After two debridements, a one-stage reconstruction was performed using iliac crest bone and the overlying skin in combination with the internal oblique muscle. Soft tissue coverage was provided for both sides of the ankle. *A,* The open wound, showing the through and thorugh defect at the time of initial debridement. *B,* Radiograph shows destruction of the distal tibia. *C,* The closed wound at three weeks with external fixation stabilization. *D,* The healed bone defect at six months with full weight bearing provided. Secondary recontouring of the bone graft for esthetic purposes is planned. (Courtesy of Dr. Neil F. Jones. From Swartz, W. M., and Mears, D. C.: Management of difficult lower extremity fractures and nonunions. Clin. Plast. Surg., *13*:633, 1986.)

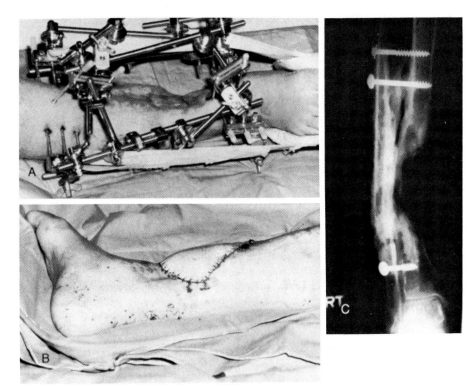

Figure 82–30. The tibia-fibula synostosis is a useful method for treating long segmental bone defects. *A*, Preoperative view of a patient with a 14 cm segmental defect of the distal tibia. The wound was initially managed with external fixation and skin grafting to obtain a closed wound. *B*, Results of a cross leg flap for obtaining soft tissue coverage after a failed latissimus dorsi free flap and free fibula reconstruction. *C*, After debridement of the necrotic fibula, a tibia-fibula synostosis was performed. Hypertrophy of the ipsilateral fibula was noted at 18 months. (From Swartz, W. M., and Mears, D. C.: Management of difficult lower extremity fractures and nonunions. Clin. Plast. Surg., *13*:633, 1986.)

a continuous granulating bed lines the defect. The defect is then filled with cancellous bone grafts and covered with a moist dressing. The wound either reepithelizes or is closed with a skin graft after granulation tissue has vascularized the bone graft. This technique has been successful even in the setting of chronic osteomyelitis.

The second technique represents the most recent development in the reconstruction of lower extremity defects. Originally described by Ilizarov (1954), a corticotomy is made proximal to the osseous defect, taking care to preserve the periosteum; after ten days in an external fixator, the external fixation device is lengthened 1 mm per day. The callus is thereby gradually lengthened and mature bone is allowed to replace the callus. The bone lengthening technique holds considerable promise for lower extremity bone reconstruction, although (like bone grafting) the time between operation and fixator-free ambulation is still long.

The principles that apply to the treatment of osseous defects also apply to the treatment of chronic non-union of the lower extremity. If infection is present, the non-union is treated in the same way as chronic osteomyelitis; radical debridement and soft tissue replacement are followed by restoration of bone integrity. In the absence of an infection, it is generally adequate to debride the ends of the bone, reduce the fracture, and reconstruct the defect with whatever soft tissue and bone elements are required.

Compartment Syndromes

Blick and associates (1986) reviewed 198 acute open fractures of the tibia and reported a 9.1 per cent incidence of compartment syndrome. It is important to realize that the soft tissue laceration accompanying an open fracture does not allow adequate decompression of the four compartments. DeLee and Stiehl

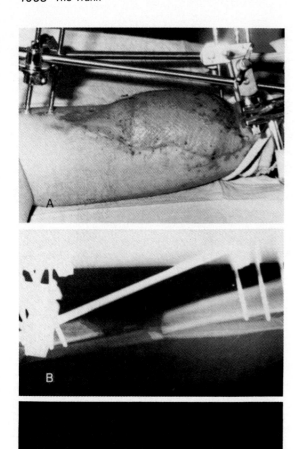

Figure 82–31. Severe traumatic injury to the lower extremity caused by a motorcycle accident. The soft tissue and bone defect measured 16 cm and was treated in two stages. First, a rectus abdominis muscle flap was transferred by microvascular anastomosis. Six weeks later, a contralateral free fibula flap was transferred. *A,* The lower extremity after transfer of the rectus abdominis flap and skin graft. *B,* Segmental bone defect before bone reconstruction. *C,* Free fibula transfer at five months, when protected weight bearing was begun. (From Swartz, W. M., and Mears, D. C.; Management of difficult lower extremity fractures and nonunions. Clin. Plast. Surg., *13*:633, 1986.)

(1981) reported a 6 per cent incidence of compartment syndrome in open tibial fractures and a 1 to 2 per cent incidence in closed tibial fractures. The development of a compartment syndrome is directly related to the degree of trauma to the soft tissues and bone.

Compartment pressures can be measured by a variety of techniques (Blick and associates, 1986). The best method of avoiding the morbidity associated with compartment syndrome, however, is to perform fasciotomies whenever a lower extremity injury is accompanied by interruption of the arterial system, or whenever there is a clinical suspicion of a compartment syndrome based on either deteriorating neurologic function or obviously tense compartments. If doubt exists, the compartment pressures can be measured and appropriate action taken, depending on the measurements.

REPLANTATION

Amputation has historically been the treatment of choice for severely injured limbs. In addition, the lack of antibiotics, adequate anesthesia, and appropriate surgical techniques precluded any complex salvage reconstructions. The concept of revascularizing an incompletely amputated extremity, or replanting a completely amputated one, was not seriously entertained until the twentieth century.

Carrel and Guthrie (1906) performed some of the earliest experimental replantation studies. Stimulated by an interest in human transplantation, they replanted canine hindlimbs by utilizing techniques gained from their pioneering work in vascular repair. Interest in replantation research waned until the 1950's, when several Russian surgeons performed numerous canine replantations with long-term limb survival. Lapchinsky (1960) reported a series of canine replantations at the midthigh level, with follow-up extending as long as six years; satisfactory function and limb survival were demonstrated. His experimental studies demonstrated the importance of cooling in the preservation of the amputated limb; some successful replantations occurred after devascularization of over 24 hours.

Clinical replantation was first achieved in the early 1960's. In 1962 Malt performed the first successful reattachment of a completely amputated arm in a young boy injured in a train accident (Malt and McKhann, 1964). The same year, Chen, Chien, and Pao (1963) reported the first successful replantation of a hand amputated at the wrist level.

Unique Surgical Problems in Replantation

Multisystem trauma or other injuries frequently coexist with amputation injuries. Head, chest, and abdominal injuries must be carefully evaluated if a lengthy replantation procedure is a possibility. Closed head injury should be evaluated by CT scan. It may be acceptable to proceed with operation if intracranial pressure monitoring is instituted. Blunt chest wall and abdominal trauma must also be carefully evaluated. Peritoneal lavage should be performed before a replantation of any magnitude on the lower extremity, since it may be necessary to heparinize the patient during the course of replantation.

Ischemia Time

Critical to the success of any replantation effort is the restoration of circulation to the amputated part before irreversible tissue changes develop. In the extremities, the most vulnerable tissue is the skeletal muscle, which can tolerate only four to six hours of warm ischemia. When a large muscle mass is involved, as in the case of lower extremity amputations, "core cooling" is not effectively achieved by surface contact cooling. It must be recognized that ischemia starts from the time of injury and ends only after successful arterial repair is accomplished. Arterial inflow can be temporarily instituted by the use of shunts in an effort to reduce the warm ischemia time.

During the interval between injury and revascularization a series of complex events must take place successfully in order to ensure a functional replantation. First, the patient must be transported to an appropriate emergency facility for the initial evaluation. He is then brought to the replantation center in preparation for surgery. Preoperative assessment, laboratory tests, anesthesia induction, preliminary debridement, and bone fixation must take place before arterial repair.

Zone of Injury

The forces resulting in amputation create injured tissues proximal and distal to the amputation site. The area must be carefully assessed and all injured tissues debrided. Damaged blood vessels and nerves must be completely excised to guarantee vessel patency and more complete nerve regeneration following replantation. Any gaps created must be bridged with appropriate vein or nerve grafts.

Nonviable muscle must be completely debrided to avoid subsequent infection. Viable but contused muscle with hemorrhage is often difficult to differentiate from nonviable muscle. In addition, when severe contamination is present in combination with contused muscle, subsequent infection may result. The individual "muscle unit" concept must be kept in mind when debriding muscle. It is of no functional value to debride either the proximal or distal muscle while ignoring the remainder of the muscle unit. "Muscle unit" debridement has the added advantage of minimizing bleeding as compared with debridement through the muscle bellies.

Large bone fragments that are attached to viable tissue may be preserved. However, periosteal blood supply to bone must be intact to avoid a late sequestrum of bone. Shortening the bone within the zone of injury may allow total debridement and subsequent primary healing of the wound edges, while at the same time minimizing nerve and vessel grafting.

It is important to keep in mind the mechanism of amputation when evaluating the zone of injury. Sharp, clean "guillotine" amputations have a minimal zone of injury, but these are seen only occasionally. Amputations involving a combination of crush and avulsion are by far the most common variety.

Replacement of Lost Tissue

The destruction of different tissue types within the zone of injury is seldom uniform. Bone shortening can be performed in order to minimize the amount of soft tissue replacement necessary. However, bone shortening in the lower extremity must be minimized to prevent gait disturbance that cannot be corrected by a heel lift, a pelvic tilt, or a subsequent bone lengthening procedure. Vein grafts, nerve grafts, skin grafts, muscle flaps, and composite free flaps are examples of available methods to maximize extremity length when bone shortening would result in an unusable lower extremity.

Traumatic amputation of the lower extremity has been successfully treated with a prosthesis for many years. Virtually normal function can be obtained in most cases of below knee amputation, because the requirements of a lower extremity substitute are relatively simple compared with those of an upper extremity.

Nature of Amputation Injury

Military injury historically accounted for most lower extremity amputations. However, today the most common causes involve crushing injury such as seen in automobile, train, and heavy farm equipment accidents. There is a high incidence of bilateral lower extremity injury because of the anatomic proximity of the legs.

Most lower extremity amputations have a wide zone of crush injury. There frequently is extensive laceration and degloving of the soft tissues. Multiple levels of injury may also occur. The amount of blood loss may be considerable.

The "bumper" injury is unique to the lower extremity. Both extremities are usually in-volved at a level just below the knee. The amputation is frequently incomplete, with possible disruption of both knee joints as well as the popliteal vessels. The associated tibial fractures are severe and reflect the explosive nature of the impact forces.

Avulsion of the plantar surface of the foot is a special type of lower extremity injury. Avulsion may occur superficial or deep to the level of the plantar fascia. The injuries are typically difficult to assess acutely. Experience has shown that despite the presence of dermal bleeding in the most distal part of the flap, it usually does not survive. The lateral plantar artery supplies most of the weight-bearing portion of the plantar surface.

Revascularization of the avulsed flap is possible with a vein graft from the intact proximal artery and vein to the lateral plantar vessels or its branches.

Indications for Replantation

After the general medical condition of the patient is deemed acceptable, replantation efforts may proceed. The time-honored adage of "life over limb" must be observed.

The condition of the amputated part must be assessed. A wide zone of injury increases the magnitude of the replantation by requiring complex soft tissue replacement or severe bone shortening. Extensive muscle or nerve loss effectively rules out replantation since a poor functional result will be the outcome. Multiple levels of injury must also be ruled out. Even though the proximal stump and the proximal end of the amputated part may appear favorable for replantation, distal contusion, bone injury, or crushed vascular components jeopardize any replantation effort.

The amount of bone shortening permissible in lower extremity amputation injuries is limited to 8 to 10 cm at maximum (Chen and Zeng, 1983). Compensating mechanisms of pelvic tilt and shoe elevation cannot effectively cope with more bone shortening. When both lower extremities are amputated, bone shortening becomes a less critical issue.

If the knee joint is severely injured, a stiff, painful lower extremity will result from replantation. In addition, the soft tissue envelope surrounding the knee is poor. Free tissue transfer will undoubtedly be necessary to achieve adequate soft tissue coverage.

Associated nerve injury is a critical factor

in determining whether to replant an amputated lower limb. Long nerve gaps or severe avulsion of nerves make favorable replantation results unlikely.

These rough guidelines must be carefully individualized when considering lower extremity replantation. A more liberal approach to replantation may be undertaken for bilateral lower extremity amputations and in younger patients.

Salvage Replantation

After the decision not to attempt replantation has been made, planning should be directed toward achieving as low a level of amputation as possible. Preservation of the knee joint, for example, simplifies rehabilitation and reduces the additional morbidity that accompanies above knee amputations.

Salvage replantation most commonly involves using portions of the foot as a microvascular free flap to provide soft tissue coverage of a below knee stump with adequate tibial length, but inadequate soft tissue coverage. A fillet of foot free flap allows transfer of the entire soft tissue envelope of the foot for proximal stump coverage (see Fig. 82–22). The heel pad can be placed over the bony stump and reinnervated, the distal tibial nerve being anastomosed to the proximal tibial nerve.

A unique type of salvage replantation is possible in certain cases of bilateral lower extremity amputation. When the amputation occurs at a different level on each side and neither side is replantable, it may be feasible to reconstruct at least one functional limb by cross leg replantation (Fig. 82–32). In this situation the best amputated part is replanted to the longer proximal stump, even though this may mean placing the foot on the contralateral side of the body. Successful subsequent ambulation has been demonstrated by Chen and Zeng (1983) and Colen and associates (1983).

Operative Technique

Lower extremity replantation involves the following techniques: debridement, bone fixation, vascular repair, nerve repair, soft tissue coverage, and fasciotomy.

Adequate debridement constitutes the first operative steps, all crushed and devitalized tissue being removed. When a major portion of a muscle is debrided and it is no longer in continuity, it makes little sense to preserve the remaining muscle. However, viable but nonfunctioning portions of muscle should be retained when they provide the only soft tissue coverage of underlying critical structures. Large bone pieces with intact soft tissue attachments should not be excised, because an intact periosteal blood supply maintains their viability. Bone shortening is performed as part of the debridement.

After debridement is complete, the replantation plan is reassessed. There may be sufficient soft tissue loss to necessitate immediate free tissue transfer, or it may be apparent that multiple secondary procedures will be needed with only a small chance of a functional result. The risks and benefits are weighed, and the plan is modified or the replantation attempt abandoned.

Bone fixation may be performed by either internal or external fixation. It must be remembered that internal fixation further compromises the bony vascular supply because of the periosteal stripping necessary to place the hardware. External fixation carries fewer acute infection risks, but the fixation is less precise. Moreover, the bone is not compressed and wound care may be more difficult. However, when dealing with contaminated crush wounds, external fixation is ideal since it allows continuous monitoring of the wound.

Vascular repair must proceed expeditiously. Vascular shunts may be used to obtain perfusion of a distal part when ischemia time is critical. Amputations of the lower extimity generally survive with only one artery being repaired. The repair of a deep vein is essential for amputations above the level of the ankle. The saphenous vein alone can provide adequate venous drainage for an isolated foot replantation.

Vein grafts must be used to overcome vessel gaps. They should be harvested from the opposite leg. Soft tissue coverage of vein grafts must be adequate, since thrombosis or wound infection risks limb loss.

Nerve repair proceeds next. Primary nerve repair should be done whenever possible. The main disadvantage is that the full extent of nerve damage cannot always be appreciated acutely. Repairs that require nerve grafts should not be done primarily except under ideal conditions. The amount of donor nerve

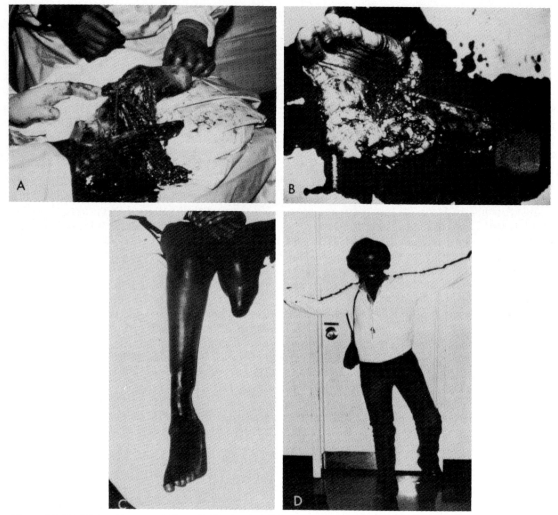

Figure 82–32. Bilateral leg amputation with "foot switch." *A, B,* Bilateral lower extremity injuries. *C, D,* Appearance ten months after replantation. (From Colen, S. R., Romita, M. C., Godfrey, N. V., and Shaw, W. W.: Salvage replantation. Clin. Plast. Surg., *10*:125, 1983.)

available is limited and conditions must be optimized before grafting.

Proper orientation of the sciatic nerve in above knee amputations is essential. The tibial and peroneal divisions should be reapproximated. Amputations through the middle of the leg should have the sural nerve repaired posteriorly as well. Amputations of the distal third should also have the superficial peroneal nerve repaired laterally. Foot amputations should proceed with repair of the tibial nerve or each of the medial calcaneal, medial plantar, and lateral plantar nerves when possible.

Adequate soft tissue coverage of underlying critical structures such as the site of bone fixation, hardware, vessels, nerves, or grafts must be provided. If local soft tissue is inadequate, free tissue transfer must accompany replantation. Local muscle flaps within the zone of injury are unreliable for coverage, particularly when wide mobilization is needed. Fortunately, sufficient bone shortening obviates the need for additional soft tissue coverage in most cases.

Fasciotomy should be routinely performed after revascularization. Four-compartment fasciotomy from a lateral approach without fibulectomy is the preferred method.

Postoperative Management

The leg should be continuously elevated throughout the postoperative period to assist venous return and reduce swelling. Vascular monitoring of the replanted part is essential. Surface temperature probes can be used, using the opposite lower extremity as a control for comparison.

Dextran is given for the first five days after replantation. Heparin is used in selective cases only when there has been extensive crush and the integrity of the vessels is unclear. It is also useful when clotted anastomoses have had to be revised. Broad-spectrum antibiotics are used for two to three days postoperatively pending operative cultures.

Complications of lower extremity replantation include extensive blood loss. Blood loss from the extremity must be controlled. A tourniquet to assist with debridement is a helpful adjunct. Dilutional coagulopathies, disseminated intravascular coagulopathies, and transfusion reactions may result from the multiple transfusions required.

Acidosis, fluid overload, and renal injury are other possible complications. Renal injury may be the result of hypotension due to blood loss or the by-products of myonecrosis, or both.

Minor wound problems are not uncommon and may require additional debridement, skin grafts, or flap procedures. Late soft tissue wound problems generally are best managed with the application of free muscle flaps.

Late complications include wound problems related to poor soft tissue coverage, nonunion, malunion, chronic osteomyelitis, foot deformities, restricted joint motion, plantar ulceration, and chronic pain.

Rehabilitation of the patient with a lower extremity replant includes a program of graded weight bearing in accordance with clinical evidence of healing at the fracture site. A brace for footdrop should be employed. Careful attention to the weight-bearing surface of the foot is essential.

PRINCIPLES OF AMPUTATION AND REHABILITATION

When a lower extremity amputation is required, the level of amputation depends on the etiology. In trauma the level of amputation is determined by the margin of devitalized tissue. In the case of peripheral vascular disease, the amputation is determined by the level at which cutaneous blood flow allows primary healing. When amputation is performed for tumor ablation, the level depends on the location, extent, and behavior of the neoplasm.

In general, the more distal the amputation, the better are the chances of successful ambulation, provided that proper prosthetic fitting can be achieved. Standard teaching dictates that below knee amputations be performed 5 inches below the knee and that above knee amputations be at the midthigh. These are acceptable levels that work well with standard prostheses (Aldredge and Murphy, 1954; Burgess, Romano, Zettl and associates, 1969). However, one must distinguish youthful traumatic amputees from elderly patients with peripheral vascular disease and diabetes. The functional requirements of the latter group are clearly different from the "high demand" requirements of younger patients.

Forefoot Level. Foot amputations are common sequelae of lawn mower accidents. Orthotic inserts can be worn within the shoe for any type or level of forefoot amputation. Because of the lack of available local flaps, foot amputations are salvaged in increasing numbers by the use of microvascular free flaps. Standard transmetatarsal amputations, if available, with a longer plantar skin closure are ideal and yield superior results to painful, cold-sensitive, dysfunctional, partial forefoot amputations.

Hind Foot–Ankle Level. Syme's amputation is the common type at this level. A broad ankle may be esthetically unpleasing when this amputation level is chosen in women. The attributes of a well-positioned heel pad for maximal weight-bearing tolerance are obvious.

Below Knee Level. The conventional below knee level is satisfactory for most patients. However, the Ertl osteomyoplasty adds the advantages of (1) closing the medullary canal, (2) increasing the surface area, (3) improving the end-bearing potential, and (4) decreasing the sometimes painful motion of a retained fibula (Keblish, 1986).

The energy requirements for a below knee amputation level are minimal compared with above knee amputations. Thus, any level of below knee amputation maintaining knee motion is preferable. Microvascular free flap reconstruction may be necessary to close the soft tissue deficit while maintaining the bone length (Gallico and associates, 1987).

Through Knee Level or Knee Disc Articulation. Prosthetists have criticized through knee level amputation, especially in women, because of the disproportionate knee lengths that complicate the design of the required prosthesis. However, recent prosthetic improvements have made through the knee amputation better tolerated.

Above Knee Amputation. A supracondylar level above knee amputation is well served with patellofemoral fusion, which provides firm bone to tendon anchorage. Knee levels can easily be equalized with prosthetic fittings, and end-bearing weight potential is excellent.

Standard Midthigh Amputation. The standard above knee level amputation, despite myoplastic closure, has proved less than satisfactory. The large thigh muscle mass tends to undergo massive disuse atrophy with a disproportionate amount of floppy skin that must be controlled by the prosthesis. Newer prostheses using suction have made the standard above knee amputation more tolerable.

Postoperative Care

After amputation it is imperative that joint contracture be avoided. The avoidance of contractures maintains proper body mechanics for subsequent prosthesis use. Range of motion exercises must be instituted early with a trained physical therapist.

Postoperative therapy must assist the amputee in the transition from inactivity to the rigorous program necessary for proper prosthetic amputation. This initially begins with simple exercises while the patient is still in bed. The program slowly advances to transfer activities such as moving from the supine to the sitting position and transferring from bed to chair. During this time careful attention must be paid to areas of potential skin breakdown, because of the new pressure points existing after the amputation.

Preprosthetic training is then instituted. Exercises are performed on the residual limb in an effort to create gross movements of the antigravity muscles. This is planned to enhance subsequent proprioception with the prosthetic limb. The principal muscle groups involved are the hip extensors, adductors, and internal rotators as well as the quadriceps and hamstrings when a below knee amputation is performed. The exercises also increase joint mobility.

Standard postural exercises are undertaken to avoid subsequent lower back pain with stressed ambulation. Mat exercises, including push-ups, sit-ups, back arching, and rolling, are used to increase trunk mobility and improve physical fitness.

The amputee must master maintaining balance after loss of a portion of one lower extremity. Once this is achieved, crutch walking is instituted.

Residual amputation stump management is begun as soon as primary healing of the wound has occurred. Serial wrappings with pressure dressings are applied in an effort to shape and shrink the stump. If a rigid dressing has been chosen by the surgeon in an attempt to prevent edema, potential pressure excess must be evaluated. The theoretical advantages of a hard shell dressing are that (1) it protects the stump from minor trauma during transfers and early mobilization, (2) it protects the tourniquet effect of wrapping, (3) it encourages shrinkage, (4) it may allow early contact conditioning, and (5) it encourages earlier pylon (practice prosthesis) ambulation.

The above knee amputee who has been given an immediate postsurgical prosthesis should begin gait training as soon as possible. Early gait training helps to reduce hip flexion contractures by requiring the residual limb to be extended at the hip joint when stepping over the prosthesis with the contralateral (normal) limb. The knee joint mechanism should be used as soon as proprioception has been established.

Ambulation should begin with the knee locked. When the foot of the prosthesis is flat on the ground, as in the standing position, the body weight is supported by the arms on the parallel bars.

After approximately two weeks the immediate postsurgical prosthesis is changed. A movable joint at the knee is now utilized for gait training. The amputee is instructed in the normal gait phases of swing and stance.

After primary healing of the stump has occurred, the amputee is fitted with an intermediate pylon approximately 3 to 4 weeks postoperatively. All skills of ambulation are now taught. The patient can make turns, go up and down stairs, and make any other movement necessary for normal ambulation. Going up stairs is performed by having the prosthetic leg reach the step after the non-amputated leg has extended, thereby lifting the prosthetic leg to the next step. Going down stairs, the prosthetic leg descends first.

Today, because of advancing technology and the gains made in rehabilitation, almost all patients with below knee amputations successfully ambulate. Rehabilitation of the below knee amputee follows the same initial steps as those for the above knee amputee patient. Weight bearing on the residual limb in a below knee amputation is performed by the thigh, the tibial condyle, and the distal end of the residual limb. As the stump molds, less weight is borne by the thigh and more weight by the tibial condyles and the distal end of the residual limb. Range of motion exercises are important to maintain motion of the knee joint and avoid any flexion contracture. Strengthening exercises are also necessary in an effort to support and stabilize the knee joint.

Ambulation in below knee amputees begins with balance training. After they have become accustomed to the prosthesis they tolerate the flexing of the knee concurrent to heel contact. The length of stride when ambulating is gradually increased as patients become more experienced.

Care of the residual limb must take high priority. Areas of potential skin breakdown, contact dermatitis, folliculitis, and stasis dermatitis must be sought. The residual limb should be washed daily and inspected carefully by the amputee. The prosthesis socket itself should also be washed and a soft liner kept clean to preserve any leather components. Any signs of a poorly fitting prosthesis should be evaluated early, otherwise they may lead to stump problems or faulty gait patterns.

The obvious goal in the management of any amputee should be to achieve the highest level of function possible. This is accomplished only by maximizing neuromuscular rehabilitation as well as addressing the psychologic needs of a patient who has lost a limb.

OSTEOMYELITIS

The development of osteomyelitis after an extensive compound fracture of the lower extremity is unfortunately not a rare sequela of the injury. Infection is the result of initial massive bacterial contamination, devascularization of soft tissue and bone, or a prolonged delay in primary wound healing (May and associates, 1982, 1984; Moore and Weiland, 1986). May and associates (1982) described five criteria for the diagnosis of chronic bone infection: (1) the presence of exposed bone with drainage for more than six weeks, (2) a positive culture from the wound at the time of debridement, (3) positive bone histology, (4) radiographic findings consistent with chronic bone infection, and (5) a bone scan consistent with chronic bone infection. Acute and subacute osteomyelitis is defined as a condition in which wounds are open for less than six weeks. There may also be persistent drainage, exposed bone, or open fistulous tracts.

Moore and Weiland (1986) defined chronic osteomyelitis as "one or more foci in bone that contain pus, infected granulation tissue, sequestra, a draining sinus and resistant cellulitis. In the depths of the chronically infected bone, there is sclerotic bone covered by a thick vascular tissue of bone scarred muscle and subcutaneous tissue."

Successful treatment of any form of osteomyelitis must first begin with an effective, radical debridement of devascularized bone, poorly vascularized surrounding soft tissue, and infected granulation tissue. The debrided wound can heal by secondary intention, be treated with a skin graft, or be covered by a flap. The work of Ger (1970, 1977) emphasized the role of local muscle and skin muscle flaps as sources of well-vascularized tissue for early wound closure. Stark (1946) described the use of muscle flaps for the surgical treatment of chronic osteomyelitis. The advent of microvascular free tissue transfer has enabled the plastic surgeon to bring well-vascularized soft tissue to distal tibial and fibular lesions in patients in whom local vascularized tissues are nonexistent. Bone management does not have to be carried out at the same time of soft tissue coverage. Staged vascularized free bone transfers (fibular or iliac) can follow. Bone lengthening according to Ilizarov (1954), Monticelli and Spinelli (1983), and DeBastiani and associates (1987) is another alternative. The authors are currently evaluating the efficiency of bone lengthening as opposed to free vascularized bone transfer in such cases.

Godina's work (1986) revolutionized the timing of free tissue transfer after extensive lower extremity trauma. In a series of over 500 cases he reported a 1.5 per cent infection rate in patients treated by free tissue transfer within the first 48 hours following injury. In contrast, cases covered more than 72 hours after the initial trauma yielded a 17 per cent infection rate. Also, bone healing was markedly prolonged compared with the healing in patients treated by early wound coverage. The average interval was 12 months in delayed cases versus six months to bone union in the immediate soft tissue transfer cases.

Chang and Mathes (1982) demonstrated in animal studies that muscle flaps are more resistant to soft tissue infection than similarly inoculated random-pattern skin flaps. They also noted that the oxygen tension of wounds covered by vascularized muscle flaps was higher than that of wounds covered by random-pattern flaps. Although the possibility of ultimate cure of chronic osteomyelitis after radical debridement and subsequent

muscle flap coverage may be questioned because of relatively limited follow-up, there is no doubt that significant gains have been made.

Conclusion

Cases of chronic osteomyelitis must be treated in a sequential manner. First, a wide radical debridement of all necrotic or infected bone and soft tissue must be performed. Bone reconstruction can be staged in cases complicated by segmental bone loss. Wound closure is accomplished by pedicled or free muscle flap procedures. The latter allow both wound closure and a well-vascularized mode for the delivery of antibiotics. Recently, antibiotic-laced beads have also been used in the depths of the wound. Once primary healing has occurred after the muscle flap transfer, bone reconstruction may be undertaken. In patients with relatively short segmental bone loss, cancellous bone grafts have been utilized. For defects larger than 6 to 8 cm in length, either vascularized fibular or iliac bone transfers are preferred. The application of bone-lengthening devices following corticotomy is another rediscovered possibility.

ULCERS

Because of the new techniques in the reconstructive surgeon's armamentarium, plastic surgeons are increasingly called upon to care for patients with lower extremity tissue loss secondary to vascular disease. Lower extremity wounds resulting from arterial insufficiency are approached in concert with a vascular surgeon in order to provide state-of-the-art care for both the arterial insufficiency and the tissue loss. Plastic surgeons who are not well trained in peripheral vascular surgery should not embark on the care of patients with these difficult problems.

The first step in the treatment of a lower extremity ulcer is to determine the etiology. The vast majority of lower extremity ulcers are the result of venous insufficiency, arterial insufficiency, or diabetes. Occasionally, they are caused by vasculitis, collagen vascular diseases, unusual infections, or malignant conditions. A careful history and physical examination, concentrating on the most common causes of lower extremity ulcers, usually reveal the etiology in the overwhelming majority of patients.

Venous stasis ulcers most often occur in the malleolar areas. Pigmentation changes related to hemosiderin deposits are common. Most venous stasis ulcers heal if the venous hypertension can be controlled, even temporarily. Bed rest with leg elevation is usually sufficient, but many patients do not comply with this regimen. Other methods of conservative management have been advertized and are occasionally successful (e.g., Unna boots).

If conservative attempts fail to result in healing of a venous stasis ulcer, surgical intervention is warranted. Occasionally, excision of the ulcer with a skin graft results in stable coverage, as long as the leg is elevated during the healing process. If the ulcer is excised, the perforating veins are ligated to provide a more hospitable environment for graft vascularization (Linton, 1953). Flap coverage of venous stasis wounds is generally unnecessary in the absence of accompanying arterial disease. In the rare event that venous stasis ulceration progresses to the point of severe disability, chronic infection, and intractable pain, amputation must be contemplated.

Newer procedures, including venous valve reconstruction and valve transplantation as well as venous bypasses, may eventually make important contributions to the care of these patients.

Small punched-out lesions on the distal extremity, accompanied by symptoms of claudication or rest pain, are generally the result of arterial insufficiency. As discussed above, the care of any patient with an arterial ulcer should be coordinated with a vascular surgeon. Physical examination and noninvasive vascular laboratory studies (pressure measurements, directional Doppler flow studies, and duplex scanning) allow the surgeon to predict with some accuracy which wounds will heal, which will not, and which are borderline. If the ankle pressure or ankle-brachial index indicates that healing is unlikely, an arteriogram is indicated to obtain the anatomic information necessary to design a surgical plan.

A relatively new role for the plastic surgeon is to provide free tissue transfer either after lower extremity revascularization or concomitantly with revascularization. Dabb and Davis (1984) reported the use of microvascular latissimus dorsi free flaps in elderly patients, some of whom had peripheral vascular disease. Colen (1987) reported ten free tissue transfers in patients with peripheral vascular disease. Seven of the ten patients underwent revascularization before the free flap procedure (Fig. 82–33) and in three patients the anastomoses were performed directly to the bypass graft. Colen and Musson (1987) described the use of the duplex system to obtain both physiologic and anatomic information. These authors were able to decide which patients required revascularization and also obtained clues as to which areas on the distal vessels were appropriate sites for microvascular anastomosis.

The interface between the vascular surgeon and the plastic surgeon is an exciting, emerging concept. As in any new field where the indications for procedures have not been defined by experience, one must choose patients with extreme care so as not to add to the morbidity that they have already suffered.

Determination of the etiology of diabetic ulcers, once thought to be related to "small vessel disease," is a complex, multifactorial problem. Current understanding is that the neuropathy related to diabetes, as well as the white blood cell dysfunction and inability to combat infection, are the most important factors in the formation of diabetic ulcers.

Treatment of diabetic ulcers varies, depending on their severity. Surgical debridement is required to evaluate the extent of the lesion. Deeper wounds are frequently hidden beneath innocent-appearing crusted areas. The surgeon attempts not to remove tissue unnecessarily, but there is nothing to be gained by leaving necrotic tissue. If loculated collections of purulent material are found, dependent drainage must be provided. The ulcers do not require antibiotic therapy unless they are accompanied by invasive infection or cellulitis. Most diabetic infections are the result of multiple organisms, and this should be kept in mind when selecting antibiotics.

After the infection has been eliminated, reconstruction can be contemplated. Because of the presence of coincident peripheral vascular disease and its predilection in diabetics for the infrapopliteal vasculature, the vascular status of the extremity must be assessed. If peripheral vascular disease accompanies the wound, interaction with a vascular surgeon, as described above, must be undertaken. In the presence of normal pedal pulses,

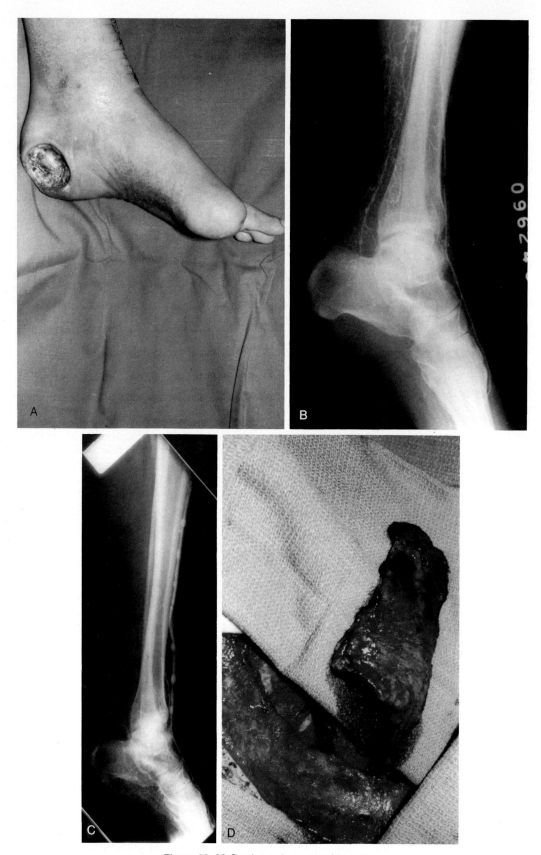

Figure 82–33 *See legend on opposite page*

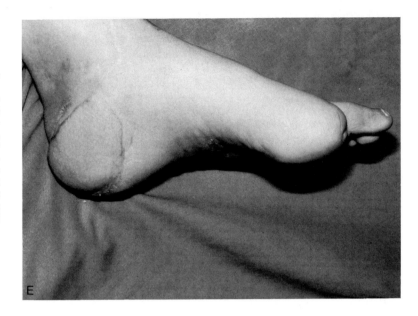

Figure 82–33. Free flap in the setting of arterial insufficiency. *A,* Heel ulcer with exposed calcaneus. *B,* Preoperative arteriogram showing severe disease in the anterior and posterior tibial arteries. *C,* Intraoperative arteriogram after in situ saphenous vein popliteal–anterior tibial bypass graft. *D,* Serratus anterior muscle with a 15 cm pedicle, allowing anastomosis to the bypass graft. *E,* Three years postoperatively the skin grafted muscle free flap is well healed.

the surgical alternatives vary from excision with primary closure to excision with free tissue transfer.

In diabetic patients with foot infections there is a 49 per cent incidence of contralateral foot infection and a 33 per cent incidence of contralateral foot amputation over an 18 month period (Kucan and Robson, 1986). In addition, once a diabetic individual undergoes an amputation, the chance of additional amputations is 50 per cent. As a result, the current trend among both vascular and plastic surgeons is to use whatever techniques are necessary to postpone amputation for as long as possible.

RECONSTRUCTION AFTER TUMOR RESECTION

Amputation was once the only ablative treatment for lower extremity malignancies, but advances in surgical oncology, chemotherapy, and microsurgery have allowed surgeons to perform more limb salvage procedures when resecting lower extremity neoplasms. Reconstruction of the lower extremity after wide resection of bone or soft tissue tumors is another area that requires close cooperation with other surgical subspecialties.

The reconstructive plan is based on the same principles that govern decision making in the trauma setting. Because reconstruction is best performed at the time of resection, the initial reconstructive strategy is formulated before the defect has been created. It is therefore imperative that the tumor surgeon estimate the magnitude of the resection so that the reconstructive surgeon can make a preliminary plan. Since the exact nature of the resection depends on the intraoperative findings, the plan must be flexible. When the resection is complete and the margins have been declared adequate by frozen section, the wound is evaluated; any exposed vital structures or open joints are noted, and other local factors (e.g., radiation) and systemic factors (e.g., age, prognosis, diabetes) are considered before the final reconstructive plan is determined.

One can employ any step on the reconstructive ladder to ensure the best possible result in an individual patient. Combined soft tissue and bone defects may be addressed by separate reconstructive stages or by composite free tissue transfer.

Gidumal and associates (1987) reported 30 patients who underwent resection of malignant or locally aggressive bone tumors, of which 12 had lower extremity lesions, with limb salvage and reconstruction by microvascular free bone flaps. Eleven of the 12 patients demonstrated primary union in an average of 6.8 months. These patients required an average of 7.6 months of immobilization and were allowed full weight bearing on the reconstructed limb after an average of 5.2 months. Other authors have reported the advantages of microvascular free bone flap re-construction after resection of lower extrem-ity neoplasms (Guo and Ding, 1981; Okada and associates, 1981; Pho, 1981; Salenius and associates, 1981; Moore, Weiland, and Daniel, 1983).

One must compare the results obtained by vascularized bone transfers with those of other available techniques such as prosthetic replacement, allografts, and nonvascularized autogenous bone grafts. In 1980 Enneking and associates (1980a) reported 65 per cent union after conventional nonvascularized bone grafting of defects greater than 7.5 cm in length. Mankin, Doppelt, and Tomford (1983) developed the use of nonvascularized allografts in lower extremity reconstruction. Although successful in some instances, the use of allografts is associated with an infec-tion rate of 13.2 per cent, a fracture rate of 16.5 per cent, and a delayed or non-union rate of 11 per cent. Custom prostheses are useful in elderly patients who do not subject the prosthesis to heavy loads over a long period; however, they are prone to loosening, implant fracture, dislocation, and exposure.

Microvascular free bone flap reconstruction compares favorably with the above alterna-tives (see Fig. 82–12). It is reasonable to employ microvascular transfer of bone for defects longer than 6 cm or for shorter defects in the setting of radiation or an unfavorable soft tissue milieu. The free flap can be fixed, depending on the situation, by using dynamic compression plates, lag screws, external fix-ators, or a combination of these techniques. Because of the relatively small diameter of the fibula, it can be dowled into the medullary cavity when larger bones such as the tibia or femur are reconstructed.

The fibula represents the most versatile free flap for osseous reconstruction (Fig. 82–34). The generous periosteal blood supply allows multiple osteotomies without compro-mising the blood supply to the bone. In fem-oral replacement, for example, the fibula can be osteotomized and folded on the intact peri-osteum to form a double-barreled, and there-fore stronger, flap that more closely approxi-mates the diameter of the femur.

SOFT TISSUE COVERAGE OF THE FOOT

The unique anatomic and functional char-acteristics of the foot merit special consider-ation. It is convenient to divide the foot into the following regions: (1) the heel and mid-plantar area; (2) the medial and lateral mal-leolus, Achilles tendon, and non–weight-bearing posterior heel; (3) the distal plantar area; and (4) the dorsum of the foot.

The difference between the cutaneous cov-erage on the plantar surface of the foot and that on the dorsum has important implica-tions for reconstruction of defects in these areas. The skin on the dorsum of the foot is mobile and thin. The skin on the plantar surface of the foot is the thickest in the body and is supported by dense subcutaneous tis-sue with vertically oriented fibrous septa that anchor the plantar skin to the underlying fascia. The extent to which these tissues can be replaced with "like" tissues determines, in large part, the success of the reconstruction.

The "team" concept is again appropriate for the management of foot injuries. An or-thopedic surgeon must be consulted for inju-ries or defects involving the bony architecture of the foot. A precisely contoured, one-stage soft tissue reconstruction of the plantar sur-face is of no benefit in the presence of an unstable ankle joint. Successful management of chronic foot problems may require preop-erative evaluation of plantar sensation, Har-ris Mat print studies, and gait analyses.

The neurovascular anatomy of the foot has been described in the section on Anatomy, but further comments are warranted. The muscles on the plantar surface of the foot are classically described in four layers. It is the first layer that is of relevance to the recon-structive surgeon; it consists of the abductor hallucis, the flexor digitorium brevis, and the

Figure 82–34. Post-ablative defect resurfaced with a composite free fibular osteocutaneous flap. *A,* Preoperative appearance; note the scar. *B,* The osseous defect in the distal tibia shown by magnetic resonance imaging. *C,* Design of flap in the contralateral lower extremity. *D,* Inset of flap.

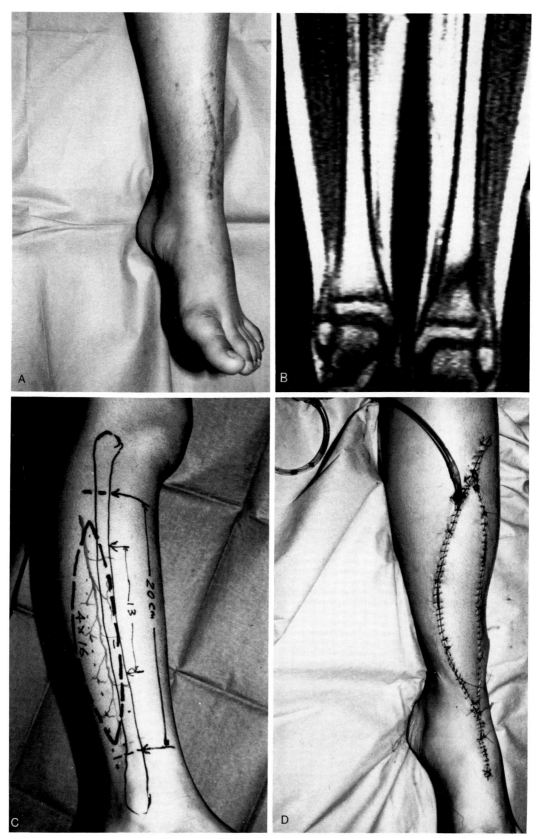

Figure 82–34 *See legend on opposite page*

abductor digiti minimi. The deeper muscle layers generally are not employed in the design of local plantar flaps. The relevant neurovascular structures lie immediately beneath this first muscle layer.

Weight-Bearing Heel and Midplantar Area

Numerous authors have identified the usefulness of the non—weight-bearing skin of the midsole for reconstruction of heel defects (Shanahan and Gingrass, 1979; Hendel and Buncke, 1980; Reiffel and McCarthy, 1980; Harrison and Morgan, 1981; Morrison and associates, 1983; Ikuta and associates, 1984; Shaw and Hidalgo, 1987). The major distinction between each of the above descriptions is the plane of dissection, which may be submuscular, subfascial, or suprafascial. The anatomic and clinical descriptions of the suprafascial flaps described by Shaw and Hidalgo (1987) have added considerably to knowledge of the subject. The "plantar subcutaneous vascular plexus" allows suprafascial flaps to be raised from the non—weight-bearing midsole area to cover heel defects without interfering with the deeper structures or risking damage to the sensory innervation of the distal foot. Shaw and Hidalgo (1986) pointed out that the flaps should be based medially so as to spare the medial calcaneal nerve (Fig. 82–35). Flaps of this design are the first choice for resurfacing defects on the weight-bearing heel up to 6 cm in diameter.

For larger defects, flaps that include the medial plantar artery either as an axial-pattern flap or an island fasciocutaneous flap are recommended. The instep island flap is elevated by making a transverse incision proximal to the weight-bearing area over the metatarsal heads (Fig. 82–36). The medial plantar neurovascular bundle is identified distally between the abductor hallucis and flexor digitorum brevis muscles. The medial plantar artery is divided distally and included in the flap as the flap is raised proximally. The entire non—weight-bearing portion of the midfoot can be raised in this fashion to reconstruct the soft tissue over the heel. The flap may be pedicled on the medial plantar artery or transferred as a microvascular free flap.

The third choice for coverage of heel defects is a local muscle flap from one of the three muscles in the superficial layer of the foot (the abductor hallucis, flexor digitorum brevis, or abductor digiti minimi) (Ger, 1975; Bostwick, 1976; Hartramp, Scheflan, and Bostwick, 1980; Shar and Pandit, 1985).

The flexor digitorum brevis muscle (Fig. 82–37) takes origin from the medial tubercle of the calcaneus and inserts into the middle phalanges of the toes. The muscle receives blood supply from both plantar arteries and is exposed through a midline plantar incision. The four distal tendons are divided and the muscle can be folded posteriorly on itself. If the muscle is mobilized to its neurovascular pedicle, it can cover the plantar surface of the heel. For coverage of the distal Achilles tendon, the origin of the muscle must be divided from the calcaneus, and for maximal mobilization the lateral plantar artery is divided distally and elevated with the overlying muscle. There are several disadvantages to this flap. The midplantar incision frequently divides the medial calcaneal nerve and therefore disrupts the sensory innervation to the lateral heel. In addition, safe elevation of the lateral plantar artery with the muscle requires dependent patency of the dorsalis pedis arterial system.

The abductor hallucis muscle arises from the medial tubercle of the calcaneus and inserts into the proximal phalanx of the great toe. Supplied by the medial plantar artery and nerve, the muscle may be useful to cover small defects on the medial aspect of the heel. It does not reliably reach the medial malleolus.

The abductor digiti minimi arises from the lateral aspect of the calcaneus and inserts into the proximal phalanx of the fifth toe. Small defects of the lateral heel may be covered with this muscle, which receives its neurovascular supply from the lateral plantar artery and nerve. The muscle does not reliably reach the lateral malleolus.

When a large defect on the weight-bearing surface of the foot or associated midplantar scarring precludes the use of local tissue, a microvascular free flap is the next option. Tube flaps and cross leg or cross foot flaps are of only historical interest. Numerous free flaps have been used to reconstruct the plantar surface of the foot. May, Halls, and Simon (1985) demonstrated that stable coverage is obtained with skin grafted free muscle flaps on the sole of the foot (Fig. 82–38). The more

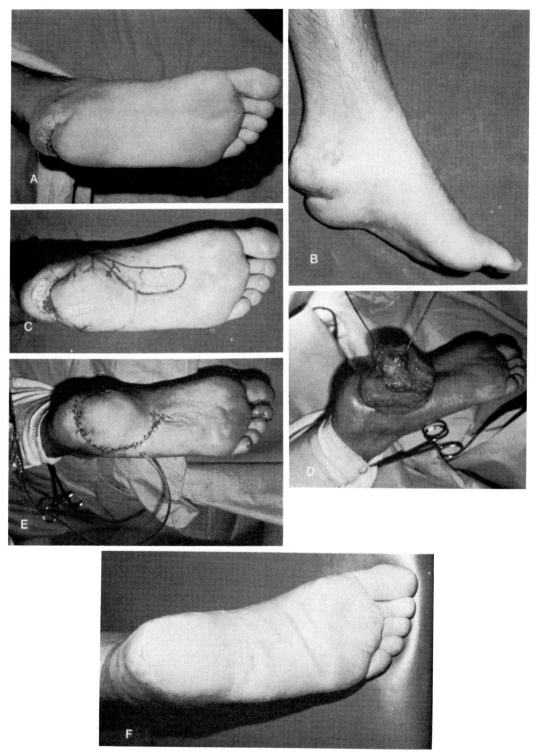

Figure 82–35. Suprafascial rotation flap for coverage of heel defect. *A, B,* Defect of the posterior weight–bearing heel. *C,* Design for the suprafascial plantar rotation flap. *D,* Flap elevation. *E,* Immediate postoperative appearance. *F,* One year postoperatively. (From Hidalgo, D. A., and Shaw, W. W.: Reconstruction of foot injuries. Clin. Plast. Surg., *13*:663, 1986.)

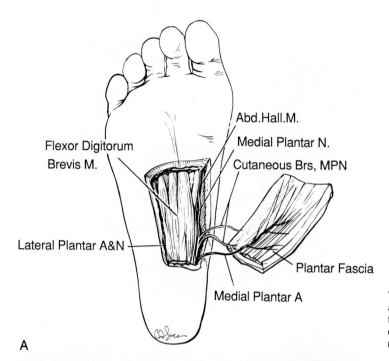

Flexor Digitorum
Brevis M.

Abd.Hall.M.

Medial Plantar N.

Cutaneous Brs, MPN

Lateral Plantar A&N

Plantar Fascia

Medial Plantar A

A

Figure 82–36. Instep island flap. *A,* The flap is raised on the medial plantar artery, sparing the medial plantar nerve to the distal foot. *B,* Flap in position. The donor site has been covered with a meshed split-thickness skin graft.

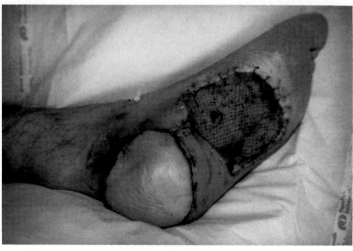

B

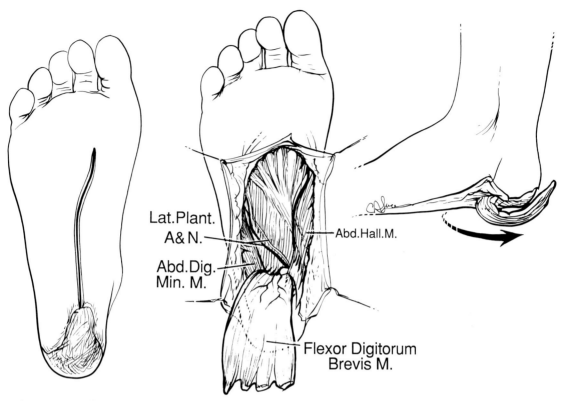

Figure 82–37. Flexor digitorum brevis muscle flap. The flap is exposed by means of a midsole incision. The muscle can be turned back over itself *(arrow)* to cover defects of the weight–bearing heel.

mobile tissue that accompanies a musculocutaneous or fasciocutaneous free flap is probably less stable and simulates the normal plantar skin less well than does a skin grafted free muscle flap.

The lateral calcaneal artery fasciocutaneous flap (Fig. 82–39) can be employed either as a transposition flap or as an island flap to cover the Achilles tendon and posterior heel (Grabb and Argenta, 1981; Holmes and Rayner, 1984; Yanai and associates, 1985). Defects with a maximal dimension of 3 cm can be closed with this flap. Between the lateral malleolus and the plantar surface of the foot, the lateral calcaneal artery (the terminal branch of the peroneal artery), the sural nerve, and the lesser saphenous vein are located. Fasciocutaneous flaps 4 to 5 cm wide can be designed over the pedicle. The donor site is skin grafted. Flaps of this type provide sensate, well-vascularized coverage of the Achilles tendon and leave a relatively innocuous donor site.

Local muscle flaps are not reliable reconstructive options in this region. In general,

the usefulness of local muscle flaps for Achilles tendon and malleolar coverage has been overestimated. The flexor digitorum brevis muscle reaches the non—weight-bearing portion of the posterior heel but requires a heel-splitting incision that disrupts the sensory innervation of the lateral heel skin, as described above. The muscle does not reach more proximally than the insertion of the Achilles tendon even if maximally mobilized with the lateral plantar artery and separated from its origin on the calcaneus. The abductor hallucis and abductor digit minimi muscles can be pedicled on their respective plantar arteries to reach the posterior aspect of the heel, but do not cover the Achilles tendon. It has been reported that the abductor muscles reach their respective malleoli but these muscles are small and are not recommended for coverage proximal to the posterior non—weight-bearing portion of the heel (Vasconez, Bostwick, and McCraw, 1974).

The extensor digitorum brevis muscle can be pedicled on the lateral tarsal artery and its parent artery, the dorsalis pedis, to reach

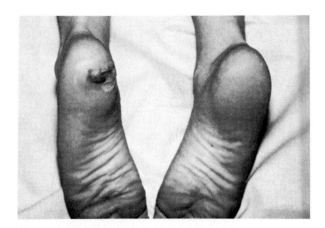

A

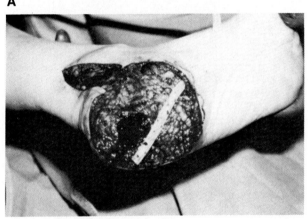

Figure 82–38. Latissimus dorsi free flap reconstruction of a heel defect. *A,* Level 5 melanoma of the left posterior heel. *B,* A 16 × 12 × 4 cm defect after melanoma resection. The posterior tibial vessels have been dissected and the circumference undermined; a deep drain has been sutured into position. *C,* Muscle flap after insetting and application of thick split-thickness skin graft.

B

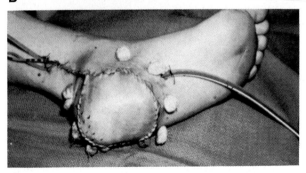

C

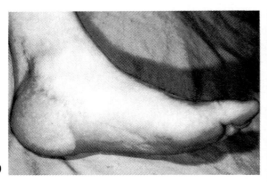

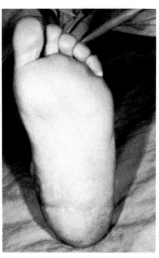

Figure 82–38 *Continued D,* Medial view demonstrating normal skin graft–heel interface with hyperkeratosis 24 months postoperatively. *E,* The well-contoured flap on plantar view. (From May, J. W., Jr., and Rohrich, R. J.: Foot reconstruction using free microvascular muscle flaps with skin grafts. Clin. Plast. Surg., *13*:681, 1986.)

the malleolus or Achilles tendon area. This flat muscle, which is approximately 5 by 6 cm in size, is innervated by a branch of the deep peroneal nerve. To raise the flap, the four tendons of the muscle are divided distally along with the dorsalis pedis artery, and the muscle is reflected proximally. If the flap is raised as a muscle flap, the donor site morbidity is not so great since the dorsal skin remains intact.

Defects over the malleoli or Achilles tendon frequently require small microvascular free flaps for coverage. The temporoparietal fascia free flap provides thin cover over the Achilles

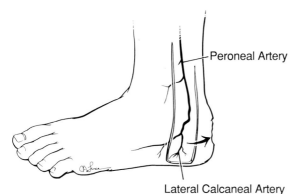

Figure 82–39. Lateral calcaneal fasciocutaneous flap. The flap is designed over the sural nerve and lesser saphenous vein, which run posterior to the lateral malleolus. The arterial supply is the lateral calcaneal artery, which is the terminal branch of the peroneal artery. The principal use of this flap is to cover defects over the distal Achilles tendon or the non–weight-bearing heel.

tendon (Brent, Upton, and Acland, 1985). Small free muscle flaps are ideal for coverage of the malleoli; they are easier, are more reliable, and involve less morbidity than attempts to stretch a local muscle flap from the sole of the foot to reach the malleoli.

Distal Plantar Area

Obtaining sensate, sturdy coverage over the metatarsal heads is frequently a difficult reconstructive problem. Plantar rotation flaps do not move well in a distal direction because the plantar nerve branches do not stretch.

Vascularized and innervated tissue from the toes can be used to cover defects over the metatarsal heads. A toe can be filleted and the bone discarded to allow transfer of the cutaneous coverage with its neurovascular supply to cover lesions over the metatarsal heads. The great toe is sufficiently large to provide transfer of lateral tissue without sacrificing the remainder of the toe.

Large defects over the distal plantar surface must be covered with microvascular free flaps. Free muscle flaps with skin graft coverage are the most durable.

Dorsum of the Foot

If the paratenon is present over the extensor tendons, the dorsum of the foot can be covered with a skin graft. If the paratenon is absent or if the extensor tendons are absent, flap coverage is required. The superficial temporoparietal fascia free flap (Brent, Upton, and Acland, 1985) is ideal for the dorsum of the foot. Most other flaps are bulky and make the wearing of normal footwear difficult.

REFERENCES

Abbott, L. C.: The operative lengthening of the tibia and fibula. J. Bone Joint Surg., *9*:128, 1927.

Acland, R. D., Schusterman, M., Godina, M., Eder, E., Taylor, G. I., and Carlisle, I.: The saphenous neurovascular free flap. Plast. Reconstr. Surg., *67*:763, 1981.

Aldea, P. A., and Shaw, W. W.: Evolution of surgical management of severe lower extremity trauma. Clin. Plast. Surg., *134*:549, 1986.

Aldredge, R. H., and Murphy, E. F.: The influence of new developments on amputation surgery. *In* Klopsteg, P. E., and Wilson, P. D. (Eds.): Human Limbs and Their Substitutes. New York, McGraw Hill Book Company, 1955, pp. 11–12.

Alho, A., Bang, G., Karaharju, E., and Aromd, I.: Filling of a bone defect during experimental osteotaxis distraction. Acta Orthop. Scand., *53*:29, 1982.

Allen, M. J., Stirling, A. J., Cranshaw, C. V., and Barnes, M. R. Intercompartmental pressure monitoring of leg injuries. An aid to management. J. Bone Joint Surg., *67B*:53, 1985.

Armenta, E., and Fisher, J.: Vascular pedicle of the tensor fascia lata myocutaneous flap. Ann. Plast. Surg., *6*:112, 1981.

Baek, S. M.: Two new cutaneous free flaps: the medial and lateral five flaps. Plast. Reconstr. Surg., *71*:354, 1983.

Barclay, T. L., Cardoso, E., Sharpe, D. T., and Crockett, D. J.: Repair of lower leg injuries with fascio-cutaneous flaps. Br. J. Plast. Surg., *35*:127, 1982.

Barford, B., and Pers, M.: Gastrocnemius-plasty for primary closure of compound injuries of the knee. J. Bone Joint Surg., 52*B*:124, 1970.

Barner, H. B., Kaiser, G. C., and Willman, V. L.: Blood flow in the diabetic leg. Circulation, *43*:391, 1971.

Barrson, B. B., and Lacy, P. E.: Diabetic microangiopathy in human toes: with emphasis on the ultrastructural change in dermal capillaries. Am. J. Pathol., *45*:41, 1964.

Bas, L., Handien, J., and May, J.: End to End Versus End to Side Microvascular Anastomosis: Patency and the Experimental Animal. Durham, NC, Plastic Surgery Research Council, May, 1983.

Benson, D. R., Riggins, R. S., Lawrence, R. M., and associates: Treatment of open fractures: a prospective study. J. Trauma, *23*:25, 1983.

Bieber, E. J., and Wood, M. B.: Bone reconstruction. Clin. Plast. Surg., *13*:645, 1986.

Blick, S. S., Brumback, R. J., Poka, A., Burgess, A. R., and Ebraheim, N. A.: Compartment syndrome in open tibial fractures. J. Bone Joint Surg., *68A*:1348, 1986.

Bosse, M. J., Burgess, A. R., and Brumback, R. J.: Evaluation and treatment of the high energy open tibia fracture. Adv. Orthop. Surg., *8*:3, 1984.

Bostwick, J.: Reconstruction of the heel pad by muscle transposition and split skin graft. Surg. Gynecol. Obstet., *143*:973, 1976.

Brent, B., Upton, J., and Acland, R. D. Experience with the temporal perineal fascia free flap. Plast. Reconstr. Surg., *76*:177, 1985.

Briedenbach, W., and Terzis, J. K.: The anatomy of free vascularized nerve grafts. Clin. Plast. Surg. *11*:65, 1984.

Brown, R. F.: The management of traumatic tissue loss in the lower limb, especially when complicated by skeletal injury. Br. J. Plast. Surg., *18*:26, 1965.

Buncke, H. J., and Colen, L. B. An island flap from the first web space of the foot to cover plantar ulcers. Br. J. Plast. Surg., *33*:242, 1980.

Burgess, E. M., Romano, R. L., and Zettl, J. H.: The management of lower extremity amputations. Prosthetic and Sensory Aid Service, Dept. of Medicine and Surgery, Veteran's Administration. Washington, August, 1969, p. 7.

Burkhalter, W. E.: Open injuries of the open extremities. Surg. Clin. North Am., *53*:1439, 1973.

Byrd, H. S.: Lower extremity reconstruction. Selected Readings Plast. Surg., *4*:1, 1988.

Byrd, H. S., Cierny, G., and Tebbetts, J. B.: The management of open tibial fractures with associated soft tissue loss: external pin fixation with early flap coverage. Plast. Reconstr. Surg., *68*:73, 1981.

Byrd, H. S., Spicer, R. E., and Cierny, G.: The management of open tibial fractures. Plast. Reconstr. Surg., *76*:719, 1985.

Cannon, B., Constable, J. D., Furlaw, L. T., Hayhurst, J. W., McCarthy, J. G., and McCraw, J. B.: Reconstructive surgery of the lower extremity. *In* Converse, J. M. (Ed.): Reconstructive Plastic Surgery. 2nd Ed. Philadelphia, W. B. Saunders Company, 1977, p. 3521.

Carrel, A., and Guthrie, C. C.: Complete amputation of the thigh with replantation. Am. J. Med. Sci., *131*:297, 1906.

Chang, N., and Mathes, S. J.: Comparison of the effect of bacterial inoculation in musculocutaneous and random-patterned flaps. Plast. Reconstr. Surg., *70*:1, 1982.

Chao, E., and Ivins, J.: Tumor Prosthesis for Bone and Joint Reconstruction: The Design and Application. New York, Thieme-Stratton, 1983.

Chen, Z. W., Chien, Y. C., and Pao, Y. S.: Salvage of the forearm following complete traumatic amputation: report of a successful case. Chin. Med. J., *82*:632, 1963.

Chen, Z. W., and Zeng, B. F.: Replantation of the lower extremity. Clin. Plast. Surg., *10*:103, 1983.

Cierny, G., and Mader, J.: Management of adult osteomyelitis. *In* Evarts, C. M. (Ed.): Surgery of the Muscular Skeletal System. New York, Churchill Livingstone, 1983.

Codivilla, A.: On the means of lengthening in the lower limbs the muscles and tissues which are shortened through deformity. Am. J. Orthop. Surg., *2*:253, 1905.

Colen, L. B.: Limb salvage in the patient with severe peripheral vascular disease: the role of microsurgical free-tissue transfer. Plast. Reconstr. Surg., *79*:389, 1987.

Colen, L. B., and Buncke, H. J.: Neurovascular island flaps from the plantar vessels and nerves for foot reconstruction. Ann. Plast. Surg., *12*:327, 1984.

Colen, L. B., and Musson, A.: Preoperative assessment of the peripheral vascular disease patient for free transfers. J. Reconstr. Microsurg., *4*, 1987.

Colen, S. R., Romita, M. C., Godfrey, N. V., and Shaw, W. W.: Salvage replantation. Clin. Plast. Surg., *10*:125, 1983.

Conrad, M. C.: Large and small artery occlusion in diabetics and non-diabetics with severe vascular disease. Circulation, *36*:83, 1967.

Cutting, C. B., and McCarthy, J. G.: Comparison of the residual osseous mass between vascularized and non-vascularized onlay bone transfers. Plast. Reconstr. Surg., 72:672, 1983.

Dabb, R. W., and Davis, R. M.: Latissimus dorsi free flaps in the elderly: an alternative to below-knee amputation. Plast. Reconstr. Surg., 73:633, 1984.

Dal Monte, A., and Donzelli, O.: Tibial lengthening according to Ilizarov in congenital hypoplasia of the leg. J. Pediatr. Orthop., 7:135, 1987.

Daniel, R., and Taylor, G. I.: Distant transfer of an island flap by microvascular anastomoses. Plast. Reconstr. Surg., 52:111, 1973.

De Bastiani, G., Aldegheri, R., Renzi Brivio, L., and Trivella, G.: Chondrodiastasis-controlled symmetrical distraction of the epifascial plate: limb lengthening in children. J. Bone Joint Surg., 68B:550, 1986.

De Bastiani, G., Aldegheri, R., Renzi Brivio, L., and Trivella, G.: Limb lengthening by callus distraction (callotasis). J. Pediatr. Orthop., 7:129, 1987.

DeLee, J., and Stiehl, J.: Open tibial fracture with compartment syndrome. Clin. Orthop., 160:175, 1981.

Duncan, M. J., Zuker, R. M., and Manktelow, R. T.: Resurfacing weight bearing areas of the heel. The role of the dorsalis pedis–innervated free tissue transfer. J. Reconstr. Microsurg., 1:201, 1985.

Edwards, E. A.: Anatomy of the small arteries of the foot and toes. Acta Anat., 41:81, 1960.

Enneking, W. F., Eady, J. L., and Burchardt, H.: Autogenous cortical bone grafts in the reconstruction of segmental skeletal defects. J. Bone Joint Surg., 62A:1039, 1980.

Enneking, W. F., Spanier, S. S., and Goodman, M. A.: A system for the surgical staging of muscular skeletal sarcoma. Clin. Orthop. 153:106, 1980.

Gallico, G. G., III, Ehrlichman, R. J., Jupiter, J., and May, J. W., Jr.: Free flaps to preserve below knee amputation stumps: long-term evaluation. Plast. Reconstr. Surg., 79:873, 1987.

Garrison, F. H.: An Introduction to the History of Medicine. 4th Ed. Philadelphia, W. B. Saunders Company, 1929.

Gebhart, M. J., Lane, J. M., McCormack, R. R., Jr., and Glasser, D.: Limb salvage in bone sarcomas—Memorial Hospital experience. Orthopedics, 8:626, 1985.

Ger, R.: Management of pretibial skin loss. Surgery, 63:757, 1968.

Ger, R.: The management of opened fractures of the tibia with skin loss. J. Trauma, 10:112, 1970.

Ger, R.: The technique of muscle transposition and the operative treatment of traumatic and ulcerative lesions of the leg. J. Trauma, 11:502, 1971.

Ger, R.: The surgical management of ulcers of the heel. Surg. Gynecol. Obstet., 140:909, 1975.

Ger, R.: Muscle transposition for treatment and prevention of chronic post-traumatic osteomyelitis of the tibia. J. Bone Joint Surg., 59A:784, 1977.

Ger, R., and Efrom, G.: New operative approach in the treatment of chronic osteomyelitis of the tibia diaphysis: a preliminary report. Clin. Orthop., 70:165, 1970.

Gidumal, R., Wood, M. B., Sim, F. H., and Shives, T. C.: Vascularized bone transfer for limb salvage and reconstruction after resection of aggressive bone lesions. J. Reconstr. Microvasc. Surg., 3:183, 1987.

Gilbert, A.: Composite tissue transfers from the foot: anatomic basis and surgical technique. In Symposium on Microsurgery. St. Louis, C. V. Mosby Company, 1976.

Godina, M.: Early microsurgical reconstruction of complex trauma of the extremities. Clin. Plast. Surg., 13:619, 1986.

Goldenberg, S., Alex, M., Joshi, R., and Blumenthal, H.: Nonatheromatous peripheral vascular disease of the lower extremity in diabetes mellitus. Diabetes, 8:261, 1959.

Gothman, L.: Arterial changes in experimental fractures of the rabbit's tibia treated with intramedullary nailing. A microangiographic study. Acta Chir. Scand., 120:289, 1960.

Grabb, W. C., and Argenta, L. C.: The lateral calcaneal artery skin flap (the lateral calcaneal artery, lesser saphenous vein and sural nerve skin flap). Plast. Reconstr. Surg., 68:723, 1981.

Gregory, C. F., Chapman, M. W., and Hansen, S. T.: Open fractures. In Rockwood, C., and Green, D. (Eds.): Fractures in Adults. Philadelphia, J. B. Lippincott Company, 1984.

Grotting, J. C., and Vasconez, L. O.: Regional blood supply and the selection of flaps for reconstruction. Clin. Plast. Surg., 13:581, 1986.

Guo, F., and Ding, B. F.: Vascularized free fibula transfer and the treatment of bone tumors: report of three cases. Arch. Orthop. Trauma Surg., 98:209, 1981.

Gustilo, R. B., and Anderson, J. T.: Prevention of infection in the treatment of one thousand and twenty-five open fractures of long bones. J. Bone Joint Surg., 58A:453, 1976.

Harii, K.: Microneurovascular free muscle transplantation for reanimation of facial paralysis. Clin. Plast. Surg., 6:361, 1979.

Harii, K., Ohmori, K., Torii, S. S., and associates: Free groin skin flaps. Br. J. Plast. Surg., 28:225, 1975.

Harii, K., Ohmori, K., and Torii, S.: Free gracilis muscle transplantation with microneurovascular anastomoses for the treatment of facial paralysis. Plast. Reconstr. Surg., 57:133, 1976.

Harmon, P. H.: A simplified surgical approach to the posterior tibia for bone grafting and fibular transference. J. Bone Joint Surg., 27:496, 1945.

Harris, W. H., Jackson, R. H., and Jowsey, J.: The in vivo distribution of tetracyclines in the canine bone. J. Bone Joint Surg., 44A:1308, 1962.

Harrison, D. H., and Morgan, D. G.: The instep island flap to resurface plantar defects. Br. J. Plast. Surg., 34:315, 1981.

Hartramf, C. F., Scheflan, M., and Bostwick, J., III: The flexor digitorum brevis muscle island pedicle flap: a new dimension in heel reconstruction. Plast. Reconstr. Surg., 66:264, 1980.

Hendel, P. M., and Buncke, H. J.: Another use for the first web space of the foot: neurovascular island flap. Plast. Reconstr. Surg., 66:468, 1980.

Hidalgo, D. A., and Shaw, W. W.: Reconstruction of foot injuries. Clin. Plast. Surg., 13:663, 1986a.

Hidalgo, D. A., and Shaw, W. W.: Anatomic basis of plantar flap design. Plast. Reconstr. Surg., 78:627, 1986b.

Holden, C. E.: The role of blood supply to soft tissue in the healing of diaphyseal fractures. J. Bone Joint Surg., 54A:993, 1972.

Holmes, J., and Rayner, C. R.: Lateral calcaneal artery island flaps. Br. J. Plast. Surg., 37:402, 1984.

Huber, J. F.: The arterial network supplying the dorsum of the foot. Anat. Rec., 80:373, 1941.

Hurwitz, D. J., Swartz, W. M., and Mathes, S. J.: The gluteal thigh flap: a reliable, sensate flap for the closure of buttock and perineal wounds. Plast. Reconstr. Surg., 68:521, 1981.

Ikuta, Y., Murakami, T., Yoshioka, K., and Tsuge, K.:

Reconstruction of the heel pad by flexor digitorum brevis muscular cutaneous flap transfer. Plast. Reconstr. Surg., *74*:86, 1984.

Ilizarov, G. A.: New principles of osteosynthesis by means of crossing pins and rings. Collection of scientific publications. Kurgin, 1954.

Keblish, P. A.: Amputation alternatives in the lower limbs, stressing combined management of the traumatized extremity. Clin. Plast. Surg., *13*:595, 1986.

Khouri, R. K., and Shaw, W. W.: Reconstruction of the lower extremity with microvascular free flaps: a 10 year experience with 304 consecutive cases. Presented at the 48th Annual Meeting of the American Association for the Surgery of Trauma, Newport Beach, CA, October 7, 1987.

Kirk, N. T.: Development of amputation. Bull. Med. Lib. Assoc., *32*:132, 1944.

Kline, D. G.: Operative experience with major lower extremity nerve lesions, including the lumbosacral plexus and sciatic nerve. *In* Omer, G. E., Jr., and Spinner, M. (Eds.): Management of Peripheral Nerve Problems. Philadelphia, W. B. Saunders Company, 1980, p. 607.

Kline, D. G.: Operative management of major nerve lesions of the lower extremity. Surg. Clin. North Am. *52*:1247, 1982.

Kojimoto, H., Yasui, N., Goto, T., Matsuda, S., and Shimomura, Y.: Bone lengthening in rabbits by callus distraction: the role of periosteum and endosteum. J. Bone Joint Surg., *70B*:543, 1988.

Kucan, J. O., and Robson, M. C.: Diabetic foot infections: fate of the contralateral foot. Plast. Reconstr. Surg., *77*:439, 1986.

LaMont, J. G.: Functional anatomy of the lower limb. Clin. Plast. Surg., *13*:571, 1986.

Landi, A., Soragni, O., and Monteleone, M.: The extensor digitorum brevis muscle for soft tissue loss around the ankle. Plast. Reconstr. Surg., *75*:892, 1985.

Lange, R. H., Bach, A. W., Hansen, S. T., Jr., and Johansen, K. H.: Open tibial fractures with associated vascular injuries: prognosis for limb salvage. J. Trauma, *25*:203, 1985.

Lapchinsky, A. G.: Recent results of experimental transplantation of preserved limbs and kidneys and possible use of this technique in clinical practice. Ann. N. Y. Acad. Sci., *87*:539, 1960.

Lau, R. S. and Leung, P. C.: Bone graft viability in vascularized bone graft transfer. Br. J. Radiol., *55*:325, 1982.

Leitner, D. W., Gordon, L., and Buncke, H. J.: The extensor digitorum brevis as a muscle island flap. Plast. Reconstr. Surg., *76*:777, 1985.

Lewis, M. M., and Chekofsky, K. M.: Proximal femur replacement for neoplastic disease. Clin. Orthop., *171*:72, 1982.

Linton, R. R.: Post-thrombotic ulceration of the lower extremity. Ann. Surg., *138*:415, 1953.

LoGerfo, F. W., and Coffman, J. D.: Vascular and microvascular disease of the foot in diabetes. N. Engl. J. Med., *311*:1615, 1984.

Macnab, I., and De Haas, W. G.: The role of periosteal blood supply in the healing of fractures of the tibia. Clin. Orthop., *105*:27, 1974.

Malt, R. A., and McKhann, C. F.: Replantation of severed arms. J.A.M.A., *189*:716, 1964.

Man, D., and Ackland, R.: The microarterial anatomy of the dorsalis pedis flap and its clinical applications. Plast. Reconstr. Surg., *65*:419, 1980.

Mankin, H. J., Doppelt, S., and Tomford, W. Clinical experience with allograft implantation: The first ten years. Clin. Orthop. *174*:69, 1983.

Martini, Z., and Castaman, E.: Tissue regeneration in the reconstruction of lost bone and soft tissue in the lower limbs: a preliminary report. Br. J. Plast. Surg., *40*:142, 1987.

Mathes, S. J., Alpert, B. S., and Chang, N.: Use of the muscle flap in chronic osteomyelitis: experimental and clinic correlation. Plast. Reconstr. Surg., *69*:815, 1982.

Mathes, S. J., and Nahai, F.: Clinical Applications for Muscle and Musculocutaneous Flaps. St. Louis, C. V. Mosby Company, 1982.

Matter, P., and Reitman, W.: The Open Fracture. Berne, Hans Huber, 1978.

May, J. W., Jr., Chait, L. A., Cohen, B. E., and O'Brien, B. M.: Free neurovascular flap from the first web of the foot in hand reconstruction. J. Hand Surg., *2*:387, 1977.

May, J. W., Jr., Gallico, G. G., III, and Lukash, F. N.: Microvascular transfer of free tissue for closure of bone wounds of the distal lower extremity. N. Engl. J. Med., *306*:253, 1982.

May, J. W., Jr., Gallico, G. G., III, Jupiter, J., and Savage, R. C.: Free latissimus dorsi muscle flap with skin graft for treatment of traumatic chronic bony wounds. Plast. Reconstr. Surg., *73*:641, 1984.

May, J. W., Halls, M. J., and Simon, S. R. Free microvascular muscle flaps with skin graft reconstruction of extensive defects of the foot: a clinical and gait analysis study. Plast. Reconstr. Surg., *75*:627, 1985.

McCraw, J. B., and Furlow, L. T., Jr.: The dorsalis pedis arterialized flaps. A clinical study. Plast. Reconstr. Surg., *55*:177, 1975.

McGregor, I. L., and Jackson, I.: The groin flap. Br. J. Plast. Surg., *25*:3, 1972.

Mears, D. C., Maxwell, G. P., Vidal, J., et al.: Clinical techniques in the lower extremity. *In* Mears, D. C. (Ed.): External Skeletal Fixation. Baltimore, Williams & Wilkins Company, 1983, p. 278.

Mears, D. C., and Stone, J. P.: The management of open fractures. Orthop. Surv., *3*:247, 1980.

Mettler, C. C.: History of Medicine. Philadelphia, Blakiston Company, 1947.

Monticelli, G., and Spinelli, R.: Limb lengthening by closed metaphyseal corticotomy. Ital. J. Orthop. Traum., *4*:139, 1983.

Moore, J. R., and Weiland, A. G.: Vascularized tissue transfer in the treatment of osteomyelitis. Clin. Plast. Surg., *13*:657, 1986.

Moore, J. R., Weiland, A. J., and Daniel, R. K.: Use of free vascularized bone grafts in the treatment of bone tumors. Clin. Orthop. *175*:37, 1983.

Morain, W. D.: Island toe flaps in neurotrophic ulcers of the foot and ankle. Ann. Plast. Surg., *13*:1, 1984.

Morrison, W. A., Crabb, D. M., O'Brien, B. M., and Jenkins, A.: The instep of the foot as a fasciocutaneous island and as a free flap for heel defects. Plast. Reconstr. Surg., *72*:56, 1983.

Ohmori, K., and Harii, K.: Free dorsalis pedis sensory flap to the hand, with microneurovascular anastomoses. Plast. Reconstr. Surg., *58*:546, 1976.

Ohtsuka, H.: Angiographic analysis of the first metatarsal arteries and its clinical applications. Ann. Plast. Surg., *7*:2, 1981.

Okada, T., Tsukada, S., Obaro, K., Yasuda, Y., and Kitayama, Y.: Free vascularized fibular graft for replacement of the radius after excision of giant cell tumor: case report. J. Microsurg., *3*:48, 1981.

Orr, H. W.: Osteomyelitis and Compound Fractures and

Other Infected Wounds. St. Louis, C. V. Mosby Company, 1929.

Orr, H. W.: Wounds and Fractures. Springfield, IL, Charles C Thomas, 1941.

Paré, A.: Les Oeuvres. Avec Les Figures et Portraits tant de L'Anatomie que des Instruments de Chirurgie, et de Plusieurs Monstres. Paris, Gabriel Buon, 1575.

Parkhill, C.: A new apparatus for the fixation of bones after resection and in fractures with a tendency to displacement, with a report of cases. Trans. M. Surg. Assoc., *15*:251, 1897.

Patzakis, M. J., Dorr, L. D., Ivler, D., et al.: The early management of open joint injuries. A prospective study of 140 patients. J. Bone Joint Surg., *57A*:1065, 1975.

Pho, R. W.: Malignant giant cell tumor of the distal end of the radius treated by free vascularized fibular transplant. J. Bone Joint Surg., *64A*:877, 1981.

Ponten, B.: The fasciocutaneous flap: its use in soft tissue defects of the lower leg. Br. J. Plast. Surg., *34*:215, 1981.

Rahn, B. A., and Perren, S. M.: Xylenol orange, a fluorochrome useful in polychrome sequential labeling of calcifying tissues. Stain Technol., *46*:125, 1971.

Rahn, B. A., and Perren, S. M.: Alizainkomplexon-fluorochrom zur Markierung von Knochen und Dentinanbau. Experientia, *28*:180, 1972.

Ramirez, O. M., Ramasastry, S. S., Granick, M. S., Pang, D., and Futrell, J. W.: A new surgical approach to closure of large lumbosacral meningomyelocele defects. Plast. Reconstr. Surg., *80*:799, 1987.

Reading, G.: Instep island flaps. Ann. Plast. Surg., *13*:488, 1984.

Reiffel, R. S., and McCarthy, J. G. Coverage of heel and sole defects: a new subfascial arterialized flap. Plast. Reconstr. Surg., *66*:250, 1980.

Riegels-Nielson, P., and Krag, C.: A neurovascular flap for coverage of distal plantar defects. Acta Orthop. Scand., *53*:495, 1982.

Rhinelander, F. W.: The normal microcirculation of the diaphyseal cortex and its response to fracture. J. Bone Joint Surg., *50*:784, 1968.

Rhinelander, F. W.: Tibial blood supply in relation to fracture healing. Clin. Orthop., *105*:34, 1974.

Rosenthal, R. E., MacPhail, J. A., and Ortiz, J. E.: Nonunion in opened tibial fractures: analysis of reasons for failure of treatment. J. Bone Joint Surg., *59A*:244, 1977.

Salenius, P., Santavirta, S., Kiviluoto, O., and Koskinen, E. V.: Application of free autogenous fibular graft in the treatment of aggressive bone tumors of the distal end of the radius. Arch. Orthop. Trauma Surg., *98*:285, 1981.

Sarrafian, S. K.: Anatomy of the Foot and Ankle. Philadelphia, J. B. Lippincott Company, 1983.

Scheflan, M., Nahai, F., and Hartrampf, C. R.: Surgical management of heel ulcers—a comprehensive approach. Ann. Plast. Surg., *7*:385, 1981.

Seddon, H. J.: Surgical Disorders of the Peripheral Nerves. Baltimore, Williams & Wilkins Company, 1972.

Serafin, D., Georgiade, N., and Smith, D.: Comparison of free flaps with pedicled flaps for coverage of defects of the leg or foot. Plast. Reconstr. Surg., *59*:492, 1977.

Serafin, D., Sabatier, R., Morris, R., and associates: Reconstruction of the lower extremity with vascularized composite tissue: improved tissue survival and specific indication. Plast. Reconstr. Surg., *66*:230, 1980.

Shaffer, J. W., Field, G. A., Goldberg, V. M., and Davy, D. T.: Fate of vascularized and nonvascularized autografts. Clin. Orthop., *197*:32, 1985.

Shah, A., and Pandit, S.: Reconstruction of the heel with chronic ulceration with flexor digitorum brevis myocutaneous flap. Lepr. Rev., *56*:41, 1985.

Shanahan, R. E., and Gingrass, R. P.: Medial plantar sensory flap coverage of heel defects. Plast. Reconstr. Surg., *64*:295, 1979.

Shaw, D. T., and Payne, R. L.: One stage tubed abdominal flaps. Surg. Gynecol. Obstet., *83*:205, 1946.

Shaw, W., Bahe, D., and Converse, J.: Conservation of major leg arteries when used as a recipient supply for a free flap period. Plast. Reconstr. Surg., *63*:317, 1979.

Shaw, W. W., and Hidalgo, D. A.: Anatomic basis of plantar flap design: clinical applications. Plast. Reconstr. Surg., *78*:637, 1986.

Shaw, W. W., and Hidalgo, D. A.: Microsurgery in Trauma. Mount Kisco, NY, Futura Publishing Company, 1987.

Sim, F. H., Bowman, W. E., Jr., Wilkins, R. N., and Chao, E. Y.: Limb salvage in primary malignant bone tumor. Orthopedics, *8*:574, 1985.

Sim, F. H., and Chao, E. S.: Prosthetic replacement of the knee and a large segment of the femur or tibia. J. Bone Joint Surg., *61A*:887, 1979.

Sommerlad, B. C., and McGrouther, D. A.: Resurfacing the sole. Long-term follow-up and comparison of techniques. Br. J. Plast. Surg., *31*:107, 1978.

Stark, W. J.: The use of pedicled muscle flaps in the surgical treatment of chronic osteomyelitis resulting from compound fractures. J. Bone Joint Surg., *28A*:343, 1946.

Steen, H., Fjeld, T. O., Bjerkrein, I., Tevik, A., Aldegheri, R., and Trivella, G.: Limb lengthening by diaphyseal corticotomy, callus distraction, and dynamic axial fixation. An experimental study in the bovine femur. J. Orthop. Res., *6*:730, 1988.

Stevenson, T. R., Kling, T. F., and Friedman, R. J.: Heel reconstruction with flexor digitorum brevis musculocutaneous flap. J. Pediatr. Orthop., *5*:713, 1985.

Strandness, D. E., Priest, R. E., and Gibbons, G. E.: Combined clinical and pathologic study of diabetic and nondiabetic peripheral arterial disease. Diabetes, *13*:366, 1964.

Swartz, W. M., and Jones, N. F.: Soft tissue coverage of the lower extremity. Curr. Probl. Surg., *22*:4, 1985.

Swartz, W. M., and Mears, D. C.: Management of difficult lower extremity fractures and nonunions. Clin. Plast. Surg., *13*:633, 1986.

Taylor, G. I.: Reconstruction of the mandible with free composite iliac bone grafts. Ann. Plast. Surg., *9*:361, 1982.

Taylor, G. I., and Daniel, R. K.: The anatomy of several free flap donor sites. Plast. Reconstr. Surg., *56*:243, 1975.

Taylor, G. I., Miller, G. D., and Ham, F. J.: The free vascularized bone graft: clinical extension of microvascular techniques. Plast. Reconstr. Surg., *55*:533, 1975.

Tessier, J., Bonnel, F., and Allieu, Y.: Vascularization, cellular behavior, and union of vascularized bone grafts: experimental study in the rabbit. Ann. Plast. Surg., *14*:494, 1985.

Trueta, J.: Treatment of war wounds and infections. New York, Paul B. Hoeber, 1940.

Trueta, J.: The Principles and Practices of War Surgery. 2nd Ed. London, H. Hamilton, 1944.

Vann, H. M.: A note on the formation of the plantar arterial arch of the human foot. Anat. Rec., *85*:269, 1943.

Vasconez, L. O., Bostwick, J., and McCraw, J.: Coverage of exposed bone by muscle transposition and skin grafting. Plast. Reconstr. Surg., *53*:526, 1974.

Vitali, M.: Amputation and Prosthesis. London, Bailliere Tindall, 1971.

Weiland, A. J., and Daniel, R. K.: Microvascular anastomoses for bone grafts in the treatment of massive defects in bone. J. Bone Joint Surg., *61A*:98, 1979.

Weiland, A. J., Moore, J. R., and Daniel, R. K.: Vascularized bone autografts. Experience with forty-one cases. Clin. Orthop., *174*:87, 1983.

Wigand, M. E., Naumann, W. H., Thormann, J., et al.: Microsurgical nerve implantation for rehabilitation of atrophied and transplanted muscles. *In* Koos, W. Th., Böck, F. W., and Spetzler, R. F. (Eds.): Clinical Microneurosurgery. Thieme-Edition, Publishing Sciences Group, 1976, pp. 271–273.

Yanai, A., Park, S., Iwao, T., and Nakamura, N.: Reconstruction of a skin defect of the posterior heel by a lateral calcaneal flap. Plast. Reconstr. Surg., *75*:642, 1985.

Yaremchuk, M. J.: Acute management of severe soft tissue damage accompanying open fractures of the lower extremity. Clin. Plast. Surg., *13*:621, 1986.

Zuker, R. M., and Manktelow, R. T.: The dorsalis pedis free flap: technique of elevation, foot closure, and flap application. Plast. Reconstr. Surg., *77*:93, 1986.

83

Leo Clodius

Lymphedema

HISTORY

Gaspar Aselli is credited with the first description of the lymphatic system: "On July 23rd of the year 1622 I had taken a healthy well-fed dog . . . when I opened the abdomen and pulled the mass of entrails and stomach downward with my hands, I suddenly saw a great number of cords which seemed to me extraordinarily thin and wonderfully white . . . I seized a very sharp scalpel and scratched one of these cords . . . when a white milk- or cream-like liquid discharged from it. I exclaimed: Eureka." After four years of work the results were published in the first anatomic work illustrated with color plates: *De lactibus sive lacteis venis,* Milano, 1627.

The lymphatic anatomy was structurally delineated in the atlas of Mascagni (1787) with accompanying plates, which look like modern lymphangiograms. John Hunter and his brother William first proposed that the lymphatics function as absorbents. Starling and Ludwig in the nineteenth century analyzed the relationship between the intravascular and tissue forces responsible for lymph formation and the lymphatic transport system. Drinker and Field (1931) demonstrated the recycling of protein molecules from the tissues into the central circulation through the lymph system and noted that blocking of the lymphatics resulted in high protein edema or lymphedema.

Indirect lymphangiography takes advantage of the unique function of the lymph circulation to absorb large molecules from the extravascular space. The first intradermal injection of a vital dye ("blue test"), which is adsorbed to protein, illustrated the superficial lymphatic network, the dynamics of lymph flow, and alterations of lymphatic permeability in inflammatory states (Hudack and McMaster, 1933). Direct lymphangiography by John Kinmonth in the 1950's started the modern era of lymphology. Nondiffusible lipid-soluble or water-soluble contrast media were slowly infused intralymphatically, permitting radiographic demonstration of the lymphatic channels, lymph nodes, and major collecting ducts. Both the formation of lymph and the flow of lymph are detectable by nuclear medicine techniques or lymphoscintigraphy (Lofferer and Mostbeck, 1983; Weissleder and Weissleder, 1988).

SURGICAL ANATOMY

The lymphatic system in extremities consists of an *epifascial* and a *subfascial* system (Fig. 83–1). Areas of dermis are drained in a

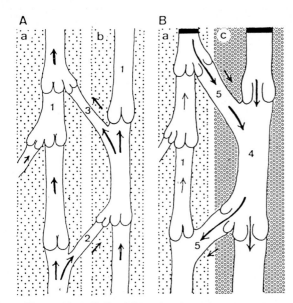

Figure 83–1. Epifascial lymph collaterals and lymphatic watersheds. *A,* Normal lymph circulation. *B,* Reversal of lymph flow in front of a lymph block. This results in dilatation of valves, valvular insufficiency, and horizontal reversal of lymph flow. a, b, c, Strips of lymphatic skin territories. In c note the secondary tissue changes associated with lymphedema. 1, Collector with normal valves. 2, Supplying and 3, draining collaterals of territory b. 4, Dilated collector with valvular insufficiency. 5, Retrograde lymph flow, resulting in "dermal backflow."

radial fashion by valveless lymphatics toward valved lymphatics at the subdermal level. The lymphatic load then drains into larger, valved trunks above the deep fascia (Fig. 83–1). These usually follow the veins and form interconnected bundles draining lymphatic skin territories, some of which are separated by lymphatic watersheds. Figure 83–2 demonstrates the importance of the epifascial collateral lymph circulation in health and in the presence of a lymph block. The deep lymphatic system lies below the deep fascia, following the main vascular structures of the extremity. Under normal conditions, as also observed in the venous system, communications exist between the epifascial and subfascial lymphatics. Unlike the veins, the perforators are fewer and the valves direct the flow from the deep to the superficial system. The perforators, however, do not function under normal conditions. The lymph reaches the filtering nodes through numerous small afferent vessels and departs via large efferent channels. At the roots of the extremities, the lymph nodes form interconnecting chain systems. Figure 83–3 demonstrates the body quadrants of superficial lymph drainage to-

ward four central draining areas: the paired axillary and inguinal lymph node systems. Mascagni's (1787) anatomic preparations (Figs. 83–4, 83–5) show the superficial and deep lymphatic systems better than present-day lymphoangiograms, the latter under normal conditions filling only a small part of the actual lymph collectors (Viamonte and Rüttimann, 1980).

Lymphatics of the Upper Extremity (see Fig. 83–4)

Most collectors of the *ulnar* (superficial) bundle, which accompanies the basilic vein, course on the medial aspect of the arm to the axillary lymph nodes. Some collectors perforate the deep fascia at the hiatus basilicus and accompany the deep lymph vessels of the upper arm. The *radial* (superficial) bundle follows the course of the cephalic vein to the lower margin of the pectoralis major muscle and crosses the upper arm ventrally to enter, together with the ulnar bundle, the axillary lymph nodes. In approximately 10 per cent of individuals a few collectors of the radial bundle bypass the axilla and, following the cephalic vein, drain directly into a supraclavicular or an infraclavicular lymph node (Kubik, 1980). Axillary lymphadenectomy should spare the infraclavicular lymphatic pathway. After axillary lymphadenectomy the remaining outflow tracts can drain the lymphatic load only via the cutaneous plexus over the lymphatic watersheds (see Fig. 83–2) or via peripheral surgical lymphovenous anastomoses (Malek, 1972). Although they have been divided into multiple groups, the axillary lymph nodes, variable in size and in number, are functionally interconnected to form a lymphatic "gyration traffic." After axillary lymphadenectomy it is essential to immobilize the dissection site under a compression dressing to allow for maximal formation of lympholymphatic anastomoses (Clodius, 1977).

Lymphatics of the Lower Extremity (see Fig. 83–5)

The *superficial* or *epifascial* system drains the skin, the subcutaneous layer, and the superficial portion of the periosteum of the anterior tibial surface and malleoli by a ven-

Text continued on page 4100

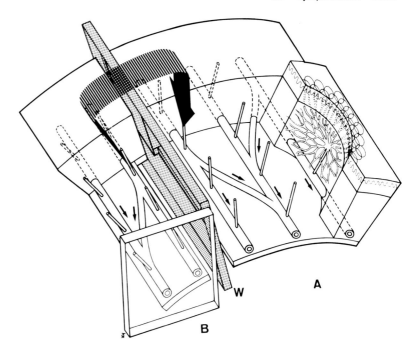

Figure 83–2. Lymph drainage of the skin from dermis toward the epifascial collectors. *A,* Territory of nonblocked epifascial lymphatics. *B,* Blocked lymphatic territory. It is separated from *A* by W, which is a lymphatic watershed acting as an obstacle to the intercommunications of the deep epifascial collectors. The block at *B* leads to a reversal of lymph flow. The lymph can escape from the blocked area *B* only by ascending from the deep lymphatics to the superficial lymphatics of the dermis. Dilatation of the lymphatics of the dermis results in the clinical development of ''peau d'orange,'' orange skin.

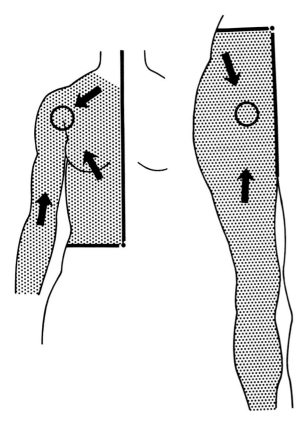

Figure 83–3. The body quadrants of superficial lymph drainage. According to Handley (1922), there is no lymph circulation across these boundaries. Forbes (1937–1938) found subcutaneous collectors, their valves directing the flow of lymph away from the quadrant edges, an important consideration in the therapeutic concept of cutaneous, metastasizing malignancies. The circles indicate the lymph node systems.

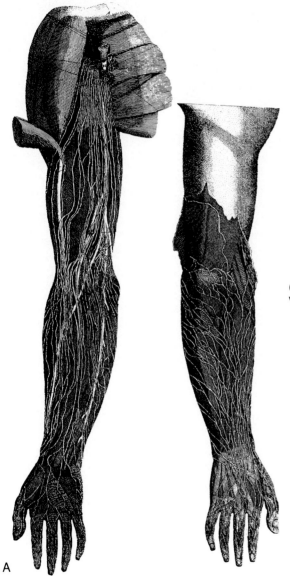

Figure 83–4. The lymphatics of the upper extremity (Mascagni, 1787). *A*, The superficial system, dorsal and ventral aspects.

A

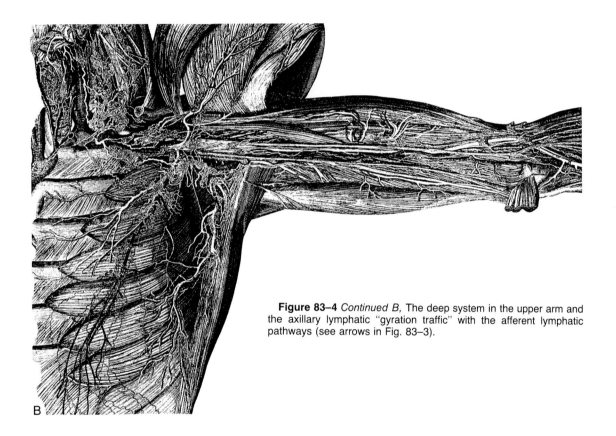

Figure 83–4 *Continued B,* The deep system in the upper arm and the axillary lymphatic "gyration traffic" with the afferent lymphatic pathways (see arrows in Fig. 83–3).

B

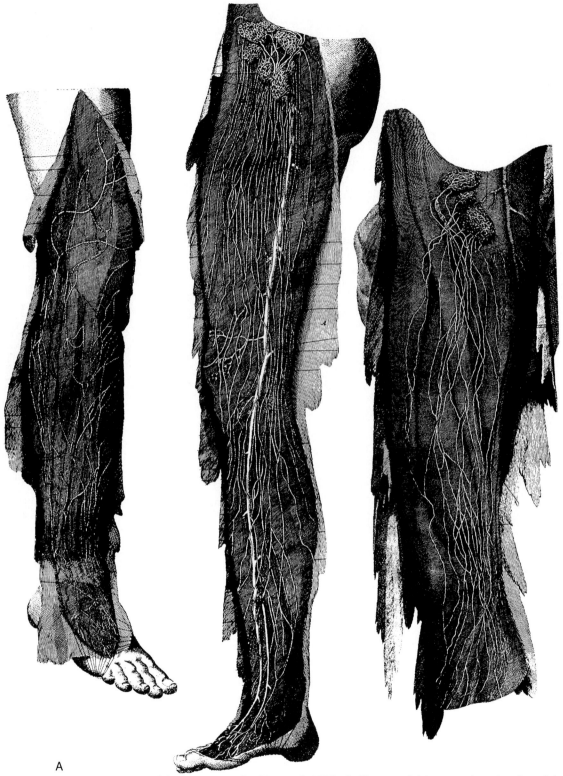

Figure 83–5. The lymphatics of the lower extremity (Mascagni, 1787). *A,* The superficial system, lateral and medial aspects and thigh area.

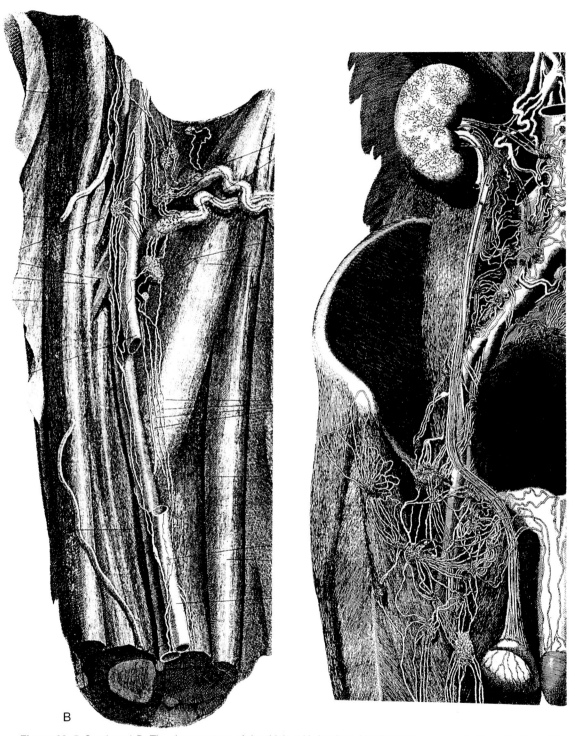

B

Figure 83–5 *Continued B,* The deep system of the thigh, with its deep lymph nodes, communicating with the pelvic lymph node system.

tromedial and a dorsolateral bundle. The lymphatics of the dorsolateral bundle, running along the lesser saphenous vein, ascend to the knee, where in a fashion similar to the ulnar bundle they continue through the popliteal nodes (three to five) as deep lymphatic trunks of the thigh. They end in the deep inguinal and occasionally directly in the anterior iliac nodes. The ventromedial bundle follows the greater saphenous vein. The course of the vessels is variable.

The *deep* or *subfascial* lymphatics collect the lymph from the muscles, fascia, joints, ligaments, bones, and periosteum. The deep collectors run along the anterior and posterior tibial artery and vein and along the fibular vessels. The lymph collectors enter directly or indirectly after passing intercalated nodes into the popliteal nodes. From there the efferent vessels course together with the collecting trunks of the thigh along the superficial femoral vessels into the deep inguinal nodes. Some of the collectors, as in the axilla, can bypass the inguinal nodes and drain directly into the pelvic or internal iliac nodes.

PHYSIOLOGY

The functions of the lymphatic system include the recycling of high molecular weight proteins, the exchanges of hydroproteins in the tissues, from the arterial end of the capillary to the junction of the thoracic duct in the neck (Fig. 83–6).

Fifty to 100 per cent of the circulating plasma proteins, approximately 20 liters of fluid, leave the blood stream each day through the wall of the arterial capillaries (Földi-Börcsök and Földi, 1973; Casley-Smith, 1976). In the arterial end of the capillary, the combined resultant forces of hydrostatic and osmotic pressures are outwardly directed into the tissues. The capillary wall controls and regulates its permeability by three types of structures: pores or junctions between the endothelial cells, vesicles in the endothelial cytoplasma, and fenestrations, which are holes through the endothelium.

The interstitial fluid performs a variety of functions, especially nourishment of the tissues. Nine-tenths of the fluid is recycled in the periphery to the blood circulation via the venous capillaries. The remaining 10 per cent are high molecular weight plasma proteins with their osmotically associated water. The latter are too large to pass readily through the venous capillary walls. Their removal from the milieu intérieur is accomplished in two ways. Some are lysed by monocyte-derived macrophages, "scavenger cells," until the fragments are small enough to reenter the capillaries. This type of tissue clearance is called the extralymphatic mastering of plasma proteins (Földi-Börcsök and Földi, 1973). The remainder is removed from the interstices by the lymphatics. The lymphatic load arrives via a three-dimensional network of channels of varying sizes called prelymphatics, formed by spaces between the gel-

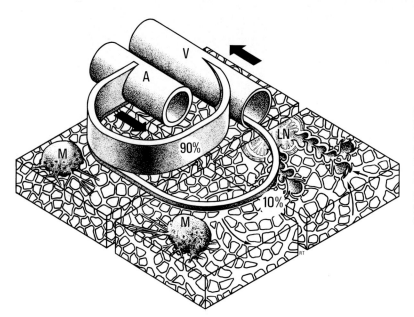

Figure 83–6. The balance of the intravascular and extravascular fluid circulation *(large arrows)* between the arterial capillary (A) and the venous capillary (V) bed, the interstices and the monocyte (M) system. LN = lymph node. The task of the lymphatic system is to process about 10 per cent of the hydroprotein vascular tissue exchange.

like ground substance, the fibers, and the cells. Through a flap valve mechanism a portion of the proteins with osmotically associated water, not lysed by the macrophages, enters the lymphatics to become lymph. The forces acting are similar to those in the blood capillaries: differences between the tissue hydrostatic pressure and the intralymphatic hydrostatic pressure, and differences between colloidal osmotic pressure within and outside the initial lymphatics. These act like millions of tiny pumps within the tissues. Their flap-valve mechanisms, operated by variations of tissue pressure in their surroundings as provided by muscle contractions and pulsatile blood flow, all propel the lymph fluid toward the collecting lymphatics. The initial lymphatics increase the formation of lymph if the water content and pressure within the interstices increase.

The collecting lymphatics can be visualized by patent blue dye and by lymphography. They possess a well-developed spiral muscle layer, and their valves provide for unidirectional flow of lymph toward the lymph nodes, the neck, and the venous system. The main propulsive force of lymph is generated by the contractions of the lymphangions, which are segments of lymphatics bordered by a distal and a proximal valve. Stretch-sensitive pacemakers situated in each lymphangion cause the lymph flow to increase automatically.

In order to understand the pathophysiology of lymphedema, the concept of the insufficiency of the lymph vascular system is here briefly outlined. The *lymph vascular system* is insufficient if the lymphatic transport capacity is lower than the lymphatic load. In one of the three forms of lymph vascular insufficiency (Table 83–1) the *lymphatic load* is not increased. The *lymphatic transport capacity,* defined as the highest total of lymph outflow channels (the anatomic element) times the power of lymphokinetic forces (the functional element), is reduced in chronic lymphedema to such an extent that multiple tissue alterations such as swelling (Table 83–2) become apparent (Altorfer, Hedinger, and Clodius, 1977).

The mechanical insufficiency of lymph flow responsible for lymphedema must be distinguished from the dynamic insufficiency of the lymph vascular system. Dynamic insufficiency arises if the lymphatic load exceeds the lymphatic transport capacity. The lymphatics are anatomically and functionally

Table 83–1. The Three Forms of Lymph Vascular Insufficiency

Mechanical insufficiency
  Lymphatic load normal
  Lymphatic transport capacity reduced
  Low lymph flow failure: tissue proteins stagnate

  Result: high protein edema (lymphedema)

Dynamic insufficiency
  Lymphatic load greater than lymphatic transport capacity
  High lymph flow failure: tissue fluids do not stagnate

  Result: low protein edema (heart/kidney failure)

Safety valve insufficiency (rare)
  Lymphatic load normal or increased
  Lymphatic transport capacity severely reduced

  Result: diffuse tissue necrosis within protein-rich edema in the extreme example

Adapted from Földi-Börcsök, E., and Földi, M.: Lymphedema and vitamins. Am. J. Clin. Nutr., 26:185, 1973.

normal but overwhelmed. A healthy lymph vascular system is able, for some time, to handle an increase of a lymphatic protein load and waterload, preventing the clinical appearance of edema. This is called the *lymphatic safety factor* against any swelling (Földi, 1969; Földi and Casley-Smith, 1983).

A rare third form of lymph vascular insufficiency occurs if the lymphatics with an already reduced transport capacity are, in addition, overwhelmed by an increased lymphatic load. This is a rare process, called *safety valve insufficiency,* leading in the extreme case to tissue necrosis, e.g., necrotizing erysipelas as a complication of lymphedema. In contrast to lymph stagnation, there is an increased stream of tissue fluid, which brings the lymphatic safety factor to a state of decompensation.

PATHOPHYSIOLOGY

Whereas an appendectomy cures the patient, surgery for lymphedema does not. Once clinically manifest lymphedema is established, reconstructive surgery is not able to produce a reversal of the lymphedematous tissue pathology (Table 83–3). The task of the lymphedema surgeon is to restore the balance quantitatively between the lymphatic load and the lymphatic transport capacity by reducing the lymphatic load and/or by increasing the lymphatic transport capacity.

Table 83–2. Mechanical Insufficiency of the Lymph Vascular System and the Consequences

Reduction of lymphatic transport capacity
Mechanical insufficiency of lymphatic transport
Overload of remaining lymphatic outflow tracts:
    remaining lymphatics
    lymphatic collaterals
    peripheral lymphovenous shunts
Lymphatic outflow tracts become incompetent
Fibrosis of lymphatic walls and of perilymphatic tissue
	Latent
	phase
	of
	lymphedema

Reduced function with radial spreading into tissues Protein and fluid accumulation, gradually replaced by fibrosclerotic tissues Disruption of normal tissue remodeling processes	Clinically manifest lymphedema
Fat deposition	
Chronic lymphedema	

In general, there are the following problems. Surgery is thought to be indicated only if conservative therapy fails, yet it would be preferable to operate during the stage of latent lymphedema and not when most of the lymphatic system is destroyed. Surgery should achieve a *permanent* and *stable* balance between the lymphatic transport capacity and the lymphatic load. It is not possible to determine in the individual patient the lymphatic load of a given lymphedematous extremity. As a rule, increasing the lymphatic transport capacity by lymphovenous shunts or lymph collector grafts does not completely *quantitatively* balance the lymphatic load. Thus, lymphedema is returned from its manifest phase only to its latent phase, and sooner or later it will recur.

In order to understand the problem of lymphedema, it is essential to realize that lymphedema not only represents tissue swelling due to an excess of fluid with an abnormally high protein content. There is also an intense tissue response, an important alteration of the functioning of the interstices with the prelymphatics, if there is failure of the

removal of protein by both the lymphatic system and by proteolysis (monocytes-macrophages). The reduced lymphatic transport capacity in primary and secondary lymphedema leads to "tissue poisoning" by the plasma proteins, further alterations of the lymphatic transport and filtration systems, changes in the direction of lymph flow, and alterations of the blood vascular system of the affected part (Altorfer, Hedinger, and Clodius, 1977; Clodius, 1977).

During the *latent phase* of edema, the initial lymphatics, the precollectors, and the collectors are massively dilated. The endothelial cells of the initial lymphatics demonstrate an intracellular edema with formation of vacuoles, dilatation of the cisternae of the endoplasmic reticulum, and increase of the osmiophilic microbodies. The interendothelial cell junctions are extremely opened to proteins, and the endolymphatically applied carbon particles can readily leave the lymphatics. Marked phagocytosis is demonstrated by the endothelial cells, which cannot be seen in *clinically chronic* edema. Similar changes are observed in the lymphatic precollectors and collectors. The walls of these structures become edematous. Protein-rich material is embedded between the cellular elements and the collagen fibers. The endothelial cells, as well as the smooth muscle cells, demonstrate an intracellular edema. During the latent phase of edema, smooth muscle cells are transformed into fibroblast-like cells. The loss of myofibrils and pinocytotic vesicles is noted, as well as the increase of granular endoplasmatic reticulum. Frequently, the lymph vessels of the epifascial and subfascial compartments are surrounded by fibrinoid material, leading to additional inflammatory reactions.

Table 83–3. Surgical Problems with Lymphedema

Latent, imperceptible stage of lymphedema
Mostly irreversible
    tissue changes
    destruction of lymphatic transport system
    destruction of lymph nodes—filter system
    changes in directions of lymph flow
        horizontal flow
        vertical flow
    blood vascular changes
Lymphatic watersheds
Body quadrants of lymph drainage

Polynucleated white blood cells, monocytes, lymphocytes, and proliferating adventitial cells migrate into the fibrinoid material formations. Many lymph capillaries are also formed. Within the lymphatics, thrombi of fibrinoid material are seen. These are organized by masses of phagocytes and by newly formed lymph capillaries. The vessel wall, adjacent to the thrombi, is usually penetrated by inflammatory infiltrates.

In *clinically chronic* lymphedema the initial lymphatics are still massively dilated. There are two additional phenomena: the basement membrane, generally discontinuous and inconspicuous, becomes enlarged and continuous. By this mechanism, large molecular substances such as protein and carbon particles are prevented from entering the lymph capillaries. In addition, the anchoring filaments of the endothelial cells are increased in number. Differentiation between the collectors and precollectors is no longer possible. The vessels are massively dilated (Fig. 83–7). Larger lymph collectors of the subfascial space demonstrate thickened and fibrosed vessel walls. The thrombi observed

during the latent phase of edema are now becoming organized and recanalized. However, a proper recanalization often cannot be observed. The layered protein deposits in the lymph vessels reveal only hyaline changes. Because of increased ectasia of the vessel walls, the lumen of such collectors remains patent, but their function is certainly diminished.

It has been stated that lymphedema is confined to the epifascial cylinder of skin and subcutaneous tissues (Kondoleon, 1912; Thompson, 1969; Kinney and Miller, 1987). The lymphedema problem thus may be solved by radical excision of the Charles (1912) type. This concept does not hold true as proved by computed tomography (CT) (Bruna, 1986) as well as by injecting radioactive lymphotropic tracers subfascially (zum Winkel, 1980). If patent blue is introduced subfascially, in experimental lymphedema as well as in the clinical case, it quickly stains the skin, demonstrating dermal lymphatic backflow from the deep to the superficial lymph draining systems.

In the *latent phase* of lymphedema, the

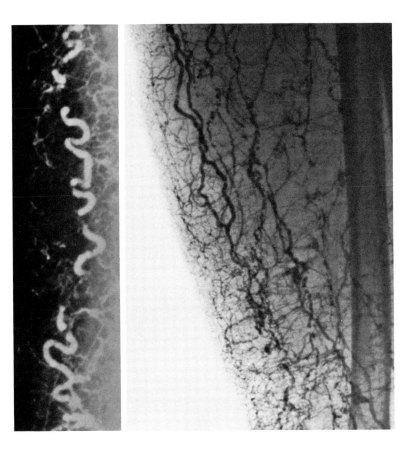

Figure 83–7. Lymphangiograms in secondary clinically manifest arm lymphedema. There is reversal of flow of the contrast medium from the deep to the superficial lymphatic system, which is not visualized in unimpaired lymph flow. Both lymphangiograms demonstrate irregular filling of dilated and extremely tortuous lymph collectors, which are functionally barely suitable for lymphovenous microvascular anastomoses.

filtration stations of the lymphatic system and the lymph nodes are also affected. Their medullary and marginal sinuses are dilated enormously. Lymph follicles are almost completely absent in some lymph nodes; in others, they are frequently present. The medullary tissue of the lymph node is reduced and replaced by the massively dilated sinus system. Opened lymphovenous shunts within the lymph nodes can be demonstrated.

During the early period of clinical lymphedema the lymph nodes, if not removed surgically or if not primarily absent, gradually start to harden and to shrink. Lymphonodovenous shunts thus should be performed early. On histologic examination the medullary sinuses of the lymph nodes are less dilated than during the latent phase. This is attributed to increased widening and sclerosis of the trabeculae and to the beginning fibrosis of the medullary tissue. An increased number of plasma cells is visible within the lymphatic medullary tissue. The lymphatic tissue of the cortex is reduced to a small marginal layer; the lymphatic tissue slowly disappears from the lymph nodes. The reduced defense against infection results in erysipelas attacks—a consequence, not a cause, of lymphedema. The regional immune insufficiency of a lymphedematous extremity may be compared with that of AIDS, both conditions leading to the development of angiosarcomas.

During operations in lymphedematous tissues, in patients as well as in animals with congenital or experimental lymphedema (Casley-Smith, Clodius, and Piller, 1980; Clodius, Piller, and Casley-Smith, 1981; Casley-Smith, Piller, and Clodius, 1986), excessive bleeding is frequently observed in the epifascial compartment. This is in accordance with the previous findings of Jacobsson (1967) in postmastectomy upper extremities affected by secondary lymphedema.

Measurements of the surface humidity of the skin of lymphedematous and normal extremities showed that in approximately 70 per cent of patients the lymphedematous extremity was drier than the normal one. A patient gave the explanation: "my swollen arm is warmer than the other, therefore the skin is dry." Thermographic studies of lymphedematous upper extremities documented this finding (Fig. 83–8). Corrosive preparations of extremities of dogs with chronic primary and secondary lymphedema demonstrated the markedly increased vascularity, leading to the temperature differences (Clodius, Piller, and Casley-Smith, 1981). Perhaps this increased vascularity is nature's way of trying to elongate the vascular span

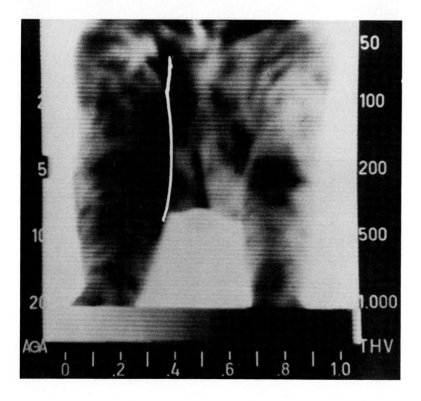

Figure 83–8. Thermography of a patient with secondary arm lymphedema of the upper extremity. The limb is up to 1°C warmer than the left.

to resorb fluid. It has also been demonstrated by serial histologic sections that lymph vessels can penetrate through the wall of blood vessels so that additional communications develop between the blood and the lymph circulation (Altorfer, Hedinger, and Clodius, 1977). Willoughby and DiRosa (1970) showed the lymphedematous changes to be very similar to the signs of chronic inflammation, as recognized almost a century ago (Winiwarter, 1892). Willoughby and DiRosa concluded that the basic cause of all inflammation is altered tissue proteins. Surgery in lymphedematous tissue thus is not without problems.

In addition to these histologic changes, there are adverse physiologic considerations in secondary lymphedema that render surgery for lymphedema difficult. The direction of lymph flow in the extremity is not only from distal to proximal, but also from the superficial to the deep lymphatic system. If, in the case of lymphadenectomy at the root of the extremity, the deep lymphatic system is interrupted, the clinical consequences or manifestations of the lymphostasis are observed in the epifascial space. When the swelling becomes clinically evident, the deep lymph collectors, which would be admirably suitable for the establishment of lymphaticovenous anastomoses, are already obliterated.

The same findings are true of primary lymphedema. If there is clinical lymphedema, the lymph vessels in the epifascial space are likely to be useless for lymphaticovenous or lympholymphatic anastomoses. In the case of other operations designed to increase the lymphatic transport capacity (e.g., enteromesenteric bridging surgery), the lymphatic system in the lymphostatic region should be capable of forming a quantitatively sufficient number of lympholymphatic anastomoses. On the basis of the histologic findings (see Table 83–2), this is probably no longer possible even in the latent phase of lymphedema.

In the deep as well as in the superficial lymphatic system the flow of lymph from a particular collector being obstructed cannot always pass over to a collateral unobstructed collector. Handley (1922) noted that lymph of a cutaneous area cannot be readily drained into another skin field. Kubik (1980; Kubik and Manestar, 1986) demonstrated these lymphatic watersheds, delineating lymph territories or "lymphangiosomes" in humans. In order to overcome these cutaneous lymphatic watersheds, the direction of the lymph flow, normally from superficial to deep, must be reversed, as shown by Gooneratne (1974).

A further obstacle to the flow of lymph from an obstructed to an unobstructed lymphangiosome is the existence of body quadrants of lymph drainage (see Fig. 83–3). The superficial lymph of each extremity, together with the adjacent lymphatics of the homolateral quadrant of the skin of the trunk, drain to the lymph nodes at the root of each extremity. The boundaries of these trunk territories are, as a rule, traversed by only valveless lymphatics (Forbes, 1937–1938).

From these anatomic findings it follows that in any surgical drainage procedure, e.g., a lymph-bearing flap for lymphedema due to a blockage at the root of an extremity (groin or axillary dissection), the new drainage system must reach the nonlymphedematous quadrant (Gillies and Fraser, 1950; Clodius and associates, 1982). It is a typical problem of local flaps, which try to bridge an area of lymphatic obstruction to which they themselves drain (Smith and Conway, 1962).

In summary, successful surgery of a vascular system is based on the following principles:

1. Patency must be restored in the damaged vascular system.

2. The direction of flow in the vascular system must be correct.

3. The flow into the reconstructed vascular system must be adequate.

4. Drainage from the reconstructed vascular system must be guaranteed.

5. Restored patency must be a permanent feature.

6. Restored patency must be quantitatively adequate.

CLASSIFICATION

It is important to differentiate between lymphedema and lymphostasis. *Lymphostasis* is a reduction of the lymphatic transport capacity. Lymphedema does not necessarily result from this, owing to the safety mechanisms against high protein edema. Interstitial fluid starts to accumulate only after the lymph flow is reduced by 80 per cent.

From the etiologic point of view, lymphedemas can be classified into primary and secondary types.

Primary lymphedema, occurring without apparent cause, is not related to a malignancy. These lymphatic malformations are radiographically divided into hypoplastic and hyperplastic (varicosis of lymph vessels) forms, the latter arising in 10 per cent of lymphatic malformations. Primary lymphedemas due to congenital disorders of the lymphatic system (hereditary or nonhereditary) may become clinically manifest as *lymphedema congenitum* (lymphedema present at birth), as *lymphedema praecox* (the disease appears before the age of 35 years), or as *lymphedema tardum* (the latent phase lasts up to 35 years and more).

Secondary lymphedema can be caused by primary or recurrent malignancies: intralymphatic tumor growth or extralymphatic compression of the lymphatics. Secondary lymphedema is iatrogenic: after surgery (block dissection, stripping of veins, peripheral vascular surgery, lipectomy) or after irradiation. Cases of *lymphedema facticium* (self-mutilation) are seen in increasing numbers. Secondary lymphedema can also result from soft tissue trauma with interruption of the lymphatic pathways, including circular constricting or amniotic bands. Bacteria, fungi, parasites (filariasis), insects, and geochemical irritants can also cause lymphangiosis and lymphangitis, resulting in secondary lymphedema.

THERAPY

The first category of patients with lymphedema includes those who manage their extremity without the help of a physician. Their family physician may once have told them that there is no cure for this condition and that they must help themselves. These patients have differences in circumferences of 2 or 3 cm between their healthy and their affected limbs. They rarely experience an attack of erysipelas. These patients still have functioning mechanisms of compensating for their reduced lymphatic transport capacity: a collateral lymphatic circulation, peripheral lymphovenous shunts (Malek, 1972), and an increased amount (up to 30 times their normal number) of activated macrophages.

The next type of patients need help. The family physician or, in the case of a secondary lymphedema, the radiotherapist or oncologist tells them what to do for the lymphedematous limb(s). He may precribe (wrongly) an elastic stocking or a sleeve, a lymphoactive drug, or a long-term diuretic, which would be illogical for treatment of a localized high protein edema.

After a while the patients discontinue this therapy because it has not reduced the extremity to normal size. After some years, the situation deteriorates. There are occasional attacks of erysipelas, and the patients seek the care of a "specialist." The compensating mechanisms are quantitatively reduced. The specialist is interested in the problem and, despite many failures with it, is determined to help. At first he will establish the most important fact prior to any therapy: the correct diagnosis—since lymphedema is only a symptom, and a late symptom at that. In making the diagnosis, a careful history and a complete clinical inspection and palpation of the patient (not only of the swollen parts) is mandatory. If doubt persists, the patent blue dye test is recommended or, if possible, microlymphangiography (Bollinger, Partsch, and Wolfe, 1985). More invasive diagnostic procedures, such as lymphangiography, can harm the remaining lymphatic system (Collard and Servais, 1978) and should be carried out only if the decision to perform a definitive surgical procedure (e.g., a lymphovenous shunting operation) (Clodius, 1977) depends on these radiologic findings. As a possible cause, even for long-standing lymphedema, a malignancy must always be considered and ruled out.

Principles

The principles of management of lymphedema must be based on the facts of lymphology as previously outlined. The aim must be to eliminate protein stagnation in the interstices and to restore normal extravascular circulation of plasma proteins from the blood circulation through the tissues and within the lymph vascular system.

Before the treatment of lymphedema is begun, a precise diagnosis is mandatory. Especially in nontropical countries, the differential diagnosis must be made to determine whether the lymphedema is due to some underlying malignant condition. The sudden onset of lymphedema (especially in the proximal part of the extremity), rapid clinical progression, frequent pain, and fast hardening of the swelling all point toward "malignant lymphedema," caused by direct tumor growth and/or metastatic disease.

Every case of lymphedema should be treated as early as possible before extensive and irreversible tissue alterations develop.

Drugs

The use of *diuretics* contradicts an understanding of the pathophysiology of lymphedema, which is not due to sodium retention. By hemoconcentration the diuretics are able to remove water held by the colloid-osmotic forces of the stagnant protein molecules. The proteins remain in the tissues, and their concentration in the remaining edema fluid increases; thus, within years, the involved tissues become even more fibrotic than they would have been without diuretics.

The *benzopyrones,* which include the flavonoids and coumarin (not to be confounded with the anticoagulant dicumarol), have been shown to be effective in the treatment of high protein edemas both experimentally and clinically (Földi-Börcsök and Földi, 1973; Bolton and Casley-Smith, 1975; Casley-Smith, 1976; Piller, 1976; Casley-Smith and Casley-Smith, 1986). In the early soft pitting stage of lymphedema, benzopyrone administration enhances protein removal from the affected area without the need of functioning lymphatics. Once in the tissues, the benzopyrones bind to abnormally accumulated protein. A situation develops that becomes more attractive to the phagocytic cells, the macrophages, which accumulate up to 30 times their normal number in the affected region. The immediate results are an enhancement of phagocytosis and an increased rapidity and completeness of protein splitting, followed by a subsequent increase of protein fragments and amino acid levels. The protein fragments can leave via the vascular system because of their reduced size, a concentration gradient directed from the tissues, their low molecular sieving, and the high diffusion coefficients. The importance of this drug-induced and controlled proteolysis is emphasized by the strong correlation existing between acid and neutral proteinase activity levels in the skin and in the edema fluid. In 92 randomized benzopyrone-treated patients with secondary arm lymphedema, the average reduction of circumference was 0.5 cm per ten months,

whereas in untreated patients the difference of circumference increased an average of 1 cm per year; in 18 per cent of patients the medication was without effect (Clodius and Piller, 1978). Thus, benzopyrone therapy is a useful adjuvant in the care of lymphedema. However, the swelling is not reduced decisively by this drug alone, since the extralymphatic mastering of plasma proteins is only an adjunctive mechanism in the lymphatic transport system.

Complex Decongestive Physiotherapy
(Winiwarter, 1892; Földi, 1983)

"Conservative management is the best approach for the majority [of lymphedemas] and surgery should be eschewed whenever possible" (Browse, 1987). In the past, for lymphedemas of irreversible, elephantiasic size, surgery was considered the treatment of choice. Figure 83–9 demonstrates the contrary.

The two-phase complex decongestive treatment consists of five parts of equal importance. During the first phase of daily therapy, decongestion is accomplished, usually on an inpatient basis. The second phase, during which the patient treats himself (like a diabetic), consists of supportive care to conserve at least the result of the first phase with the goal to further improve the lymphedematous extremity.

The five steps are summarized below:

1. Hygienic measures and the eradication of fungal affections are mandatory. In most cases, this suffices to abolish attacks of erysipelas. If not, antibacterial treatment, eventually lifelong, must be started.

2. Manual lymph drainage. The first goal of this special massage technique, commenced over the contralateral quadrant of the trunk that is free of lymphostasis, is to increase lymphokinetic activity in the normal lymphatics. It is known that lymphangions increase their output if subjected to mild mechanical stimuli. The lymphatics should start to drain the lymphostatic quadrant across the lymphatic watershed. The decongestion of the lymphostatic trunk quadrant then allows edema fluid to pass through dilated tissue channels (and, if present, lymphatics) from the limb, first into the ipsilateral, and then into the contralateral trunk quadrant. This

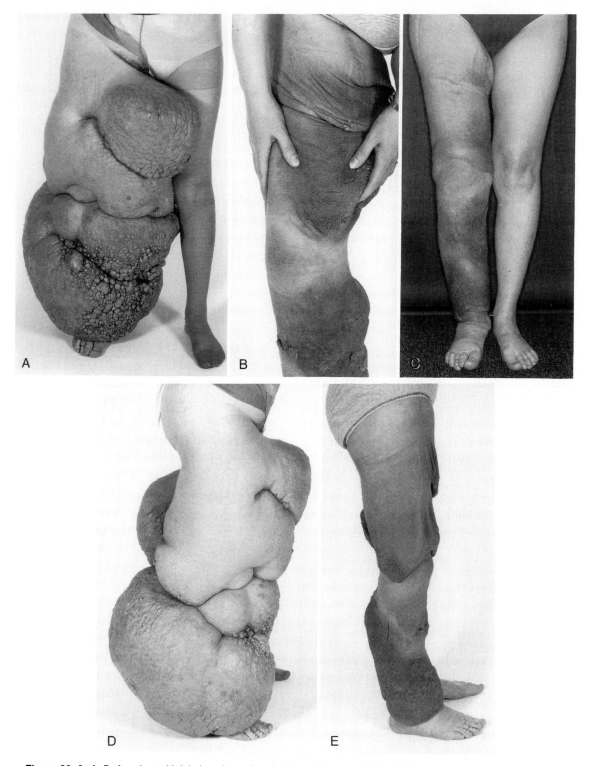

Figure 83–9. *A, D,* A patient with lobular primary lymphedema. Excess of 55 kg of "lymphedema" was contained within the affected leg. The skin between the lobular parts of the lymphedematous tissues revealed multiple foci of infection; the patient was in a subseptic state. Surgery at this stage would have been associated with a high rate of complications. Therefore, the patient was referred for complex decongestive physiotherapy. *B, E,* The result after conservative management of five months, now hampered by the excess of loose skin, which was excised. *C,* The patient eight years after the beginning of therapy. There has been no recurrence of the swelling, and resection of loose skin at the thigh and above the ankle is possible.

phenomenon will of course start centrally, the decongestion finally arriving in the tips of the fingers and toes. Pecking and associates (1985) showed that the speed of the lymphatic transport of a tracer injected into the edematous hand of a patient suffering from postmastectomy lymphedema increases immediately if the contralateral normal quadrant is treated by "manual lymph drainage." The second step in "manual lymph drainage" consists in pushing edema fluid gently from the lymphostatic quadrant into the normal one, the healthy lymphatics of which have previously been stimulated. The upper arm (thigh) will be evacuated if the ipsilateral quadrant of the trunk is already free of edema. Treatment of the lower arm (leg) begins later; the latest step consists in the treatment of the hand (foot).

3. From the beginning of the treatment, bandages are applied over the lymphedematous limb. One of the first pathologic consequences of lymphedema is a destruction of elastic fibers. Consequently, the elastic insufficiency of the connective tissue of the subcutaneous layer adds to the effect of the decrease of tissue pressure brought about by the evacuation of edema fluid by manual lymph drainage. If tissue pressure decreases, effective ultrafiltrating pressure increases. Without bandaging, the edema fluid would reaccumulate. Bandages not only counterbalance the elastic insufficiency but also increase tissue pressure. It has been shown that there is a positive correlation between tissue pressure and lymph flow.

4. Remedial exercises, performed while the bandages are worn, enable muscle and joint pumps to exert their lymphokinetic effects.

5. At the end of the treatment, which lasts approximately four weeks, an elastic support, as strong as can be tolerated by the patient, must be prescribed. The goal of the elastic support is not to compress the lymphedematous limb but to prevent the reaccumulation of edema. It has often been said that after the first phase of decongestion lymphedema recurs sooner or later. In West Germany all patients treated as described obtained their individually fitted elastic stocking from the same company, which stored the names and the concomitant measurements. It was therefore possible to verify the late results of the initial treatment of 726 patients over a period of six years. The extremity of 672 patients (92.6 per cent) remained stable, 36 (5 per cent) continued to improve, and 18 (2.4 per cent) had a relapse of the lymphedema (Clodius and Piller, 1978).

A word of caution is required concerning the use of pneumatic compression devices. It was demonstrated experimentally that any form of vigorous massage is deleterious to the functioning of the remaining lymphatics (Casley-Smith, 1977). The pneumatic compression machines should never be used to replace complex decongestive physiotherapy. If one readily expresses the edema fluid without preparing the homolateral quadrant by manual evacuating massage, the limb may be evacuated but the edema stagnates as a ring of fluid immediately above the expressive device. At this site edema may increase or even be created. Its stagnation induces fibrosis and further obstructs lymph drainage.

As after surgery, the lymphedema patients treated conservatively are not cured. Treatment for lymphedema is a lifelong process (Table 83–4). There is, however, no contrain-

Table 83–4. Rules and Hints for Lymphedema Patients

In General

Take good care of the lymphedematous extremity and avoid clothes that are constricting

Nail care is important; do not pick or cut cuticles

Do not use irritant cosmetics

Maintain your weight; avoid undue intake of salt

Sauna is contraindicated

During Daily Activities

Do not dig in the garden or work near thorny plants

Be careful with the kitchen knife; do not reach into a hot oven

Do not carry heavy bags

Wear loose-fitting rubber gloves when washing dishes; wear a thimble when sewing

Elevate, when possible, the lymphedematous extremity

Avoid direct sun or heat to the lymphedematous extremity

Avoid scratches from cats

With the Physician

Do not permit injection or withdrawal of blood specimens from the lymphedematous extremity; no acupuncture is allowed

Do not permit a lymphophlebogram or arteriogram without therapeutic indications

Do not permit biopsies or removal of (remaining) lymph nodes without clear therapeutic indications

Avoid blood pressure recordings on a lymphedematous arm

Avoid pressure stockings or sleeves that are not individually fitted

Avoid any pressure-type massage on the affected extremity

dication for the described conservative treatment and, in contrast to surgery, no complications have been observed.

Heat and Bandage Treatment
(Zhang and associates, 1984)

Local limb hyperthermia is a traditional method of Chinese medicine. An electrocontrolled heating chamber, now a microwave oven with a temperature of up to 120°C, elevates the temperature of the extremity by 6° to 7°C up to one hour once a day for 20 days. Three to five courses of therapy are recommended, with an interval of seven to ten days, during which time tightly fitting bandaging is applied. Zhang and associates (1984) reported clinical improvement in over two-thirds of the patients with this technique, without long-term follow-up. There was a sixfold reduction of the attacks of erysipelas; the lymphographic picture improved, as well as the clearance of radioiodinated albumin from the lymphedematous tissues.

Surgery

Plastic surgical treatment for lymphedema has undergone considerable changes (Table 83–5). New surgical techniques have been developed and applied (Olszewski and Nielubowicz, 1966; Kaye, Smith, and Acland, 1980; Baumeister and associates, 1981; Ho, Lai, and Kennedy, 1983; O'Brien, 1985). However, because of the progress of conservative therapy for lymphedema during the past 20 years, the author rarely recommends surgery as the primary treatment at present. Nahai and Stahl (1984) concurred with this: "Classically, the treatment of congenital lymphedema is nonoperative." The surgeons Esmarch and Kulenkampff (1885) stressed that no surgery be initiated before conservative therapy (hygienic measures, compression, elevation) had been fully explored.

However, in other parts of the world, there may be good reasons for different opinions. For example, in a tropical climate the lymphatic load increases, making the lymphedematous skin situation more difficult to control. The finesse of conservative therapy unfortunately may not be available to many lymphedematous patients. This is one reason why, in addition to conservative therapy, sur-

Table 83–5. Principal Surgical Techniques

Procedures to Reduce Load for Lymphatic Clearance
Resection of epifascial lymphedematous tissue:
Successive removal of ellipses of skin and subcutis with primary closure (Sistrunk, 1918, 1927; Ghormley and Overton, 1935; Miller, 1975, 1977)
Excision with wound closure by local skin flaps (Homans, 1936; Pratt and Wright, 1941; Brunner, 1969)
Radical resection of epifascial lymph space
Suction lipectomy of epifascial lymph space (Teimourian, 1987)
Wound closure by split-thickness skin graft (Charles, 1912; Macey, 1940, 1948; Mowlem, 1948)
Wound closure by full-thickness skin graft (Gibson and Tough, 1954, 1955; Barinka, 1977, 1984)
Ligatures of arterial blood supply (Carnochan, 1854; Esmarch and Kulenkampff, 1885; Winiwarter, 1892; Mayall, Mayall, and Ferreti, 1979; Jaju, 1976, 1987)

Procedures to Increase Lymphatic Transport Capacity
Reconstruction of new "lymph vessels" with threads and tubes (Handley, 1908, 1910; Lenggenhager, 1961; Zieman, 1962; Weber and Steckmesser, 1982)

Drainage
Drainage through strips of fascia or through tensor fascia lata (Martorell, 1958; Chitale, 1987)
Drainage through omental transfer (Dick, 1935; Mowlem, 1948; Kirikuta, 1963; Goldsmith, 1974)
Drainage through skin flaps (Rosanow, 1912; Gillies and Fraser, 1950; Pratt and Wright, 1941; Standard, 1942; Mowlem, 1948; Smith and Conway, 1962; Thompson, 1969; Hirshowitz and Goldan, 1971; Clodius and Gibson, 1979; Clodius and associates, 1982)
Drainage through enteromesenteric bridging surgery (Kinmonth, 1982; Hurst, Kinmouth, and Rutt, 1981)
Drainage through peripheral lymphaticovenous anastomoses
Lymphonodovenous anastomoses (Olszewski and Nielubowicz, 1966; Nielubowicz and Olszewski, 1968; Jamal, 1981)
Anastomoses between lymph collectors and veins (Laine and Howard, 1963; Sedlacek, 1969; Yamada, 1969; Degni, 1974; Gilbert and associates, 1976; O'Brien, 1985; Huang and associates, 1985; Nieuborg, 1982)
Bridging of localized obstructions of lymphatic drainage by transplantation of lymph collectors (Baumeister and associates, 1981; Ho, Lai, and Kennedy, 1983) by transplantation of veins (Mandl, 1981)

gical approaches are discussed. A patient with severe lymphedema that has lasted ten years or more has a 10 per cent chance of being affected with the worst complication of lymphedema: lymphangiosarcoma (Woodward, Ivins, and Soule, 1972).

From a physiologic standpoint, surgery must reduce the lymphatic load or increase the lymphatic transport capacity. The ideal time to increase lymphatic drainage, particularly after an axillary or inguinal lymph node resection, is the early latent period as described above. Since the remaining lymphatics degenerate progressively, therapeutic relief should be instituted before tissue and vascular changes become irreversible and drainage operations are futile. From the patient's standpoint it seems essential that a thin and soft extremity of normal color, contour, and texture be restored.

PROCEDURES REDUCING THE LOAD FOR LYMPHATIC CLEARANCE

Excisional operations are designed to remove as much of the edematous subcutaneous tissue as possible and are of two types: (1) procedures in which skin flaps are retained to close the wound after excision and (2) those in which both skin and subcutaneous tissue are excised and the wound is covered, either with the original skin prepared as a free graft, or with split-thickness skin grafts from other donor sites. Each has its advantages and disadvantages. The techniques can improve the patient's situation. The functional aspect consists of reducing the lymphatic load from the epifascial compartment. In addition, the distance over which the lymph must flow from the deep to the superficial lymphatics is reduced, possibly an explanation for the lowered incidence of subsequent erysipelas attacks. Repeated debulking by suction assisted lipectomy (SAL) (Teimourian, 1987) obviated the problem of skin reconstruction.

For the author, the indications for a reducing procedure are twofold: (1) when there is an elephantiasic deformity and no complex decongestive therapy is available; and (2) when there has been successful conservative treatment (Fig. 83–9) and excessive skin prevents adequate bandaging and manual evacuating massage, and the wearing of compressive sleeves is an esthetic problem. "Reducing operations do not cure the underlying condition. They are palliative and leave the patient with unsightly scars. These aspects of the operation must be clearly explained to the patient before the operation. When a patient with mild swelling presses for an operation the author tries to introduce them to a patient who has had a reducing operation. This usually diminishes their enthusiasm for surgery" (Browse, 1987).

There are two varieties of excisional procedures: the ones using skin flaps and those employing skin grafts.

Skin Flap Procedures. Sistrunk (1918, 1927) modified Kondoleon's (1912) technique to include as large as possible an excision of skin and subcutaneous tissue but still allowing primary closure. Although there are better procedures for the lower extremity, excisional techniques of this type are valuable for the thigh and for some cases of arm lymphedema. If adequate postoperative care is taken, the results may remain stable for a long time (Ghormley and Overton, 1935). Homans (1936) reduced elephantiasic lower legs in four steps. Pratt and Wright (1941) went further and excised three-quarters of the edematous tissue in one procedure by extensive undermining; they recovered any skin loss with flaps from the abdomen, an undesirable necessity.

Skin Graft Operations. Radical excision followed by split-thickness skin grafting has been described by multiple authors. Macey (1940, 1948), Mowlem (1958), and Campbell, Glas, and Musselmann (1951) harvested the graft from the abdomen or thigh. Others removed the grafts from the edematous lower leg before excising the mass (Hergenroeder, 1938; Poth, Barnes, and Ross, 1947; Farina, 1951). The use of split-thickness skin grafts for this purpose on the lower leg, often erroneously called the Charles procedure, is a poor choice for two reasons: (1) it is not possible to cut a large enough skin graft to cover the whole area, and multiple sheets and strips are needed; and (2), more important, such thin grafts are unstable, and eczema and breakdown are common postoperative sequelae. It is possible to use a single sheet of full-thickness skin harvested from the mass of skin and fat resulting from the excision.

The technique was developed from the multiple-stage operation described by Homans (1936) in which long flaps of full-thickness skin were elevated, the underlying edematous mass was excised, and the flap was replaced. Invariably there was congestion with necrosis along the edge of the flap. Better results were obtained when the flap was completely detached before being replaced as a full-thickness skin graft, and the next logical step was to deal with the whole circumference of the leg in this way (Gibson and Tough, 1954, 1955).

The results are stable for many years and the incidence of erysipelas is greatly reduced, although not invariably totally abolished.

Thinning or debulking of the areas over the malleoli at a second procedure often allows the patient to wear ordinary shoes. Barinka (1977, 1984) used this approach as a two-stage procedure, including the distal half of the thigh and the knee.

Ligation of Arterial Blood Supply. It has been mentioned that the flow of blood in the epifascial compartment was found to be increased (Jacobsson, 1967; Clodius, Piller, and Casley-Smith, 1981). For this reason and on the basis of arteriographic findings, Jaju (1976, 1987) and Mayall, Mayall, and Ferreti (1979) resorted to arterial ligation as introduced in 1854 (Carnochan). Postoperatively, no signs of arterial insufficiency were observed, the subcutaneous edematous tissues were reduced substantially, the skin was hanging in loose folds, and keratotic changes cleared up. Jaju (1976, 1987) attributed the improvement following reducing operations with flaps and skin grafts also to the reduction of the blood supply due to the ligatures of musculocutaneous perforators.

No long-term statistics are available on these arterial ligation techniques. It is the author's opinion that an increased blood supply to the tissues, as seen in vascular malformations and tumors, does not lead to an increase of the formation of lymph across the capillary wall. The increased blood flow through the epifascial lymphedematous extremity cylinder (with no elevation of the total blood supply) (Jacobsson, 1967) is the consequence of the secondary aseptic inflammatory reactions in lymphedema leading to angiogenesis (Willoughby and DiRosa, 1970).

PROCEDURES INCREASING LYMPH DRAINAGE

Although ablative surgery yields the greatest reduction in the size of a limb, "the surgery of ablation is but a poor substitute for the ability to restore normality" (Mowlem, 1958). The many fascinating trials listed in Table 83–5, aiming to reconstruct the lymphatic circulation, have led to increased knowledge of the lymphatic system experimentally and clinically (Clodius, 1977; Olszewski, 1982), including the immunologic aspects of lymph (Galkowska and Olszewski, 1986).

Creation of "New Lymphatics." Handley (1908) introduced silk threads across the lymphatic barrier with the idea that their capillary action would enable them to replace the missing lymphatics and to transfer the excess fluid to regions with normal circulation. However, Handley wrote in 1910: "To my mind lymphangioplasty has failed to establish its position in the treatment of elephantiasis." Histologic findings presented in 1912 (Madden, Ibrahim, and Ferguson) were of dense fibrous tissue around the sutures, effectively preventing any absorption of fluid. In the light of today's knowledge about the elaborate function of the lymphatic system, i.e., that lymphedema is high protein edema, it is difficult to understand why this procedure is still in use (Lenggenhager, 1961; Zieman, 1962). Believing that the operative trauma is the main cause of scar formation around the implanted threads of his nylon net, Degni (1974) advocated postoperative use of corticosteroids. He claimed an average edema reduction of 61 per cent in a follow-up period of one to 12 months. The concept that scar tunnels around implanted threads and tubes might replace the complicated function of the interstices and of the canalicular lymph system must be considered science fiction.

It is, however, important to mention the unspecific effect of any procedure on lymphedema. With regard to the thread and tube drainage lymphatic substitute (Silver and Puckett, 1976), Winiwarter stated in 1892: "Different surgeons repetitiously made the peculiar observation that elephantiasis was to be decisively improved by any larger operation, even when it was deemed impossible to have any effect upon the condition and even when surgery took place in an entirely different part of the body!"

Drainage Through Strips of Fascia or Tensor Fascia Lata (Martorell, 1958; Chitale, 1987). It is doubtful whether a sufficient number of lymphatics could grow along the fascia lata, which is carried in two strips underneath the inguinal ligament, one on the surface of the psoas muscle and one placed subcutaneously to the opposite abdomen. From the studies of Gray (1939) and Odén (1960), it seems unlikely that newly formed valved lymph collectors are able to bridge such a distance. Chitale (1987) used the homolateral tensor fascia lata flap for drainage, based on the concept of the lymphatic quadrants of the body. It follows, however, that the contralateral would have been preferable (Clodius and associates, 1982).

Drainage Through a Flap of Omentum.

Dick (1935) used the omentum pedicled on its gastroepiploic vessels for successful drainage in two cases of scrotal lymphedema. As one patient developed an incarcerated hernia at the site of exit of the omentum through the abdominal wall, the omental pedicle had to be severed and the lymphedema recurred. Mowlem (1948) used the omentum in two patients with lower extremity lymphedema, and Kirikuta (1963) and Goldsmith, De los Santos, and Beattie (1968) popularized the method for treatment of lymphedemas of the upper and lower extremities. The omentum has a relatively rich lymph system; one or two longitudinal lymph collectors run parallel to the major branches of the gastroepiploic arcades to drain toward the inferior gastric and the pancreaticosplenic lymph nodes. As in all such drainage procedures, the question is whether a sufficient number of lympholymphatic anastomoses form for adequate drainage of the edematous area. For the treatment of scrotal lymphedema this was apparently the case, but Goldsmith (1974) obtained only moderate improvement with lymphedema of the arms and legs. When he weighed these results against the magnitude of the operation and such complications as hernias, intestinal obstruction, and gastric dysfunction, he abandoned the procedure.

There is a second problem: when the omentum is lengthened on its distal vascular arcade to reach into an extremity, its proximal lymphatics are by necessity divided. Whether and if so how many vertical lymphatic cross connections exist in the omentum, the author has not been able to determine. Since 1973, in 12 cases of irradiation damage to the brachial plexus, the omentum has been grafted to the axillary region with end to side anastomoses to the axillary vessels (Clodius, Uhlschmid, and Hess, 1984). All patients also suffered from various degrees of secondary arm lymphedema. Only the progression of the lymphedematous swelling was halted, but the patients became and remained free of pain.

Drainage Through Skin Flaps. It has been shown by lymphangiography that when a pedicle flap is transferred to a new site, lymphatics in the flap link up with lymphatics in the recipient bed (Clodius, 1977). This possibility had earlier inspired Gillies and Fraser (1935) to transfer a long, narrow flap of skin from the arm to the lateral side of the thigh and abdomen to promote lymph drainage from a lymphedematous leg to the axilla, bypassing the presumed block in the inguinal region. In this case of moderate lymphedema, this "lymphatic wick" provided adequate lymph drainage on long-term follow-up (Gillies and Fraser, 1950). However, the arm from which the flap was taken subsequently became lymphedematous.

Although its success was qualified by the arm complication, this procedure showed that a lymphatic barrier could be bridged. A variety of other flaps were used about this time (Pratt and Wright, 1941; Mowlem, 1948; Smith and Conway, 1962) and on the whole the results were poor. Many, such as tube pedicles, required multiple-stage procedures, and the scarring may well have inhibited lymphaticolymphatic anastomoses.

The best skin flaps to serve as lymphatic wicks thus appear to be local transposed flaps containing axial lymphatics, not dilated and with their proximal pedicle, the lymphatic outlet, as close to the axilla or groin as possible. In selected patients they may be well worthwhile (Fig. 83–10) (Clodius and associates, 1982).

Sappey (1874) was the first to notice that in congenital and acquired lymphedema the swelling seemed to be restricted to the skin and subcutaneous compartment of the extremity. The deep fascia was found to be thickened and thus was considered as a barrier across which no lymph could flow from the superficial compartment to be absorbed by the deep compartment. As mentioned above, the concept of the fascial lymph barrier function has been disproved (Watson, 1953; Gibson and Tough, 1954; Crockett, 1965; Clodius, 1977; Bruna, 1986). Therefore, so-called physiologic operations that resect strips or all of the deep fascia (Kondoleon, 1912; Peer and associates, 1954) or implant strips of it (Lanz, 1911), triangles of subcutaneous tissue (Rosanow, 1912), or shaved skin flaps (Thompson, 1969) between extensor and flexor muscles are based on a false concept.

Lymphatic-Vein Anastomoses. When Edwards and Kinmonth in 1969 performed lymphangiography on a patient with bilateral lymphatic deficiency but only one swollen leg, they visualized a lymphovenous shunt in the normal-appearing leg. Besides the formation of a collateral lymphatic circulation, the opening of lymphovenous shunts is one of nature's methods of bypassing a surgical block; this has been confirmed in man under

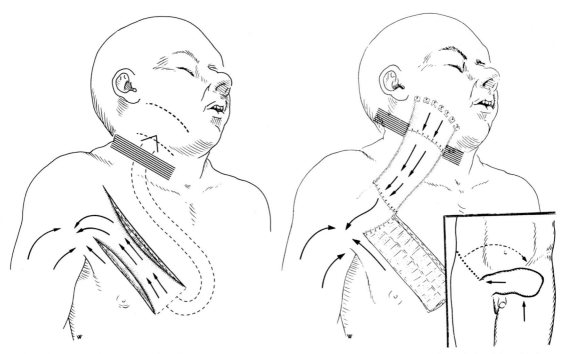

Figure 83–10. The principle of lymph drainage by a flap as demonstrated in a rare case of unilateral cheek lymphedema. A relatively broad deepithelized flap with a lymphatic transport capacity as large as possible, draining directly to a confluence of lymphatics at the root of an extremity, is transferred through a subcutaneous tunnel to the base of the cheek. Thus, at only one site, lympholymphatic anastomoses are left to form spontaneously. The inset shows the same principle for lymphatic groin drainage. The arrows demonstrate the direction of lymph flow postoperatively.

normal conditions (Frautschi, 1948; Kubik, 1952; Threefoot and Kossover, 1966; Rusznyak, Földi, and Szabo, 1967; Pressman, Dunn, and Burtz, 1967) and in lymphedema (Picard, Arvay, and Charbit, 1966).

This natural phenomenon has stimulated others to create, surgically, anastomoses between the lymphatics in lymphedematous tissues and suitable veins. This may be achieved in two ways: (1) by inserting part of a lymph node into a vein and (2) by direct linkage of a lymphatic to a vein by microsurgical anastomosis.

Lymphonodovenous Anastomosis. This technique was first performed for lymphedema of the lower limb by Olszewski and Nielubowicz (1966) who, in their experimental studies, proved histologically that the anastomosis remains patent if there is an increased lymphatic pressure (Nielubowicz and Olszewski, 1968; Olszewski, 1977, 1982). Kinmonth (1982) confirmed the patency of such an anastomosis by a lymphangiogram two years postoperatively in a patient with primary hyperplastic lymphedema. For best results, as many lymph nodes as possible should be anastomosed to the femoral vein.

The indications for this operation are reflected in the results: optimal results are seen in patients with secondary lymphedema (carcinoma of the uterus). Half of Olszewski's (1977, 1982) patients had good results at two

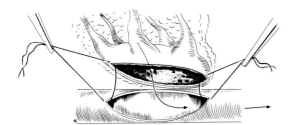

Figure 8–11. Lymphonodocapsular-venous shunt. The arrows point to the direction of lymph flow.

years; in primary hyperplastic lymphedema, good results were obtained in 43 per cent at three years postoperatively; but in hypo- or aplastic lymphedema, improvement was present in only 16 per cent at three years. If lymph nodes are palpable, the author considers lymph node–vein shunts as the operative procedure of choice. It does not reduce an elephantiasic lower leg, but combined with excisional operation it also reduces the lymphatic load and the thigh is softer and somewhat thinner. One of the author's patients with primary lymphedema, when elevating her leg for lymph drainage, experienced severe pain in the groin. This was relieved by lymph node–vein shunts. If the lymph nodes cannot be palpated with certainty, suprailiac lymphangiography (Bruna, 1973) is advised. Unfortunately, lymph node–vein anastomoses are not available for secondary arm lymphedema.

The earlier techniques consisted of transplanting a section of the node into an incision in a vein. However, the development of intranodal fibrosis in the pulp caused resistance to flow (Papp, 1969). The present technique removes as much of the pulp as possible, with the aid of magnification, and the part of the capsule carrying the cortical sinus is carefully sutured into a defect tailored to fit in the wall of the vein (Fig. 83–11).

Lymphovenous Anastomosis. When there are no available lymph nodes, direct anastomosis of the lymphatic collectors to suitable veins is a possible alternative. The earliest attempts (Laine and Howard, 1963; Sedlacek, 1969; Degni, 1974) were of end to side anastomoses, and although some were successful, the patency rate was moderate. Yamada (1969) anastomosed lymphatics end to end with veins at canine ankles, suturing them over a temporary polythene catheter. Two-thirds remained patent for up to three months. O'Brien (1977) reported similar experimental results without the need for a polythene splint (Gilbert and associates, 1976). Antibiotic prophylaxis and impeccable technique are required if reliable patency is to be achieved; the more anastomoses performed, the better is the result. However, the clinical problems are more difficult than those in the laboratory. The author has explored lymph collectors, visualized by lymphangiography in secondary lymphedema, but found them to be unstretchable, rendering an anas-

tomosis impossible. The use of lymphovenous shunts must be regarded as an early or even prophylactic measure. In primary lymphedema they may be used only in the rare hyperplastic form.

Nieuborg (1982) in his monograph on this procedure for postmastectomy lymphedema reports a volume decrease of over 50 per cent after one year. O'Brien (1985), during an average follow-up time 17 months, found in 58 per cent of 116 patients a decrease of the excess volume exceeding 10 per cent. The author's patient with forearm lymphedema, reported in 1977 to demonstrate a good result, suddenly suffered a massive return of the swelling nine years after the operation.

Bridging of Localized Obstructions of Lymph Drainage by Transplantation of Lymph Collectors. This technique was developed experimentally and introduced clinically by Baumeister and associates in 1981. The single collectors are harvested from the inner aspect of the patient's thigh up to a length of 30 cm and are used to bridge a postsurgical lymph block in the axilla or groin (Fig. 83–12). Ho, Lai, and Kennedy (1983) reported a similar microlymphatic bypass technique of removing a compound composite graft from the thigh, including three lymph collectors and the saphenous vein. Baumeister's five year results (1985) indicate a volume reduction of up to 70 per cent, with better results for the arm than for the leg. Pre- and postoperative lymphoscintigrams showed a significant improvement of the transport capacity.

The early use of a lymphovenous shunt in front of a lymph block or the early replacement of resected lymph collectors is the most logical surgical approach to overcome a localized obstruction of lymph flow.

Unfortunately for the microvascular surgeon today, it cannot be determined how many lymph collectors are missing in the area of the lymph block in the individual patient. If the lymph collector grafts are used to bridge the gap, and three lymph collectors are missing (Fig. 83–12), the patient has been cured. But if six were missing, the lymphedema has been returned at best into its latent phase, after which it will recur, unless the patient is treated with complex decongestive physiotherapy. A lymphatic load that is too high for a given number of remaining or grafted lymph collectors, unfortunately, with

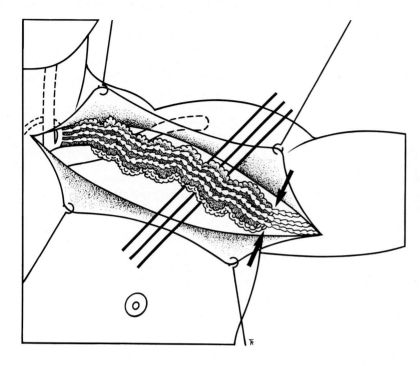

Figure 83–12. The three bars schematically demonstrate the axillary lymph block, bridged by three lymph collectors, anastomosed end to end in the upper arm *(arrows)* and end to side to the thoracic duct in the neck.

Figure 83–13. Lymphangiogram of a dog with secondary manifest lymphedema. The two arrows divide the picture into two sections, corresponding to the site of the partial lymphatic blockade, traversed by a few remaining healthy lymph collectors. In the lower part of the picture the typical signs of obstructive lymphedema are present. The upper part visualizes the problem of any type of microlymphatic surgery that fails to balance lymphatic transport capacity against the lymphatic load completely. Within unobstructed, healthy tissue the remaining healthy lymph collectors have decompensated, at which time the latent phase of lymphedema comes to an end.

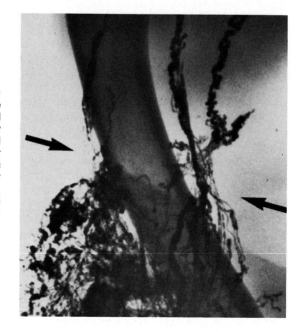

time, forces them to decompensate (Fig. 83–13).

Chylous Reflux

The cause of chylous reflux to the lower extremities and the external genitalia is an anatomic obstruction or malfunction of the cisterna chyli, leading to dilatation and incompetence of the lymphatics draining the legs and the external genitalia. Etiologic factors include primary lymphatic malfunction, infections such as filariasis, trauma including operative trauma, and malignant disease (Kinmonth, 1982). A malabsorption syndrome may also be present, indicating hypertension in the intestinal lymphatics. The diagnosis is easily ascertained by the ingestion of Sudan red III dye mixed with milk or butter; approximately one hour later the vesicles of skin will be stained, indicating dilated lymphatics. Chylous reflux may present more problems to the patient than the lymphedema, but it can be stopped by radical excision and ligation of all enlarged incompetent retroperitoneal lymphatics leading to the area of peripheral chylous reflux. It sometimes is also possible to perform a supplemental lymphovenous shunt between a large collector and a pelvic vein. Kinmonth (1982) reported his results in 15 patients with chylous reflux treated by excision and ligation of incompetent abdominal pathways. Four were cured by a single procedure, nine experienced alleviation of their condition, and there were two failures.

REFERENCES

Altorfer, J., Hedinger, C., and Clodius, L.: Light and electron microscopic investigation of extremities of dogs with experimental chronic lymphostasis. Folia Angiol. I (Berlin), *25*:141, 1977.

Barinka, L.: The technique of the excisional operation for lymphedema of the lower extremity using a new instrument. *In* Clodius, L. (Ed.): Lymphedema. Stuttgart, Thieme, 1977.

Barinka, L.: Surgical Treatment of Lymphedema of the Extremities. Vol. 85. Brno, Acta Facultatis Medicae Universitatis Brunensis, 1984.

Baumeister, R. G.: Five years of autogenous lymph vessel transplantation. Progress in Lymphology: Proceedings of the Tenth International Congress of Lymphology, Adelaide, Australia. University of Adelaide Press, 1985, p. 250.

Baumeister, R. G., Seifert, J., Wiebecke, B., and Hahn, D.: Experimental basis and first application of clinical lymph vessel transplantation of secondary lymphedema. World J. Surg., *5*:401, 1981.

Bollinger, A., Partsch, H., and Wolfe, J. H.: The Initial Lymphatics. New York, Thieme-Stratton, 1985.

Bolton, T., and Casley-Smith, J. R.: An in vitro demonstration of proteolysis by macrophages and its increase with coumarin. Experientia, *31*:271, 1975.

Browse, N.: Reducing Operations for Lymphedema of Lower Limb. London, Wolfe Medical Publications, 1987.

Bruna, J.: Suprailiac lymphography. Acta Radiol. [Diagn.] (Stockh.), *14*:157, 1973.

Bruna, J.: Diagnostik des Lymphödems durch die Computertomographie. Oedem., *1*:117, 1986.

Brunner, U.: Das Lymphödem der untern Extremitäten. Bern, Huber, 1969.

Campbell, D. A., Glas, W. W., and Musselmann, M. M.: Surgical treatment of massive lymphedema of lower extremities. Surgery, *30*:763, 1951.

Carnochan, M.: Elephantiasis des Arabes, siégeant au membre inférieur droit. Guérison par la ligature de la fémorale, puis de l'iliaque externe. Gaz. Hôp. (Paris), *27*:228, 1854.

Casley-Smith, J. R.: The actions of the benzopyrones on the blood-tissue-lymph system. Folia Angiol., *24*:7, 1976.

Casley-Smith, J. R.: The structural basis for the conservative treatment of lymphedema. *In* Clodius, L. (Ed.): Lymphedema. Stuttgart, Thieme, 1977.

Casley-Smith, J. R., and Casley-Smith, J. R.: High Protein Oedemas and the Benzopyrones. Sydney, J. B. Lippincott Company, 1986.

Casley-Smith, J. R., Clodius, L., and Piller, N. B.: Tissue changes in chronic experimental lymphedema in dogs. Lymphology, *13*:130, 1980.

Casley-Smith, J. R., Piller, N. B., and Clodius, L.: Fine structural observations on two congenitally lymphedematous dogs. Eur. J. Plast. Surg., *9*:122, 1986.

Charles, R. H.: Elephantiasis scroti. *In* Latham, A., and English, T. C. (Eds.): A System of Treatment. Vol. III. London, Churchill, 1912.

Chitale, V. R.: Use of tensor fascia lata myocutaneous flap in lymphedema of congenital, tubercular and filarial origin. *In* Transactions of the Ninth International Congress of Plastic and Reconstructive Surgery. New Delhi, McGraw-Hill Book Company, 1987.

Clodius, L.: The experimental basis for the surgical treatment of lymphedema. *In* Clodius, L. (Ed.): Lymphedema. Stuttgart, Thieme, 1977.

Clodius, L., and Gibson, T.: Lymphedema. *In* Rob, C., and Smith, R. (Eds.): Operative Surgery. 3rd Ed. London, Butterworths, 1979.

Clodius, L., and Piller, N. B.: Conservative therapy for the postmastectomy lymphedema. Chir. Plast. (Berlin), 193, 1978.

Clodius, L., Piller, N. B., and Casley-Smith, J. R.: The problems of lymphatic microsurgery for lymphedema. Lymphology, *14*:69, 1981.

Clodius, L., Smith, P. J., Bruna, J., and Serafin, D.: The lymphatics of the groin flap. Ann. Plast. Surg., *9*:447, 1982.

Clodius, L., Uhlschmid, G., and Hess, K.: Irradiation plexitis of the brachial plexus. Clin. Plast. Surg., *11*:161, 1984.

Clodius, L., Uhlschmid, G., and Hess, K.: Irradiation plexitis of the brachial plexus. Clin. Plast. Surg., *11*:161, 1984.

Clodius, L., Uhlschmid, G., Smahel, J., and Altorfer, J.: Microsurgery and lymphatics. *In* Daniller, A. I., and Strauch, B. (Eds.): Symposium on Microsurgery. St. Louis, C. V. Mosby Company, 1976.

Collard, M., and Servais, M. F.: The lymphography enters in agony. Lymphologie, *2*:96, 1978.

Crockett, D. J.: Lymphatic anatomy and lymphoedema. Br. J. Plast. Surg., *18*:12, 1965.

Degni, M.: New technique of drainage of the subcutaneous tissue of the limbs with nylon net for the treatment of lymphedema. Vasa, *3*:329, 1974.

Dick, W.: Über die Lymphgefässe des menschlichen Netzes, zugleich ein Beitrag zur Behandlung der Elephantiasis. Beitr. Klin. Chir., *162*:296, 1935.

Drinker, C. K., and Field, M.: The protein content of mammalian lymph and the relation of lymph to tissue fluid. Am. J. Physiol., *97*:32, 1931.

Edwards, J. M., and Kinmonth, J. B.: Lymphovenous shunts in man. Br. Med. J., *4*:579, 1969.

Esmarch, F., and Kulenkampff, D.: Die elephantiastischen Formen. Hamburg, J. F. Richter, 1885.

Farina, R.: Elephantiasis of the lower limbs. Plast. Reconstr. Surg., *8*:430, 1951.

Földi, M.: Lymphedema. *In* Kugelmass, I. N. (Ed.): Diseases of Lymphatics and Lymph Circulation. Springfield, IL, Charles C Thomas, 1969.

Földi, M.: Lymphedema. *In* Földi, M., and Casley-Smith, J. R. (Eds.): Lymphangiology. Stuttgart, Schattauer, 1983.

Földi-Börcsök, E., and Földi, M.: Lymphedema and vitamins. Am. J. Clin. Nutr., *26*:185, 1973.

Forbes, G.: Lymphatics of the skin, with a note on lymphatic watershed areas. J. Anat., *72*:399, 1937–1938.

Frautschi, W. C.: Lymphovenous anastomoses. Surgery, *2*:12, 1948 (Russian).

Galkowska, H., and Olszewski, W. L.: Cellular composition of lymph in experimental lymphedema. Lymphology, *19*:139, 1986.

Ghormley, R. K., and Overton, L. M.: The surgical treatment of severe forms of lymphedema (elephantiasis) of the extremities: a study of end results. Surg. Gynecol. Obstet., *61*:83, 1935.

Gibson, T., and Tough, J. S.: The surgical correction of chronic lymphoedema of the legs. Br. J. Plast. Surg., *7*:195, 1954.

Gibson, T., and Tough, J. S.: A simplified one stage operation for the correction of lymphedema of the leg. Arch. Surg., *71*:809, 1955.

Gilbert, A., O'Brien, B. M., Vorrath, J. W., and Sykes, P. J.: Lymphaticovenous anastomosis by microvascular technique. Br. J. Plast. Surg., *29*:355, 1976.

Gillies, H. D., and Fraser, F. R.: The treatment of lymphoedema by plastic operation. Br. Med. J., *1*:96, 1935.

Gillies, H. D., and Fraser, F. R.: The lymphatic wick. Proc. R. Soc. Med., *43*:1054, 1950.

Gillies H. D., and Millard, D. R., Jr.: The Principles and Art of Plastic Surgery. Boston, Little, Brown & Company, 1957.

Goldsmith, H. S.: Long-term evaluation of omental transposition of chronic lymphedema. Ann. Surg., *180*:847, 1974.

Goldsmith, H. S., De los Santos, R., and Beattie, E. J., Jr.: Omental transposition in the control of chronic lymphedema. J.A.M.A., *203*:1119, 1968.

Gooneratne, B. W. M.: Lymphography—Clinical and Experimental. London, Butterworths, 1974.

Gray, H. J.: Studies of the regeneration of lymphatic vessels. J. Anat., *74*:309, 1939.

Handley, W. S.: Lymphangioplasty; new method for relief of brawny arm of breast-cancer, and for similar conditions of lymphatic oedema. Lancet, *1*:783, 1908.

Handley, W. S.: Hunterian lectures on the surgery of the lymphatic system. Br. Med. J., *1*:853, 1910.

Handley, W. S.: Surgery of the lymphatics. *In* Burghard, F. F., and Kanavel, A. B. (Eds.): Oxford Surgery I. New York, Oxford University Press, 1920, p. 537.

Handley, W. S.: Cancer of the Breast. London, Murray, 1922.

Hergenroeder, F.: Results of surgical therapy for elephantiasis of the lower extremity. Total excision of the skin of the lower leg, defect closure by Thiersch grafts. Vestn. Khir., *55*:603, 1938.

Hirshowitz, B., and Goldan, S.: Bi-hinged chest-arm flap for lymphedema of upper limb. Plast. Reconstr. Surg., *48*:52, 1971.

Ho, L. C., Lai, M. F., and Kennedy, P. J.: Microlymphatic bypass in the treatment of obstructive lymphoedema of the arm: case report of a new technique. Br. J. Plast. Surg., *36*:350, 1983.

Homans, J.: The treatment of elephantiasis of the legs. N. Engl. J. Med., *215*:1099, 1936.

Homans, J.: Lymphedema of the limbs. Arch. Surg., *40*:232, 1940.

Huang, G-K., Hu, R-Q., Liu, Z-Z., Shen, Y-L., Lan, T-D., and Pan, G-P.: Microlymphaticovenous anastomosis in the treatment of lower limb obstructive lymphedema: analysis of 91 cases. Plast. Reconstr. Surg., *76*:671, 1985.

Hudack, S. S., and McMaster, P. D.: Lymphatic participation in human cutaneous phenomena: study of minute lymphatics of living skin. J. Exp. Med., *57*:751, 1933.

Hurst, P. A., Kinmonth, J. B., and Rutt, D. L.: The entero-mesenteric bridging operation for bypassing lymphatic obstructions. *In* Weissleder, H., Bartos, V., Clodius, L., and Malek, P. (Eds.): Progress in Lymphology: Proceedings of the Seventh International Congress of Lymphology, Florence, 1979. Avicenum, Czechoslovak Medical Press, 1981.

Jacobsson, S.: Studies of the blood circulation of lymphedematous limbs. Scand. J. Plast. Reconstr. Surg. [Suppl.], *3*:1, 1967.

Jaju, J. R.: Elephantiasis—lymphedema. A new concept in management based on physiological observations. *In* Marchac, D. (Ed.): Transactions of the Sixth International Congress of Plastic and Reconstructive Surgery. Paris, Masson, 1976.

Jaju, J. R.: Communication at the Ninth International Congress of Plastic Surgery, New Delhi, 1987.

Jamal, S.: Lymphonodovenous shunt in the treatment of filarial elephantiasis. *In* Weissleder, H., Bartos, V., Clodius, L., and Malek, P. (Eds.): Progress in Lymphology: Proceedings of the Seventh International Congress of Lymphology, Florence, 1979. Avicenum, Czechoslovak Medical Press, 1981, p. 250.

Kaye, J., Smith, P., and Acland, R.: Experimental end to end anastomosis of lymphatic trunks in the canine hind limb. Chir. Plast., *5*:163, 1980.

Kinmonth, J. B.: The Lymphatics. London, E. Arnold, 1982.

Kinney, B. M., and Miller, T. A.: Lymphedema of the extremities. *In* Georgiade, N. G., Riefkohl, R., and Barwick, W. J. (Eds.): Essentials of Plastic, Maxillofacial, and Reconstructive Surgery. Baltimore, Williams & Wilkins Company, 1987.

Kirikuta, I.: L'emploi du grand épiploon dans la chirurgie du sein candéreux. Presse Méd., 71:15, 1963.

Kondoleon, E.: Die operative Behandlung der elephantiastischen Oedeme. Zentralbl. Chir., 39:1022, 1912.

Kondoleon, E.: La pathogénie et le traitement de l'éléphantiasis. Arch. Ital. Chir. (Bologna), 51:464 (Donati Festschr. 2), 1938.

Kubik, I.: Die hämodynamischen und mechanischen Faktoren in der Lymphzirkulation. Acta Morph. Hung., 2:95, 1952.

Kubik, S.: Drainagemöglichkeiten der Lymphterritorien nach Verletzung peripherer Kollektoren und nach Lymphadenektomie. Folia Angiol. (Berl.), 28:228, 1980.

Kubik, S., and Manestar, M.: Anatomische Grundlagen der Therapie des Lymphödems. Oedem., 1:19, 1986.

Laine, J. B., and Howard, J. M.: Experimental lymphatico-venous anastomosis. Surg. Forum, 14:111, 1963.

Lanz, O.: Eröffnung neuer Abfuhrwege bei Stauung im Bauch und unteren Extremitäten. Zentralbl. Chir., 38:153, 1911.

Lenggenhager, K.: Zur Behandlung der Elephantiasis nostras. Helv. Chir. Acta, 28:175, 1961.

Lofferer, O., and Mostbeck, A.: Nuclear medicine technique in diagnosis and differential diagnosis of swollen arms and legs. In Földi, M., and Casley-Smith, J. R. (Eds.): Lymphangiology. Stuttgart, Schattauer, 1983.

Macey, H. B.: A new surgical procedure for lymphedema of extremities; report of a case. Proc. Staff Meet. Mayo Clin, 15:49, 1940.

Macey, H. B.: Surgical procedures for lymphedema of the extremities. J. Bone Joint Surg., 30A:339, 1948.

Madden, F. C., Ibrahim, A., and Ferguson, A. R.: On the treatment of elephantiasis of the legs by lymphangioplasty. Br. Med. J., 2:1212, 1912.

Malek, R.: Lymphaticovenous anastomoses. In Handbuch der Allgemeinen Pathologie. Berlin, Springer-Verlag, 1972.

Mandl, H.: Experimentelle Untersuchungen zur mikrochirurgischen Rekonstruktion von Lymphgefässdefekten. Z. Plast. Chir., 5:70, 1981.

Martorell, F.: Un nuevo tratamiento del linfedema: la linfangioplastica pediculada. Angiologica, 10:151, 1958.

Mascagni, P.: Vasorum lymphaticorum corporis humani historia et ischonographia. Senis. Ex. Typ. Pazzini Carli, 1787.

Mayall, R. C., Mayall, J. C., and Ferreti, U. R.: Treatment of lymphedemas of the lower leg—new concepts. Progress in Lymphology: Proceedings of the Sixth International Congress of Lymphology. Stuttgart, Thieme, 1979, p. 391.

Miller, T. A.: Surgical management of lymphedema of the extremity. Plast. Reconstr. Surg., 56:633, 1975.

Miller, T. A.: A surgical approach to lymphedema. Am. J. Surg., 134:191, 1977.

Mowlem, R.: The treatment of lymphedema. Br. J. Plast. Surg., 1:48, 1948.

Mowlem, R.: Lymphatic edema—an evaluation of surgery in its treatment. Am. J. Surg., 95:216, 1958.

Nahai, F., and Stahl, R. S.: Congenital deformities of the lower extremity. In Serafin, D. and Georgiade, N. G. (Eds.): Pediatric Plastic Surgery. St. Louis, C. V. Mosby Company, 1984.

Nielubowicz, J., and Olszewski, W.: Surgical lymphaticovenous shunts in patients with secondary lymphoedema. Br. J. Surg., 55:440, 1968.

Nieuborg, L.: The Role of Lymphaticovenous Anastomoses in the Treatment of Post Mastectomy Edema. Alblasserdam, Kanters, 1982.

O'Brien, B. M.: Microvascular Reconstructive Surgery. Edinburgh, Churchill Livingstone, 1977.

O'Brien, B. M.: Microlymphatic surgery in the treatment of lymphedema. Progress in Lymphology: Proceedings of the Tenth International Congress of Lymphology, Adelaide, Australia. University of Adelaide Press, 1985, p. 235.

Odén, B.: A micro-lymphangiographic study of experimental wound healing by second intention. Acta Chir. Scand., 120:100, 1960.

Olszewski, W.: Surgical lympho-venous shunts for the treatment of lymphedema. In Clodius, L. (Ed.): Lymphedema. Stuttgart, Thieme, 1977.

Olszewski, W.: What is lymphology—prospects in human studies. Lymphology, 15:74, 1982.

Olszewski, W., and Nielubowicz, J.: Surgical lymphaticovenous communication in the treatment of lymph stasis. Paper read before the Forty-Third Congress of Polish Surgeons, Lodz, 1966.

Papp, M.: Cit. from Rusznyak, J., Földi, M., and Szabo, G.: Lymphologie. Stuttgart, G. Fischer, 1969.

Pecking, A., Cluzan, R., Desprez-Curely, J. P., and Guérin, P.: Functional study of limb lymphatic system. In Progress in Lymphology: Proceedings of the Tenth International Congress of Lymphology, Adelaide, Australia. University of Adelaide Press, 1985, p. 135.

Peer, L. A., Shahgholi, M., Walker, J. C., and Mancusi-Ungaro, A.: Modified operation for lymphedema of the leg and arm. Plast. Reconstr. Surg., 14:347, 1954.

Picard, J. D., Arvay, N., and Charbit, A.: Les communications lympho-veineuses. (Suppl.) Presse Med., 74:42, 1966.

Piller, N. B.: Drug-induced proteolysis: a correlation with oedema-reducing ability. Br. J. Exp. Pathol., 57:266, 1976.

Poth, E. J., Barnes, S. R., and Ross, G. T.: A new operative treatment for elephantiasis. Surg. Gynecol. Obstet., 84:642, 1947.

Pratt, G. H., and Wright, I. S.: The surgical treatment of chronic lymphedema. Surg. Gynecol. Obstet., 72:244, 1941.

Pressman, J. J., Dunn, R. F., and Burtz, M.: Lymph node ultrastructure related to direct lymphaticovenous communication. Surg. Gynecol. Obstet., 124:963, 1967.

Rosanow, N. W.: Lymphangioplastik bei Elephantiasis. Arch. Klin. Chir., 99:645, 1912.

Rusznyak, I., Földi, M., and Szabo, G.: Lymphatics and Lymph Circulation. London Medical College, Pergamon Press, 1967.

Sappey, M. P. C.: Anatomie, Physiologie, Pathologie des Vaisseaux Lymphatiques Considérés chez l'Homme et les Vertebrés. Paris, A. Delahaye & E. Lacrosnier, 1874.

Sedlacek, J.: Lymphovenous shunt as supplementary treatment of elephantiasis of lower limbs. Acta Chir. Plast., 11:157, 1969.

Silver, D., and Puckett, C. L.: Lymphangioplasty: a ten year evaluation. Surgery, 80:748, 1976.

Sistrunk, W. E.: Further experiences with the Kondoleon operation for elephantiasis. J.A.M.A., 71:800, 1918.

Sistrunk, W. E.: Contribution to plastic surgery. Ann. Surg., 85:185, 1927.

Smith, J. W., and Conway, H.: Selection of appropriate surgical procedures in lymphedema: introduction of the hinged pedicle. Plast. Reconstr. Surg., *30*:10, 1962.

Standard, S.: Lymphedema of the arm following radical mastectomy for carcinoma of the breast; new operation for its control. Ann. Surg., *116*:816, 1942.

Teimourian, B.: Suction Lipectomy and Body Sculpturing. St. Louis, C. V. Mosby Company, 1987.

Thompson, N.: The surgical treatment of advanced post-mastectomy lymphedema of the upper limb. With the late results of treatment by the buried dermis flap operation. Scand. J. Plast. Surg., *3*:54, 1969.

Threefoot, S. A., and Kossover, M. F.: Lymphaticovenous communications in man. Arch. Intern. Med., *117*:213, 1966.

Viamonte, M., and Rüttimann, A.: Atlas of Lymphography. Stuttgart, G. Thieme, 1980.

Watson, J.: Chronic lymphoedema of the extremities and its management. Br. J. Surg., *31*:31, 1953.

Weber, E. G., and Steckenmesser, R.: Die Behandlung des chronischen Lymphödems unter Verwendung von Silikonschläuchen nach der Methode von Schrudde. Z. Lymphol., *6*:103, 1982.

Weissleder, H., and Weissleder, R.: Lymphedema: evaluation of qualitative and quantitative lymphoscintigraphy in 238 patients. Radiology, *162*:729, 1988.

Willoughby, D. A., and DiRosa, M.: A unifying concept for inflammation. *In* Immunopathology in Inflammation. Excerpta Med. Int. Congr. Series, *229*:28, 1970.

Winiwarter, A.: Die Elephantiasis. *In* Deutsche Chirurgie. Stuttgart, F. Enke, 1892.

Woodward, A. H., Ivins, J. C., and Soule, E. H.: Lymphangiosarcoma arising in chronic lymphedematous extremities. Cancer, *30*:562, 1972.

Yamada, Y.: Studies on lymphatic venous anastomosis in lymphedema. Nagoya J. Med. Sci., *32*:1, 1969.

Zhang, T. S., Huang, W. Y., Han, L. Y., and Liu, W. Y.: Heat and bandage treatment for chronic lymphedema of extremities. Chin. Med. J., *97*:567, 1984.

Zieman, S. A.: Lymphedema. New York, Grune & Stratton, 1962.

zum Winkel, K.: Scintigraphy. *In* Viamonte, M., and Rüttimann, A. (Eds.): Atlas of Lymphography. Stuttgart, G. Thieme, 1980.

84

John B. McCraw
Charles E. Horton
Charles E. Horton, Jr.

Basic Techniques in Genital Reconstructive Surgery

BASIC PRINCIPLES

A clear understanding of the plastic surgical principles of tissue transfer is necessary for the successful management of both simple and complex genitourinary reconstructions. Although this recognition of principles sometimes takes the form of a deference to the techniques of Z-plasties, grafts, and flaps, the proper requisite should be the broad principles of plastic surgery as they relate to tissue transfer. In the case of genitourinary reconstruction, the cornerstone of these principles must include the basic sciences of anatomy, embryology, wound healing, and flap physiology. Without this foundation, no amount of technical knowledge about flaps and grafts will produce predictable, positive results.

The layered structures of the penis offer an example of the importance of the pertinent regional anatomy. The skin of the penis glides on the dartos fascia, which contains the primary blood supply to the overlying skin. This relationship of the skin to the dartos fascia becomes critically important when "island" preputial flaps or Z-plasties are designed, since the skin of the penis cannot be safely mobilized without the dartos fascia. The important sensory nerves of the penis reside in Buck's fascia, the next layer of the penis. The deepest layer is the easily palpable tunica albuginea, which surrounds the plexiform vascular structures known as the corporeal bodies. It is the tunica that becomes fibrotic and constricted in Peyronie's disease. Release of this contracture requires the replacement of the tunica with a dermis graft, but this must be done without injury to the sensory nerves above or the vascular structures below. The paired internal pudendal neurovascular bundles provide the dominant blood and nerve supply to the penis and scrotum. Knowledge of their location, distribution, and physiologic functions is essential to the proper performance of reconstructive penile surgery.

The embryology of the most common congenital anomalies of the penis and scrotum should be understood, so that the failure of fusion can be recognized in the anatomic arrangement of the abnormally located structures. In the case of penoscrotal hypospadias, the nature of the remaining midline epithelium, the splitting of the corpora spongiosum, the chordee, and even the elevated testicles are matters to be not just observed, but understood. Associated anomalies should be sought, and genetic counseling must be part of the overall treatment program.

The physiology of wound healing bears on nearly every surgical act in reconstructive genitourinary surgery. Epithelization of the margins of a neourethra must occur rapidly and provide an end to end seal as the first line of defense against fistula formation. This first requires perfect dermal to dermal approximation, so that the epithelial "gap" can be bridged within one or two days. The new epithelium provides essentially all the wound strength from the time it is completed (one to two days) until collagen appears at the wound margin at about the fifth day. The absorbable sutures that effect this seal must have two contradictory attributes of (1) continuous strength and (2) rapid dissolution. On the one hand, the sutures must be sufficiently strong to fix the structures in the proper position for a long enough time to avoid suture line disruption. On the other hand, the sutures must dissolve before they can act as a "wick" for epithelization along a suture tract. This suture tract epithelization, which would only cause a "stitch mark" on the surface, may be the genesis of an epithelized sinus that eventually expands into a frank fistula of the neourethra.

Wound healing contraction must constantly be controlled, even if subconsciously. For example, a urethral stent must remain in place for at least six weeks, and possibly six months, if it is to overcome the forces of scar contraction that contribute to a urethral stricture. Any stent left in place for less than six weeks cannot be there for reasons of overcoming these contractile forces. In the case of an early postoperative fistula, the placement of either a urethral stent or a Foley catheter serves only to overcome the forces of wound contraction that might facilitate the closure of a small fistula. Rather than allowing the urethra to collapse and to epithelize, the stent stops the contraction of the wound, and in this case may be harmful. Once the contraction of the wound is stopped by the catheter, the wound has no other means of healing besides further epithelization, which only serves to enlarge the fistula.

Surface losses must be repaired by either epithelization, contraction, or replacement of the lost skin, and the surgeon should make this choice consciously. If there is enough surrounding skin laxity for wound contraction to take place, epithelization must be thwarted until contraction is complete. This wound contraction allows the dermal margins to touch, and results in a finer scar than the scar of epithelization. If there is too little skin laxity for contraction to occur, or if wound contraction would result in a wound contracture, replacement of the lost tissue is the preferred method of closure. A longitudinal incision and scar on the ventral surface of the penis can also cause a contracture, since the ventral surface of the penis heals as though it is a flexor surface of an extremity. Because all scars shorten, a Z-plasty should be used to redirect the forces of wound contraction in the closure of the ventral penis.

The inflammatory or substrate phase of wound healing is the least understood of all the phases. It is probably the most important in this surgery, because if a wound healing delay occurs in this phase, all the subsequent wound healing events will fail similarly. The wound must be cleared of dead tissue, debris, and foreign material by the acute and chronic inflammatory cells before epithelization and collagen deposition occur, because neither epithelial cells nor fibroblasts will enter a dirty, "hostile" area. Once the area is "cleared" by the inflammatory cells, a proper environment is established, including a mucopolysaccharide gel substrate and a fibrin network that facilitates the ingrowth of capillary buds and fibroblasts. Collagen deposition can occur at the wound site only after the arrival of the fibroblasts and capillary buds, and the strength of the wound is directly related to the amount of collagen deposition and the collagen crosslinkage. Any prolongation of the inflammatory phase delays the progression of the wound strength, so that a minor traumatic event at the wound margin, e.g., the removal of a catheter, may disrupt the fragile, inflamed wound. Rapid passage through this phase includes the avoidance of foreign bodies in the wound, such as dead and traumatized tissue and large sutures, as well as attention to the technical details of suturing and dead space management.

The physiology of flap transfers is related to the basic considerations of wound healing, but on a larger scale. Although the current fundamental understanding of the microcirculation is rudimentary, recent developments in axial flaps, "island" flaps, and musculocutaneous and fasciocutaneous flaps have provided a macroscopic understanding of flap manipulation. Every axial flap is composed of a "self-contained vascular territory" that is in constant flux with the other adjacent vascular territories; i.e., the physiologic limits of one vascular territory expand as the adjacent territory contracts. The neurovascular bundle that forms the "dangling vessels" of the island flap serves as the trunk of this vascular tree, and acts as the rotational axis of the flap. When more than one neurovascular bundle supplies an axial flap, one of these bundles serves with relative dominance over the other bundles. In skin flaps, the arborization of this vascular tree is through direct cutaneous perforators or fasciocutaneous perforators to the skin. In musculocutaneous flaps, this arborization first passes through the intramuscular vascular connections, which interconnect the deep perforating systems, and then pass through the deep fascial system as muscular perforating vessels entering the skin. The arc of rotation of the flap can then be determined from the known location of the flap axis and the expected length of the viable flap.

Certain factors that affect the delicate physiologic balance between flap viability and flap death are under the control of the surgeon. Vascular compromise of the flap may be preexisting and caused by, for example, irradiation of the dominant vascular pedicle, nicotine sensitization of the microcirculation, denervation, or diabetes. However, most of the recognized causes of vascular compromise are a direct result of technical errors by the surgeon. For instance, it is necessary to include the appropriate vasculature in the dartos fascia pedicle in order for the island preputial flap to survive. It is also imperative that the surgeon not devascularize the "donor" skin from which the dartos vasculature has been removed, in the process of this dissection. This donor skin must survive on just the subdermal plexus, after the removal of the dartos fascia, and any additional vascular insult can be fatal to the donor skin. Another common example of devascularization is the improper elevation of the gracilis musculocutaneous flap. The cutaneous segment must be placed directly over the gracilis muscle, and the skin island cannot be extended into the distal thigh without a "delay." Incorrect flap designs such as this devascularize the flap even before the flap elevation is completed.

Mechanical factors can also be a source of technical flap necrosis. Torsion and crossing tension of cutaneous flaps can physically occlude the capillary flow. Torsion is caused by twisting the flap at the site of inset, and crossing tension is caused by obliquely occluding a strip of the capillary circulation. Vascular spasm of the dominant vessel of an island flap can be caused by clumsy dissection of the vascular pedicle or torsion at the arc of rotation. This normally protective mechanism (spasm), which exists to stop bleeding, can effectively shut off the blood flow to a flap and is difficult to reverse when it occurs. Compression of a muscle flap beneath a tight skin bridge is the most common cause of muscle flap necrosis. It is recognized that all muscle flaps swell and that this swelling requires space for expansion. If the muscle swelling is constrained, it will be transmitted back to the surface of the muscle and cause a sequence of events similar to the Volkmann's ischemic event—venous compression, more swelling, and finally arterial compression. Although the physiologic nature of these observed events is not completely understood, it is important to learn from these empirical observations.

PREOPERATIVE STUDIES AND PATIENT PREPARATION

Before undertaking a reconstructive procedure, the anatomy and functional status of the genitourinary system must be examined. Specific studies are directed to pertinent questions, such as reflux, bladder volume and drainage, continence, and erectile functions. Cystoscopy is performed routinely since it may help to identify unsuspected diverticula, strictures, and urethral hair growth that cannot be seen by indirect inspection. The route of urinary diversion is chosen preoperatively, depending on previous scarring and the need for either total or partial diversion. A mechanical bowel preparation may be performed in advance of the surgery, so that bowel movements will not be necessary for three to five days. Antibiotic preparation of the bowel, in an effort to prevent infection, is not required, but prophylactic systemic antibiotics are used before surgery and continued until all urinary catheters are removed. Patients or their families are also instructed about the special precautions in regard to postoperative erections, swelling, dressings, bowel and bladder needs, bed cradles, bladder "spasm," and pain relief.

The short-term goals and long-range objectives must be clearly understood by all involved parties. Each operative session has a goal, which must fit into the overall long-range plan. Once agreed upon, the patient's expectations of achievement should not cause a deviation from the plan. For instance, the creation of a structural neourethra with an island preputial flap can be the goal. A better goal is the creation of a structural neourethra, whether this is done with a flap or a graft. Further, the goal can still be achieved, i.e., structurally, even though a fistula or leak happens to mar the beauty and function of the new structure. The goal may be as simple as "repair the fistula" or as complex as "do what is needed to try to bring the meatus to the tip of the glans," but it should be an agreed goal.

The complications of reconstructive genitourinary surgery are now well recognized. The patient should accept the fact that fistulas occur in at least 10 per cent of new cases of hypospadias, even in the best of hands. This need not be perceived as something bad, but rather viewed as a "gift" if it does not happen. In case a "one-stage" hypospadias repair takes two stages because of a complication, it must be pointed out beforehand that a "two-stage" procedure always takes two stages without a complication. Only the catastrophic complications, such as the loss of a flap, cannot be anticipated. Other predictable events need to be put into context for all to ponder before the time of surgical intervention.

TECHNICAL CONSIDERATIONS

Special instruments are necessary to the performance of these delicate procedures, including Castroviejo forceps, Webster needleholders, two millimeter hooks, and a variety of sharp and dull scissors. The microscope has been used for the initial hypospadias repair, but it has not proved its added value over loupes to this point. The Wood's light and fluorescein are occasionally useful whenever the viability of a flap is in question. The Reese or Padgett dermatome is used for split-thickness sheet grafts, but most full-thickness grafts are taken with a No. 10 blade.

The choice of an atraumatic suture is even more important than the choice of instruments, because the suture penetrates and resides in the wound during healing. Most sutures used in genitourinary reconstruction are absorbable, with the exception of nylon, which may be used in the skin of adults. Nonabsorbable suture is never used on a mucosal surface, such as the lumen of the bladder or the urethra, since it acts as a nidus for stone formation. Even Vicryl and Dexon may not dissolve properly when exposed intraluminally, so they are considered in the same category as permanent suture when used within a lumen. Since suture strength is so critical, it should be remembered that PDS suture is stronger than Vicryl, and Vicryl is stronger than catgut, for the given size of suture. Plain catgut is never used, because it is much more reactive than chromic catgut and its holding strength is less predictable. In the past, Prolene and nylon sutures were used to secure dermal grafts to the tunica albuginea, because of their inherent strength. These sutures have been replaced with PDS sutures, which are almost as strong, because the permanent sutures remain palpable to the patient. Taper needles are used only in the PDS suture (5–0 RB-1 and 6–0 BV). All other suture is used with a cutting needle (6–0 G-1 and 5–0 P-3). Coloring the suture improves its visibility, and this is used for both the 6–0 chromic (blue) and the 5–0 PDS (violet).

The suture technique used must be atraumatic and precise. The structures being sutured should not be grasped with forceps, and a nearly perfect dermal to dermal match must be achieved without tension. In the repair of uroepithelial surfaces, care should be taken to invert the epithelium toward the internal surface of the lumen. A second layer is always placed above this, using fine chromic or PDS sutures, and "key" deep sutures are always placed with PDS suture. The integrity of the suture line is checked with dilute methylene blue, which is instilled through the urethra, and any leaks are repaired before the second layer is completed. Corporeal erection can be stimulated with saline injection into one of the corporeal bodies, using a No. 23 needle and normal saline. This is done to confirm the complete release of the chordee and to examine the dermal graft closure of the tunica. It is always necessary to double-check the injection solution, since the penis has been lost completely owing to the injection of hypertonic (3 per cent) saline.

Siliconized urinary drainage catheters are used routinely. Bladder "spasms" are a common problem; the surgeon must decide from his own experience whether a Foley balloon catheter or a disposable straight catheter is better in this respect. Foley catheters are used only for urinary drainage, rather than stenting, since the balloon may disrupt the suture line at the time of its removal. The authors' preferred pediatric-sized stent is the 0.078 × 0.125 (10 French) Silastic tubing made by Dow Corning. This stent is large enough for a No. 5 feeding tube to be passed through its inner lumen, and the combination is frequently used for both stenting and drainage. The stent can also be slit along one margin, allowing it to collapse partially, to increase the softness of the stent.

Incisions are preferably placed along natural lines; properly placed incisions in the penis, scrotum, and vulva heal quite well. The ventral surface of the penis and the junction between the penis and the pubic area heal like "flexor" surfaces in the extremity, so vertical incisions in these areas should always be broken with a Z-plasty. A longitudinal incision with an added Z-plasty gives excellent direct access to the underlying penile shaft. The circumcision type of incision is also commonly employed by elevating the skin and the dartos layer together and "peeling" down to the base of the penis.

SKIN GRAFTING

Split-thickness sheet grafts, full-thickness grafts, and dermal grafts are relatively new developments in genitourinary surgery. Their impact on reconstructive surgery in this anatomic area has certainly been as significant as the recent developments of axial and musculocutaneous flaps. Split-thickness grafts were first described, independently, by Ollier (1872) and Thiersch (1874). A split-thickness graft was first used to create a neourethra by Nové-Josserand in 1897. Unfortunately, the high incidence of fistula and stricture formation caused this technique to be discarded for urethral reconstruction until McIndoe introduced it again in 1937. The problem of graft shrinkage and stricture formation was countered with prolonged stenting lasting six months or more, but this was only a partial solution for this biologically recurring event. Other uses of the split graft proved to be more fruitful. The "sheet" graft was a major advance over the "pinch" graft described by Davis (1919). In 1929 Blair and Brown de-

scribed the sheet graft and a method to harvest it with a special knife. The sheet graft was then applied to the problems of elephantiasis (Muller and Jordan, 1933), traumatic denuding of the penile shaft (Owens, 1942), and congenital absence of the vagina (McIndoe, 1949). Sheet grafts are still used for surface problems in which some graft shrinkage is acceptable, including lymphedema, hidradenitis, and burns.

Full-thickness grafts have had an even more profound effect on genitourinary reconstructive surgery than split-thickness grafts. The first full-thickness tube urethroplasty was described by Horton and C. J. Devine, Jr. in 1958. P. C. Devine and associates (1963) successfully used full-thickness grafts for urethral strictures, and Horton and C. J. Devine, Jr. (1973) described dermal graft replacement of the diseased tunica albuginea in Peyronie's disease. Full-thickness grafts are useful for reconstruction of the urethra in hypospadias, epispadias, and strictures because the grafts maintain their elasticity and shrink very little. Clinically, the full-thickness graft appears to grow at the same rate as the patient. Baran and Horton (1972) first experimentally demonstrated this parallel growth (of both the graft and the patient) in minipigs.

There are several special considerations for the use of full-thickness grafts. Hairless skin must be used for urethral reconstruction to avoid later encrustation and stone formation. The preputial skin offers the ideal donor site because it is thin, elastic, and hairless. Only a few other relatively hairless donor sites exist, including the areas of the iliac crest, the inner arm, the dorsum of the foot, and the lower neck.

The full-thickness tube graft should be completed with an elliptic anastomosis to prevent a circular scar and a stricture. Full-thickness grafts are just as useful as split grafts for resurfacing the shaft of the penis, and the "take" of the graft is comparable. This is particularly useful in the hypospadias "cripple" or the epispadias patient with deficient shaft skin. In these cases, a full-thickness graft can give both a durable and an esthetic result. Full-thickness grafts can also be used to reconstruct the umbilicus, and their application to reconstruction of the congenitally absent vagina has been advocated by Sadove and Horton (1988). Unlike the split-thickness graft vaginoplasty, which requires the use of a stent or mold for six to 12 months, the full-thickness graft becomes supple more quickly and requires only a short period of stenting.

Dermal grafts offer an elastic material for replacement of the scarred tunica albuginea in Peyronie's disease, hypospadias, epispadias, and traumatic deformities of the corpora. A normal erection is associated with symmetric elongation and expansion of the tunica albuginea. Shortening in one dimension results in a bent penis, much like a pinch in the side of an expanding balloon. The elasticity of the tunica can be replaced by the dermal graft, which is made approximately twice the needed size to allow for graft shrinkage. The formation of buried epidermal cysts might be expected, but has not been observed.

FLAPS

Local axial flaps are preferentially chosen whenever possible, because local "random" flaps in the perineum have an unpredictable blood supply. These axial flaps are based on known vessels, rather than the subdermal plexus blood supply. Examples of small flaps include the posterior vulvar flap based on the labial and perineal vessels, and the "island" preputial flap based on the dorsal artery and vein of the penis. Some useful large axial flaps include the posterior thigh flap, which is based on the inferior gluteal vessels, and the standard groin flap.

In the past the perineal area was thought to have a propensity to poor healing, because of a presumed deficiency of the blood supply. In fact, the perineum is no different from the hand, foot, or trunk in its healing capacity. It is true that none of these areas is as vascular as the face, where very long and narrow flaps can be raised in any direction because of the rich subdermal plexus vasculature. The previous problems with healing have been more closely related to a poor understanding of the blood supply of flaps.

The concept of the axial flap with its self-contained vascular territory was first described by McGregor and Jackson in 1972, using the standard groin flap as a model. Before this description of the groin flap, the only recognized "axial" flaps in the trunk and extremities included the vertical groin flap (Shaw and Payne, 1946) and the medially based deltopectoral flap (Bakamjian, 1965).

The posterior thigh flap has proved to be quite useful in resurfacing the perineum, because of the excellent color match, contour restoration, and sensibility. The standard groin flap has been used in the past for total penile reconstruction, because of its ability to be immediately tubed and transferred. It has been used very little otherwise in perineal problems, since its pale color contrasts with the darkly pigmented perineal structures, and because of its bulkiness.

Color match has been the primary limiting factor in the use of local axial flaps. The pigmentation of the perineal structures is unique and can be distinctly different over a distance of a few millimeters. The melanin content is highest in the scrotum and vulva, and decreases progressively from the perineal surface to the penis or clitoris, and finally to the suprapubic area and thigh. As an example, a flap transferred from the suprapubic area to the penis is too pale, and a flap transferred from the scrotum to the penis too dark. These are not minor differences; they may appear so to the observer, but they are esthetically disturbing to the patient.

The most commonly used local axial flap in genitourinary reconstructive surgery is penile skin supplied by the dorsal artery and vein within the dartos fascia. In its purest form of "island" flap design, the island preputial flap is a primary flap source for the initial reconstruction of the neourethra in hypospadias. Since the dartos fascia contains the primary blood supply to the penile skin, a variety of other "subcutaneous" flap designs are possible. This allows the penile shaft skin to be immediately tubed for the formation of a partial or total neourethra, or buried for the closure of a urethral fistula. As a general rule, if the penile skin is viable in situ, it can be elevated and moved on the basis of the dartos blood supply.

Muscle flaps are thought of as recent developments in reconstructive genitourinary surgery, but Kanavel reported the use of the inferiorly based rectus abdominis muscle flap in 1921 to repair a combined pelvic and lower abdominal wall defect, and Pickrell and associates described the use of the gracilis muscle flap for anal incontinence in 1954. In 1977 McCraw and Dibbell described the "island" musculocutaneous vascular territories of the gracilis, biceps femoris, rectus femoris, gluteus maximus, and rectus abdominis musculocutaneous flaps. Many other new descriptions of flaps in the perineal area followed in the late 1970's and early 1980's, including the tensor fascia lata (TFL) fasciocutaneous flap and the vastus lateralis muscle flap.

These are discussed in detail later in the chapter.

The individual characteristics of each of these flaps differ, but the principles of application do not. A sound knowledge of anatomy is the starting point, beginning with the surface markings and the flap design. Each flap has a vascular axis that acts as the rotation point of the flap. In the case of multiple vascular pedicles, the relative dominance of each pedicle must be known. The arc of the flap is dependent on its length and axis, and this determines whether the flap reaches the defect. The vascular territory of each flap has been determined empirically, and varies only with the changes in the surrounding vascular territories. For instance, a given territory can be expanded by a flap delay that effectively expands this territory at the expense of an adjacent one.

The functional inset of each flap, i.e., the contacting surface of the inset flap, determines its applicability to a given problem. Skin is useful to replace skin, but the functional surface of a skin flap is fat, which is not helpful in eradicating infection in the area of inset. Fascia is primarily transposed because of its structural strength, but it may also act as a "carrier" of the skin of the flap, as in the case of a fasciocutaneous flap. Muscle is usually transposed because of its bulk or vascularity. The intense vascularity of muscle flaps is a useful adjunct in the revascularization of ischemic defects, such as irradiation ulcers, infection, or a scarred bed of inset.

The two different factors of simplicity and quality are the primary determinants in the choice of flap. In accordance with the guiding axiom of "keeping it simple," the ascending approach of the reconstructive ladder is suggested, in which the operative procedure is chosen primarily because of its simplicity. In this scheme, a skin graft is chosen before a local flap, and a local flap before a distant or free flap. This is not to suggest that a skin graft is necessarily better than a local flap, but if it is simpler it is to be considered first in this logical progression. The question of the quality of the reconstruction is not addressed by the reconstructive ladder, and these factors include the esthetics of the contour and color match, the functional replacement of muscle, the sensibility, the revascularization capabilities, and so forth. For instance, a free flap may be at the end of the line in the reconstructive ladder, but it may be the only source of sensibility, the proper thinness, and the appropriate color match. These considerations of quality and simplicity are good for our thinking processes, but the pertinent input data in choosing flaps should not be limited to these few factors.

Finally, there are several fundamental questions to pose before the final commitment: (1) will the flap survive?; (2) will it cover the defect?; (3) what do you do when it fails?; and (4) what about the patient? These major reconstructions are major investments for both the patient and the surgeon, and both need to face reality squarely before the fact. If the flap will not survive or cover the defect, there is very little reason to pursue it as an option. Since any flap can fail, a "back-up" flap must be chosen with the same care as the initial one. What to do when the flap fails is a matter of judgment, but this question should also be answered in advance of surgery. Finally, the tolerance of the patient for the rigorous nature of many of these extensive reconstructive procedures must be assessed, because the ultimate goal is to cure the patient, not the disease.

Certain technical requisites are essential to the performance of reconstructive genital surgery, including the essential techniques for the split-thickness sheet graft, the full-thickness tube graft, the Z-plasty, and the "island" muscle and musculocutaneous and axial flaps. Without the availability of the "island" muscle flap, there would be no safe and effective method of reconstructing the irradiated vesicovaginal and rectovaginal fistulas; without the "island" musculocutaneous flap, total vaginal reconstruction would involve the use of either the large or small bowel.

SPECIFIC FLAP APPLICATIONS

The anatomy of the several local muscle flaps of the pelvis and perineum has been adequately described, but the applications of these flaps are constantly evolving, and are influenced by current understanding of anatomy and microcirculatory physiology. One of the fundamental aspects of the clinical use of local muscle flaps in this region is the logic of the choice between the available flaps. The order of desirability of each flap may change with time, but the basic reasons for this order do not change.

Gracilis

USES

If any flap is the mainstay of perineal and pelvic reconstruction, it is the gracilis muscle flap. This muscle is totally expendable from a functional standpoint, and the gracilis muscle flap is one of the few that can be considered completely reliable. It has dramatically improved our capabilities to correct vesicovaginal and rectovaginal fistulas, as well as hemivaginal defects. It is the most accessible muscle flap for these low defects, and the additional blood supply converts these ischemic, nonhealing wounds into a predictably healed condition. The gracilis muscle flap is just as useful for the revascularization of full-thickness skin grafts of the urethra, and in cases of dense scarring and ischemia associated with long-standing urethral strictures (Figs. 84–1 to 84–5). In any low pelvic or

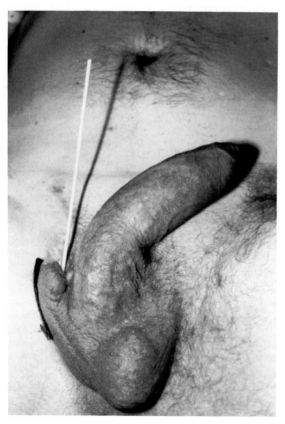

Figure 84–1. A 45 year old man with a recurrent periurethral fistula from Crohn's disease. An applicator stick is placed in the fistula that exists on the thigh. Half of the scrotum has already been removed in previous attempts to eradicate the fistula.

perineal situation in which primary healing is problematical, such as the abdominoperineal defect, the gracilis muscle flap should be considered as a matter of routine (Figs. 84–6 to 84–9).

The gracilis musculocutaneous flap is primarily recognized as a useful source of replacement tissue for partial and total vaginal reconstructions. It is also useful for the correction of rectal and vaginal fistulas within the pelvis, and for small perineal surface defects. Bilateral gracilis musculocutaneous flaps are generally used for major vaginal reconstructions, such as pelvic exenteration defects. Unilateral gracilis musculocutaneous flaps are more often used for partial vaginal defects, e.g. when the bladder mucosa is still remaining, or for large rectovaginal fistulas. In the latter situation, the skin of the flap can be placed either within the rectal lumen or within the vagina, depending on the need for soft tissue replacement of one of the mucosal surfaces (Figs. 84–10 to 84–15). The addition of both skin and muscle to these scarred defects helps to tip the balance in favor of a primarily healed wound in several ways: (1) it adds the vascularity of the muscle flap, (2) it removes the tension of the closure, and (3) it physically separates the adjacent hollow cavities.

Bilateral gracilis musculocutaneous flaps can be used to resurface standard radical vulvectomy defects or other major surface defects of the central perineum. The gracilis musculocutaneous flap can also be used to resurface the medial two-thirds of the groin, as well as the immediate suprapubic area. It is seldom considered for penile reconstruction, since it is less versatile than either the inferiorly based rectus abdominis muscle flap or several other flaps that can be transferred via microsurgical techniques.

DISADVANTAGES

The gracilis muscle flap is a very reliable flap in the authors' experience. The musculocutaneous flap has a justifiable reputation for being technically demanding, but its reliability in the authors' hands exceeds 95 per cent. A gracilis musculocutaneous flap has not been lost in any application during the past eight years in the authors' unit, whether through skill or luck. It is true, however, that the flap must be carefully designed, by placing the cutaneous segment directly over the

Text continued on page 4136

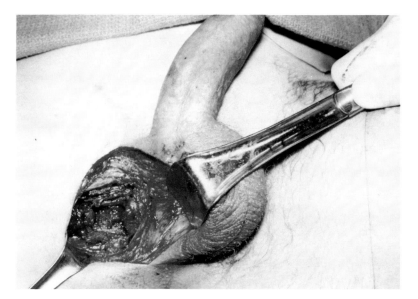

Figure 84–2. The wide excision of the fistula resulted in a 10 cm by 10 cm defect adjacent to the scrotum.

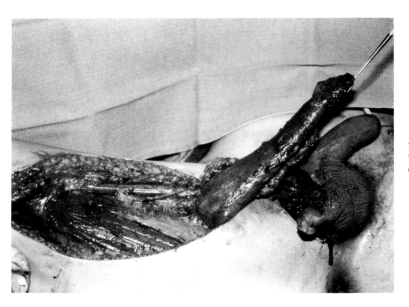

Figure 84–3. A gracilis muscle flap is elevated and will be used to vascularize the urethra and obliterate the dead space.

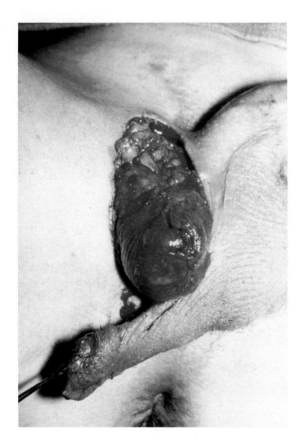

Figure 84–4. A gracilis muscle flap filling the excisional defect of the thigh. The remaining scrotum is retracted with a hook and will be used to cover the muscle flap.

Figure 84–5. Completed closure of the surface defect with the scrotal flap. The wound has remained healed for five years.

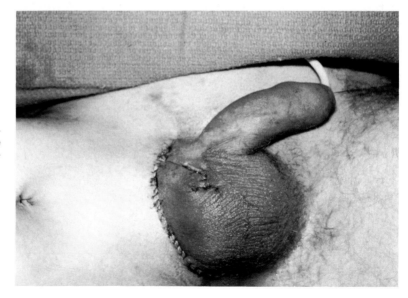

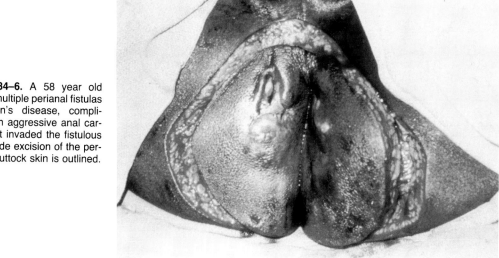

Figure 84–6. A 58 year old male with multiple perianal fistulas from Crohn's disease, complicated by an aggressive anal carcinoma that invaded the fistulous tracts. A wide excision of the perineal and buttock skin is outlined.

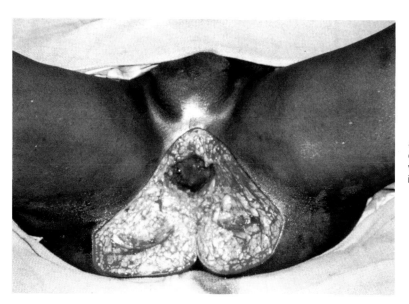

Figure 84–7. The same patient as in Figure 84–6. Completed abdominoperineal resection and wide excision of the posterior perineum.

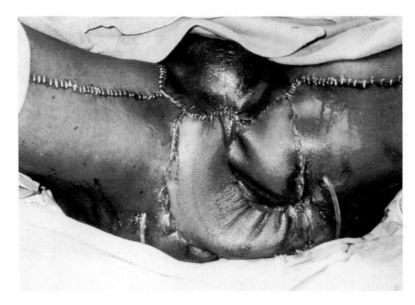

Figure 84–8. The same patient as in Figure 84–6. An immediate reconstruction was performed using bilateral gracilis musculocutaneous flaps. The right flap was used for surface cover of the central and posterior perineum. The left flap was partially deepithelized and used for both surface cover and obliteration of the pelvic dead space.

Figure 84–9. The same patient as in Figure 84–6. Healed gracilis flaps two years after resection of the anal carcinoma. The patient is alive and well eight years after surgery.

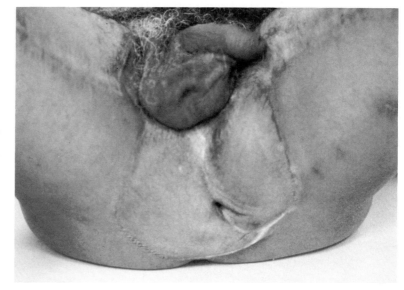

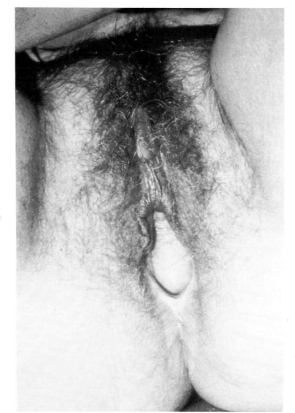

Figure 84–10. A 40 year old female after an abdomino-perineal resection that included the posterior half of the vagina. Only the anterior vaginal mucosa on the surface of the bladder is still present.

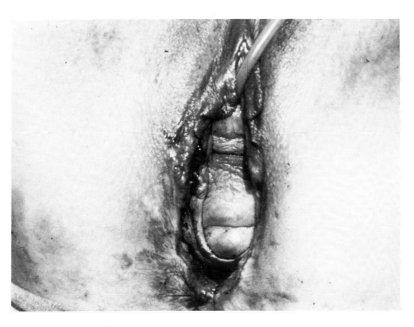

Figure 84–11. The same patient as in Figure 84–10. The remaining vaginal mucosa is separated from the surrounding perineal skin contracture. This case is of historical interest because this is the first reported case in which an undelayed "island" musculocutaneous flap was used.

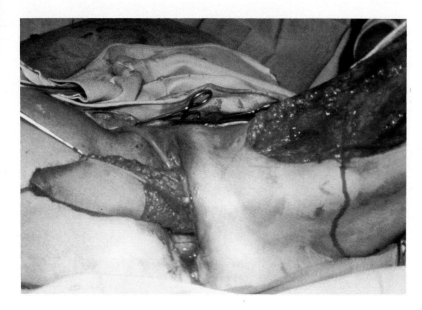

Figure 84–12. The same patient as in Figure 84–10. A left gracilis musculocutaneous flap is transposed into the perineal defect. The proximal portion of the skin segment has been deepithelized, and will be buried for soft tissue "fill."

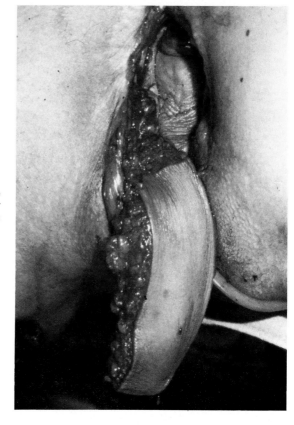

Figure 84–13. The same patient as in Figure 84–10. The proximal margin of the gracilis flap is inset into the posterior margin of the existing vaginal mucosa. The flap will then be rotated distally to replace the posterior wall of the vagina.

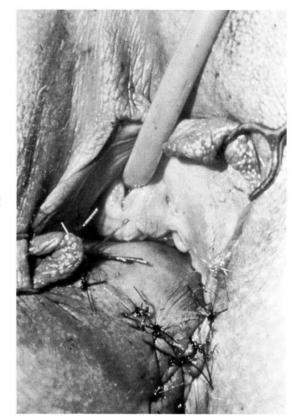

Figure 84–14. The same patient as in Figure 84–10. A close-up view of the inset gracilis flap replacing the posterior one-half of the vagina.

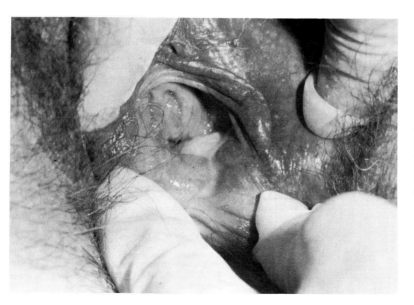

Figure 84–15. The same patient as in Figure 84–10. The healed flap (white) at one year. Although the musculocutaneous flap was in contact with secreting vaginal mucosa, it did not become macerated.

muscle, and by not extending the cutaneous portion of the flap into the distal one-third of the thigh. Acute vascular "spasm" of the dominant vascular pedicle is the most commonly recognized cause of flap necrosis, but this should be an avoidable problem in most situations. It is clear that the technical manipulations of the dominant pedicle should be performed with the utmost care, since vascular "spasm" may be an irreversible cause of flap necrosis. It is interesting that the muscular portion of the flap usually survives this vascular insult, but the cutaneous segment does not (Figs. 84–16 to 84–19).

ADVANTAGES

The gracilis musculocutaneous unit provides muscle, skin, and bulk, each of which can be used for a number of different reconstructive problems. Even though bulk is sometimes perceived as disadvantageous, there are times when it is beneficial. For instance, the fundamental reason for reconstructing the vagina with musculocutaneous flaps in pelvic exenteration defects is to obliterate the pelvic "dead space." This is truly a life-saving maneuver, since unrepaired pelvic dead space can be equated with a 20 per cent body burn, which carries its own lethality.

The gracilis musculocutaneous flap reaches a higher point in the pelvis than any local musculocutaneous flap of the thigh. Only the inferiorly based rectus abdominis flap, as a local flap, reaches a higher point in the pelvis. A common reason to choose the gracilis musculocutaneous flap, rather than a local fasciocutaneous flap, is the ability to revascularize an ischemic or scarred bed of inset with the gracilis muscle at the same time that the cutaneous segment is used to resurface either the vaginal wall or the central perineum.

The donor site is associated with a scar of the medial thigh, but overall it is rarely a source of postoperative complications, and the functional loss of the gracilis muscle is inconsequential.

REGIONAL FLAP COMPARISONS

For surface defects the gracilis musculocutaneous flap is usually compared with the posterior thigh fasciocutaneous flap based on the inferior gluteal vessels. The posterior thigh flap has the advantage that it is less bulky than the gracilis flap, and thereby offers more of an "in kind" replacement of perineal skin. This excellent restoration of the perineal surface does routinely require secondary revision for the "dog-ear" that remains at the base of the flap after rotation and inset. The innervation of the posterior thigh flap, through the incorporation of the posterior cutaneous nerve of the thigh, is an even more significant contribution to perineal reconstruction, since it provides sensibility to an area that is uniquely important for both sitting and sexual arousal.

The tensor fascia lata (TFL) flap is more commonly used for groin coverage, because it resurfaces a larger area, particularly in the lateral half of the groin. For this reason, it is

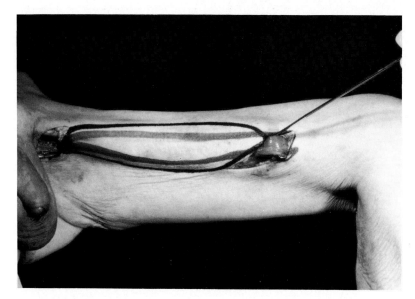

Figure 84–16. Cadaver dissection of a gracilis musculocutaneous flap. The gracilis muscle is retracted through an initial incision in the distal thigh to locate the proper position of the skin island. The adductor longus tendon has already been identified in the proximal incision. (From McCraw, J. B., and Arnold, P. G.: Atlas of Muscle and Musculocutaneous Flaps. Norfolk, VA, Hampton Press, 1986.)

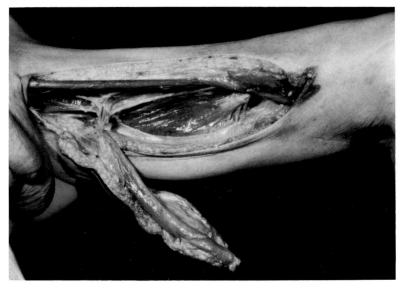

Figure 84–17. Completed elevation of the gracilis musculocutaneous flap. The neurovascular pedicle can be seen passing between the adductor longus and the adductor brevis muscles. Stretching the vascular pedicles, as illustrated, is the primary cause of vascular "spasm," which results in flap necrosis. (From McCraw, J. B., and Arnold, P. G.: Atlas of Muscle and Musculocutaneous Flaps. Norfolk, VA, Hampton Press, 1986.)

the standard flap of choice for repair of radical groin dissection defects. For massive surface defects of the groin area, the inferiorly based rectus abdominis flap is chosen because of its size and more extensive arc of rotation.

For problems requiring revascularization, the gracilis muscle flap is primary compared with the inferiorly based rectus abdominis flap. Even though the gracilis muscle flap is smaller, it is more accessible to low pelvic defects. It is also easier to retrieve and has a less consequential donor site. The rectus abdominis muscle flap can be used for exactly the same defects as the gracilis flap, but it is more difficult to manipulate and requires a laparotomy for inset of the flap into the lower region of the pelvis. Nevertheless, the rectus abdominis musculocutaneous flap is clearly the flap of choice for high pelvic defects, because of its dependability, larger size, and versatility of design.

Rectus Abdominis

USES

The inferiorly based rectus abdominis muscle flap is supplied by the deep inferior epigastric vessels that arise from the common femoral vessels and enter the rectus abdominis muscle approximately 6 to 7 cm above its insertion in the pubis. When this flap is employed as a "pure" muscle flap, its arc includes the iliac crest, the groin, the central and posterior perineum, and the entire sur-

face of the internal pelvis. This wide arc of rotation is the result of both the extensive length of the rectus abdominis muscle and a vascular axis that lies near the pubic symphysis. Through incision of the posterior rectus fascia, the rectus abdominis muscle flap can be transposed directly into the pelvis for a vesicovaginal or rectovaginal fistula, as well as coverage of the iliac vessels. Bilateral rectus abdominis muscle flaps can also be used to resurface the entire perineum.

The inferiorly based rectus abdominis musculocutaneous flap is the largest single local flap available for both pelvic and perineal reconstructions. The vertical skin design is usually employed for surface problems of the perineum or groin, while the horizontal (TRAM) design is more commonly used for total vaginal reconstructions and other intrapelvic space problems (Fig. 84–20).

The arc of rotation of both the vertical and horizontal flaps includes the perineum and the groin. The longer vertical flap also reaches the lateral flank of the abdomen, and distally reaches the midthigh. Because some of these massive wounds are associated with vascular insufficiency of the iliac vessels, it may be necessary to use the opposite common iliac vessels to supply the rectus abdominis flap. The rectus abdominis musculocutaneous flap can also be designed as relatively smaller bilateral flaps, as a means of increasing the area of coverage and decreasing the size of the individual donor sites (Figs. 84–21, 84–22). This provides the additional benefit of "splitting" the coverage of the entire perineum into two separate flaps (Fig. 84–23).

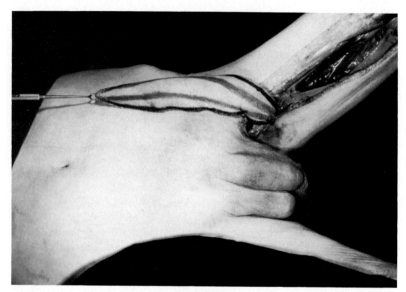

Figure 84–18

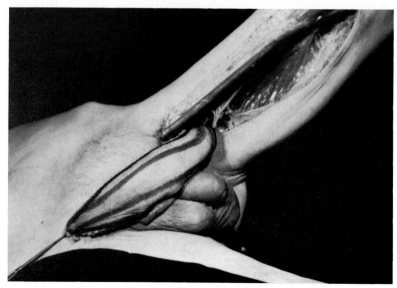

Figure 84–19

Figures 84–18, 84–19. Counter-clockwise arc of rotation of the gracilis flap, passing through the medial groin, the suprapubic area, and the central perineum. (From McCraw, J. B., and Arnold, P. G.: Atlas of Muscle and Musculocutaneous Flaps. Norfolk, VA, Hampton Press, 1986.)

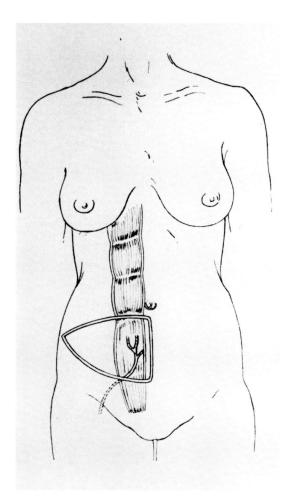

Figure 84–20. Outline of the horizontal design of the deep inferior epigastric TRAM flap. The vessels enter the posterior surface of the muscle approximately 6 cm above the pubis.

DISADVANTAGES

The anterior rectus fascial donor site closure is the major disadvantage of the rectus abdominis musculocutaneous flap, but it is not a disadvantage of the "pure" muscle flap, since the anterior fascial defect can easily be primarily closed without any tension. In the case of the horizontal (TRAM) flap, an anterior fascial defect of only 3 to 4 cm in width should be expected, and this can be primarily closed, with few exceptions. This fascial closure may still require reinforcement with a Gore-Tex patch, when it is closed under any tension or in obese patients. A tense closure may also be caused by nitrous oxide inhalation during the anesthetic or by an inadequate bowel preparation.

Almost all vertically oriented rectus abdominis musculocutaneous flaps require an end to end artificial patch closure, because the full width of the anterior fascia must be taken with the overlying skin to protect the direct cutaneous perforators passing between the muscle and the flap skin. This "cookie cutter" donor defect is the result of transferring skin, fascia, and rectus abdominis muscle in an en bloc fashion. The nature of the abdominal closure needs to be clearly understood by all the surgical specialists involved with the reconstruction, since the anatomy of this closure will be foreign to many of them. The closure may be threatening in its magnitude and may even lead to doubts about the advisability of the procedure itself, unless this is recognized and accepted in advance.

The rectus abdominis flap is generally associated with significant donor site discomfort, but this should last for only a day or two. For some reason, the inferiorly based TRAM flap is not as sensitive to cold as the superiorly based flap, but it should be protected in the course of a long operative procedure.

The horizontal flap may interfere with stomal formation at the time of the Wertheim hysterectomy, unless it is carefully designed. The location of the proposed neostomal site should be estimated preoperatively, so that the vertical approximation of the donor site skin does not adversely affect the desired stomal site location.

For low vesicovaginal and rectovaginal fistulas it is necessary to enter the abdominal cavity to inset the rectus abdominis muscle flap properly. This is not a disadvantage if an intra-abdominal approach is already planned. It *is* a disadvantage when the same fistula can be safely repaired from below with a gracilis muscle flap without the need to enter the abdominal cavity.

ADVANTAGES

Both the inferiorly based rectus abdominis muscle and musculocutaneous flaps are predictable in their reliability. The rectus abdominis muscle itself is approximately 8 to 10 cm in width, compared with the 4 cm width of a gracilis muscle. The musculocutaneous flap can also be designed in dimensions that resurface the entire perineum with a single flap, or two flaps can be used to reconstruct the perineum and vagina simultane-

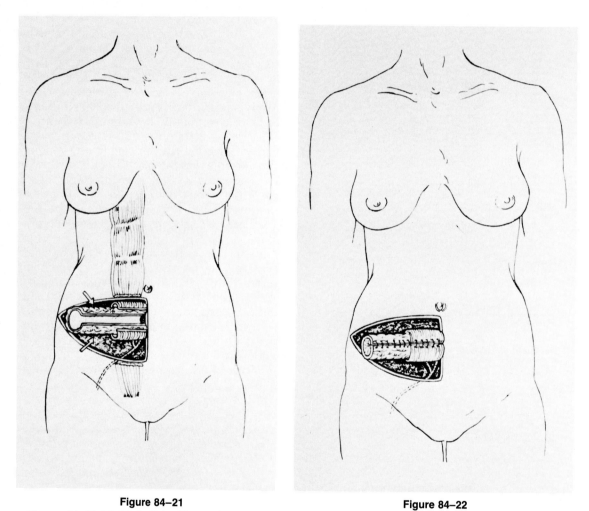

Figure 84–21   **Figure 84–22**

Figures 84–21, 84–22. An "island" musculocutaneous flap is created by dividing the rectus abdominis muscle proximally and distally. The skin segment *(arrows)* is tubed in the distal flap, which will form the introitus. Both skin and muscle are tubed in the proximal flap.

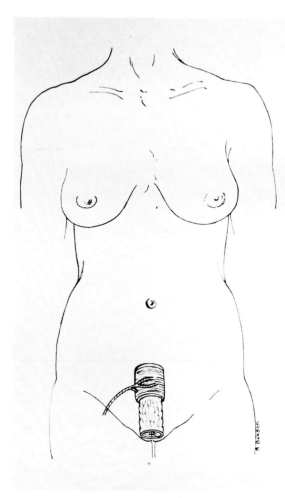

Figure 84–23. The inferiorly based TRAM flap is passed into the pelvis through the posterior rectus sheath. Total vaginal reconstruction with a single flap requires a vertical flap dimension of 13 cm to provide an introital diameter of 5 cm. For this reason, smaller bilateral flaps are sometimes used, so that the abdominal skin can be closed without any undermining.

ously. The versatility of various rectus abdominis flap applications for defects of the upper pelvis and lower pelvis is unmatched by any other flap. Although the donor site considerations are formidable, the rectus abdominis flap can in fact reduce the multiplicity of operations for some of the complex problems of genitourinary reconstructive surgery.

REGIONAL FLAP COMPARISONS

The horizontal rectus abdominis musculocutaneous flap is the preferred flap for total vaginal reconstruction when it is available and can be used. It is a totally reliable flap,

accessible for both high and low pelvic defects, and effectively obliterates the entire pelvic dead space (Figs. 84–24 to 84–27). The gracilis musculocutaneous flap is reasonably reliable and convenient, but does not reach the upper pelvis. Unlike the gracilis flap, the flap dissection necessitates an interruption in the abdominal portion of the Wertheim procedure while the flap is being elevated. The vertical rectus abdominis flap is useful for either small or massive perineal defects, and two (bilateral) flaps can certainly cover any perineal defect.

Most groin defects can be easily covered by a simple transposition of the TFL fasciocutaneous flap, as in the case of a radical groin dissection. Occasionally the supplying vessels of the TFL flap will have been injured, and it becomes reasonable to consider an inferiorly based rectus abdominis flap. At the present time, the inferiorly based rectus abdominis flap is primarily employed for massive defects of the perineum, pelvis, and groin, but improved operative applications will encourage its use for smaller defects.

Posterior Thigh

USES

The posterior thigh flap is primarily used for surface defects of the perineum, rather than for pelvic problems. Major perineal defects require bilateral posterior thigh flaps, since each flap measures only 7 to 8 cm in width. The flap is not usually considered for vaginal defects, because of its limited excursion above the level of the introitus.

DISADVANTAGES

The posterior thigh flap is quite well vascularized, but carries no muscle for the purpose of revascularization of the ischemic or irradiated wound. The subfascial vascularization of the flap is adequate to support a "fresh" full-thickness neourethral graft. It is primarily used in situations that do not require muscle revascularization, such as simple surface replacement of the perineum. The flap is not so useful for vaginal reconstructions as the rectus abdominis and gracilis musculocutaneous flaps, since it extends above the introitus for only 5 to 8 cm.

The most common patient complaint is the dog-ear that is left at the base of the flap

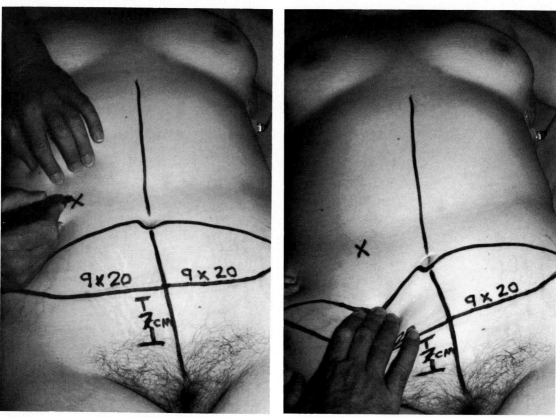

Figure 84–24
              Figure 84–25

Figures 84–24, 84–25. A 30 year old female with a diethylstilbestrol-caused carcinoma of the vagina that invaded the bladder. Bilateral horizontal TRAM flaps are outlined for total vaginal reconstruction, which will be performed at the time of the total vaginectomy and cystectomy. The narrower (9 cm versus 13 cm) vertical dimension of the bilateral flaps was chosen to avoid distortion of the planned urinary stoma, which is marked with an "X." The abdominal skin will be closed primarily without any undermining.

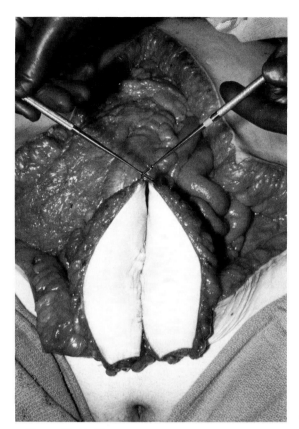

Figure 84–26. The same patient as in Figure 84–25. The inferior margins of the TRAM flaps are approximated to form the posterior wall of the neovagina. The "dome" of the neovagina is retracted by the skin hooks.

when it is rotated onto the perineum. This can be easily remedied, but it is associated with an unsightly bulge until a secondary revision can be made. There is some loss of sensation in the posterior thigh after the retrieval of the posterior cutaneous nerve of the thigh with the posterior thigh flap, but this is an acceptable price to pay in transferring this sensation to a new location.

ADVANTAGES

The posterior thigh flap is one of the favored flap choices for contour replacement of the perineal surface. It is less bulky than any other adjacent flap, and the transfer of related sensibility from the thigh is an important addition to the sitting surface. The transfer of the flap from the posterior thigh to the perineum is made by simple transposition, and the donor site usually is primarily closed and heals without incident (Figs. 84–28 to 84–33).

REGIONAL FLAP COMPARISONS

The usual flap comparisons of the posterior thigh flap have already been discussed in the sections on the gracilis and rectus abdominis flaps. There is one application that cannot be accomplished by any other local flap: the combination of the posterior thigh flap with the inferior gluteus maximus musculocutaneous flap. Both of these flaps are supplied by the inferior gluteal vessels, and the elevation of a true "island" flap dramatically improves their central and upward excursion. This maneuver enables the posterior thigh flap to be rotated 180 degrees and transferred to the sacrum or the opposite buttock. This also improves the excursion of the posterior thigh flap above the level of the introitus for vaginal applications. Difficulties with positioning of the patient still remain when this flap is used for vaginal reconstructions, because the flap elevation is preferably performed with the patient in the prone position, while the supine position is best for the flap inset.

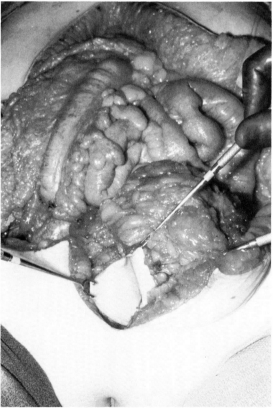

Figure 84–27. The same patient as in Figure 84–25. A view of the introitus of the neovagina following the formation of the anterior wall. Note the proximity of the flap to the perineum, before its inset. This young patient returned to sexual activity and is alive and well two years after surgery.

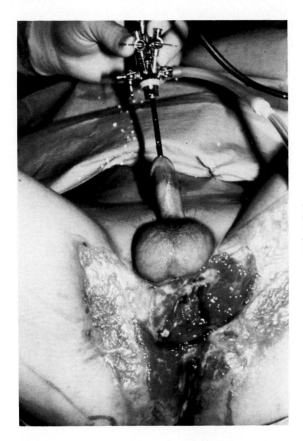

Figure 84–28. An 11 year old boy who sustained a fourth degree burn of the perineum while pinned beneath a hot car muffler. The urethra was totally lost between the bladder neck and the scrotum, and the anus was not definable in the dense perineal scar. A colostomy had been created previously to protect the perineal burn.

Figure 84–29. The same patient as in Figure 84–28. Initial debridement and elevation of an inferior gluteal fasciocutaneous flap from the right thigh. The posterior cutaneous nerve of the thigh is visible on the deep fascial surface of the flap, and the inferior gluteal vascular bundle is pointed out.

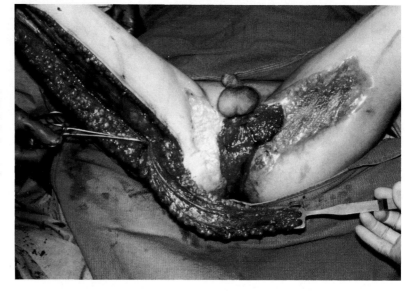

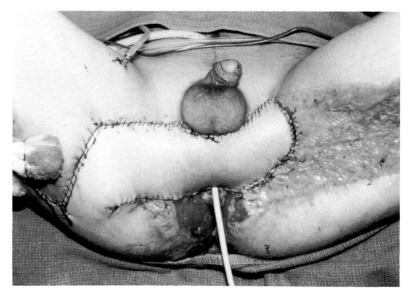

Figure 84–30. The same patient as in Figure 84–28. Transposition and inset of the right posterior thigh flap. A perineal urethrostomy is in place. Note the healed skin graft in the left thigh.

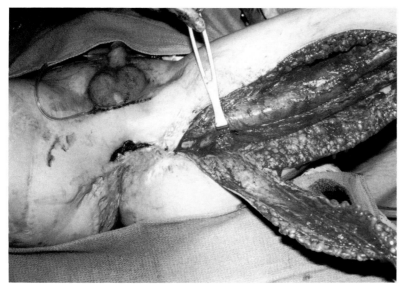

Figure 84–31. The same patient as in Figure 84–28. Even though the "base" of the inferior gluteal fasciocutaneous flap in the left thigh had been grafted, the distal sensation and Doppler pulses were intact. The inferior gluteal neurovascular bundle was explored before the recreation of the posterior perineal deformity.

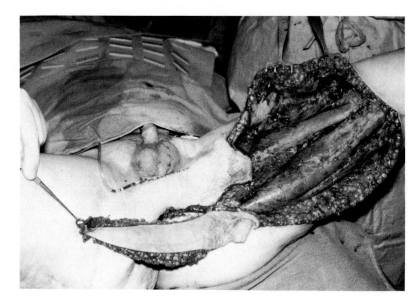

Figure 84–32. The same patient as in Figure 84–28. Transposition of the fasciocutaneous flap from the left thigh. Note the skin grafted surface of the proximal portion of the flap.

Figure 84–33. The same patient as in Figure 84–28. The anterior half of the perineum was resurfaced by the right flap, and the posterior perineum was covered by the left flap. Urinary continence was reestablished with a full-thickness tube graft. Anal incontinence was corrected by a local plastic procedure on the anus, and the colostomy was removed. The patient continues to do well eight years after the surgery.

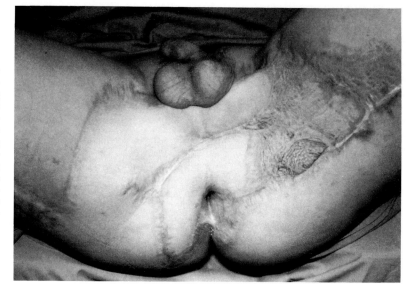

V-Y Biceps Femoris

USES

The V-Y biceps femoris flap is primarily used and is the usual flap of choice for ischial pressure sores. It provides the necessary muscle revascularization of the deep ischial cavity, as well as simultaneous surface skin replacement. In the case of a recurrent ischial ulceration at the margin of the transposed flap, the entire reconstructive procedure can be repeated by simple readvancement of the flap.

The V-Y biceps femoris flap can also be advanced into the central perineum. The usual indication for this application is a radical vulvectomy defect in patients with pendulous posterior thigh skin. When it can be used, it offers a simple correction of radical vulvectomy defects or repeated simple vulvectomy defects.

DISADVANTAGES

Because the posterior nerve of the thigh is included with the V-Y flap and is necessarily divided distally, this may be a source of painful neuromas. Current understanding of the reasons for neuroma formation is incomplete, but it is a recognized problem with the saphenous nerve, the lateral femoral cutaneous nerve, and the posterior cutaneous nerve of the thigh. The donor site is otherwise quite favorable and leaves no functional deficit.

ADVANTAGES

The V-Y biceps femoris musculocutaneous flap is the most suitable for ischial pressure sores, because of its ease of elevation, the muscle bulk, and the surface replacement with flap skin. It can also be used initially as a musculocutaneous flap, and later separated into a biceps femoris muscle flap and a posterior thigh fasciocutaneous flap. For major defects of the lower buttock, it can be incorporated with the other hamstring muscles and used to carry the entire skin of the posterior thigh for purposes of superior advancement. Occasionally, this "hamstring" musculocutaneous flap is large enough to repair ischial and trochanteric ulcerations simultaneously.

REGIONAL FLAP COMPARISONS

The TFL flap is usually compared with the V-Y biceps femoris flap. The latter has the distinct advantage of carrying muscle to the ischial defect, while the TFL flap is primarily used to replace the surface skin loss. Further, the arc of rotation of the TFL flap includes only the ischium and usually requires a skin grafted donor site. As a generalization, the overall experience with the biceps femoris flap has been much more satisfactory than that with the TFL flap in solving difficult ischial problems: primary healing is more difficult to obtain with the latter and the wound is less stable over the long run.

In the pendulous thigh, the hamstring modification of the biceps femoris flap can be used to cover the greater trochanter and the ischium at the same time, if a wide cutaneous segment is designed and all the hamstring muscles are moved in combination. This particular flap necessitates division of the distal insertions of the posterior thigh muscles in the flap, in order to facilitate the upward excursion of the musculocutaneous unit.

In the perineum, either the posterior thigh flap or the gracilis musculocutaneous flap is usually chosen for small perineal defects, and the inferiorly based TRAM flap is selected for large defects, for the reasons already mentioned. A simple V-Y biceps femoris flap can also be used for lateral defects of the perineum if the thigh skin is somewhat pendulous. This is particularly good for the remaining perineal contracture that follows multiple simple vulvectomies in elderly patients.

The V-Y biceps femoris musculocutaneous flap is associated with more morbidity than the gracilis flap, probably because of the larger extent of the dissection. It has the advantages of simple elevation by fascial release, and primary closure of both the donor and recipient sites by V-Y advancement. The proximal tip of the flap can usually be advanced 10 cm if both the long and the short heads of the biceps femoris tendon are divided. When the posterior cutaneous nerve of the thigh is protected during flap elevation, it is also possible to raise the flap as an innervated flap.

Because of the variations in upward mobility of the biceps femoris flap, it may still be necessary to use the gracilis musculocutaneous flap at the same time or later. The previous elevation of a biceps femoris V-Y advancement flap does not preclude the later elevation of a gracilis flap. In fact, the V-Y flap can be returned to its site of origin and a gracilis musculocutaneous flap can be used instead during the same operation.

Tensor Fascia Lata

USES

The TFL fasciocutaneous flap is primarily used for replacement of groin skin after radical groin dissections. Because of the fragility of the "native" groin dissection skin flaps, the transposition of a TFL flap is a reasonable consideration for routine replacement of this compromised skin. The TFL donor site can be primarily closed, and this flap replacement significantly enhances the ability to obtain a promptly healed wound. Another common application of the TFL fasciocutaneous flap is in combination with the vastus lateralis, rectus femoris, and biceps femoris muscle flaps, since the TFL flap does not provide deep muscular coverage for purposes of revascularization. In some patients with meningomyelocele the lateral thigh sensation is intact, so that the TFL flap can be used to transfer sensible skin to the ischium.

The tensor myofascial flap is primarily used for upper abdominal wall reconstruction, since the tensor fascia can be extended to the level of the xiphoid. The myofascial flap can also be used for lower abdominal wall defects, but this is usually accomplished with the more easily dissected rectus femoris muscle flap.

DISADVANTAGES

The donor site of the TFL flap represents its biggest disadvantage because of recurrent seroma formation. It can be primarily closed in dimensions of 9 to 10 cm or less, but a skin graft closure of the donor site is remarkably unsightly. The fasciocutaneous flap does not provide muscle coverage of exposed groin vessels, but it does provide well-vascularized skin to the area.

It was once logically presumed that the TFL donor site would be less significant than the rectus femoris muscle flap donor site from a functional standpoint, but this choice has been empirically proved to offer even chances. The use of the rectus femoris muscle flap does

weaken terminal knee extension temporarily, but this has not been observed as a permanent problem if the vastus lateralis and medialis muscles are redirected into the midline to replace this function. Conversely, the tensor fascia is an important lateral knee stabilizer, and on at least one occasion it has been necessary to replace this function with a transfer of a rectus femoris muscle into the distal stump of the tensor fascia at the knee. This should be an infrequent problem, but it deserves consideration.

ADVANTAGES

The TFL flap is a simple transposition flap for groin coverage. It is supplied by the same vessels that supply the rectus femoris and vastus lateralis muscle flaps, so it is possible to use these three flaps simultaneously. This is occasionally done when there is exposure of the femoral vessels, and muscle coverage is required. In this case, either a rectus femoris or a vastus lateralis muscle flap can be used to cover the exposed vessels, and the TFL flap can be employed for skin coverage. Beside the standard McGregor groin flap, this is the only local fasciocutaneous flap that is accessible for coverage of the entire groin. Further, the transfer of the TFL to the "sitting area" in patients with meningomyelocele can offer permanent protection. The rectus femoris muscle flap is easier to use for lower abdominal wall structural defects, but only the tensor fascia reaches the upper abdomen as a local myofascial flap.

REGIONAL FLAP COMPARISONS

The TFL fasciocutaneous flap is the most accessible flap for the replacement of groin skin, and this is the main indication for its use. The gracilis musculocutaneous flap can be used for small medial groin defects, but is more fragile than the TFL flap. The inferiorly based rectus abdominis musculocutaneous flap is usually reserved for massive groin defects, even though it is reasonable to use it for smaller groin and perineal defects in which muscle coverage is necessary. The vastus lateralis muscle flap is also supplied by the lateral femoral circumflex vessels and is large enough to resurface the entire groin, but the dissection is much bloodier than that of the TFL flap.

Since the tensor fascia can also be "carried" by the rectus femoris muscle flap as a vascularized fascial flap without including the tensor muscle, the rectus femoris muscle serves as an alternative flap for both upper and lower abdominal fascial replacement. Using the rectus femoris muscle flap to carry the tensor fascia involves less tedious dissection than the creation of an "island" tensor myofascial flap, and it provides the added benefit of the strong rectus femoris muscular fascia for the repair of the lower abdominal wall.

The TFL flap was initially designed as a method of transferring skin to ischial and greater trochanteric pressure sores. It is still used for those purposes, but it is more often employed in combination with the rectus femoris muscle flap (for the trochanter) or the vastus lateralis muscle flap (for the ischium). These combinations remove the disadvantage of the TFL flap's lack of muscle, and offer the apparent advantage of flap skin coverage rather than that of a skin grafted muscle flap.

Rectus Femoris

USES

The rectus femoris muscle flap is easily transposed into suprapubic and lower abdominal wall defects. The rectus femoris musculocutaneous flap is also useful for resurfacing ischemic ulcerations of the suprapubic area (Figs. 84–34 to 84–38). The rectus femoris muscle can be used to carry skin to the margins of the perineum, but it is not useful for vaginal reconstructions. The tip of the cutaneous segment can be extended for 4 to 5 cm above the introitus, which is usually inadequate for a total vaginal reconstruction. Either the rectus femoris musculocutaneous flap or the skin grafted rectus femoris muscle flap can be used to resurface the vulva.

DISADVANTAGES

The stated disadvantage of the rectus femoris flap is the potential for loss of terminal knee extension. This has not occurred in the authors' experience, when the vastus medialis and vastus lateralis muscles have been reapproximated in the midline of the thigh. The most common criticism of this flap is its lack of upward mobility because of the low level of entry of the dominant vascular pedicle. This limits the superior excursion of the tip of the rectus femoris muscle to the area of the umbilicus, so that it cannot be used as a single flap for upper abdominal structural reconstructions without including the adjacent tensor fascia.

ADVANTAGES

The rectus femoris muscle flap is one of the easiest flaps to manipulate and is one of the

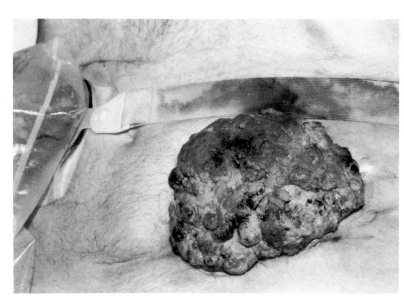

Figure 84–34. A 60 year old man with a fungating adenocarcinoma arising from the left colon and invading the abdominal wall. The patient had previously undergone a right colectomy for a primary carcinoma of the right colon. The tumor of the left colon represented a second primary tumor.

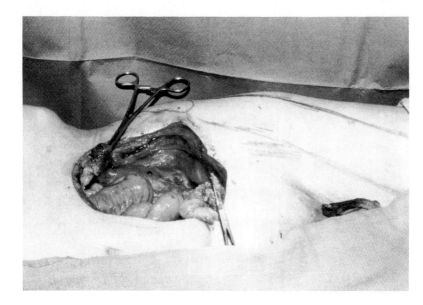

Figure 84–35. The same patient as in Figure 84–34. An en bloc resection of the left colon and the abdominal wall was carried out. The 15 cm by 20 cm defect of the abdominal wall extended from the inguinal ligament to a point 5 cm above the level of the umbilicus. A rectus femoris musculocutaneous flap is outlined in the left thigh.

Figure 84–36. The same patient as in Figure 84–34. The rectus femoris muscle was used to "carry" an 8 cm by 30 cm skin segment from the anterior thigh.

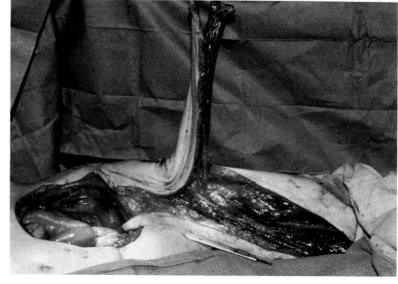

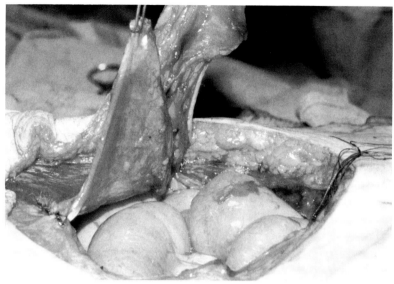

Figure 84-37. The same patient as in Figure 84-34. The strong fascia on the posterior surface of the rectus femoris muscle was used to repair the abdominal wall defect without the use of artificial mesh.

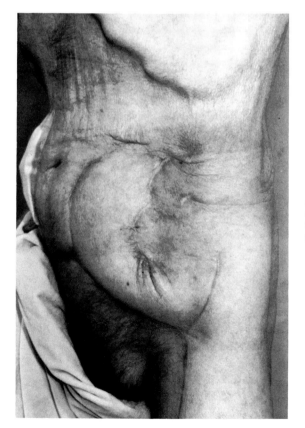

Figure 84-38. A healed rectus femoris musculocutaneous flap and stable abdominal wall in this patient with severe chronic obstructive lung disease. The patient was free of disease at the time of his death in a motor vehicle accident two years after surgery.

most reliable. It can also withstand a great deal of torsion and tension. If the dominant vessels are not stretched to the point of causing vascular "spasm," the muscle flap can be safely used for tense closures of large abdominal defects.

REGIONAL FLAP COMPARISONS

Although the tensor myofascial flap can also be used for structural defects of the lower abdomen, the rectus femoris muscle flap provides a stronger fascia and is more easily transposed into this area. The rectus femoris musculocutaneous flap can be transposed to the suprapubic area just as easily as the TFL flap, but with a less consequential donor site. The rectus femoris muscle flap that "carries" the tensor fascia is the authors' current preference for most structural replacements of the abdominal wall.

Free Microvascular Transfers

There are only a few indications for the use of free flaps in reconstructive perineal surgery, and almost none in reconstructive pelvic surgery. At the present time, free flaps are used for a few specialized functions. The dorsalis pedis, lateral arm, and forearm flaps have been employed in total penile reconstruction to provide a thin and sensate flap for the surface of the new penis. The latissimus dorsi flap has been used in cases of massive replacements that could not be accomplished as effectively with multiple local flaps or multiple-staged procedures. The deep inferior epigastric, inferior gluteal, and femoral vessels offer excellent recipient sites for free flaps, and applications will be found only after the operative time consumed by the vascular anastomosis is reduced.

REFERENCES

Bakamjian, V. Y.: A two-stage method for pharyngoesophageal reconstruction with a primary pectoral skin flap. Plast. Reconstr. Surg., 36:173, 1965.

Baran, N. K., and Horton, C. E.: Growth of skin grafts, flaps and scars in young mini pigs. Plast. Reconstr. Surg., 50:487, 1972.

Blair, V. P., and Brown, J. B.: Use of large split skin grafts of intermediate thickness. Surg. Gynecol. Obstet., 49:82, 1929.

Davis, J. S.: Plastic Surgery—Its Principles and Practice. Philadelphia, Blakiston, 1919.

Devine, P. C., Horton, C. E., Devine, C. J., Sr., Devine, C. J., Jr., Crawford, H. H., and Adamson, J. E.: Use of full-thickness skin grafts in repair of urethral strictures. J. Urol, 90:67, 1963.

Horton, C. E., and Devine, C. J., Jr.: Hypospadias—A One Stage Repair. Norwich, NY, Eaton Medial Film Library, 1958.

Horton, C. E., and Devine, C. J., Jr.: Peyronie's disease. Plast. Reconstr. Surg., 52:503, 1973.

Kanavel, A. B.: Plastic procedures for the obliteration of cavities with noncollapsible wall. Surg. Gynecol. Obstet., 32:453, 1921.

McCraw, J. B., and Dibbell, D. G.: Experimental definition of independent myocutaneous vascular territories. Plast. Reconstr. Surg., 60:212, 1977.

McGregor, I. A., and Jackson, I. T.: The groin flap. Br. J. Plast. Surg., 25:3, 1972.

McIndoe, A. H.: Treatment of hypospadias. Am. J. Surg., 38:176, 1937.

McIndoe, A. H.: The treatment of congenital absence and obliterative conditions of the vagina. Br. J. Plast. Surg., 2:254, 1949.

Muller, G. P., and Jordan, C. G.: Elephantiasis nostra. Am. Surg., 97:226, 1933.

Nové-Josserand, G.: Traitement de l'hypospadias; nouvelle methode. Lyon Med., 85:198, 1897.

Ollier, L.: Greffes cutanée ou autoplastique. Bull. Acad. Med., 1:243, 1872.

Owens, N.: Reconstruction for traumatic denudation of the penis and scrotum. Surgery, 12:88, 1942.

Pickrell, K. L., Masters, F. W., Georgiade, N., and Horton, C. E.: Rectal sphincter reconstruction, using gracilis muscle transplant. Plast. Reconstr. Surg., 13:46, 1954.

Sadove, R. C., and Horton, C. E.: Utilizing full-thickness skin grafts for vaginal reconstruction. Clin. Plast. Surg., 15:443, 1988.

Shaw, D. T., and Payne, R. L.: One stage tubed abdominal flaps. Surg. Gynecol. Obstet., 83:205, 1946.

Thiersch, K.: Über die feineren anatomischen Veränderungen bei Aufheilung von Haut auf Granulationen. Verh. Dtsch. Ges. Chir., Third Congress, 1874, pp. 67–75.

85

Charles E. Horton
Richard C. Sadove
Charles J. Devine, Jr.

Reconstruction of
Male Genital Defects:
Congenital

EMBRYOLOGY

Normal Development

The sex of the developing embryo is determined by the chromosome content of the spermatozoon that fertilizes the ovum. A sperm containing an X chromosome yield an XX individual (female), and a sperm containing a Y chromosome yields an XY (male).

The embryonic disc lying beneath the amnion consists of two cell layers at the end of two weeks of development. These consist of ectoderm and endoderm. The primitive streak is formed by proliferation of ectodermal cells at the caudal end of the disc and produces a midline groove. From this groove, the embryonic mesoderm forms between the ectoderm and endoderm. Mesodermal cells proliferate and migrate peripherally, separating the endodermal and ectodermal layers.

Ectoderm and endoderm fuse and form the cloacal membrane just caudal to the primitive streak. The allantois develops as an outpouching of the posterior wall of the yolk sac into the connecting yolk stalk. Owing to increasing proliferation and migration of mesodermal cells, the embryonic disc grows and elongates. At the fourth week the primitive streak has regressed. The cell layers in the cloacal membrane are inseparable, so the migrating mesodermal cells pile up around it and form the cloacal ridge.

The embryo buckles upward and begins to overgrow its slower-growing margins. Head and tail folds form, and the embryo assumes a more or less cylindric shape. By day 21 the tail fold has formed, and the cloacal membrane and the allantois become part of the ventral wall. The hindgut terminates in a blindly ending sac (the cloaca) that terminates at the relocated cloacal membrane.

The external genitalia and anus are formed by developments about the cloacal membrane. Migrating mesodermal cells continue to be blocked by the fused membrane, and the cloacal folds continue to grow. A mound (the genital tubercle) builds up between the membrane and the allantois. A midline depression (the urethral groove) persists in the genital tubercle and extends to its tip. An epithelial tag forms from proliferating ectodermal cells. The tubercle lengthens, carrying the groove with it and maintaining the tag at its tip.

The cloacal cavity is divided into the ventral portion, which becomes the bladder, and the dorsal portion, which becomes the rectum. By six to seven weeks this urorectal septum meets the cloacal membrane, where lateral tissues have formed a transverse bar dividing it into urogenital and anal membranes. Urogenital folds are formed from the ventral portions of the cloaca. The anal folds are formed from the dorsal parts. As the genital tubercle elongates and swells, the urogenital membrane grows and creates the urogenital ostium. The anal membrane forms in a deep pit (the proctodeum) and then ruptures, establishing an outlet for the rectum.

At this stage external genitalia may show hints of sexual differentiation, such as the extent of the urethral groove, but this stage is essentially the same for both sexes. If testes did not develop, the external genitalia would grow into a normal female configuration. The genital tubercle would become the clitoris, the urogenital folds would become the labia minora, and the labioscrotal swellings would enlarge to form the labia majora. The fetal testis secretes a hormone necessary to direct development into the male structure.

Lateral to the axis of the embryo, proliferating mesoderm differentiates into three parts: the paraxial mesoderm, the lateral plate, and a portion between these called the intermediate mesoderm. The nephrogenic cord is formed at the caudal end of this structure. At about five weeks the gonadal ridge appears between the midline dorsum mesentery and the nephrogenic cord, which has by this time developed into the mesonephros.

The primordial germ cells that have formed in the wall of the yolk sac migrate into the germinal ridge through the dorsal mesentery of the hindgut, and form the gonads. Primitive sex structures surround the germ cells in the mesenchyme.

In males the primitive sex cords continue to proliferate and become separated from the surface epithelium by the tunica albuginea during the sixth to eighth weeks. The interstitial cells of Leydig develop from mesenchyme located between the cords. Testosterone secreted by the testes causes the external genitalia to develop a male configuration. The genital tubercle grows rapidly and assumes a more cylindric shape until it is identifiable as a phallus. Distally a definite circumferential groove appears, delineating the glans.

The phallus is now growing perpendicular to the abdominal wall. As it enlarges, the urethral groove deepens. The urethral folds become quite prominent. At the end of three months the urethral folds begin to close. The original urogenital ostium closes, and the urethral grooves seam together. A tube forming the urethra progresses distally, with the urogenital ostium advancing before it. The seam remains as a prominent median raphe. The consolidated mesenchyme in the dorsal portion of the phallus divides in the midline to form the two corpora cavernosa. Mesenchyme around the developing urethra becomes the corpus spongiosum.

Urethral closure continues to the glans penis, where the urogenital ostium can be identified as a diamond-shaped opening. The glans enlarges, deepening its urethral groove; it then closes over the groove but does not fuse at this stage. The deep, epithelium-lined trough is still open, filled with desquamated epithelial cells.

A roll of skin arises on either side of the urethral opening at about the third month. This ridge extends to encircle the shaft of the penis and forms the prepuce, which extends to sheath the glans. As the prepuce grows, the edges of the glans seal the glandular urethra until the urethral meatus reaches its final location at the site of the former epithelial tag. The deep epithelial tract in the glans now forms the navicular fossa of the urethra.

The genital tubercle elongates and the labioscrotal swellings appear at about eight weeks. Sharply separated from the penis by the lateral phallic grooves, they migrate posteriorly and around the phallus to form the scrotum. The median raphe is a septum that maintains two separate compartments. The testes descend into the scrotum by nine months, completing development of the male external genitalia.

Hypospadias and Chordee

Hypospadias is probably due to incomplete masculinization of the genitalia. Interstitial cells of the testis hypertrophy over a limited time, which coincides with the period during which the urethra is formed. It is likely that an inductor substance is generated by these cells; without this inductor, the development would be female. In hypospadias, we frequently see the results of interruption of androgenic stimulation after normal development. This is probably due to premature involution of the interstitial cells. It is possible that receptor cells in the embryonic phallus are unable to receive the message sent by the normal production of an inductor substance, or that the inductor substance may be present but flawed.

If any deviation from normal occurs, the urethral meatus remains on the ventral surface of the shaft of the penis, and the penis distal to this continues to form in a female fashion. The urethral groove remains as a shallow depression in the skin extending out to the groove in the glans. The glans is flattened. The mesenchyme, which would have formed the corpus spongiosum, Buck's fascia, and the dartos fascia, does not differentiate and becomes a layer of inelastic fibrous tissue that extends in a fan shape from around the urethral meatus to insert along the ventral aspect of the glans penis, thus causing chordee.

The prepuce develops as a hood and is deficient ventrally, only a groove being present in the ventrum of the glans. The fibrous band causing the chordee extends from one edge of the hooded prepuce to the other.

Chordee can occur without hypospadias in three types. As the urethral groove deepens, the edges of the skin come together to form the urethra, which is separated from the skin. If mesenchyme does not form any of the structures around the urethra, a fibrous band forms and causes chordee (Type I). If the corpus spongiosum forms, but Buck's fascia and the dartos fascia do not differentiate, chordee will be present (Type II). In both Types I and II, fibrous dysgenetic tissue will be found deep to the urethra. If the corpus spongiosum and Buck's fascia form, but the dartos fascia does not, the fibrous tissue causing the chordee will be found lateral to the urethra and superficial to Buck's fascia (Type III).

Epispadias and Exstrophy

The defect causing hypospadias occurs late in embryologic development. The developmental defect causing exstrophy and epispadias occurs early, because it is associated with the formation failure of the cloacal membrane. These abnormalities therefore are usually present in more severe forms.

Mesodermal cells form at the primitive streak and migrate outward, separating the endoderm and the ectoderm. The first cells that move peripherally are the cells that surround the cloacal membrane and form the cloacal ridges. About 20 days after fertiliza-

tion, the paraxial mesoderm has formed two broad strips lateral to the notochord and begins to segment into somites. About 40 pairs of somites have formed by the end of the fourth week. The cells of the ventromedial part (the sclerotome) drift toward the midline and form the connective tissue, cartilage, and bone of the axial skeleton. The remainder of the somites divide into a medial (myotome) portion and a lateral (dermatome) portion. Cells from the dermatome migrate laterally between the ectoderm and the somatic mesoderm to form the deep structures of the skin and subcutaneous tissues. The cells from the myotome become the muscles of the body wall. When layers from both sides have joined in the midline, the abdominal wall is complete. If the cloacal membrane extends too far cranially, it will interfere with penetration of the mesodermal cells into the ventral abdominal wall. Thus, when the membrane ruptures, the interior surface of the bladder will be exteriorized and exstrophy of the bladder will be present.

The precise mechanism that causes exstrophy and epispadias has not been delineated. It can occur because the somatic mesoderm did not penetrate far enough to finish the abdominal wall. The cloacal membrane itself could be too large, thus acting as a wedge to hold the two edges apart. The presence of epispadias indicates that the mesoderm piling up in the cloacal ridge has bridged the cloacal membrane to form a genital tubercle caudal to the urogenital diaphragm. The urethral groove is formed on the dorsal surface of the phallus, resulting in epispadias. Complete exstrophy with epispadias is the most common form of this abnormality. Epispadias alone is seen much less frequently, as are the more severe types of lesion with gastrointestinal involvement and cloacal formation, or duplication of the penis or clitoris.

HYPOSPADIAS

Hypospadias, a congenital anomaly in which the urethra ends on the ventral surface of the penile shaft or in the perineum, occurs in one of 350 live male births in the United States. It ranges in severity from the most frequent type involving the glans, through the less frequent penile shaft types, to the rarer and more severe scrotal or perineal forms. Ninety per cent of all forms of hypospadias are in the distal shaft or glans.

Normal Anatomy

The structures that form the bulk of the substance of the penis are three erectile bodies consisting of the paired corpora cavernosa and the corpus spongiosum, which lies ventrally in the groove between the two corpora cavernosa. Each is surrounded by the tunica albuginea. Central arteries are located in the corpora cavernosa and bring blood into these structures. The urethra traverses the penis through the corpus spongiosum and emerges at the distal end of the conical enlargement of the corpus called the glans penis. Below the penile skin is the dartos fascia, a loose layer of connective tissue in which run superficial lymphatics and the superficial dorsal veins. Buck's fascia is located beneath the dartos fascia and extends distally to the prepuce. It surrounds the corpora cavernosa and splits to contain the corpus spongiosum separately.

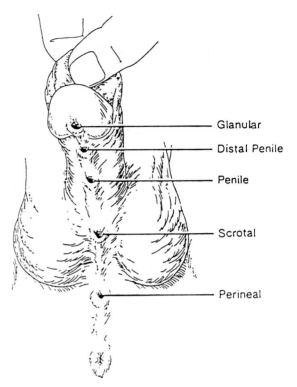

Figure 85–1. The anatomic locations of the meatus.

Description of Deformity

Various classifications of hypospadias have been described. However, elaborate classifications are not essential. The authors use the following categories: glanular, distal penile, penile, penoscrotal junction, scrotal, and perineal (Fig. 85–1). These are significant because they may determine the type of reconstruction.

In most but not all patients with hypospadias, there is a downward curvature of the penis, noted especially during erection. This chordee, as it is called, is caused by fibrous tissue that extends from the hypospadiac meatus to the glans penis. Rarely, chordee may occur without hypospadias. In these patients, fibrous tissue around and under the urethra causes the tunica albuginea of the corporal bodies to be inelastic and in certain cases to restrict growth of the ventral tunica. Even though the meatus may be normally placed in the glans, bending occurs (tunica disproportion).

The glans of the hypospadiac penis is usually spatulate and flattened, and the prepuce is deficient ventrally. In addition, the hypospadiac penis differs from the norm in the absence of the distal urethra and corpus spongiosum.

Undescended testicles, kidney abnormalities, hernias, and other congenital anomalies are found more frequently in patients with hypospadias than in the general population. This makes systemic evaluation of the patient essential in every case.

A cystoscopic examination is performed before each operation for hypospadias. Special care is taken to diagnose valves or a large utriculus that may later cause difficulty with catheterization. In severe cases of hypospadias, the external appearance may leave the sex in doubt. Buccal smears, sex chromatin studies, and occasionally laparoscopy or laparotomy may be necessary for a definite diagnosis.

The midline raphe of the penis may deviate to one side or the other, in association with torsion or twisting of the penile skin. Rarely, blind urethral channels may be found distal to the existing meatus; such congenital urethral duplications or fistulas are associated with hypospadias. Occasionally a portion of the base of the scrotum may be found anterolateral to the base of the penis (engulfment) and needs to be corrected for esthetic purposes. In proximal cases, the scrotum is cleft.

Preoperative Considerations

If the sex is misdiagnosed preoperatively or if associated anomalies are undetected, the patient may suffer irreparable harm from indiscriminate surgery. Obstructive uropathy should be corrected, and plans formulated for the correction of the other anomalies at appropriate times. Pre-urethroplasty circumcision should never be performed in patients with hypospadias, even though the degree of hypospadias may be slight. Occasionally, more chordee becomes evident as the penis grows, and patients who are initially thought not to require surgery, may later need correction. This hazard should have been resolved by the age of 4 years.

The urethral meatus in hypospadias patients is usually patulous and allows a good urinary stream. Occasionally, however, the meatus is small, causing the patient to strain during micturition. A meatotomy is not usually necessary because the meatus will dilate; if it is stenotic, a ventral meatotomy may be necessary. Insertion of a triangular flap of glans epithelium into a dorsal meatal slit has been found to be the most efficient way to correct meatal stenosis; occasionally an incision just at the distal part of the meatus can be made in a longitudinal fashion and closed in a transverse direction, thereby enlarging the meatus.

Operative Care

One-stage repairs are preferable to multiple-stage procedures because they reduce hospitalization, minimize physical and mental trauma, and allow completion of repair before the age of memory recall. Successful one-stage operations require more attention to detail and more delicate surgical technique than multiple-stage procedures. In this area of the body where the function of the organ is so dependent on the psyche of the patient (which in turn is influenced by the appearance of the penis), perfection in surgical planning and technique is mandatory. One-stage repairs are offered as a better, not an easier, way to repair hypospadias. However, it is important to be conversant with the older types of multiple-stage repairs.

TWO-STAGE REPAIRS

In the past, only multiple-stage repairs of hypospadias were made, because surgeons believed that chordee was caused by growing tissue that could recur after resection. To repair a urethra in a penis that may have a recurrent curvature would be imprudent. It has been proved, however, that the tissue causing chordee is static and fibrous, and does not recur if it is adequately excised.

It was also thought imprudent to bring the meatus to the tip of the glans. The occurrence of meatal stenosis and stricture was so common that any operations attempting to extend the meatus to the tip of the penis were found to have unacceptable rates of complication. It was surmised that meatal stenosis was due to the circumferential contracture of the scar at the urethral opening. Tissue is cored out of the glans in the proper tissue plane. By the development of a flap to interpose in the circular distal meatal opening, the problem of meatal stenosis has been overcome.

Every hypospadias surgeon should be familiar with four popular multiple-stage techniques for the repair of this deformity. More than 250 different techniques have been described in the literature; the four described below have been the most popular.

All these repairs share the correction of chordee as a first stage (Fig. 85–2). After the penis has been straightened, the dorsal prepuce and penile skin is used to cover the ventral skin deficit. The technique of release of chordee is described later in the chapter. The second stage of the hypospadias repair is that of urethroplasty, and it is in this area that authors differ in their approach to the problem.

The second stage of the two-stage repair is usually carried out after allowing at least six months for healing. The urethra can be constructed in this second stage by using either a free graft or local flaps. A full-thickness graft has normal growth potential and does not contract. If a split-thickness graft is used, it must be splinted for at least 12 months to overcome the tendency toward contracture. Either graft can be inserted through a subcutaneous tunnel to the top of the glans, where it can be anastomosed to a V-shaped glanular flap. The anastomosis between the graft and the urethra can be completed at this second stage of surgery, or can be deferred for a third stage.

Duplay Technique. The Duplay (1880) technique consists of an incision around the urethral meatus extending distally to the coronal sulcus so that the ventral surface of the penis is exposed. All tissue causing chor-

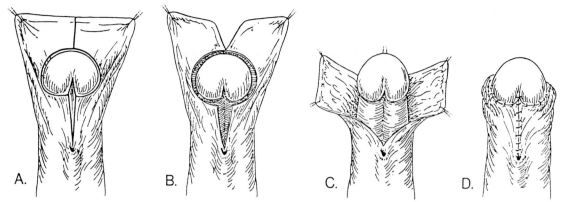

Figure 85–2. A to D, Correction of chordee: dorsal prepuce and penile skin used to cover the ventral surface of the penis.

dee is then resected or released. Skin flaps are next brought ventrally from the abundant prepuce either by splitting the prepuce (Byars, 1964) or by perforating the prepuce in the midline. Six months after the transfer of preputial skin to the ventral surface, the second stage of surgery is performed. The urethroplasty is completed in the Duplay (Byars) technique by making parallel incisions on each side of the urethra to the glans, and tubing the midline strip of skin to form a urethra (Fig. 85–3). The lateral adjacent penile shaft skin is advanced ventrally and closed in the midline to cover the newly tubed and reconstructed urethra. The deficiency of this method is that it can never extend the urethral meatus to the tip of the glans.

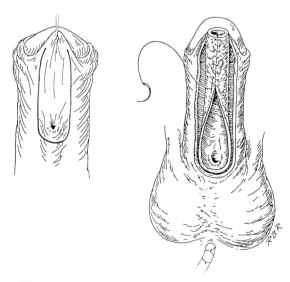

Figure 85–3. Thiersch-Duplay (Byars) technique of tubing midline skin to form a urethra to the glans.

Denis Browne Technique. The first stage of the Denis Browne (1946) technique is similar to the Duplay. The chordee is released and preputial tissue is transferred to the ventral surface. At the second stage, approximately six months after the first, similar parallel incisions are made on the ventral surface of the penis (Fig. 85–4). This midline strip on the penis is not tubed; instead the lateral skin flaps are drawn over the strip of midline skin, burying the strip of skin. Epithelization begins from each edge of the strip, eventually epithelizing a tube of skin that forms the urethra. In principle this technique is simple, but multiple fistulas and strictures frequently result.

Cecil-Culp Technique. As in the two above described techniques, the first stage of the Cecil-Culp operation is the release of chordee (Cecil, 1932; Culp, 1959). At the second stage, performed approximately six months after the first, a midline strip is tubed into a urethra (Fig. 85–5). Instead of using penile skin to cover the ventral urethra, the phallus is buried in the scrotum. An incision is made in the scrotum. The penis is folded downward, and the lateral edges of the penile wound are sutured to the lateral edges of the scrotal wound, thereby burying the ventral surface of the penis in the scrotum. At a third stage, three months later, the penis is released from its attachment to the scrotum, completing the operation.

In patients whose lateral penile skin is insufficient for ventral coverage, the technique may be valuable even today.

Nové-Josserand and McIndoe Technique. Free grafting was first described by Nové-Josserand (1897) and later modified by

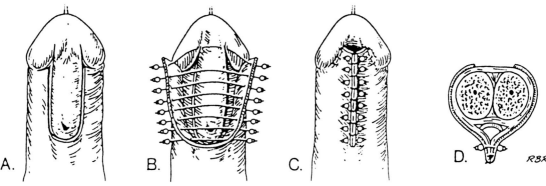

Figure 85–4. Denis Browne techique of burying midline skin. *A,* Parallel incisions. *B,* Mobilization of shaft skin. *C,* Midline closure. *D,* Native skin forms the dorsal aspect of the urethra, and the ventral urethra forms by epithelization.

McIndoe (1937). In this operation, the first stage of release of chordee is identical to that previously described. Six months after the release of chordee, a urethra is made by undermining beneath the ventral skin of the

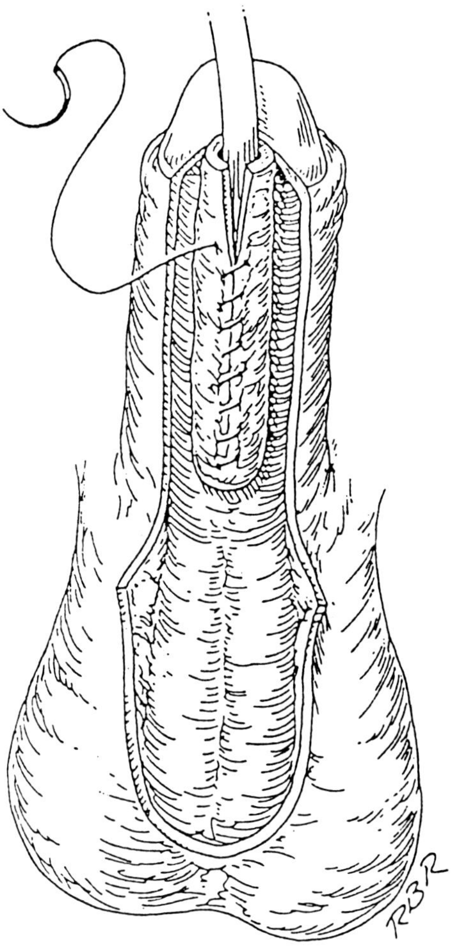

Figure 85–5. Three-stage Cecil-Culp technique: (1) correction of chordee, (2) urethroplasty as in the Thiersch-Duplay technique with closure of the ventral shaft to the scrotum, and (3) penile release from the scrotum.

penis from the existing urethral meatus to the subglanular area. A strip of split-thickness skin is used to form a urethral tube. A stent is kept in place in the new skin graft urethra for six to 12 months to reduce graft contracture. The new urethra and the old urethra may be connected at the second stage of surgery, but this is usually deferred until the neourethra has matured, so that a third stage is required. In spite of prolonged splinting, urethral stenosis and stricture are common in this technique.

The authors are firmly committed to the principle that hypospadias is best repaired in one stage of surgery, and prefer to operate on these children by their second birthday. However, if a multiple-stage repair is planned, the ventral defect is best repaired by unfolding the prepuce, splitting it in the middle and transferring the two flaps of prepuce ventrally. The Ombrédanne type of hood, in which a buttonhole is made in the unfolded prepuce and transferred to the ventral surface of the penis, is mentioned only to be condemned. This buttonhole flap produces unsightly dog-ears laterally, and has not been used as a procedure of choice for many years.

ONE-STAGE REPAIRS

In 1955 the authors began a series of one-stage hypospadias repairs, using full-thickness skin grafts from the prepuce. Many other surgical techniques followed to complete hypospadias repair in one stage. The evolution of a one-stage philosophy for hypospadias seems assured, since Broadbent, Woolf, and Toksu (1961), DesPrez, Persky, and Kiehn (1961), Toksu (1970), Hodgson (1970), Hinderer (1968), Mustardé (1965), Duckett (1981a), Standoli (1982), Hendren (1981), and others have reported successful one-stage procedures for this congenital anomaly. The combined advantages of completely correcting the chordee and reconstructing the urethra in a single operation, together with the associated low morbidity rate, are responsible for the growing acceptance of various one-stage repairs for hypospadias. A satisfactory appearance, with a normal urinary stream and normal sexual function, is obtainable in every case.

Recently, we have been advocating the use of loupes, the operating microscope, or both for hypospadias operations. These procedures call for more attention to delicate technique, but ensure a watertight urethral reconstruction and make certain that all epithelial edges are inverted into the urethral lumen.

In the authors' experience, no one operation is suitable for every case of hypospadias. The surgeon is obliged to have a variety of techniques available for use as dictated by the anatomic circumstances of the deformity.

The first requisite of any good hypospadias repair is to straighten the penis by resecting or releasing all the tissues causing the chordee. The fibrous tissue of the chordee does not continue to grow.

To release chordee, the authors recommend an incision around the meatus extending distally in the midline on the ventral shaft of the penis to and around the coronal sulcus. The lateral skin flaps are elevated at the level of Buck's fascia, and all abnormal tissue in the ventral area of the penis is excised down to the normal tunica albuginea. Bleeding from the venae profundae penis, which lie immediately adjacent to Buck's fascia, may mislead the surgeon into believing that he has inadvertently entered the corpora. These veins are in fact some distance from the tunica albuginea, and the dissection should be continued to a deeper plane until the normal tunica albuginea has been completely uncovered. Dissection must be carried around the existing meatus at the end of the corpus spongiosum. If this structure is entered, excessive bleeding will be encountered. The authors extend the dissection under the glans where the abnormal fibrous tissue inserts into the glanular tissue. If the tunica albuginea of the corpora cavernosa is inadvertently entered in this dissection, it is repaired with 6–0 chromic gut suture.

Acute dorsiflexion of the penis over an assistant's finger aids the dissection and helps to control bleeding. Palpation of the tunica albuginea may reveal small strands of fibrous tissue that may be hard to visualize. Bleeding can best be controlled with electrocautery, using fine-tipped forceps to grasp each individual bleeding point. Once all the abnormal fibrous tissue is removed, the penile shaft should remain straight and have no visible ventral curve.

In the occasional patient, even though it appears that all the tissue causing chordee has been released, the penis may continue to remain slightly curved on erection. The use of an intraoperative artificial erection test with normal saline is essential (Fig. 85–6). Sterile injectable saline is injected into the corpora while venous outflow is occluded. Rather than perform a urethroplasty on a curved penis, the authors prefer to incise the ventral tunica albuginea to release the curvature. A dermal graft applied to this deficit

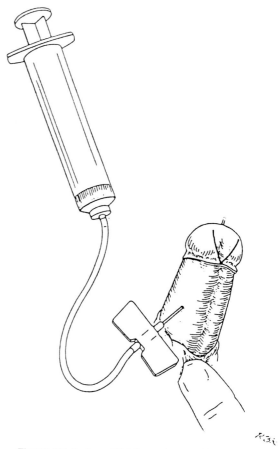

Figure 85–6. An artificial erection test is performed by injecting normal (injectable) saline into the corpora cavernosa while venous outflow is digitally occluded. A 25 gauge butterfly needle is used.

elongates the expansile tunica albuginea on the ventral surface. This technique then obviates the use of a free full-thickness graft for the urethroplasty: a graft cannot be placed on a dermal graft, and vascularization from either structure could not be expected to aid the other. This would mandate a vascularized urethral flap reconstruction. Rarely, if a vascularized island flap is not used for urethroplasty, a small wedge of tunica albuginea from the dorsal surface can be resected to straighten the penis. Care must be taken not to injure the dorsal vessels and nerves to the glans.

Meatal Advancement and Glansplasty (MAGPI). For patients who have the meatus in the glans and who do not have chordee, this is an ideal technique (Duckett, 1981b). Skin hooks are placed on the lateral edges of the glanular urethral groove (Fig. 85–7). Retraction laterally is used to expose a band of mucosa on the dorsal wall of the urethral groove. This band of mucosa is incised longitudinally in the midline. It is then closed transversely with interrupted 6–0 chromic catgut sutures. A circumcising incision is made around the glans adjacent to the coronal margin. The ventral portion of the glans is

freed from the corporeal caps. At the most inferior portion of the existing meatus, a hook is placed for traction to pull the meatus distally. This forward pull on the meatus forces the lateral glanular wings to swing together. As the wings are closed above the extended urethra, the meatus is advanced further to the tip of the penis. The epithelium is closed with 6–0 chromic catgut sutures. The excess prepuce can be removed as in a routine circumcision, or if necessary the preputial skin can be transferred to the ventral portion of the penis for resurfacing. The penile skin is approximated with 6–0 chromic catgut. Urethral diversion usually is not necessary. The wound is dressed with loosely applied Bioclusive dressings, and cold compresses are recommended for the first 24 hours. This operation is usually done on an outpatient basis.

Flip-Flap Hypospadias Repair for Patients Without Chordee. This procedure is suitable for distal shaft hypospadias without chordee when there is an adequate-sized distal meatus (Fig. 85–8). A ventral flip-flap based on the urethral meatus is elevated to reconstruct the ventral surface of the new urethra. From the meatus, parallel incisions

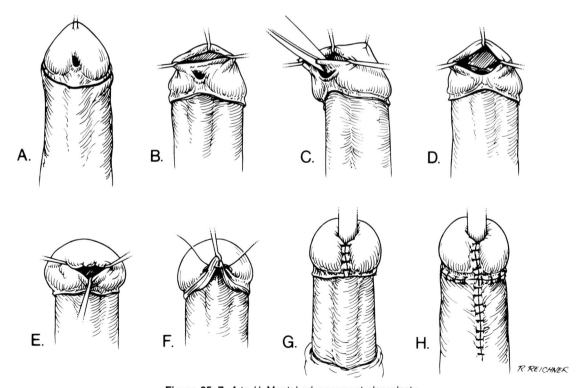

Figure 85–7. *A* to *H,* Meatal advancement glansplasty.

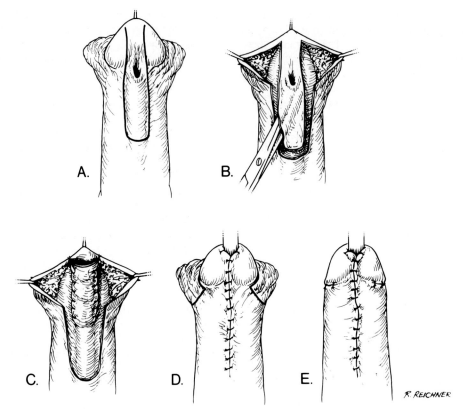

Figure 85–8. *A* to *E,* Flip-flap hypospadias repair without chordee.

are then made distally on the ventral surface of the glans to its tip. This strip of glanular epithelial tissue is used for dorsal urethral reconstruction. The absence of chordee makes subcutaneous access unnecessary. Therefore, parallel incisions suffice.

The lateral glanular wings are dissected and elevated. The flip-flap is then advanced distally and the urethral reconstruction completed by suturing the flip-flap to the dorsal urethral skin. The authors prefer to use subcuticular 6–0 or 7–0 PDS sutures, inverting the epithelium into the urethral lumen and producing a watertight anastomosis. As the final sutures are placed in the distal meatus, a sound is placed in the urethra. This ensures a meatal opening that is adequate in size and leaves the urethra divergent at the meatus. When the new urethra has been constructed, the anastomosis is tested with methylene blue–dyed saline to make sure it is watertight. The lateral glans flaps are then approximated with one or two sutures of 5–0 PDS subcutaneously and 6–0 chromic interrupted sutures through the glans epithelium. The flip-flap is sutured to the glans epithe-

lium with 6–0 interrupted chromic catgut. The resulting ventral skin defect is covered by advancing dorsal preputial skin to the ventral surface of the penis. This is best done by splitting the prepuce in the midline and choosing the flap that has the best vascularity to rotate into the defect. Subcutaneous sutures of 6–0 PDS and skin sutures of 6–0 chromic complete the procedure. Redundant skin is excised. In order to avoid ventral pressure upon the closure of the two lateral glanular wings, it is recommended that a catheter should not be used.

Flip-Flap Associated With Distal Shaft Chordee. This procedure is utilized for patients with distal shaft hypospadias who also exhibit ventral chordee (Fig. 85–9). A meatally based flip-flap is marked on the ventral skin of the penis in a similar fashion. A midline triangular glans flap is made approximately one-third the size of the existing glans. It is necessary to raise this flap in order to gain access to the underlying dysgenetic tissue. It is this glans flap that distinguishes the technique.

The lateral glanular wings are elevated.

The midline glans flap is raised, and all excess tissue beneath the midline glans flap is removed to thin the flap so that it will not encroach on the distal urethra. All tissue causing curvature of the penis is released and resected. A circumcising incision is then made around the coronal sulcus approximately 1 cm proximal to the corona. The incision is continued distal to the urinary meatus and exposes the tissue that is causing the chordee. The lateral skin flaps are elevated from the penis, and the prepuce is unfolded. By means of an artificial erection test, the total correction of chordee can be determined. If the resection of abnormal tissue is adequate, the penis should be straight and the urethroplasty can be started. To begin the procedure, the midline glans flap is secured to the tunica albuginea with 6–0 PDS sutures and is advanced into a meatotomy performed on the dorsal surface of the existing meatus. The midline glans flap is sutured into the meatus with 5–0 or 6–0 chromic interrupted sutures. The flip-flap is then turned forward and sutured to the midline glans flap, inverting the epithelium edges

into the urethral lumen and completing the urethra. Again, a sound is placed in the distal meatal opening to prevent stenosis during the suturing. To provide ventral resurfacing of the penis, preputial skin is unfolded and divided in the midline. In most cases, closure is performed as described for patients who do not have chordee.

One-Stage Repair of Proximal Shaft, Scrotal, and Perineal Hypospadias: Full-Thickness Skin Graft. In these types of hypospadias, the required length of the flip-flap cannot be constructed so that it is viable. It is therefore necessary to construct a urethral tube that will bridge the area (between the meatus and the glans) (Fig. 85–10). A circumcising incision is made around the coronal sulcus, down the ventral midline, and around the urethral meatus. The skin is elevated from the shaft of the penis, the prepuce is unfolded, and all elements of tissue causing chordee are released and/or excised. The midline glans flap and lateral glanular wings are formed in the fashion previously described. A full-thickness skin graft for the urethroplasty is taken from unfolded preputial skin, and all

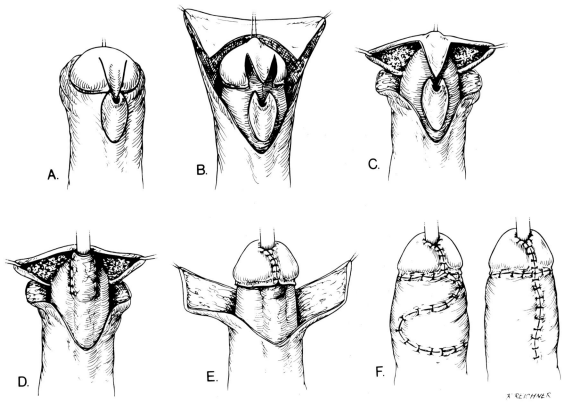

Figure 85–9. *A* to *F,* Flip-flap hypospadias repair with chordee.

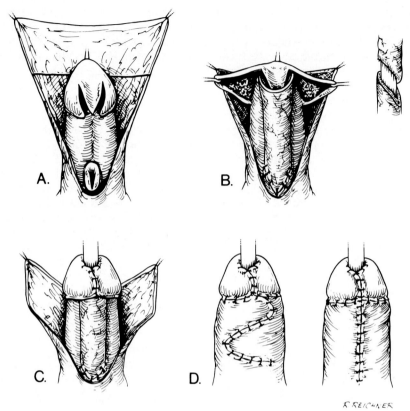

Figure 85–10. A to D, Proximal shaft hypospadias repair with a full-thickness skin graft.

excess subcutaneous tissue is removed. The tissue is formed into a tube with a long "tongue" on each end. It must be adequate in length. In most pediatric patients operated at 1½ to 2 years of age, the skin is tubed over a No. 12 French stent using a running 7–0 PDS suture. The stent is then placed in the proximal urethral opening, and the tongue of the skin tube is sutured to the existing urethra with interrupted 7–0 PDS sutures in the subepithelial tissue. The distal end of the graft is sutured to the midline glans flap with the same suture material. A ventral meatotomy in the existing meatus is made to provide for a large tongue-in-groove anastomosis between the tubed full-thickness skin graft and the existing urethra.

The lateral glanular wings are brought inferiorly to cover the distal portion of the urethra; 5–0 PDS sutures are used subcutaneously in the glans and 5–0 or 6–0 interrupted chromic sutures in the glans epithelium. Blue-stained saline from a bulb syringe is instilled into the neourethra to ensure a watertight closure. The skin graft is anchored to the tunica with multiple sutures along

each side of the tube. The prepuce can then be divided in the manner already described.

Urinary diversion in these patients is usually effected by a suprapubic catheter. In cases of scrotal and perineal hypospadias, this operation can be modified when there is a strip of hairless skin in a cleft scrotum. A tube of this hairless skin is formed, extending the site of the original meatus 2 to 3 cm more distally. Once it is extended to the base of the penis, the preputial graft is long enough to reach the tip of the penis. The scrotal cleft is corrected with the addition of a Z-plasty in the midline.

Vascularized Preputial Island Flap. A preputial vascularized island flap may be useful in certain cases. The incisions to release the tissue causing the chordee are similar in this operation to those previously described. After the penis is straightened, a meatotomy is made in the existing meatus. A midline glans flap and lateral glanular wings or a tunnel through the glans may be constructed. Instead of using a full-thickness graft to complete the urethroplasty, a vascularized preputial pedicle flap is constructed based on subcutaneous tissue (Fig. 85–11). Asopa (1971), Standoli (1979), Hinderer (1971), Broadbent, Woolf, and Toksu (1961) and DesPrez, Persky, and Kiehn (1961) described variations of this operation, which was later popularized by Duckett (1980). To make this flap, the prepuce is unfolded and the length and breadth of the prepuce are evaluated to determine whether adequate tissue is present to construct the desired length and caliber of urethra. In most cases of penile shaft hypospadias, there is adequate tissue. Incisions are placed in the preputial skin after careful caliber measurement. The rectangular flap is marked transversely on the prepuce. Dissection, proximally, must be done with care to preserve vessels that vascularize the preputial island. Once mobilization is satisfactory, the adequacy of the blood supply to the flap can be tested with fluorescein: if fluorescence is not noted, the flap should be excised and used as a full-thickness graft. If fluorescence is seen, the new urethra can be formed around an appropriately sized sound or stent, using fine, subcuticular 6–0 PDS sutures. The vascularized graft is tubed and managed as the nonvascularized graft described above.

Postoperative Care

The penis is wrapped with a clear Biocclusive dressing. The transparency of the dressing allows inspection of the vascularity of the skin flaps. The immobilization and support it provides is comforting to the patient. The foot of the bed is elevated when possible to reduce edema. The patient is not allowed out of bed for three days, because ambulation would cause dependency of the operated area and result in edema. The dressing is left in place for about five days. If bladder spasms occur, belladonna and opium rectal suppositories may be indicated. Warm baths may also be of some assistance. All patients must be carefully evaluated for possible urinary infection.

Erections may be a problem in teenagers or adults, causing postoperative bleeding and dehiscence of suture lines. Amyl nitrite pearls are kept at the bedside of all adult patients, so that they can crush and inhale the fumes; this immediately reduces the erection. Erotic materials are avoided. Nocturnal erections without conscious control by the patient present a serious problem.

In the postoperative period, the intravenous fluids are discontinued as soon as the patient is able to tolerate oral fluids. Edema of the tissues is minimized with the use of a rolled towel beneath the scrotum. Broad-spectrum antibiotics are continued orally for several days. An appropriate dosage of diazepam by mouth on a p.r.n. basis helps to reduce the incidence of erections and to sedate older patients. Appropriate dosages of oral acetaminophen with codeine and intramuscular meperidine hydrochloride (Demerol) are prescribed in the immediate postoperative period for pain control. Appropriate orders are written for care of the drains, usually small vac-

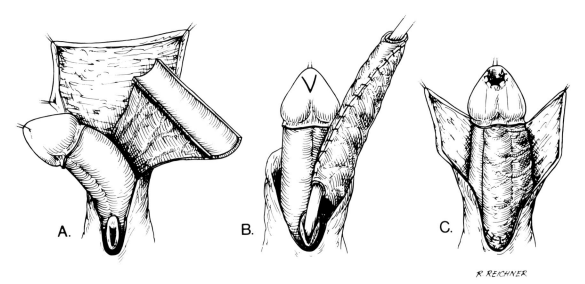

R. REICHNER

Figure 85–11. *A* to *C,* Preputial flap hypospadias repair.

uum-tube systems. Finally, the orders specifically request that the physician be notified if there is persistent bleeding. Three days postoperatively, it is recommended that the patient be soaked three times a day in a clean tub to help decrease edema and to clean the area. Bandages are not removed manually but allowed to soak off in the tubbing process. The meatus should be gently cleaned and (when not stented) dilated frequently with an antibiotic ointment from an ophthalmic tipped tube. The tip of the tube is gently placed in the meatus to remove all crusts, so that plugging does not occur. In the absence of urinary symptoms, postoperative calibration or instrumentation is not necessary. If symptoms indicative of stricture or infection are noted, the urethra should be calibrated and dilated as necessary. Urethroscopic evaluation may be necessary.

CATHETERS

In the past perineal diversion was used in most hypospadias repairs, but the authors now have changed this philosophy and rarely do so for such repairs. For the distal MAGPI repair, no urinary diversion is required; these patients may urinate through the repair without harm. For cases of distal hypospadias, when lateral glanular flaps are closed in the midline, it is better to avoid pressure from exerting a catheter force ventrally, which may cause a dehiscence of the wound. The authors therefore use a soft silicone tube through the length of the repair, through which the patient may void. A suprapubic catheter diversion is preferable for most cases in which glanular flaps are present.

For midshaft and proximal hypsopadias, a small stent is used extending 1 cm distally to the new urethral meatus and 1 to 2 cm proximally to the anastomosis with the native urethra. Suprapubic diversion has proved to be desirable in most of these cases. At postoperative day seven, the suprapubic diversion is closed and a voiding trial is allowed. If the latter reveals evidence of leakage of the repair, the suprapubic diversion is opened and the patient is not allowed to void through the repair for three or four more days. This cannot be done with a perineal diversion.

Complications

In the authors' series of one-stage hypospadias repairs, 90 per cent or more of all cases have healed primarily and required no further surgery. No complications have ensued from a one-stage hypospadias repair that would not be expected in a comparable series of multiple-stage repairs. No irreversible complications have occurred in the authors' series; in our last reported series of 56 cases, a 6 per cent complication rate was encountered.

Regardless of the type of surgery utilized, urethrocutaneous fistulas and strictures occur after all hypospadias repairs. The basic principles of atraumatic tissue handling must be observed to prevent crushing of the skin edges and delayed healing. All flaps and grafts used in the formation of the urethra should be adequate in width. The original urethral meatus must be patulous before the new urethra is constructed. Any anastomosis should be created with a long ellipse; a circular anastomosis would contract.

Perioperatively, complications are concerned either with infection or skin necrosis due to avascularity of flaps. If infection or wound dehiscence occurs, local and symptomatic treatment should be provided. No attempt should be made to resuture the damaged tissue in the immediate healing phase. The wound should be allowed to heal and secondary surgical procedures performed several months later. If hematoma occurs in the immediate postoperative phase, the flaps should be opened and the hematoma evacuated.

Complete breakdown of the hypospadias repair has not occurred in the authors' series. The most frequent complication of one-stage repairs consists of small fistulas, usually measuring 1 to 2 mm in size; occasionally these heal spontaneously without surgical intervention. It is recommended that no attempt at fistula repair be made until six months after the initial surgery, to allow tissue softening and healing. Local treatment with silver nitrate or trichloroacetic acid sometimes stimulates healing. If surgical repair of the fistula is required, the urethra should be calibrated to make certain that there is no obstruction distal to the fistula. If a distal obstruction is present, it must be corrected before the fistula is repaired.

Fistula repair is accomplished by careful dissection of the track to the uroepithelium. The latter is then closed with multiple sutures that are placed outside the lumen. If the channel of the urethra is diminished by direct closure of the fistulous opening, a small portion of flip-flap skin based on the side of the fistula can be placed to provide epithelial lining for the urethra. When the uroepithelial surface has been reestablished, the surrounding skin should be undermined widely and closed in multiple layers over the urethra. If excess tissue is present on the ventral surface of the penis, it is preferable to sacrifice normal skin from around the fistula repair and to rotate a wide flap over the repair, taking care not to superimpose the suture lines of the flap over the uroepithelial closure.

Rarely, diminution in the size of the urethra occurs postoperatively. These patients should be observed for graft growth maturation, because occasionally, as softening occurs, the narrowed urethra may dilate as a result of the physiologic stretch of voiding. If an intractable stricture occurs, a direct incision should be made over the area and the strictured segment opened. Reconstruction of an adequate urethral channel can be accomplished by a patch graft of full-thickness skin with the epithelial surface placed inside the lumen, or by using a lateral flap of penile skin based on subcutaneous tissue. After wide undermining, the skin can be closed in layers over this repair.

Meatal stenosis has been a common complication in procedures that attempt to bring the urethra to the tip of the penis. The stenosis can be caused by (1) contraction of the circular anastomosis of the urethral tube to the glans or (2) failure to remove a core of the glanular tissue during the creation of the new tunnel to the tip of the glans. Meatal stenosis is treated with a V-shaped dorsal glans flap. It is important that this flap is sutured to the tunica of the corpora cavernosa to prevent its being pulled out of the meatus. The flap can be advanced (on the dorsal side of the meatus) as far proximally as necessary to correct the stenosis. As the wider portion of the triangle is advanced into the stenotic areas, the caliber of the meatus increases. Another rare complication is the development of a diverticulum. When distal obstruction occurs, the proximal urethra may dilate with the formation of a small epithelial pouch. If this occurs, the distal obstruction should be corrected before the diverticulum is excised. The entire sac of diverticulum can be excised and the uroepithelium closed. The overlying tissues should be closed in layers and an indwelling urinary catheter maintained in position for approximately five days for urinary diversion; a suprapubic catheter may be preferable.

PRIMARY EPISPADIAS AND EXSTROPHY

Epispadias and exstrophy of the bladder are congenital deformities in which there is failure of normal development of the dorsal surface of the penis, abdomen, and anterior bladder wall. Although these defects are not completely understood embryologically, they represent varying degrees of a single disorder. Exstrophy of the bladder with complete epispadias (or bifid clitoris) is the form most commonly seen, but cases have been reported in which the penis is normal. In epispadiac deformities distal to the bladder neck, urinary continence is not a problem. A cosmetically satisfactory and functional reconstruction is possible. A thorough preoperative work-up is necessary for incontinent patients.

Exstrophy with complete epispadias occurs in approximately one in 30,000 births, and is three to four times more common in males. Epispadias alone occurs much less frequently than exstrophy of the bladder, the ratio being approximately 1:4. The frequency is the same for males and females.

Description of Deformity

The extent of associated deformity is highly variable, ranging from minimal in distal cases to severe in cases of complete proximal epispadias and exstrophy. In both males and females with severe proximal epispadias and exstrophy, the hair-bearing skin of the escutcheon is lateral and inferior. The umbilicus is commonly absent and the rectus abdominis muscles are divergent inferiorly. The fascia may be absent in the midline between the separate halves of the pubic rami. The pubic symphysis is absent in the midline and the lateral pubic bone is rotated, causing lateral displacement of the hips and anterior positioning of the anus. The bladder is opened and exposed on the anterior abdomen. If lesser bladder neck deformity is present, it may range from incompetency to bladder neck competency and only a split phallus or clitoris.

In females the clitoris is divided into two separate portions by a strip of mucosa leading anteriorly to a flattened mons veneris. The labia minora are displaced by the separation of the pubic ramis, and the urethra is very short and wide.

In males the corpora cavernosa are separated, and normal dorsal neurovascular bundles are divided and displaced laterally. Separate neurovascular bundles are located on the lateral side of each corporeal body. The corpus spongiosum may be present only as a triangular mass of vascular tissue between the proximal ends of the corpora cavernosa. The penis appears short and tethered to the anterior abdominal wall, and the penoscrotal angle is broad and obtuse.

Reconstruction

Distal epispadias should be treated with the exact reversed technique used for hypospadias repair in the same anatomic position. The epispadias reconstruction is on the dorsal surface of the penis, while the hypospadias reconstruction is on the ventral surface. In epispadias a large prepuce is present on the ventral surface of the glans, and can be used in the reconstruction. Prepuce remaining after urethral reconstruction is divided in the midline and brought to the dorsal surface of the penis, where it is used to cover the dorsal defect. The length of urethral tissue is usually deficient and, if left unaddressed, will continue to cause dorsal curvature. When the urethral meatus is on the distal third of the penile shaft, a flip-flap type of repair is used.

In more proximal cases of epispadias, when the midline glans flap cannot reach the epispadiac meatus, a free full-thickness graft of preputial skin is used. Occasionally, the prepuce in patients with epispadias is deficient and inadequate for tube graft reconstruction. The ventral surface of the penis and prepuce may be used as a vascularized preputial flap to be transferred to the dorsal side of the penis. The urethral plate is usually short and causes chordee; it must be divided to correct the curvature. Construction of the urethra is carried out just as in the hypospadias repairs described above, but on the dorsal surface.

Epispadias that extends to the bladder neck may be associated with urinary incontinence. This can be repaired functionally by releasing the bladder from the scarring of the midline and creating wedges of anterior bladder neck to elongate the urethra. After closure of the mucosa, the surrounding tissue-containing sphincter muscle fibers are imbricated about it. After the sphincter has been reconstructed, the distal urethra is created with a full-thickness graft. If the ureters are implanted in a low position so that the lower bladder muscle cannot be easily dissected without injuring the ureters, the ureters must be replanted into a higher position. If bladder capacity is inadequate, a colonic augmentation may be necessary. The scrotum can be advanced on the ventral surface of the penis to provide more skin to the area. The rectus abdominis muscle is taken as a muscle flap on the inferior epigastric vessels and is used to fill the pelvic space over the bladder neck and proximal urethra.

Occasional cases of epispadias involve separate corporeal bodies, and two artificial erection devices are necessary; in distal cases, one may suffice. Postoperative care is the same as for patients with hypospadias.

Exstrophy of the Bladder

In exstrophy of the bladder, there is separation of the symphysis pubis and a defect in the abdominal wall. The anterior bladder wall is absent and the bladder is everted. The ureters enter the bladder at right angles and are therefore incapable of preventing reflux. This may be accompanied by incompetence of the upper urinary tract. If this condition is not corrected it results in pain, infection, ureteral dilatation, and renal destruction. An occasional patient whose exstrophy has not been corrected has lived to adult life, but this is unusual. Carcinoma of the bladder frequently develops in older untreated patients.

The magnitude of multiple defects presented by congenital epispadias with bladder exstrophy has been a problem area for reconstructive surgeons. Classically, closure of the abdominal defect and genital reconstruction have been neglected while attention has been focused on urinary diversion. In recent years, surgical advances have offered more functional and esthetic reconstructive alternatives. Development of a urinary conduit can no longer be accepted as the end point.

An estimated 100 to 150 newborn infants with exstrophy are born each year in the U.S. Exstrophy rarely occurs in more than one member of a family. Even though the exstrophy is almost always complete, minor variations of an abdominal wall defect with a superior or inferior vesical fissure may be seen. Simple layered closure of these defects is usually considered adequate treatment.

It may be acceptable to use any available closure in difficult cases of exstrophy, but it is unacceptable to allow the abnormal escutcheon or the bent penis to remain as the permanent result.

The best treatment for exstrophy of the bladder remains a controversial subject. There are two schools of thought. One advocates excision of the bladder and urinary diversion. An ileal or colon conduit may be used. The bladder is excised and the abdominal wall defect is closed with local flaps of muscle, fascia, and skin. Other surgeons advocate functional closure of the bladder in an attempt to provide continence without obstruction or vesicoureteral reflux. Repair of the associated deformities of the external genitalia can be made simultaneously or later. No method of treatment for this congenital anomaly is entirely satisfactory.

Ureterocolic urinary diversion may provide continence, but a moderate percentage of patients with exstrophy of the bladder also have rectal incontinence. Incontinence cannot be assessed in infants. Long-term results of this procedure have shown that it is not always satisfactory even in patients with rectal continence. Many die early from infections and their complications. Carcinoma has been reported at the implantation site. Ileal or colon loop diversion is an alternative, because it provides better protection to the kidneys, but it requires an external collection device. Sigmoid diversion was thought to be better tolerated in young patients. Recently, an isolated continent ileal or sigmoid loop diversion has been recommended.

The disadvantages of older flap closures are numerous. A typical midline closure divides the escutcheon with a wide, hairless scar, frequently tethering the penis to the abdominal wall. Multiple-stage procedures not only lead to further morbidity, but often create unesthetic donor sites.

RECONSTRUCTION

In recent years, a "functional closure" for exstrophy of the bladder has become popular. This should be done immediately after birth. **Operative Technique.** The total correc-

tion of the exstrophy-epispadias deformity is made in stages. The authors prefer to carry this out in two stages, with bladder and abdominal wall closure within 48 hours of birth.

The everted bladder is freed from its attachment to the abdominal wall, and the edges are approximated with a two-layer closure. The abdominal wall is closed in layers. Flaps of rectus muscle and/or rectus fascia can be raised to provide anterior wall support. A catheter is left in as a suprapubic drain. A simple, reliable W-flap with hair-bearing tissue is used to reconstruct the normal escutcheon, elongate the inferior abdominal wall, and allow penile release. These paired inguinal groin flaps described by the authors correct the shortness of skin and the deficiency of the escutcheon.

Bilateral iliac osteotomies to bring the symphysis pubis together in the midline, simplifying the closure, are recommended by some authors. The authors do not consider this necessary. Some consider that osteotomy shortens the penis. Others recommend the use of nonabsorbable materials to hold the pubis together under tension.

Vesicoureteral reflux is frequent in these patients. An antireflux procedure such as ureteral replantation is often necessary, either at the time of primary closure or later. Because of the distorted nature of the bladder wall and the irregularity of the mucosa, it is usually better to delay this procedure. If it is done at the primary stage, reimplanting the ureter is preferable to an intravesical reinforcing procedure. The corpora are not released at this stage. At about the age of 2 years the genitalia have grown sufficiently for repair.

At the second stage, the penis is released and lengthened, the dorsal penile curvature corrected, and a urethra constructed. When necessary, lower abdominal wall reconstruction, correction of vesicoureteral reflux, and a bladder neck plication to achieve continence are performed.

POSTOPERATIVE CARE

When the repair is carried out primarily, it is necessary to continue the suprapubic drainage for six to eight weeks to avoid damage to the ureteral repair by increased intravesical pressure.

COMPLICATIONS

The degree of continence to be expected depends in part on the sex of the patient. Females have a better chance of being continent after functional closure. Males can expect improvement in continence at puberty as a result of prostatic growth. All patients may develop urinary tract infection and must be maintained on urinary antiseptics or antibiotics. If obstruction becomes a problem, severe, uncontrollable infection and dilatation or destruction of the upper urinary tract may follow. Diversion should be carried out in these patients in an effort to preserve renal function. This is the primary objective of treatment, and other esthetic considerations are secondary.

SECONDARY RECONSTRUCTION OF EPISPADIAS AND EXSTROPHY

The genital defect in patients with exstrophy and epispadias results in esthetic, functional, and psychologic problems, which may be worse in patients who have undergone urinary diversion and are required to wear a stomal appliance. In mature males, a penis that has been lengthened and straightened greatly improves the body image and should enable them to perform sexually. The closure of congenital epispadias and exstrophy of the bladder has been described previously. In patients who receive only urinary diversion and no penile reconstruction, secondary reconstruction is necessary, and provides a unique challenge to the plastic surgeon. Most patients will have had reconstructive surgery to the bladder with little attention paid to the esthetics or function of the external genitalia. Nearly all these patients seek to normalize the appearance of their perineum and abdominal wall; puberty heightens their realization that they are "different" (Fig. 85–12).

Description of Deformity in Older Patients

The deformity caused by the primary epispadias-exstrophy complex has been described in detail, and the reader is encouraged to refer to the above discussions in order to

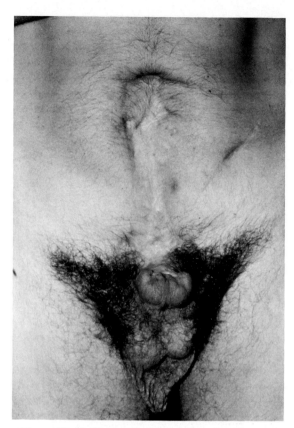

Figure 85–12. Preoperative view of an epispadiac penis that has undergone previous reconstruction without release and lengthening of the affected structures.

fully understand the following material. Deformity in patients with the epispadias-exstrophy complex is variable. Such diversity is dependent on the extent of the primary deformity and the extent of the previous surgical correction.

The primary goal is to attain a phallus that dangles when flaccid and is straight when erect (Fig. 85–13). Once this has been achieved, the patient is concerned with the correction of numerous additional deformities.

The hair-bearing skin of the escutcheon is lateral and inferior to the base of the penis. It may be separated either by the open bladder or by heavy scars from previous surgery. The subcutaneous fat may be excessive laterally and absent in the midline, creating a marked contour deformity. The bladder neck may be patulous with heavy scar tissue attachments to the overlying skin. Partial or total bladder incontinence may be concomitant.

EXSTROPHY/EPISPADIAS

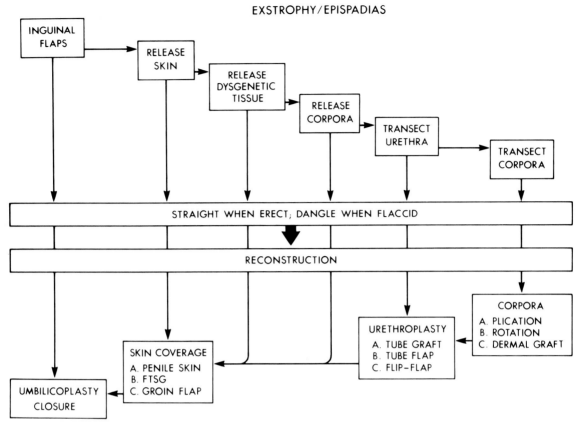

Figure 85–13. The systematic approach to operative care of the epispadias deformity. FTSG = full-thickness skin graft.

The penis may appear short and tethered to the anterior abdominal wall. The corpora are of normal size, but the penis appears broader because of widely separated attachments of the corpora. The penoscrotal angle is broad and obtuse. The dorsal penile skin appears tight and may be scarred from previous attempts at reconstructive surgery. There is usually no umbilicus.

The factors that prevent the penis from dangling may be one or more of the following: (1) skin, native and/or scarred; (2) congenital fibrous bands between the penis and the splayed symphysis; (3) divergent corpora with abnormal attachments to the pubic bone; (4) a short urethral plate; and (5) a short or inelastic dorsal tunica albuginea.

From this spectrum of multiple severe deformities, all degrees of epispadias and exstrophy may exist, extending from minor urethral or chordee problems to scars and deformities from numerous previous operations. Unfortunately, most of these patients are seen after they have been through puberty. It is not uncommon for them to have

undergone as many as ten operative procedures by this age.

Reconstruction

The time at which genital surgery is performed is ideally around the age of 2 years. The child is less traumatized psychologically at this time, especially with parental rooming-in during hospitalization and modern nursing supportive techniques.

Operative Care. A systematic approach to releasing, lengthening, and straightening the penis during urethral and lower abdominal wall reconstruction in patients with exstrophy and epispadias allows the surgical team to achieve a satisfactory esthetic result. This systematic approach consists of progressively increasing the extent of surgical dissection (Fig. 85–14) until the goal (a phallus that is straight when erect and dangling when flaccid) is achieved. The dissection begins with skin, progressing as necessary to underlying dysgenetic tissue, urethra, and corpora. At

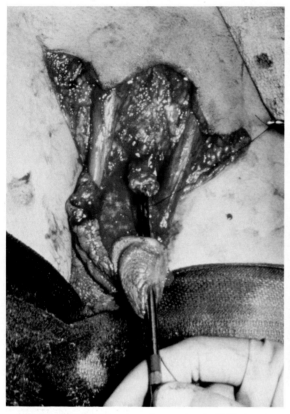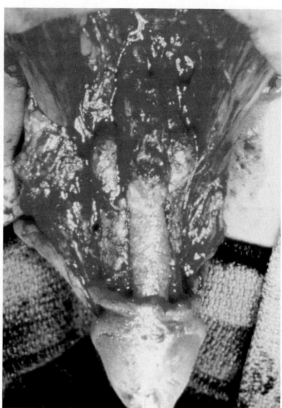

Figure 85–14. The epispadiac urethra is divided and reconstructed with an interpositional full-thickness skin graft.

any point in this continuum when the primary goal is achieved, the reconstructive phase begins without further dissection. For example, if the primary goal is reached after urethral transection, the surgeon proceeds to urethroplasty followed by skin reconstruction without progressing to corporaplasty. The abdominal wall and ejaculatory system may also require reconstruction.

Skin Coverage. Usually the surgical approach is through a circumcising incision for dissection of the phallus and a W incision over the pubis for access to underlying structures. After the systematic disection of the phallus, three basic options exist for phallic coverage: "reverse Byars flaps," a full-thickness skin graft, or a preputial flap. Local dorsal coverage may be achieved with rotation of ventral skin in a "reverse Byars' flap" fashion. When a full-thickness graft urethroplasty is not present on the dorsal surface, full-thickness skin grafts may be used for coverage of the phallus. When a graft urethroplasty is necessary for the urethra (a full-thickness skin graft being contraindicated), there are two alternatives: (1) the urethra

may be rerouted between the two corporeal bodies in order to lie on the ventral surface, after which the dorsum may be grafted; or (2) a preputial flap based on the subcutaneous tissues may be rotated to the dorsal surface for coverage. Considerations for additional skin coverage include umbilicoplasty and escutcheon correction.

Ideally, the penis is covered with redundant penile skin, which is hairless and of appropriate pigmentation, texture, and elasticity, and also provides sensation. Deficiencies in penile skin coverage can be corrected with a hairless full-thickness skin graft. Neurotization of the skin graft should eventually provide sufficient sensation. The appearance of the skin graft will not match the pigmentation of the genital skin and therefore is more noticeable. However, esthetic appearances may be improved by keeping skin grafts and suture lines to the ventral aspect of the penis.

Many younger patients are particularly self-conscious regarding their absent umbilicus. The umbilicoplasty is performed by placing an appropriately sized semicircular incision midway between the xiphisternum and the upper margin of the symphysis. A plug of subcutaneous fat is removed and the rostral skin edge sutured to the midline rectus fascia. Remaining defects in this wound are covered with a full-thickness skin graft.

The escutcheon can be reconstructed by rotation of W-shaped skin flaps to bring the lateral and inferior hair-bearing skin superiorly and medially. Simultaneous removal of midline scars and contouring of the suprapubic area can also be carried out. The incision that exposes optimally the genital area for correction of the anomaly and simultaneously allows normalizing of the escutcheon is the W incision. These paired groin flaps allow wide penopubic dissection for partial release of the corpora and lengthening of the penis. Approximation of these skin flaps during wound closure permits hair-bearing skin to be rotated superiorly and medially in order to normalize the escutcheon.

The apices of the paired inguinal skin flaps (W-shaped flaps) extend to points lateral and inferior to the base of the penis. Markings are begun at a point inferior and lateral to the anterior superior iliac spine, and extended inferiorly in the groin crease to a point well below the penile base, usually at a mid-scrotal level. The marking is then continued superiorly, including a small portion of the scrotum to the superior penile border where it is joined by mirrored markings from the opposite groin.

The vascular supply of these superiorly based flaps is from the perforating vessels of the inferior epigastric vessels. The flaps are elevated at the fascial level, just superficial to the external oblique aponeurosis.

After repair and release of deeper structures as indicated, the flaps are closed bilaterally in a V to Y fashion. The flaps may be further rotated to close in a Z configuration, but this leaves a significant suprapubic skin defect.

A great advantage of this approach is the exposure provided for reconstruction of deeper structures. The urethra, corporeal bodies, pubic ramus, midline diastasis, and bladder are all made accessible to complete systematic evaluation of the individual problem. The crura of the corporeal bodies can be freed easily from the pubic bone. Release of chordee, particularly important in epispadiac patients, is made convenient.

Flap design allows excision of unattractive midline scarring. The tissue brought into the suprapubic region is hair-bearing and produces an esthetic escutcheon. Elongation of the lower abdominal midline mobilizes skin that, in combination with procedures for the deeper structures mentioned above, significantly enhances penile length. The donor defect is a well-hidden inguinal scar.

After full release of chordee, corporeal bodies, and the urethra, there may rarely remain a skin deficit at the penile base. Since maximal penile lengthening is desirable, closure of this area must be tension free. A full-thickness skin graft may be used if the soft tissue defect is limited to skin only. Typically, however, if a deficit exists, underlying repairs to the urethra or tunica corporeal bodies may necessitate vascularized flaps. An island groin flap tunneled subcutaneously, a rectus abdominis flap, or a rectus femoris musculocutaneous flap have been used to close the defect.

Artificial erection tests are used to identify the site and degree of penile curvature. These are repeated several times while chordee is corrected until penile straightness is confirmed. The technique requires injection of sterile normal physiologic saline into each corpus (unlike the normal penis), because the corpora usually do not communicate.

All dysgenetic tissue on the dorsal surface of the corpora midline is resected, with care taken to preserve the lateral neurovascular bundles. Dysgenetic bands on the corpora are resected and the corpora mobilized. Often the penis is seen to dangle by this stage.

After release of the skin, attention is directed to the release of subcutaneous scar and dysgenetic tissue that may be tethering the phallus. In the penopubic dissection, it is important to release the corpora from the ischial tuberosities except for their most proximal portions. It is here that the pudendal artery enters, and total mobilization may devascularize the corpora. Dissection must be meticulous to preserve first the midline ejaculatory ducts on the prostate between the corpora, and second the pudendal nerves running laterally on the corporeal bodies. Damage to the ejaculatory ducts may result in impotence. Overmobilization of the corpora may also displace the penis further below the symphysis, while midline approximation of the corpora may restrict the corpora rather than providing length. The aim of corporeal release is to create a penis that dangles.

Urethral Reconstruction. Once chordee

has been corrected completely, urethral reconstruction may be contemplated. It is futile to consider such reconstruction before the penis has been released and lengthened and chordee has been corrected. The neourethra may be tethering the penis. In these cases, the urethra is transected proximally and reconstructed with an interpositional graft. For distal shaft epispadias, the urethra may be reconstructed in a fashion similar to the flip-flap procedures for hypospadias correction. Usually, however, the urethroplasty takes the form of a tubed full-thickness graft, ideally taken from redundant ventral preputial skin. Unfortunately, penile skin is often deficient in patients who have undergone previous attempts at genital repair. Alternatively, a tube graft is constructed from full-thickness skin taken from a hairless area adjacent to the anterior superior iliac spine. The graft is tubed about a silicone stent and the urethroplasty completed with elliptic anastomoses. The proximal anastomosis is done first, and the distal anastomosis completed after creating the glans wings and the ventral midline glans V-flap. The neourethra can be secured further along its length with interrupted 5–0 or 6–0 PDS (polydioxanone, Ethicon) sutures to the corpora. If adequate dorsal skin coverage is present, no attempt is made to bring the urethra ventrally, since this does not appear to improve esthetic results.

The tube graft urethroplasty requires special considerations in two situations: (1) when a dermal graft has been used to correct dorsal chordee and (2) when a full-thickness skin graft may be needed to cover the penis because of insufficient native penile skin. The problem is that one graft cannot be laid on another, or acquisition of vascularity between the grafts will be compromised. When a dermal graft has been used to correct chordee, the urethroplasty may be done as a staged procedure, or the new skin graft urethra can be routed inferiorly beneath the corporeal bodies from the dermal graft to emerge at the ventral tip of the penis. If there is insufficient penile skin to cover the penis and a dermal graft has been used to correct chordee, or a full-thickness skin graft to construct the urethra, penile skin coverage may be completed with a ventrally based penile flap, or the penis may be buried within scrotal flaps and revised at a later date.

Curvature that persists after transection and mobilization of the proximal and distal urethra is usually due to a congenital deficiency or to inelasticity of the dorsal corporeal tunica. This can be corrected in one of three ways: (1) the length of the corpora may be plicated in the ventral midline to induce an outward rotation and straightening; (2) an ellipse of ventral tunica may be removed and the tunica reapproximated; or (3) a dermal graft may be inserted into the dorsal surface of the tunica to correct the disproportion between the dorsal and ventral surface, and to allow straightening. Care must be taken to preserve the lateral neurovascular bundles.

Ideally, the penis should also serve as a conduit for urine and sperm. This function may be difficult to achieve in patients who have undergone urinary diversion and in whom the urethra is not being periodically dilated through the process of urination. Such patients may therefore be at increased risk of stricture formation in the neourethra.

Children who have undergone urinary diversion are also offered urethral reconstruction at a later date, since the chances of ensuring permanent urethral patency are fewer. The aim of urethral reconstruction in these patients is to connect the neourethra to the ejaculatory ducts on the prostate, to create a conduit for the ejaculate. These patients may require prolonged periodic urethral dilations after urethroplasty and may be at risk of developing infections such as epididymo-orchitis. Alternatively, a neourethra may not be constructed and the ejaculatory ducts may be left to open as a sinus in the penopubic area. A urethra can always be created at a later date when the patient wishes to ejaculate from the penis. In a penis that functions with the prostatic sinus, conception may be brought about by collecting the ejaculate for artificial insemination. Patients with exstrophy and epispadias are normally potent and fertile. Penile prostheses do not usually have a part in the reconstruction of the penile deformity.

Patients with the exstrophy-epispadias complex may have a variety of complaints relative to the urinary bladder. The urinary bladder may be small in size and dysgenetic, and the ureters may be low-lying or subject to reflux. These problems may be addressed through bladder augmentation or ureteral replantation at the time of reconstruction. Flaps of rectus muscle or rectus fascia can be raised to provide anterior wall support or coverage of bladder reconstruction.

When there are abdominal wall hernias, the repair may be dependent on whether or not urinary tract surgery is performed. When urethral mucosa has not been violated, prosthetic materials such as mesh may be used for its repair. When urethral mucosa *has* been violated, the risk involved in the use of prosthetic materials is too great and fascial flaps may be created to close the defect.

When there are wide bone gaps in the pubic symphysis, the patient may desire their correction; this is particularly true of females. The bone correction may be addressed in two different ways:

1. A large inner table iliac crest bone graft up to 12 cm in length may be harvested and secured to the freshened ends of the pubic bones.

2. Osteotomies may be performed on either side of the pubis in such a manner as to preserve the periosteum on one edge and allow the bone to be rotated in a turn-over fashion. The blood supply is based on the intact periosteum. The bone flaps are then secured together.

In either case, bone healing is required for stability of the pubis.

Iliac osteotomies do not enhance penile length. In fact, closure of the symphysis through iliac osteotomies may decrease penile length because of a downward tilting of the pubic rami.

In females, in addition to the deformities already discussed, there may be a bifid clitoris and separation of the labia minora. This is corrected by removing the abnormal central portion and by approximation in the midline. A Z-plasty may be added to avoid scar contracture over the pubis.

The interior rotation of the hips and anus provide minimal systemic and cosmetic deformity. Surgical correction of these deformities is not considered.

Postoperative care is the same as that for hypospadias.

PENILE CURVATURES

Penile curvature is not well recognized by most physicians. Chordee, or bending of the penis, was most commonly associated with infection following gonorrhea, but this is rarely seen today.

The normal flaccid penis is usually worn in the left pant leg. The erect penis is expected to be straight in the average male. If on erection noticeable curvature is present, the male may suspect that he is abnormal and unacceptable to female or male partners. Thus, the condition may become a problem both functionally and emotionally.

During an erection, the tunica albuginea stretches and elongates. If all surfaces have equal expansion, the penis extends lengthwise in a straight direction. Curvature occurs if a lack of expansion restrains a certain portion of the penis while the remainder elongates. Normally, the penis curves toward the inelastic tunica. If an inflatable balloon is taped on one side, the inelastic taped side will not expand. The untaped side has normal expansion and continues to enlarge, which causes a curvature toward the fixed inelastic surface. If the inelastic penile surface is circumferential, the phallus will be small but straight. If the unstretchable portion is on the dorsal surface, the curve will be upward; if on the ventral surface, downward; and if on the lateral surface, lateral.

The causes of penile curvature may be varied. Congenital curvatures occur at birth and are associated with hypospadias, epispadias, chordee without hypospadias, and congenital short urethra. Tunica albuginea disproportion can occur in conditions that restrict growth in one area of the penis. It does not change in severity, nor is it painful. This produces one corporeal body longer than the other and causes a lateral curvature with erection.

In hypospadias or epispadias with severe uncorrected chordee, the congenital fibrous tissue bands can cause tunica disproportion due to restriction of growth. The tunica, although expansile, simply has been restrained in growth and cannot elongate normally.

Any abnormal pathologic condition that causes inelasticity of the external shaft skin can cause a curvature. A burn scar or another kind of traumatic scar may cause tethering. An asymmetric circumcision causing absolute shortness in one area can result in a curvature.

Penile curvatures can be due to scarring from previous surgery. Trauma to the deeper tissues of the penis can also cause curvature by producing inelastic scarring in the tunica albuginea. A falling upon an erect penis can rupture the tunica albuginea, which will heal with an inelastic scar.

Peyronie's disease is characterized by a replacement of the normally elastic tunica albuginea with fibrous, hyalinized, and sometimes ossified tissue that has no elasticity.

These patients usually have no curvature until 40 to 60 years of age, when either an acute or a slowly developing curvature is first noted.

Differential Diagnosis of Penile Curvature

If the condition has persisted since birth, it is assumed to be congenital in origin. External deformities of the genitalia make the diagnosis obvious. More difficult to diagnose is the condition of congenital chordee without hypospadias. The penis and prepuce appear normal and the urethra emerges at the tip of the penis. Although this condition was once called "congenital short urethra," it is not usually due to a short urethra. The true cause is the occurrence of inelastic congenital fibrous tissue between the spongiosum and the corporeal bodies in the urethral groove, which result in a shortened penis on the ventral surface. When the inelastic layers of the dartos fascia and Buck's fascia are adequately removed, the penis can straighten and the urethra will stretch. The curvature is usually corrected, although sections of the tunica occasionally need to be removed from the dorsal surface. Very rarely is there a true congenital short urethra. When this does occur, in addition to resection of the congenital inelastic tissue, the urethra must be sectioned and reconstructed.

When there is a history of post-traumatic

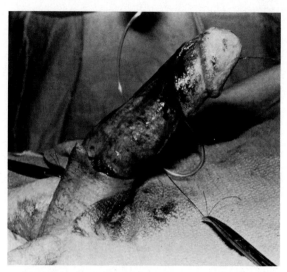

Figure 85–16. A second test performed intraoperatively demonstrates a successful repair.

curvature, it is obviously due to scar. If the condition occurs later in life and the penis was previously straight, Peyronie's disease must be suspected. The disease usually occurs on the dorsum of the penis, and the thickened tunica can be palpated as a mass when the penis is stretched.

A Polaroid photograph is obtained to show the penis during erection to aid proper diagnosis. An artificial erection test may be performed without anesthesia on an outpatient basis. The base of the penis is compressed and intravenous saline is injected into the corporeal body. With this technique, the true state of the penis can be assessed. Artificial erection tests are performed during surgery both before and after corrective treatment (Figs. 85–15, 85–16).

Surgery

The authors do not recommend that minor curvatures be treated. If sexual activity is hampered, surgical correction is indicated. If skin scarring is present, it can be excised and released. In overzealous circumcisions, when circumferential skin deficiency exists, skin can be added to the shaft with a graft. A circumferential graft at the base of the penis can produce edema of the distal penile skin, so it is better to graft the distal portion of the penis just proximal to the coronal sulcus. When a deficiency of skin is demonstrable only in one contracture band, Z-plasties in

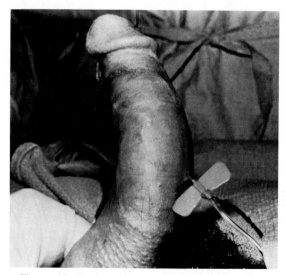

Figure 85–15. An artificial erection test using normal injectable saline demonstrates a dorsal surface curvature.

the band can correct the problem adequately. A traumatic scar of the tunica can be excised or strengthened with a dermal graft.

When chordee is associated with hypospadias or epispadias, proper treatment corrects the problem. Occasionally, small curvatures persist after the excision of all tissue external to the tunica albuginea. A ventral longitudinal incision between the corporeal bodies usually releases the last portion of the curvature. Scarring from surgery may cause iatrogenic inelasticity of the tunica and a curvature. The tunica scar should be replaced with a dermal graft.

When there is tunica disproportion, the shortened tunica may be incised and opened, and a dermal graft inserted to add length. It may be necessary to go to the elongated side of the penis and excise a portion of the normal expansile tunica to adjust the expansibility.

In chordee without hypospadias, an incision is made around the coronal sulcus, and the skin is retracted to the base of the shaft. After mobilization of the urethra, the congenital bands beneath the urethra are resected.

Rarely, it becomes necessary to insert a dermal graft to the tunica albuginea on the ventral surface. Excision of the normal tunica albuginea is frequently the best and simplest treatment. In certain patients the excised tunica has been used as a graft to the shortened surface of the tunica, thereby adjusting both surfaces for a more perfect result.

In congenital short urethra, the urethra must be divided, its tethering action released, and the urethra reconstructed. The authors prefer a one-stage operation, constructing the urethra with a full-thickness graft.

Adjunctive Diagnostic Techniques

As for all patients who have severe genital problems, the services of a sex therapist are recommended and have proved invaluable in predicting and ensuring patient cooperation. A healthy, realistic postoperative outlook can be more readily achieved. Many patients expect a perfect penis after surgery, but perfection cannot be obtained. Slight curvatures may persist. The goal of surgery is to restore normal function by correcting the curvature, and to keep the remaining slight curvature within acceptable limits. Therapy is an adjuvant to the restoration of the patient's abil-ity to function through adequate sexual performance.

HIDDEN PENIS

The unusual congenital anomaly of hidden penis is characterized by abnormal dartos fascia, which is abnormally thickened and attached to the penile shaft, and which allows prolapse of the skin distally over the phallus. This conceals the true length of the penis, because it restricts the elongation of the phallus and the exposure of the shaft is restrained by the abnormal fascia. Usually there is a prominent suprapubic fat pad in association with this anomaly. The penile skin and corporal bodies are normal, although because of the retrusion of the penile shaft, circumcision will usually have been attempted several times in order to expose the shaft of the penis by removing the abnormal-appearing penile skin. Unfortunately, the circumcision accentuates the problem of the hidden penis and does not solve it.

The suprapubic fat pad that rests over the pubic area obscures the length of the penis and affects the length of the functional penile shaft. This suprapubic fat contains fibrous tissue that is somewhat different from abdominal fat. The suprapubic fat rests on the deep fascia of the abdomen and extends into the scrotum and perineum. Laterally, in this fat are the spermatic cords, which must be protected when this condition is treated. Second, in the true concealed penis there are abnormal, thick, dysgenetic bands of dartos fascia attached to the penis. These bands, which are continuous with the dartos and scarpus fascia, tether the corporeal bodies proximally, while the penile skin, being untethered, drapes distally over the shaft.

No statistics are available to document the incidence of hidden penis. The authors have seen many such cases, which include numerous instances of repeated circumcision in ill-fated attempts to correct the condition. Many infant boys have baby fat surrounding the penile shaft. These should not be considered instances of true hidden penis, because most of these patients develop normally and the excessive baby fat regresses (Fig. 85–17). Surgery is not recommended for suprapubic obesity in infant boys. It *is* recommended if penile concealment fails to resolve after school age. Concurrent problems such as con-

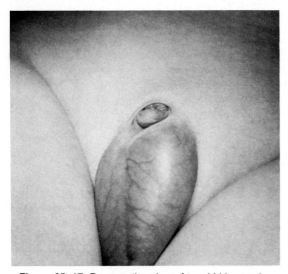

Figure 85–17. Preoperative view of true hidden penis.

genital anomalies of epispadias, hypospadias, chordee without hypospadias, and penile torsion may be present in patients with hidden penis. If these other conditions are present, earlier surgery may be necessary to correct the primary problem.

For the ordinary concealed penis, a suprapubic defatting is approached through a transverse incision above the base of the penis. The incision should be contained in the area where pubic hair is expected to grow, thereby disguising the scar after puberty. If the patient has not been excessively circumcised, the skin of the lower abdomen can be undermined and the subcutaneous fatty tissue removed to the level of the rectus fascia. The spermatic cords are identified and the scrotal fat is excised and removed (Fig. 85–18). During the excision, the fat pad and dense strands of dartos fascia are identified and removed. Traction on the dysgenetic tissue demonstrates that the penile body has been tethered by this abnormal tissue. Care is taken to preserve the penile dorsal neurovascular bundles. By pulling on the glans after section of the abnormal dartos bands, it can be readily demonstrated that the penis has been lengthened. If necessary, the penile suspensory ligament can be divided to assist the penile release, but this is not often required. The penile shaft skin can then be sutured to the base of the penis, while the suprapubic skin is sutured to the rectus fascia

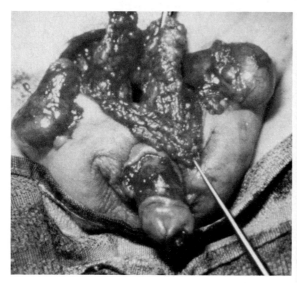

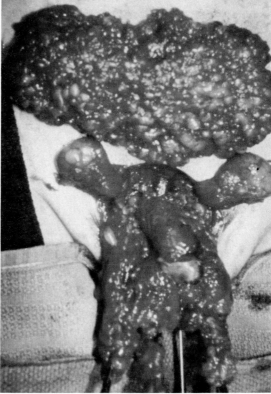

Figure 85–18. Intraoperative views identifying the spermatic cors.

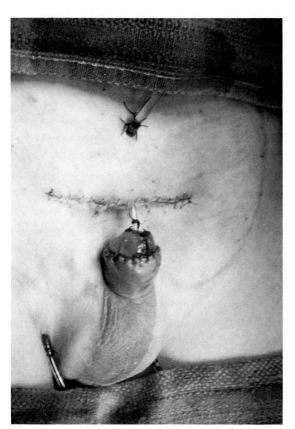

Figure 85–19. Postoperative view of repair of hidden penis.

with nonabsorbable material (Fig. 85–19). Liposuction may help to contour the adjacent abdominal fat, but is not effective in removing the more fibrous scrotal and pubic fat pad.

For patients who have been circumcised previously, a Z-plasty incision at the penopubic angle is recommended. If, when the penis is elongated by release of the dense bands, there is inadequate skin coverage of the shaft, a full-thickness skin graft can be used to complete the penile coverage. A circular incision around the base of the penis is avoided, to minimize the risk of penile edema.

The differential diagnosis between micropenis and hidden penis is determined by deep palpation to ascertain whether the corporeal bodies hidden within the pubic fat and beneath the skin are normal in size. If the stretched penile length is normal, the hidden penis can be expected to grow and an adequate penis will be present after puberty. The procedure of removing the suprapubic and pubic fat pad and cutting the suspensory ligament has also been used in adults in whom the distal portion of the penis has been

destroyed by either cancer or trauma. In patients who desire a more prominent penis, this procedure allows more protrusion of a short but functioning penis and obviates a major reconstruction.

Children with the hidden penis syndrome also require psychologic support. Counseling before and after the surgery is extremely valuable.

REFERENCES

Asopa, H. S.: One stage correction of penile hypospadias using a foreskin tube. Int. Surg., *55*:435, 1971.

Broadbent, T. R., Woolf, R., and Toksu, E.: Hypospadias: one-stage repair. Plast. Reconstr. Surg., *27*:154, 1961.

Browne, D.: An operation for hypospadias. Lancet, *1*:141, 1946.

Byars, L. T.: Hypospadias and epispadias. *In* Converse, J. M. (Ed.): Reconstructive Plastic Surgery. 1st Ed. Philadelphia, W. B. Saunders Company, 1964.

Cecil, A. B.: Surgery of hypospadias and epispadias in the male. J. Urol., *27*:507, 1932.

Culp, O. S.: Experiences with 200 hypospadias: evolution of a therapeutic plan. Surg. Clin. North Am., *39*:1007, 1959.

DesPrez, J. D., Persky, L., and Kiehn, E. L.: One-stage repair of hypospadias by island flap technique. Plast. Reconstr. Surg., *28*:405, 1961.

Duckett, J. W.: Transverse preputial island flap technique for repair of severe hypospadias. Urol. Clin. North Am., *7*:423, 1980.

Duckett, J. W.: The island flap technique for hypospadias repair. Urol. Clin. North Am., *8*:503, 1981a.

Duckett, J. W.: MAGPI (meatoplasty and glanuloplasty): a procedure for subcoronal hypospadias. Urol. Clin. North Am., *8*:513, 1981b.

Duplay, S.: Sur le traitement chirurgical de l'hypospadias et de l'épispadias. Arch. Gén. Méd., *5*:257, 1880.

Hendren, W. H.: The Belt-Fuqua technique for repair of hypospadias. Urol. Clin. North Am., *8*:431, 1981.

Hinderer, U.: Hypospadias. Rev. Esp. Chir. Plast., *1*:53, 1968.

Hinderer, U.: New one-stage repair of hypospadias (technique of penis tunnelization). *In* Hueston, J. T. (Ed.): Transactions of the 5th International Congress of Plastic and Reconstructive Surgery. Sydney, Butterworths, 1971, p. 283.

Hodgson, N. B.: A one-stage hypospadias repair. J. Urol., *104*:281, 1970.

McIndoe, A.: The treatment of hypospadias. Am. J. Surg., *38*:176, 1937.

Mustardé, J. C.: One-stage correction of distal hypospadias: and other people's fistulae. Br. J. Plast. Surg., *18*:413, 1965.

Nové-Josserand, G.: Traitement de l'hypospadias; nouvelle méthode. Lyon Méd., *85*:198, 1897.

Standoli, L.: Correzione dell'ipospadias in tempo unico: tecnica dell'ipospadias con tempo ad isola prepuziale. Rass. Italia Chir. Pediatr., *21*:82, 1979.

Standoli, L.: One-stage repair of hypospadias: preputial island flap technique. Ann. Plast. Surg., *9*:81, 1982.

Toksu, E.: Hypospadias: a one-stage repair. Plast. Reconstr. Surg., *45*:365, 1970.

86

Charles E. Horton
Gerald H. Jordan
Michael R. Spindel

Reconstruction of Male Genital Defects: Acquired

LYMPHEDEMA

Lymphedema of the penis and scrotum is a condition that, although uncommon in countries not experiencing endemic filariasis, remains important because of the associated profound physical and psychologic sequelae. Minor degrees of this disorder can generally be treated conservatively, but chronic, unremitting lymphedema requires definitive surgical therapy. Since the first report of the diagnosis and treatment of penoscrotal lymphedema by the ancient Indian surgeon Sushruta, the long search for an effective surgical method of management has continued.

Etiology

A satisfactory classification of the etiology of penoscrotal edema was formulated by Bulkley (1962) as follows:
A. Primary or idiopathic
    1. Congenital (Milroy's disease)
    2. Lymphedema praecox (developing at puberty)
B. Secondary or obstructive
    1. Inflammatory
        a. Filarial (tropical, leading to elephantiasis)
        b. Lymphogranuloma, chancroid, tuberculosis, syphilis, erysipelas, leprosy
    2. Surgical
        a. Lymph node dissection of the inguinal region
        b. Scars in the groin
    3. Carcinoma with blockage of the lymphatics
    4. Postirradiation destruction of the lymphatics
    5. Medical
        a. Cardiac or renal failure
        b. Venous thrombosis
        c. Hypoproteinemia
To Bulkley's classification may be added, under surgical causes, obstruction of the lymphatics secondary to paraffin injections (used to ablate hydroceles and to simulate hernia to avoid selective service) and subcutaneous silicone injections into the penile shaft to enhance size.

The vast majority of worldwide cases of genitourinary lymphedema are postinflammatory in nature as a result of filarial infection. Although in the continental United States other causes of lymphedema are the rule, a reservoir of residual filarial disease remains in veterans of the Armed Forces (the Pacific Theater), and immigration from endemic areas adds to this pool.

Primary lymphedema of the penis and scrotum is a disease of childhood and early adulthood. Lymphedema praecox develops at puberty and represents approximately 80 per cent of all cases of the idiopathic form of this disease.

Anatomic Considerations

The anatomic bases of the pathology of, and surgical approach to, lymphedema of the male genitalia are related to the pattern of lymphatic drainage, which is divided into two systems. The superficial network (Fig. 86–1) derives from lymphatics of the prepuce and penile shaft coverings down to Buck's fascia. These lymphatics coalesce into a dorsal lymphatic trunk and ultimately drain into the superficial inguinal lymph nodes. A separate and deeper network accommodates the urethral and glanular lymphatics. This network of lymphatics flows deep to and within Buck's fascia, and ultimately drains into the caudal group of superficial inguinal nodes. In patients with genital lymphedema, only the tissues drained via the superficial system are affected, and excising them does not disturb lymphatic drainage of the glans and deep shaft structures. This configuration also makes it imperative that only a small cuff of subcoronal skin be left after dissection, otherwise lymphedema will recur in the residual penile shaft skin.

Lymphatics of the scrotal skin and subcutaneous tissues drain laterally into the inguinal nodes from the median raphé (Fig. 86–1). The primary lymph node chains of the testes and cord are para-aortic, and these structures are unaffected in the lymphedematous process. Although the matter is controversial, many investigators describe a collateral lymphatic drainage system of the nonrugose posterior scrotal skin via perirectal lymphatics. This area is consistently less involved than the remaining scrotum and may be used to reconstruct a neoscrotum after dissection of lymphedematous skin is complete.

Pathology

Obstruction of lymph flow is the common denominator in the group of patients manifesting lymphedema of the penis and scrotum. The histopathology of chronic lymphedema reveals marked dermal fibrosis and ectasia of the lymphatics and small blood vessels. An increased number of endothelium-lined vascular spaces devoid of red blood cells may be present. Lymphatic hypoplasia, aplasia, or hyperplasia can be observed in congenital forms of lymphedema along with varicose ectasia of the lymphatic channels.

The gross picture is one of significant hypertrophy of the skin, which may range from 2 to 4 cm in thickness. The affected areas may become covered with flat wartlike or nodular excrescences (varicose variant). The skin may be chronically infected owing to the presence of static, protein-rich fluid that acts as an excellent culture medium. Although in extreme cases the penis may be completely buried, there generally is no obstruction of urinary flow.

Therapy

Medical and infectious causes of penoscrotal lymphedema are managed by first treating the underlying disease process. Surgical

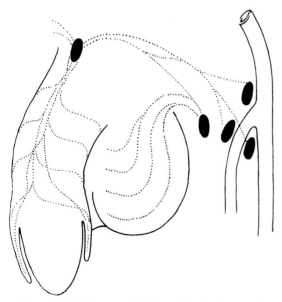

Figure 86–1. The superficial lymphatic drainage system of the penis and scrotum. The glans penis is drained by a separate deep system.

therapeutic options fall within two major categories: (1) procedures that recreate normal lymph flow away from affected areas (lymphangioplasty) and (2) procedures in which lymphedematous tissue is excised, followed by either primary closure or skin grafting (lymphangiectomy).

LYMPHANGIOPLASTY

Attempts have been made to create normal local lymph flow by diverting lymph away from affected areas, using foreign material such as silk, nylon, and polyethylene implanted into the dermis to form fibrous drainage channels. Natural shunts have been created with omentum and skin flaps, but all produced only marginal improvement. Success through the creation of lymphaticovenous shunts using microsurgical technique has been reported by Gong-Kang, Ru-Qi, and Zong-Zhas (1985). Using a scrotal-inguinal approach, vessels 0.5 mm in diameter have been anastomosed, creating a shunt of sufficient longevity to effect a clinically significant reduction in the amount of lymphedema. These findings have been qualified by the authors, who state that the best results occur in patients operated on before fibrosis occurs.

LYMPHANGIECTOMY

Opinion regarding excisional approaches to penoscrotal lymphedema is divided into two basic groups, one using the skin overlying affected areas as coverage, and the other believing that both skin and subcutaneous tissues are involved in the process and therefore need to be removed. The work of Feins (1970) is representative of the first group. He developed a procedure whereby all subcutaneous tissue is carefully debrided, leaving full-thickness penile and scrotal skin flaps in place. One contraindication for this procedure is the presence of chronically damaged skin. A variation of the above theme is the use of the inner layer of preputial skin by Khanna (1970). He states that this layer of skin is generally not involved, and that it can be used for penile shaft coverage while posterior scrotal skin flaps are configured into a neoscrotum.

The authors believe that the skin overlying lymphedematous areas becomes intimately involved in the process of chronic inflammation and fibrosis, and therefore favor the approach of complete excision with skin grafting and the use of flaps where indicated. Patients are treated with a parenteral cephalosporin if active superinfection is present, and an aminoglycoside plus a cephalosporin are initiated eight hours before surgery, to be continued through the fifth postoperative day. The surgical procedure is performed with the patient in the "frog-leg" position unless there is massive scrotal involvement, in which case the lithotomy position is used.

Dissection begins with a circumcising incision, leaving minimal subcoronal shaft skin. The skin of the shaft and scrotum is then incised ventrally in an inverted T configuration (Fig. 86–2), which allows for complete stripping of all affected skin and subcutaneous tissue down to Buck's fascia on the penile shaft. A Foley catheter is placed for identification of the urethra and is used postoperatively until day five while the patient is immobilized. The dorsal neurovascular bundle is protected by keeping the surgical plane above Buck's fascia. The inverted T incision allows for careful dissection around the testes and cord structures, as well as removal of all affected tissue.

After dissection and debridement are completed, a decision is made regarding the method of scrotal reconstruction. If sufficient normal posterior scrotal skin remains, it can be configured into a neoscrotum. The literature on trauma supports the findings that even a small scrotal remnant will eventually stretch to form an adequate pouch. The testes

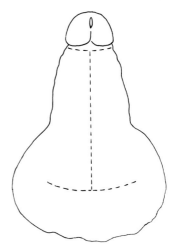

Figure 86–2. The initial circumcising incision is followed by an inverted T incision giving access to all necessary tissue planes and underlying structures.

are attached together in the midline, and a vacuum drain is placed beneath the flaps to avoid accumulation of fluid.

Penile shaft coverage is achieved by the use of an appropriately sized split-thickness skin graft (15 thousandths of an inch) harvested from a hairless area. If the scrotal skin remnant is inadequate for formation of a pouch, the testes are also covered with split-thickness grafts at this time. Although spiraling the graft around the penile shaft leads to satisfactory functional results, the authors prefer to interdigitate the graft edges, placing the suture line along the ventral aspect of the penis to yield a more normal cosmetic result. A bolster dressing is applied over Vaseline gauze to be removed on postoperative day five. Graft "take" is usually close to 100 per cent, and grafted areas are kept covered with the gauze until postoperative day 14.

General Considerations

As in all reconstructive surgery, there are many ways to accomplish the task. The surgeon must be ready to adjust the procedure to the individual circumstance. The authors believe that excision of involved skin and subcutaneous tissue provides the most satisfactory surgical resolution to penoscrotal lymphedema. The penis has characteristics that make split-thickness skin grafting a satisfactory method of coverage, and graft contraction is not a problem.

The lymphatic drainage of the penis (see Fig. 86–1) is such that unless only a thin rim of subcoronal shaft tissue is left, there is potential for the formation of a recurrent ring of lymphedema. This anatomic configuration also makes the use of the inner layer of foreskin for shaft coverage somewhat risky (unless this skin is unaffected and therefore draining into the deep lymphatic system).

Although there has been some question concerning the impact of the use of thigh pouches on fertility, the major issue appears to be the restoration of the normal configuration of the scrotum (the "hanging bag"). Therefore, it is considered that either posterior scrotal flaps or skin grafting should be used in the initial reconstruction. Malloy, Wein, and Gross (1983) and Raghavaiah (1977) described the recurrence of lymphedema in pouches formed from posterior scrotal flaps, but other authors, including our group, have had success with this technique. The solution to this dilemma most likely lies in proper patient selection. If the tissue in question appears to be involved in the disease process, it cannot be used without risk.

Finally, the use of microsurgical lymphaticovenous shunting techniques merits discussion. Obviously, better results may occur as the learning curve exerts its effect; the technique described by Gong-Kang, Ru-Qi, and Zong-Zhas (1985) has a place in the algorithm of treatment of penoscrotal lymphedema, most likely in the early stages of the disease or in a congenital defect with minimal to moderate skin change. Once significant fibrosis of the skin and subcutaneous tissues has occurred, the condition is probably permanent, and excisional therapy (lymphangiectomy) should be undertaken.

PEYRONIE'S DISEASE

Etiology

Although the cause of Peyronie's disease is unknown, it was first reported in 1743 by de la Peyronie, who described a patient who "had rosary beads of scar tissue to cause an upward curvature of the penis during erection." It is primarily seen in 40 to 60 year old patients, although it has been reported in younger and older individuals. Approximately 10 per cent of patients with Peyronie's disease also have Dupuytren's contracture of the palmar fascia.

There is no known medication that is effective for Peyronie's disease. Vitamin E therapy may help patients in the early stages of the condition. The authors use this medication routinely in all cases, but make no claim that this is a specific medication to cure the disease. The etiology of Peyronie's disease is probably related to trauma in which the fibrous strands of the septum are detached from the corporeal tunica, and a deposition of scar tissue occurs in the traumatized area. In younger patients, the more elastic tissues of the penis allow better healing and more stretching of the elastic tissue; in the older 40 to 60 year group, when the penis is bent or traumatized, the unyielding fibrous tissue snaps, bleeding occurs, elastin and collagen are deposited in the area, and a thick plaque of scar tissue results. Peyronie's disease is characterized by a loss of elasticity in the tunica albuginea of the corporeal bodies. A thickening of the dorsal tunica usually occurs in which the normal elastic fibers become hyalinized and thickened with deposits of fibrin, elastin, calcium, and occasionally even bone. The involved tunica is thickened in an irregular fashion and, when cut, feels gritty with occasional small spicules of bone or calcium present. Most frequently, the plaque is on the dorsal midline of the penis. The septum sometimes is involved, and rarely the Peyronie's plaque is located ventrally or laterally. Many patients state that the disease occurred with trauma, or associated a particular injury during sexual activity with the onset of the disease. Others can recall no beginning of the process, and in half the patients the disease, when first discovered, is as bad as it will ever be. Occasionally, Peyronie's disease may resolve and disappear completely. When pain occurs early, the pain may diminish until only a curvature remains, or may persist with erection.

It is normal for 40 to 60 year old patients to have diminishing sexual desire and ability. When something is wrong with the penis, they fear to engage in sexual activity and begin to wonder if they will ever be normal. Impotence may occur with Peyronie's disease, but the disease itself does not cause impotence.

Evaluation

Impotence may be attributed to the onset of Peyronie's disease by many patients who seek medical advice regarding this condition. Many other systemic diseases are related to impotence, such as hypertension (and its medication) and diabetes. We do not believe that Peyronie's disease can cause impotence, since there is no way for the plaque to block the flow of blood into the penis and physically cause erectile failure. However, the psychologic changes that a patient may experience when a severe curvature occurs may cause psychologic impotence, or venous outflow disease may occur in this age group, causing an inability to obtain an erection. Most patients undergo a nocturnal penile tumescence study before surgery for Peyronie's disease. All patients and their partners should see the sex therapist, who can explain in the same detail as the surgeon that the disease is not malignant, that it can be helped with surgery, and that psychologic support during and after the

surgery can help to avoid psychologic impotence postoperatively. Surgical treatment is not recommended if intercourse can be performed without too much difficulty. If, on the other hand, the patient or his partner experience pain, and if the positioning for sexual intercourse becomes impossible, correction of the inelastic tunica albuginea is necessary. For patients with a mild or moderate curvature who are still able to have intercourse, Vitamin E therapy and observation are recommended. Reassurance that the disease is not malignant may be adequate to allow these patients to continue with the physical ability remaining, and not to seek surgery. However, if intercourse is impractical or if there is pain with the disease, the authors believe that surgical treatment is desirable.

Treatment Options

Radiation therapy has been recommended for Peyronie's disease. The authors do not believe this to be satisfactory, since it causes endarteritis and fibrosis in an already fibrotic condition. Other surgeons recommend the placement of a penile prosthesis down the corporeal bodies of each side of the penis in order to physically straighten the penis with this firm rod support. The authors have not been impressed with this treatment; it destroys the patient's ability to have normal erections in the future, since it scleroses and fibroses the vascular and muscular tissue of the corporeal bodies. It does not treat the Peyronie's disease and simply straightens an already deformed and shortened penis to some degree. Penile prostheses carry complications: they can erode, may be uncomfortable, and are never normal in feeling or appearance to the partner. The overall acceptance of a penile prosthesis is not universal either by the patient or the partner, and the satisfaction produced by the penile prosthesis is not as great as that of patients who have had surgery to remove the fibrotic plaque and replace it to allow normal erections to occur. The authors therefore consider that if a penile prosthesis is contemplated, it should be used after surgery for removal of the plaque has been completed and after a trial period to determine whether the patient can have a normal erection. Potassium *p*-aminobenzoate (Potaba) has been recommended to treat Peyronie's disease, but the authors have never seen a patient helped with this medication.

Surgical Procedure

Once the patient has been evaluated by the sex therapist and determined to be a good candidate for treatment, he is admitted to the hospital and a circumcising incision is performed, 1 to 2 cm proximal to the coronal sulcus. The incision is made through Buck's fascia and the dorsal neurovascular bundle is removed free from the tunica, exposing the fibrotic area of the plaque of Peyronie's disease (Fig. 86–3). The majority of this plaque is excised, although if it is an extremely large plaque encompassing the whole dorsal surface on the sides of the penis, some of the inelastic tissue is occasionally allowed to remain. Incisions are made along each side of the deformity that is created by the excision, and relaxing incisions made so that no restriction of the straightness of the penis will occur with the inelastic tunica albuginea (Fig. 86–4). After removal of the plaque and incision of the tunica laterally, the resultant defect is always four to six times larger than the plaque removed (Fig. 86–5). The defect is measured, placing the penis on a stretch, and the size of the dermal graft to be used in the reconstruction determined.

A dermal graft is taken from the groin and defatted. It is sutured to the defect while the penis is on stretch, first along one lateral side of the defect; it is attached to the septum between the corporeal bodies and then to the opposite side of the septum. Two separate corporeal bodies are thereby constructed as a result of the reconstruction of the septal attachment. This gives stability to the graft site and to the penis. An artifical erection test is performed in which the penis should be straight. If the penis is still curved dorsally, additional dermal graft should be used, since it is not possible for a penis demonstrated to be curved at surgery after dermal grafting to become straight in the healing phase; it must be straight at surgery.

General Considerations

Erections are discouraged for the first two to four postoperative weeks, and sexual activity is discouraged for at least six weeks to allow the dermal graft to become securely attached to the tunica defect. After six weeks, the patient is told that normal erections will hurt but will not be harmful in the healing phase of the disease. The partner is asked to massage the area with lubricating oil, to understand that the penis will be fibrotic and sore for two to three months after the surgery, and that it will be six months before the penis has a normal appearance. The patient will continue to improve for six months after the surgery, and should have normal erections and normal sensation. A few patients have noted some anesthesia of the glans or the penis, which usually diminishes in the postoperative phase. Statistically, a total of 110 patients with at least one year of follow-up experience have been evaluated. Over a period of 20 years the authors have seen more than 1000 patients with Peyronie's disease.

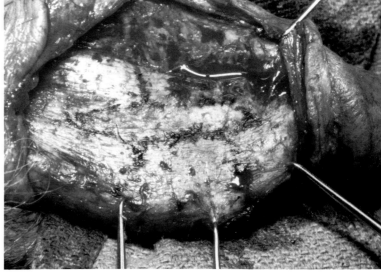

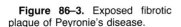
Figure 86–3. Exposed fibrotic plaque of Peyronie's disease.

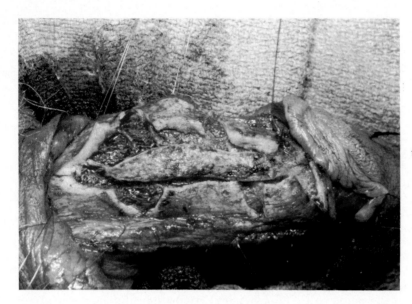

Figure 86–4. Relaxing incisions to prevent restriction upon erection.

Surgical treatment by excision of the plaque of inelastic tissue, and replacement of this pathologically involved tissue with a dermal graft, has corrected curvature and pain in approximately 85 per cent of the patients surveyed. Patients who had received radiation therapy or steroid injections did less well. Painful erections were completely eradicated postoperatively. The authors believe that Peyronie's disease can be successfully treated with a surgical excision and the proper use of dermal grafting to reconstruct the defect of the tunica. Steroid injections, radiation therapy, vitamin E, and Potaba are treatments of secondary choice and should be used only in patients who are not candidates for surgical correction. If the patient is not having normal erections before the correction of Peyronie's disease, a simultaneous dermal graft and implantation of a Silastic penile rod as a stiffener may be performed. For those who are having normal erections, it is preferable to carry out the surgery of excision of the diseased tunica and correction with a dermal graft; six months afterward, if the patient is not having normal erections, a prosthesis can be used. Less than 5 per cent of the authors' patients with Peyronie's disease have had to resort to this therapy.

Careful postoperative evaluation is neces-

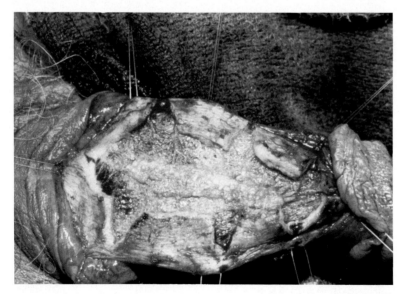

Figure 86–5. The resultant defect after removal of the Peyronie's plaque.

sary to make certain that patients with minimal disease and minimal complaints are not operated on for a condition that usually will stabilize and not progress. If a patient becomes incapacitated sexually, excision and dermal grafting of the defect is a procedure that may be expected to give good results. In certain selective cases, a prosthesis is necessary. Intraoperative artificial erections are required to allow the surgeon to correct the disease and to anticipate normal straightening of the penis during erection. Pre- and postoperative sexual therapy has proved of inestimable value in managing these patients and preventing their becoming psychologic cripples.

URETHRAL STRICTURES

Etiology

The urethra is customarily divided into anterior and posterior parts. Posterior urethral strictures are usually the result of trauma and are frequently associated with pelvic trauma. Anterior urethral strictures can be caused by trauma, inflammation, or both. Most anterior urethral strictures presenting to the reconstructive surgeon today have undergone attempts at "conservative" management, i.e., internal urethrotomy or dilation. Thus, many of these strictures are long in length, with extension of the primary stricture process resulting from intervention by dilatation and internal urethrotomy or from peristrictural inflammation.

Urethral injury associated with fracture of the pelvis usually involves the urethra immediately distal to the prostate gland or urogenital diaphragm. As a distinct anatomic entity, the urogenital diaphragm really does not exist. We have come to think of the urogenital diaphragm as those tissues surrounding the membranous portion of the urethra. Because of that concept, the posterior urethral stricture associated with fracture of the pelvis has been compared with "plucking an apple off the stem." In fact, the disruption of the urethra can occur at the prostatomembranous junction, directly through the membranous urethra, or at the membranobulbous junction. The last-named seems to be the most common situation encountered.

Although urethral disruption occurs in only a small percentage of males with injuries sufficient to cause a fracture to the pelvis, distortion or distraction of these points of fixation may result in a shearing force that traumatizes the urethra. When the pelvic fracture causes displacement of the pubis, the prostate gland, mobilized by its ligamentous attachments, rises into the pelvis with the bone fragments, thus disrupting the urethra below it. In most cases, the symphysis is displaced momentarily and quickly returns to a reasonably normal anatomic position. Urethral disruption can be partial or total, the difference being of academic interest only. Contrast studies merely show that the integrity of the urethra has been disrupted, and the extent of disruption is not usually ascertainable.

Treatment Options

It is emphasized that the immediate management for posterior urethral strictures is designed to limit the further sequelae of the injury. The formation of stricture, per se, is determined at the time of impact. Some controversy exists in the literature, but all agree that the immediate placement of a suprapubic cystostomy tube works best in the hands of most surgeons.

Virtually all posterior strictures can be handled by excision of the stricture, with primary anastomosis of the bulbous urethra to the anterior surface of the apical prostatic urethra. Anterior strictures can seldom be managed with excision and primary anastomosis. There is no question, however, that any stricture that can be managed with excision and a primary tension-free anastomosis of normal urethra to normal urethra represents the best form of urethral reconstruction for stricture.

For most anterior urethral strictures, reconstructive surgeons are forced to transfer tissue into the urethral deficit. Not all strictures are alike, and the technique of transfer best suited to a situation is largely dictated by the anatomy of the stricture. The components necessary to define the anatomy of a stricture are easily remembered with the mnemonic LLDD: length, location, density, and depth. The length and location of a stricture are easily defined by the information attained with urethroscopy and antegrade and retrograde contrast urethrography (Fig. 85–6). The density and depth of the stricture

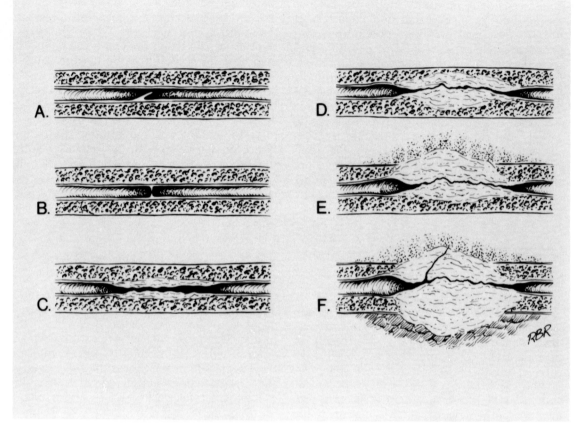

Figure 86–6. Classification (Devine) of urethral stricture disease according to the anatomy of the stricture. (From Jordan, G. H.: Management of anterior urethral stricture disease. Probl. Urol., *1,* 2:199–225, 1987.)

(spongiofibrosis) are somewhat more difficult to determine precisely. Much information is gained by the appearance of the urethra on contrast studies and at urethroscopy. High resolution real time or gray scale B-mode ultrasonography is also useful in providing information about the depth of spongiofibrosis. Once the anatomy of the stricture is defined, the best technique of tissue transfer can be selected.

The reconstructive ladder concept is as out of date when applied to urethral reconstruction as it is for general reconstructive procedures. The tendency to offer all patients multiple dilatations and internal urethrotomies before pursuing a course of open reconstruction must be avoided. Internal urethrotomy and dilatations can be predictably curative for strictures with insignificant or minimally deep spongiofibrosis. Likewise, the strictures are usually of extremely short length and in most cases represent either an iris or an exaggerated mucosal fold. In the case of the

patch graft urethral reconstruction procedure, the literature supports a diminished chance of success in patients who have had multiple dilatations. The authors feel that a corollary must exist for patients who have had multiple internal urethrotomies. In summary, the reconstructive surgeon is forced to consider the ultimate quality of the result to be paramount. With such an approach, most anterior urethral strictures can be managed in the knowledge that a 93 to 95 per cent chance of cure is attainable. In the case of posterior urethral strictures, the excision and primary anastomosis procedure yields excellent or good results in more than 95 per cent of patients.

Anatomic Considerations

No discussion of reconstruction for urethral stricture can proceed without a description of the anatomy of the genitalia and associated skin structures (Fig. 86–7). The urethra in the male is divided into four parts: prostatic, membranous, bulbous, and penile/pendulous. The urethra as a conduit channels the products of the urinary and genital systems. The prostatic and membranous portions are commonly thought of as those portions comprising the posterior urethra. Embryologically, this concept is incorrect, because the prostatic urethra represents the only true posterior urethra. The bulbous and pendulous portions make up the anterior urethra. The anterior urethra, apart from the membranous urethra, is invested by the spongy erectile tissue of the corpus spongiosum and the glans penis. In many cases the division of the urethra may be best described as the proximal urethra, composed of the posterior and membranous, and the distal portion, composed of those portions of the urethra invested by the corpus spongiosum. Anterior urethral stricture disease occasionally extends into the membranous urethra, but most strictures of

the anterior urethra are confined to the urethra caudal to the area of penetration of the urethra through the triangular ligament. The triangular ligament is formed by the transverse perineal muscles posteriorly and the ligamentous attachments of these muscles across the decussation of the corpora cavernosa. In the nontraumatized urethra, the concept of its being fixed firmly in these ligamentous attachments is not correct. The concept of a defined diaphragm comes from observations at posterior urethral reconstruction. However, the dense formation of scar in the triangular ligament and space immediately beneath it is deceptive. Thus, the membranous urethra is incarcerated in the scar.

The fascial planes of the genitalia and genital skin are closely associated with the urethra and its adjacent structures. These fascia, and the potential spaces that they bound, determine many of the clinically observed phenomena with complicated urethral stricture disease. The inferior fascia of the

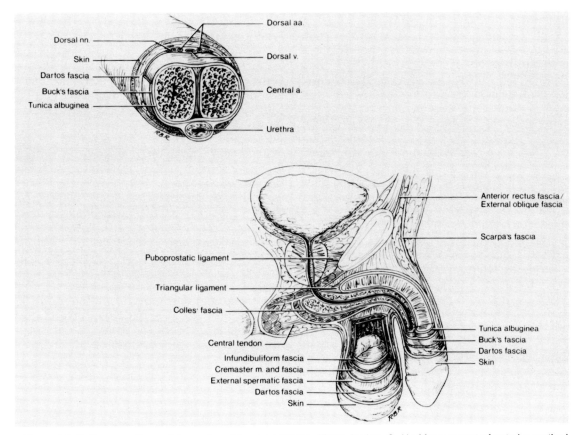

Figure 86–7. Cross sections of the male pelvis and genitalia. (From Jordan, G. H.: Management of anterior urethral stricture disease. Probl. Urol., *1*, 2:199–225, 1987.)

"urogenital diaphragm" fuses with Colles' fascia, which then continues over the abdomen anteriorly as Scarpa's fascia. The dartos fascia of the scrotum and penis are merely an extension of the Colles' fascia as it surrounds the genital structures anteriorly. The fascia lata of the thigh is also an extension of Colles' fascia. Colles' fascia forms a limiting barrier of great importance in the case of extravasation, abscess, or hematoma. Buck's fascia invests the three corporeal bodies of the penis; it becomes confluent with the glans penis and continues into the perineum, where it fuses posteriorly with Colles' fascia. Buck's fascia, except when eroded by infection or acutely disrupted by trauma, forms an almost impenetrable membrane against extravasation, or hematoma from the bulbous or pendulous portion of the urethra.

The arterial supply of the anterior urethra emanates from terminal branches of the internal pudendal vessels. The anterior urethra is supplied by the artery to the bulb and the circumflex cavernosal arteries. Some arterial flow is supplied in a retrograde fashion through the glans penis, and hence represents the terminal blood flow from the dorsal arteries of the penis. Either supply can by itself adequately support the urethra, and this fact is capitalized on in many urethral stricture repairs. The concept of wide mobilization of the urethra must be carefully addressed, however. Patients have been encountered who show evidence of disruption of the pudendal arteries proximally, and in these wide mobilization of the corpus spongiosum can be disastrous. Likewise, if the anterior urethra is being mobilized proximally, the blood flow that one depends on is via the terminal flow of the dorsal artery of the penis through the spongy erectile tissue of the glans and the spongy erectile tissue of the corpus spongiosum. Since anterior urethral stricture disease is part and parcel with spongiofibrosis, in the case of the patient with coexisting anterior stricture disease, the proximal portions of the anterior urethra may not be reliably mobilized: the extent of spongiofibrosis may limit the blood flow proximally in the corpus spongiosum, and hence lead to ischemic damage to the corpus spongiosum and proximal anterior urethra. Likewise, in the case of the hypospadiac patient, most repairs divide the communication of the bifid corpus spongiosum with the glans penis. Not uncommonly, hypospadiac patients present with iatrogenically induced stricture, and radical mobilization of the distal urethra is not a good option for reconstruction of these individuals. The division of the attachments to the glans having been done at hypospadias repair, the urethra then survives only on the proximal arteries, i.e., the circumflex cavernosa and the deep arteries of the bulb. The veins of the urethra and associated corpus spongiosum eventually empty into Santorini's plexus.

The preputial, penile, and scrotal skin receive blood flow via the superior external and deep pudendal arteries. These arteries arise from the femoral artery before the departure of the profunda femoris. These arteries end as axial branches in the fascial layers immediately beneath the dermal aspect of the genital skin, and as the subdermal and intradermal plexus in the genital skin. The arteries enter the preputial and scrotal skin from the posterolateral aspect. There is rich arborization across the midline of both the superficial plexus and the deeper axial vessels. The veins draining this region are likewise dual in arrangement. The veins from the deeper tissues contained in the dartos layer drain into the internal deep pudendal veins, whereas the more superficial veins drain into the external superficial pudendal veins. This dual arrangement of vascularity is important for the development of many of the new preputial and scrotal flaps in skin island procedures.

Posterior urethral strictures are associated with a marked amount of periurethral inflammation and scar. Because of this, tissue transfer techniques must be performed very carefully. Fortunately, the vast majority of these injuries can be managed by primary excision of the stricture with a precise approximation of the bulbous urethral epithelium to the prostatic urethral epithelium. As with all strictures, a knowledge of the anatomy of posterior strictures is essential. Obtaining this information is often difficult, because most of these patients have competent bladder necks, and thus the prostatic urethra is not well demonstrated on cystograms. If a patient strains during the cystogram phase, spasm is occasionally bladder stimulated, so that contrast material fills the prostatic urethra. In these cases, the precise length of the urethral defect can be ascertained. Most patients, however, are unsuccessful in attempts to fill the prostatic urethra. Fortunately, most have indwelling suprapubic cystostomies, and thus cystoscopy through the suprapubic sinus is possible. The cystoscope can be advanced through the bladder neck, down the prostatic urethra to the level of the verumontanum, and often to the level of the external sphincter. With this knowledge, combined with the position of the prostate on rectal examination, the length of the defect can be estimated.

Surgical Procedure

The vast majority of these strictures can be reconstructed by placing the patient in the exaggerated lithotomy position and approaching the stricture via a perineal exposure. It is essential that the lithotomy position be as exaggerated as that contemplated for a radical perineal prostatectomy. In this position the urethra and the anterior surface of the prostate can be well exposed (Fig. 86–8).

There are several instruments to assist in getting the patient into the proper position. General anesthesia with paralysis is a necessity. The Chick table combined with Allen stirrups are invaluable for positioning of the patient. Likewise, the Denis Browne retractor makes exposure, once the incision is created,

much easier, because the exaggerated lithotomy position makes it difficult for more than one assistant to approach the perineal wound (Fig. 86–9). An inverted Y- or lambda-shaped incision very nicely exposes the central tendon of the perineum, which is then divided. The underlying adipose tissue is dissected (Fig. 86–9A), revealing the midline fusion of the ischial cavernosus muscles (bulbocavernosus muscles). The dissection can then be carried beneath the scrotum beyond the ischial cavernosus musculature, where the "bare" corpus spongiosum is encountered. The ischial cavernosus muscles can then be carefully dissected off the corpus spongiosum and divided in their midline (Fig. 86–9B to D). The urethra is dissected from its attachments to the triangular ligament and the corpora cavernosa (Fig. 86–9E). The amount of mobilization of the anterior urethra depends on the length of defect to be spanned. Generally, mobilization is not carried farther than the penoscrotal junction; mobilization beyond that point can be associated with foreshortening of the penis or ventral chordee. If it is necessary to mobilize the corpus spongiosum beyond the penoscrotal junction, it is preferable to mobilize the urethra completely to the attachment of the glans, thus avoiding chordee. Placement of the Denis Browne attachment at the point of dissection of the muscles

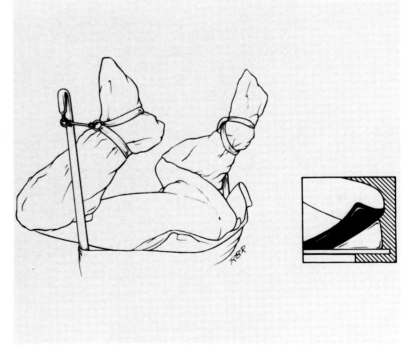

Figure 86–8. A patient in exaggerated lithotomy position. Care must be taken to elevate the hips and buttocks, thus exaggerating the position. The patient should not be forced into the position by pulling up the legs. The legs and feet should be stabilized by the stirrups after the exaggerated position is achieved by elevation of the buttocks.

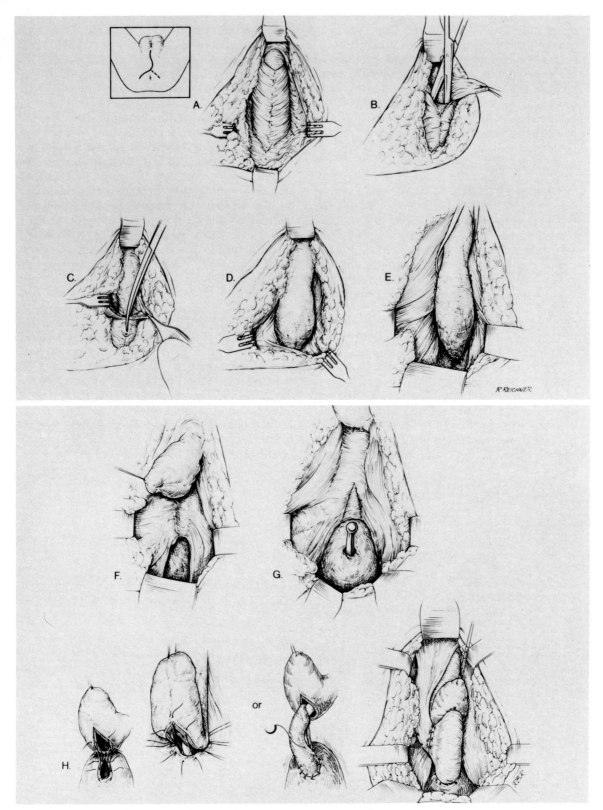

Figure 86–9. *A* to *H*, Diagrammatic detail of the dissection of a membranoprostatic stricture with direct reanastomosis or a full-thickness skin graft interposition with a dartos fascial flap *(H)*. See text for details.

allows good exposure. Care must be taken when retracting the muscles to avoid tearing, because the muscles are important for the limitation of scar after reconstruction. The anterior urethra is completely dissected down to the point of the stricture, which is usually encountered at the departure of the urethra from the bulbospongiosum. The latter must be detached from the perineal body. It is at this point that the deep arteries to the bulb are encountered. Generally, these arteries can be visualized and hemostasis obtained using the bipolar electrocautery forceps. While the bulbospongiosum can be amputated beyond the point where the bulbous urethra departs from the corpus spongiosum, total dissection of the bulb from its attachments to the perineal body is not difficult and limits bleeding. The corpus spongiosum now remains attached distally by the urethra as it exits the bulbospongiosum. The urethra can be divided at that point (Fig. 86–9*F*). The corpus spongiosum should be placed in a moist sponge and retracted from the field.

At this point, a Haygrove sound or a flexible cystoscope is introduced through the suprapubic sinus tract and manipulated through the bladder neck. The tip of the sound or cystoscope is palpated. The triangular ligament of the perineum is opened down to the pubis. Immediately superficial to the pubis are found the crural and deep dorsal veins of the penis. These veins are easily ligated and retracted from the field. With the tip of the sound or cystoscope palpated, one can now cut down onto the tip of the sound into the proximal portion of the disrupted urethra (Fig. 86–9*G*). The division of the triangular ligament, along with mobilization of the corpora off the pubis, makes it possible to place a Gelpi retractor, thus greatly improving the exposure of the anterior prostatic urethra. Once the proximal urethra is located, the urethrotomy should be enlarged to the point where a cystoscope can be advanced through the incision, allowing inspection of the prostatic urethra and bladder neck. This endoscopic step is essential; many patients have been referred who inadvertently had anastomosis of the anterior urethra to the bladder directly, or to the midportion of the prostatic urethra, the latter situation leaving a blind-ending prostatic urethral segment distal to the point of the anastomosis.

The scarred tissue must now be totally excised. In some cases it is essential to carry the dissection up beneath the pubis, thereby releasing the puboprostatic ligaments. For a good, tension-free anastomosis it is imperative that the prostate be mobilized and allowed to descend into the wound. In some cases a partial infrapubectomy is needed. This removal of the lower aspect of the pubis is easily accomplished with Kerrison rongeurs. The corporeal bodies must be carefully mobilized off the pubis before infrapubectomy is performed. The resection of the pubis can be as vigorous as required to obtain exposure of the apical anterior prostate.

The division of the triangular ligament, coupled with the mobilization of the corpus from the pubis and infrapubectomy, all serve to limit the radius of the curve that the anterior urethra must traverse to the apical prostate. These maneuvers allow the surgeon to span quite sizable urethral defects and still accomplish a secure anastomosis. If these maneuvers fail to provide a tension-free anastomosis, the urethra can be routed around the corporeal body, thus shortening the course by an additional 1 to 1.5 cm. If the urethra is to be rerouted around the corporeal bodies, vigorous infrapubectomy must be performed.

It is essential that the apical prostatic urethra be anastomosed to the epithelium. If appropriate, a button of prostatic tissue must be excised along with the scar. The bulbous urethra must be widely spatulated (Fig. 86–9*H*), and the anastomosis can then be performed. The authors currently use interrupted sutures of an absorbable material placed full thickness through the epithelium. Before these sutures are seated, a No. 24 French silicone catheter is placed through the repair under direct vision. The sutures can then be seated, thus approximating the epithelial surfaces (Fig. 86–9*H*). The urethra is reattached to the corporeal bodies with interrupted absorbable sutures. The bulbospongiosum can be splayed to surround the reanastomosis, thus limiting scarring in the area with the interposition of the vascular bulbous spongiosum.

The perineum is closed in layers. The ischial cavernosus muscles are closed with interrupted sutures, allowing the escape of collections from beneath to a suction drain, which is placed deep to the central tendon of the perineum but superficial to the ischial cavernosus muscles.

The suprapubic cystostomy tube is then

placed to gravity drainage. The No. 24 French catheter is customarily changed to a smaller No. 16 or 18 French catheter on the seventh postoperative day. The urethral catheter remains in place as a stent up to postoperative day 21. At that time, the catheter is removed and a voiding study with contrast material is performed. In the absence of extravasation, the suprapubic tube is left clamped and the patient is allowed to continue voiding per urethra. The suprapubic cystostomy tube, barring complications, can be removed within the ensuing five to seven days.

If the above procedures for shortening the course of the urethra coupled with the innate elasticity of the urethra are not sufficient to allow primary anastomosis, a tissue transfer interposition technique can be applied. A tubed full-thickness skin graft is seldom successful, because the pronounced scarring in the area of the apical prostate does not provide a good vascular graft host bed. If a full-thickness skin graft is used, a dartos fascia flap must be mobilized to surround the graft (Fig. 86–9*H*). Another option is that a fascial flap with a skin island can be mobilized. The specifics of the various local genital fascial island flaps are discussed later. These flaps can be employed very successfully in the reconstruction of long-segment posterior urethral strictures.

The technique of full-thickness skin graft urethroplasty as applied to the anterior urethra is the most versatile of all open urethral reconstructive procedures. The best results of full-thickness urethroplasty are obtained in patients with very superficial spongiofibrosis. The behavior of the full-thickness skin is determined by the thickness of the dermis (Fig. 86–10). Full-thickness skin taken from the penile or preputial areas is thought to be the best. Extra gonadal, hairless full-thickness skin can be used as a graft for urethral reconstruction, but this skin clearly behaves differently from genital full-thickness skin grafts. Split-thickness skin is never applicable for use in urethral reconstruction, with the exception of the mesh graft urethral reconstruction technique described by Noll and Schreiter (1987). By and large, full-thickness skin grafts are best applied to reconstruct bulbous urethral strictures in patients who have not had previous open urethral reconstruction. The proximal anterior urethra and the bulb are covered by the midline fusion of the ischial cavernosus musculature. These muscles provide a good vascular bed for the full-thickness skin graft. In the penile or distal pendulous urethra, the dartos layer serves as the graft bed and probably is a more tenuous one.

The urethra lies eccentrically in the corpus spongiosum, tending to be located toward the anterior surface (Fig. 86–11). In patients with known deep spongiofibrosis, the urethrotomy is created on the lateral aspect of the urethra; however, this lateral placement precludes spongioplasty (Fig. 86–11*B*). In patients with superficial spongiofibrosis, the urethrotomy is created on the ventral surface of the corpus spongiosum, in anticipation of the performance of a spongioplasty after the full-thickness skin is in place (Fig. 86–11*A*). The spongioplasty procedure has two advantages: (1) the spongioerectile tissue offers a rich graft bed and (2) the full-thickness skin graft is supported by the reapproximated spongioerectile tissue and adventitia of the corpus spongiosum. It is emphasized, however, that spongioplasty can be performed only when spongiofibrosis is superficial. If deep spongiofibrosis exists and spongioplasty is attempted, one merely reapproximates the stricture over the full-thickness skin graft.

It is essential that the urethrotomy be carried through the entire length of the stricture and into the adjacent normal urethra and corpus spongiosum. This allows for spatulation of the full-thickness graft patch into the normal urethra, and thus avoids "anastomotic" stricture recurrences. The graft is first secured by a number of interrupted chromic sutures, allowing for careful tailoring and symmetric distribution of the graft. Once the graft is tacked in place, a running absorbable suture is placed in a subepithelial fashion, creating a watertight suture line. Extraepithelial placement of the suture allows use of the newer generation of absorbable sutures. These sutures are associated with less inflammation when placement of the suture avoids the epithelial surface. A second advantage of extramucosal suture placement is that such a suture line tends to invert the mucosa. Mucosa does not heal to mucosa, and hence apposition of the dermis to the urethral lamina propria hastens healing.

After the graft suturing has been completed, a stenting or diverting urethral catheter can be placed through the repair. In most cases suprapubic urinary diversion is preferred, with a urethral catheter or a thin-walled silicone tube placed as a stent. In cases of strictures with superficial spongiofibrosis, spongioplasty is performed by reapproximating the superficial spongy tissue and adventitia of the corpus spongiosum over the graft (Fig. 86–11A). This closure of the superficial corpus spongiosum must be watertight to limit hematoma formation. When a urethrotomy has been created laterally, care must be taken to include both the adventitial layer of the corpus spongiosum and the immediate subepithelial layer of the closure (Fig. 86–11B); failure to do so leads to troublesome bleeding in the postoperative period. Absolute hemostasis is a necessity before closure. In addition to the obvious effects of hematoma on graft "take," hematomas are known to create a vasospastic phenomenon in flaps. In all cases of urethral reconstruction, hemostasis is achieved by the use of bipolar electrocautery forceps. When the urethral reconstruction has been in the bulbous urethra, the ischial cavernosus muscles are carefully reapproximated with individually placed sutures. Again, individual sutures allow for escape of serous or bloody collections in the space between the muscle and the full-thickness graft. A suction drain is placed superficial to the closed muscle.

In the case of pendulous urethral stricture,

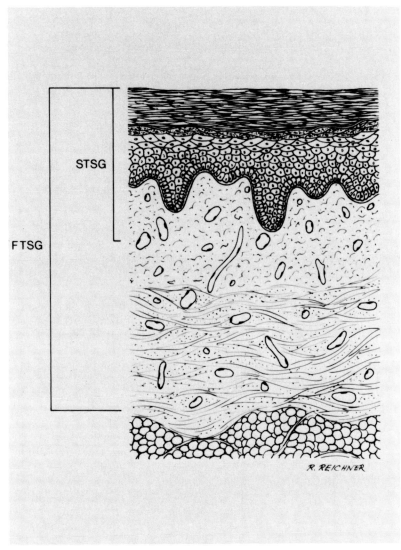

Figure 86–10. Cross section of skin showing the layers that are included in the split-thickness (STSG) and full-thickness (FTSG) skin grafts. (From Jordan, G. H.: Management of anterior urethral stricture disease. Probl. Urol., *1, 2*:199–225, 1987.)

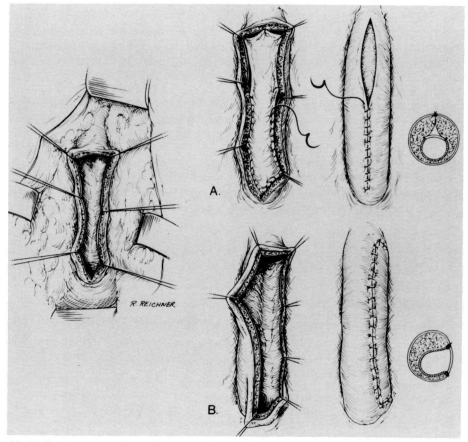

Figure 86–11. Urethrotomies with grafting; closure is in accordance with the site of the incision. *A,* Midline ventral incision, the graft sutured to the mucosa and spongioplasty performed. *B,* The urethra opened on the lateral aspect, and the graft sutured into place. (From Jordan, G. H., and Devine, C. J.: Surgery following the failed urethral reconstruction. *In* McDougal, W. S. (Ed.): Difficult Problems in Urological Surgery. Chicago, Year Book Medical Publishers, 1987, p. 289. Copyright 1987, Year Book Medical Publishers. Reproduced with permission.)

a longitudinal ventral island flap of penile skin, originally described by Orandi (1968, 1972), works well (Fig. 86–12). Orandi's procedure has been greatly modified. When the use of this flap is contemplated for repair of distal anterior urethral stricture, the incision in the ventral penile skin is placed lateral to the midline and carried sharply through Buck's fascia, revealing the underlying tunica albuginea of the corpus cavernosum and the corpus spongiosum. Dissection is carried over the corpus spongiosum by reflecting Buck's fascia from the tunica albuginea and the adventitia of the corpus spongiosum (Fig. 86–12*A*). This ensures that the dartos fascia with its vessels is elevated without damage to the vessels.

The urethrotomy is created on the lateral aspect of the corpus spongiosum contralateral to the original skin incision but ipsilateral to

the side of the flap dissection (Fig. 86–12*B*). The urethrotomy is extended into normal urethra proximally and distally. Tacking sutures are placed to stabilize the mucosa and thus limit problems with false passage. These genital fascial flaps with skin islands are axial flaps, and as such have no limitations with regard to length to width ratios. The ventral longitudinal flap must be carefully tailored and measured with the preputial skin expanded, thus avoiding the placement of an oversized flap with attendant diverticulum.

With the incision completed as described, the flap and flap pedicle have already been elevated; cutaneous continuity is then interrupted with a superficial incision on the contralateral aspect of the flap (Fig. 86–12*C*). Thus, the adjacent skin and the superficial subdermal and intradermal plexus are ele-

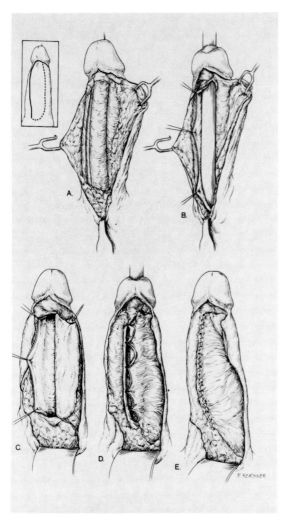

Figure 86–12. Orandi urethroplasty. *A,* The flap is developed in the layer immediately beneath Buck's fascia. *B,* Urethrostomy is performed on the lateral aspect of the urethra contralateral to the original incision in the penile skin. *C,* The flap is sutured into position with a running submucosal suture. *D,* The flap is inverted to the urethrotomy defect with tacking sutures. *E,* The submucosal suture line is completed. (From Jordan, G. H.: Management of anterior urethral stricture disease. Probl. Urol., *1,* 2:199–225, 1987.)

vated from the flap pedicle. With the flap developed in the midline as described, torsion of the penis is greatly limited and the flap is easily inverted into the urethrotomy defect (Fig. 86–12*D*). The flap is sutured into place in the same way as the full-thickness skin graft (Fig. 86–12*E*).

With the flap in position, a stenting catheter is placed. Urethral catheters are never used for urinary diversion in distal stricture repair.

The dorsal transverse preputial island flap as described by Duckett (1981) can be used as a patch island flap for strictures as far back as the midproximal penile urethra (Fig. 86–13). For these cases, a ventral midline incision is carried to the level of Buck's fascia where it overlies the corpus spongiosum. This incision can be extended into the anterior surface of the scrotum through the raphé. With the stricture identified and the urethrotomy created as described, the preputial skin is elevated in a layer immediately superficial to Buck's fascia. In a patient who is already circumcised, care must be taken to ensure that the dissection is in the correct plane immediately superficial to Buck's fascia. The urethrotomy defect is carefully measured, and a flap conforming to these measurements is marked transversely on the dorsal surface of the penile-preputial skin (Fig. 86–13). Superficial incisions just through the skin are then created on the outer aspects of the flap, and a fascial flap with the skin island is dissected. This island flap can then be transposed around the penis and placed in the urethrotomy (Fig. 86–13). The flap is not easily employed for more proximal urethral strictures because of the dorsal position of the vascular pedicle.

For cases of proximal urethral stricture disease, a ventral longitudinal or transverse island preputial flap can be used (Fig. 86–14). Quartey (1983) described a flap similar to the one used by the authors. For relatively short strictures, the flap is elevated from the ventrum of the penis in a longitudinal aspect. By mobilizing the flap in the midline, as opposed to the ventrolateral aspect as described by Quartey, less of the remaining skin must survive as a random flap. The vascular pedicle is dissected from the ventrolateral aspect of the penis. The pedicle is elevated in the same layer as is the pedicle of the Orandi flap. In this case, the flap pedicle is based inferiorly on the dartos layer as it extends onto the scrotum (Fig. 86–14*A*). For longer strictures, the skin island can be designed in a fan or hockeystick shape so that the flap is designed with the longitudinal limb on the ventral aspect of the penis, turning laterally as the flap approaches the frenulum and coronal margin. This flap is also developed from the midline tissue, thus limiting the amount of remaining penile skin that must be nourished by the superficial vessels. Quite sizable flaps can be mobilized in this fashion, up to

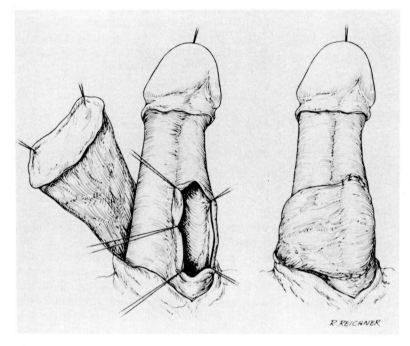

Figure 86–13. The Duckett (dorsal transverse preputial island) flap as applied to a stricture of the penoscrotal urethra. (From Jordan, G. H.: Management of anterior urethral stricture disease. Probl. Urol., *1,* 2:199–225, 1987.)

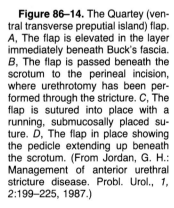

Figure 86–14. The Quartey (ventral transverse preputial island) flap. *A,* The flap is elevated in the layer immediately beneath Buck's fascia. *B,* The flap is passed beneath the scrotum to the perineal incision, where urethrotomy has been performed through the stricture. *C,* The flap is sutured into place with a running, submucosally placed suture. *D,* The flap in place showing the pedicle extending up beneath the scrotum. (From Jordan, G. H.: Management of anterior urethral stricture disease. Probl. Urol., *1,* 2:199–225, 1987.)

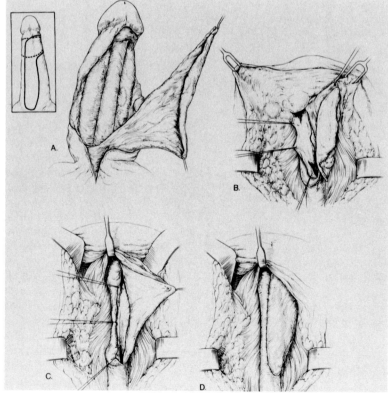

11 × 3 cm. This flap can be widely mobilized and is of great use for both anterior and posterior urethral strictures. In most cases, stenting catheters are used for these procedures, diversion being accomplished by a suprapubic cystotomy catheter.

Many men have significantly large hairless areas on the scrotum. The scrotum has proved to have the same kind of dual vascularity as the penile and preputial skin. The authors have used what is termed a "hairless scrotal island flap" (Fig. 86–15). If applicable, this has the advantage of requiring minimal mobilization and dissection when applied to the bulbous urethra. In patients with hairless scrotal skin, development of this tissue as a flap offers an alternative requiring less dissection yet allowing reconstruction of the urethra with vascularized hairless skin. The hairless areas most frequently lie immediately adjacent to the raphé; however, significantly large hairless areas have been identified completely overlying one hemiscrotum. Obviously, this flap cannot be used in prepubertal males, and scrotal flaps are inadvis-

able for urethral reconstruction in children. The dartos vessels extend onto the scrotum from the lateral aspect. These flaps must be based laterally (Fig. 86–15B). The tendency to base these flaps on the septum must be avoided, since the vascularity in the septum of the scrotum is not reliable. Careful tailoring of these scrotal skin flaps is paramount. Because the flap pedicle is dissected laterally from the scrotum, a laterally placed urethrotomy is used to allow for easy transposition and inversion of the flap into the urethrotomy defect. As in all the flap procedures described, the scrotal island flap maintains complete compliance and distensibility, and will develop into a urethral diverticulum if not carefully measured and tailored.

In patients with deep complex stricture disease, two-stage procedures are used. In these individuals, the area of the urethral stricture is almost completely excised. A relatively hairless full-thickness skin graft is then transferred to the area of the genitalia and perineum, and tubularized in a second stage. The grafts are positioned open faced in

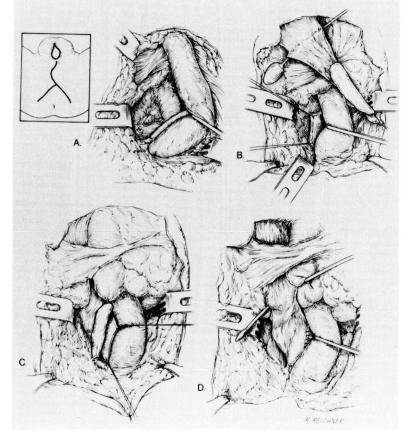

Figure 86–15. The hairless scrotal island flap. *A,* Dissection of the bulbomembranous portion of the urethra. *B,* The flap is elevated on the dorsolateral pedicle with a lateral urethrotomy created on the lateral aspect of the bulbomembranous portion of the urethra. *C, D,* The flap is sutured into the urethrotomy defect. Note the probe beneath the vascular pedicle. (From Jordan, G. H.: Management of anterior urethral stricture disease. Probl. Urol., *1,* 2:199–225, 1987.)

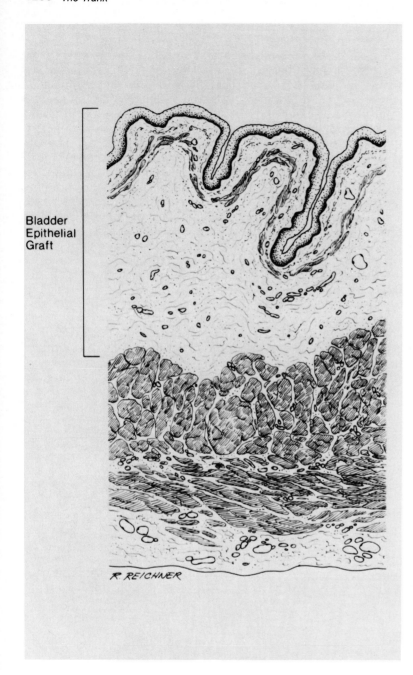

Bladder
Epithelial
Graft

R REICHNER

Figure 86–16. A bladder epithelial graft.

the midline; the patient voids through a proximal urethrotomy or the stream is diverted via suprapubic cystostomy. The grafts are allowed to mature free from the passage of urine. After three to six months of graft maturation, a second stage Thiersch-Duplay type of tubing procedure is performed.

Noll and Schreiter (1987) described a similar procedure. In this case, however, a meshed-split thickness graft is placed into the perineum. The graft is allowed to mature for approximately six to eight weeks and the

tissue is then tubed by the Thiersch-Duplay procedure. The procedure seems to defy the rules of tissue transfer for urethral reconstruction, but these authors have described excellent results in a large series of patients.

In two patients full-thickness skin has been transposed to the area of the scrotum, tubularized, and wrapped in the dartos layer. The full-thickness tube is left out of continuity with the urethra and allowed to mature for four to six months. After graft maturation, the tube is mobilized as a tube island flap and placed in the urethral defect. Bladder epithelium serves as a good source of hairless epithelium (Fig. 86–16). The authors have tended to use bladder epithelium only in cases in which cystostomy was required for other reasons at the time of urethral reconstruction. The bladder epithelial graft is usually very reliable; with maturation, it is truly hairless and maintains good compliance. A major problem with bladder epithelium is the subsequent formation of diverticulum. The graft is placed on the assumption that it is virtually noncontractile, and thus far there have been no problems with stenosis or diverticulum formation. Care must be taken in handling the graft to avoid desiccation, because bladder epithelium appears to be especially prone to injury from this cause. Likewise, if urethral reconstruction needs to be carried to the urethral meatus, a cuff of full-thickness skin graft must be interposed between the meatus and the bladder epithelium. The latter tends to undergo hypertrophic changes at the meatal interface, leading to poor cosmetic and functional results.

Strictures of the fossa navicularis represent an entirely different challenge. The procedures described by Blandy (1980), Cohney (1963), and Branon and associates (1976) have all resulted in rather good functional results but less than optimal cosmetic results. Because of the poor cosmetic results, patients were often reluctant to allow early reconstruction and thus underwent frequent dilatations or internal urethrotomies. The frequent instrumentation of these patients probably led to iatrogenic extension of the urethra proximally. A technique of island flap urethroplasty was described that represents a modification of the Branon (1976) procedure. The authors prefer a different island flap procedure described by Jordan (1987) (Fig. 86–17), which uses a ventral transverse fascial flap with a skin island and has yielded good functional and cosmetic results. The procedure, as with all others for fossa reconstruction, is useful only for isolated strictures of the fossa navicularis and meatus. The flap is developed from the ventral skin immediately proximal to the frenulum and elevated on a broad-based pedicle, a feature that is

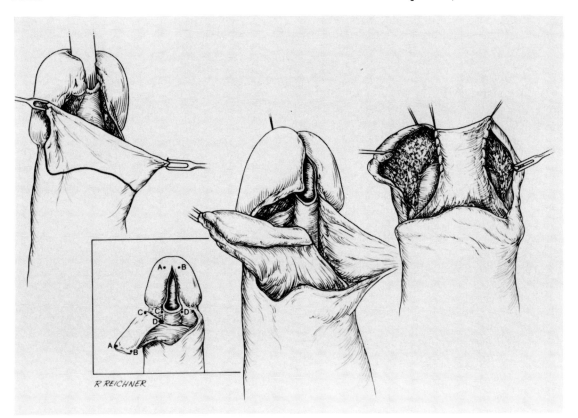

R REICHNER

Figure 86–17. Technique of ventral transverse preputial island flap for reconstruction of the fossa navicularis. See text for details. (From Jordan, G. H.: Reconstruction of the fossa navicularis. J. Urol., *138*:102, 1987. © 1987 by Williams & Wilkins.)

believed to be superior to the procedure described by DeSy (1984). The flap is easily mobilized in the layer immediately superficial to Buck's fascia. It can then be easily transposed and inverted into the urethrotomy defect, requiring minimal mobilization of the broad-based pedicle. Ventral closure of the glans is accomplished by elevating the lateral glans tissue broadly from the tips of the corpora. The interface between the tips of the corpora and the overlying spongy erectile tissue of the glans is a relatively avascular space and is easily developed. Care must be taken to elevate the lateral glans flap sufficiently for the glans flaps to be reapproximated ventrally around the island flap without limitation of the lumen or excess tension on the flaps. The island flap is designed to create a 28 to 30 French meatus and fossa. With a No. 28 French sound placed through the repair, the lateral glans flaps are reapproximated in the ventrum, using a subcutaneous stitch placed in the erectile tissue with the skin edges approximated with chromic vertical mattress sutures. The defect of the ventral skin is easily closed primarily. Burow's triangles can be used at the corners of the defect to eliminate dog-ears. For the repair of fossa strictures, the distal urethra is opened ventrally until normal tissue is found. The strictured urethra is totally excised and the glans flaps are developed as described above. A skin graft is then obtained from the penile skin. The graft can be closed over a sound to form a tube, and the glans wings are brought around as described above. This procedure has also been very useful for many forms of fossa stricture. It probably should not be used in patients with fossa strictures resulting from balanitis xerotica obliterans. The authors believe that flap and graft procedures such as those described above should be performed when obstruction has reached a point at which a urethral meatotomy would once have been carried out. These patients can be offered optimal functional and cosmetic results without the risk of iatrogenic injury to the urethra more proximally.

Urethral strictures provide a challenge to the reconstructive surgeon. In the past, strictures were managed and often not cured. The advent of modern tissue transfer techniques, however, allows the reconstructive surgeon to approach these cases with confidence, knowing that cure is possible in more than 90 per cent of patients.

REFERENCES

Asopa, H. S.: One stage correction of penile hypospadias using a foreskin tube. Int. Surg., 55:435, 1971.
Blandy, J. P.: Urethral stricture. Postgrad. Med. J., 56:343, 1980.
Branon, W., Ochsner, M., Fuselier, H., and Goodlet, J.: Free full-thickness skin graft urethroplasty for urethral stricture: experience with 66 patients. J. Urol., 115:677, 1976.
Bulkley, G. J.: Scrotal and penile lymphedema. J. Urol., 87:422, 1962.
Cohney, B. C.: A penile flap procedure for the relief of meatal stricture. Br. J. Urol., 35:183, 1963.
DeSy, W. A.: Aesthetic repair of meatal stricture. J. Urol., 132:678, 1984.
Duckett, J. W.: The island flap technique for hypospadias repair. Urol. Clin. North Am., 8:503, 1981.
Feins, N. R.: A new surgical technique for lymphedema of the penis and scrotum. J. Pediatr. Surg., 46:481, 1970.
Gong-Kang, H., Ru-Qi, H., and Zong-Zhas, L.: Microlymphaticovenous anastomosis for treating scrotal elephantiasis. Microsurgery, 6:36, 1985.
Jordan, G. H.: Reconstruction of the fossa navicularis. J. Urol., 138:102, 1987.
Khanna, N. N.: Surgical treatment of elephantiasis of male genitalia. Plast. Reconstr. Surg., 46:481, 1970.
Malloy, T. R., Wein, A. J., and Gross, P.: Scrotal and penile lymphedema: surgical considerations and management. J. Urol., 130:263, 1983.
Noll, F., and Schreiter, F.: Meshgraft urethroplasty. Presented at the Genitourinary Reconstructive Surgeons Annual Meeting, Hotel St. Francis, San Francisco, October 16, 1987.
Orandi, A.: One stage urethroplasty. Br. J. Urol., 40:77, 1968.
Orandi, A.: One stage urethroplasty: 4 year followup. J. Urol., 107:977, 1972.
de la Peyronie, F.: Sur quelques obstacles qui s'opposent a l'ejaculation naturelle de la semence. Mem. Acad. Roy. Chir., 1743, p. 425.
Quartey, J. K.: One stage penile/preputial cutaneous island flap urethroplasty for urethral stricture: a preliminary report. J. Urol., 129:284, 1983.
Raghavaiah, N. V.: Reconstruction of scrotal and penile skin in elephantiasis. J. Urol., 118:128, 1977.
Standoli, L.: Hypospadias one stage repair—preputial island flap. Alpine Workshop, Sestriere, Italy, February, 1977.

87

Charles E. Horton
Richard C. Sadove
John B. McCraw

Reconstruction of Female Genital Defects

Reconstruction of the female perineum is appropriate for congenital absence of the vagina, lymphedema, vaginal fistulas, and ablative defects. Genital wound coverage involves special problems such as fecal contamination, difficult immobilization, and adjacent rectal and urethral repairs. Vaginal reconstruction after ablative surgery must, of necessity, take into account wound conditions different from those found in congenital absence of the vagina or created by transsexual surgery. Local abundance of well-vascularized tissue allows for grafting techniques in cases of congenital absence and transsexuality. Such is not the case following ablative surgery, in which large, bulky, well-vascularized flaps must be brought into the pelvic region.

CONGENITAL ABSENCE OF THE VAGINA

History

The history of attempts to form a vagina dates back to ancient times. Hippocrates described "membranous obstruction" of the vagina. Realdus Columbus in 1572 described vaginal aplasia. Dupuytren reported an attempt at surgical correction in 1817. The rectum and colon were first used to form a vagina by Sneguireff in 1892 (reported in 1904). In 1904 Baldwin described an operation in which an ileal flap was used to function as a vagina. In 1904 labial grafts were first used by Jewett. Graves used the method of two thigh flaps and two labial flaps over a glass mold in 1908. These early attempts were associated with high rates of morbidity and mortality.

The nonoperative technique of intermittent perineal pressure was described by Frank in 1938. Wells (1935) and Kanter (1935) popularized the method of spontaneous reepithelization of the vaginal tract over a stent placed in the rectovesical septum after blunt dissection of the space.

Skin grafting techniques to reconstruct the vagina were used by Abbé in 1898. Much later, McIndoe (1938) achieved excellent results with split-thickness skin grafts inverted over a stent, and this has remained the most popular technique to date.

The concept of using thicker grafts can be

traced to a publication by Burian in 1935. In 1953 Conway and Stark emphasized the importance of thick grafts, recommending a thickness of 20/1000ths of an inch. They noted the relationship between thicker grafts and decreased graft shrinkage: "A free graft of thick split skin contains sufficient dermis to afford resiliency. Hence, the likelihood of contraction of the graft is lessened," they wrote. Fara, Vesely, and Kafka (1972) described the use of thick grafts harvested with a dermatome from the buttocks; however, this necessitated split-thickness grafting of the donor site.

Diagnosis

The diagnosis of congenital absence of the vagina is frequently missed at birth and often does not become apparent until puberty (Fig. 87–1). Estimates of the incidence vary from one in 4000 to one in 80,000. If this diagnosis is made, the parents may desire counseling.

Occasionally a patient presents with an abdominal mass. The parents of a pubertal child will not be aware of the true diagnosis. On exploration the mass is determined to be blood in the uterus, and on examination the patient proves to have congenital absence of the vagina. In the past it was recommended that these patients undergo hysterectomy, since if the cervix is not competent and if a vagina is made, infection will cause endometriosis to such a degree that the mortality rate is unacceptable. However, new theories have provided an additional answer to this problem. If a vagina can be constructed to the cervix, and if the cervix has an endocervical canal and is competent, the patient can bear children successfully. On the other hand, if the cervix has no canal, the problem still exists of endometrial proliferation in the uterus with hematocolpos. The solution may lie in the new in vitro fertilization techniques pioneered by the Jones Institute. If the uterus is kept intact and suppressive hormones are given to control endometrial proliferation, in vitro fertilization can occur after marriage and the potential for intrauterine pregnancy remains. Cesarean section can then deliver a normal pregnancy. For this reason alone, a vagina should be constructed and the uterus retained until such time as the desirability, advisability, and practicality of pregnancy can be determined.

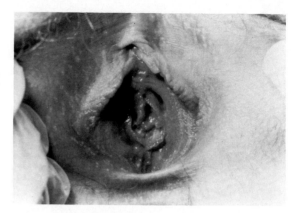

Figure 87–1. Congenital absence of the vagina. (From Sadove, R. C., and Horton, C. E.: Utilizing full-thickness skin grafts for vaginal reconstruction. Clin. Plast. Surg., *15*:443, 1988.)

A careful physical examination of patients with congenital absence of the vagina should reveal evidence of secondary sexual characteristics. Internal genital anatomy must be determined before surgery. The high incidence of associated renal tract anomalies makes intravenous pyelograms a necessity, and further studies such as ultrasonography, nuclear magnetic resonance, cystoscopy, and retrograde pyelography may be needed. Buccal smears for karyotype will differentiate between the testicular feminization syndrome and simple congenital absence of the vagina.

Surgical Techniques

FULL-THICKNESS SKIN GRAFTS

The authors have found full-thickness skin grafts for vaginal reconstruction to be superior for certain types of deformity. They reduce the amount of time required for postoperative stenting, allow reconstruction at an earlier age, and minimize the risk of vaginal stenosis by decreasing postoperative vaginal contraction. Full-thickness skin grafts grow proportionately with the remainder of the body. This technique is applied primarily to vaginal aplasia, but is also useful in cases of male to female transsexualism, unsuccessful transsexual operations resulting in vaginal stenosis, and certain other intersex conditions and cases of iatrogenic disease.

When split-thickness grafts were used to construct the vagina, the cavity needed to be stented, dilated, and used sexually over a period of years to prevent stenosis. Therefore,

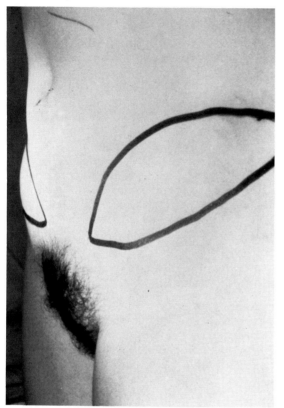

Figure 87–2. Bilateral inguinal donor sites for full-thickness skin grafts, which are later closed primarily. (From Sadove, R. C., and Horton, C. E.: Utilizing full-thickness skin grafts for vaginal reconstruction. Clin. Plast. Surg., 15:443, 1988.)

in the past, vaginal reconstruction was not recommended until the patient was planning marriage. The diminished stenosis rates of the authors' technique allow vaginal reconstruction at an earlier age. It is recommended that congenital absence of the vagina be treated anytime after puberty when the anomaly is recognized. The patient can then have the psychologic reassurance that she is externally normal as she develops into adulthood.

Preoperatively, a full mechanical and antibiotic bowel preparation is made. Full-thickness skin grafts are obtained from the lateral hairless groin areas bilaterally or from the gluteal crease. The groin donor site may extend from the pubis, parallel to the inguinal ligament, to beyond the lateral line (Fig. 87–2). The donor sites are closed primarily. All extra fat is removed from the undersurface of the grafts which are sutured together over a stent. The stent is carved

from a block of foam rubber and placed in a condom. Commercially available stents do not appear to conform well to the internal contours of the new vagina. The end of the condom is left open to facilitate its placement in the neovagina. The patient's labia are sutured to the lateral thigh skin to expose the introitus. A V-shaped, inferiorly based incision is used to dissect a flap made of introitus mucosa. This is later inserted into the new vaginal cavity and sutured to the grafts. The flap prevents a circular scar contraction at the opening of the vagina.

The new vaginal pocket is dissected above the rectum and below the bladder to the peritoneal cavity (Fig. 87–3). The cavity is made with blunt and sharp dissection so that an ample vaginal size is established. Care must be taken to avoid injury to the urethra and rectum. A finger in the rectum helps to identify the proper place for dissection. A catheter in the urethra assists in identification of the urethra, to avoid injury. The inferiorly based V-flap of vaginal mucosa is turned inward into the new cavity, and sutured as far cephalad as possible. The foam rubber stent covered by the full-thickness grafts is then inserted into the new tract, and the proximal open edge of the skin graft is sutured to the vaginal mucosa and the V-flap with 3-0 interrupted sutures. The labial tissue is sutured together with two 2-0 nylon mattress sutures to prevent extrusion of the stent and graft. Suprapubic urinary drainage

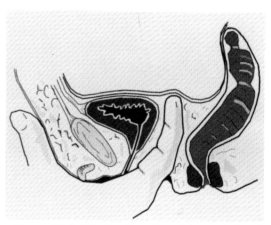

Figure 87–3. Site for dissection of the vaginal cavity, between the rectum and the bladder, extending to the peritoneum. (From Sadove, R. C., and Horton, C. E.: Utilizing full-thickness skin grafts for vaginal reconstruction. Clin. Plast. Surg., 15:443, 1988.)

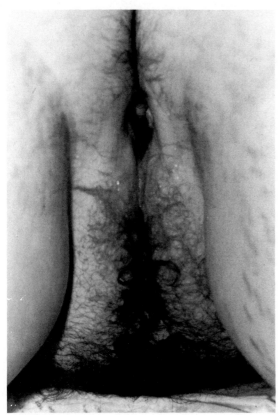

Figure 87–4. Postoperative appearance of vaginal reconstruction with full-thickness skin grafts. (From Sadove, R. C., and Horton, C. E.: Utilizing full-thickness skin grafts for vaginal reconstruction. Clin. Plast. Surg., *15*:443, 1988.)

is used instead of urethral catheter drainage to prevent pressure necrosis of the urethra.

Bed rest is prescribed for four or five days. On the fifth day the patient is returned to the operating room where, under general anesthesia, the stent is removed, the cavity is cleaned and irrigated, and the grafts are inspected. The stent is replaced and held stationary with a firm girdle. The labia are not resutured. After the first dressing change, most patients tolerate subsequent changes without anesthesia. The patient is given instructions on stent removal, daily sitz baths, and povidone-iodine (Betadine) douches and then discharged to continue this regimen.

After the first month, a stent of balsa wood covered with a condom or hollow acrylic is given to the patient to wear at night for three months. A trial period with total removal of the stent is then suggested. After the full-thickness graft is stabilized, there is no further need for stenting (Fig. 87–4).

SPLIT-THICKNESS SKIN GRAFTS: MCINDOE TECHNIQUE

Preoperative preparation and intraoperative dissection are the same as for full-thickness grafts. In this technique, however, a full dermatome drum of split-thickness skin is taken from the buttock or lateral hip area. The thickness is usually 0.016 or 0.018 inch. The graft is sewn with its epithelial surface around a vaginal stent. The patient is kept at bed rest for seven days. Once confident of self-care, the patient is discharged. Sexual intercourse is permitted after six weeks. The patient is instructed to wear the stent continuously for at least six months, except during intercourse and douches.

INTERMITTENT PERINEAL PRESSURE: FRANK TECHNIQUE

In the Frank technique, intermittent perineal pressure is applied with vaginal dilators graduated in size to create and stretch the vaginal canal. The smallest dilator is placed at the dimple between the anus and the urethra, and pressure is applied until the patient feels mild discomfort. The pressure is relieved and then applied again. This process is continued over a period of weeks until the largest vaginal dilator can be introduced and worn comfortably. Independent corroboration of the success of this procedure is not widespread.

INTESTINAL FLAPS

Intestinal segments have been used in the creation of a vagina with varying degrees of success; portions used have included the small intestine, ascending colon, sigmoid colon, and sigmoid and lower rectum.

The patient should be in the hospital two days before the operation in order to prepare and sterilize the bowel adequately. With the patient in a lithotomy position, a vaginal tract is first dissected from the perineum into the peritoneum and the tract widened laterally. When hemostasis is satisfactory, the vaginal tract is packed and the abdomen opened. The sigmoid is generally mobile enough to allow a satisfactory vascular pedicle to develop. With proper planning, an adequate length of intestine (12 to 15 cm) can be isolated, an oblique end to end anastomosis performed, and the bowel segment drawn through the vaginal tract. The patient is returned to a lithotomy position. The end of the bowel is scalloped to gain additional room, and then attached to the introitus.

Complications and Comparisons

Failures with the split-thickness technique are frequently due to hematomas, resulting in graft loss, or early removal of the stent by noncompliant patients. This causes excessive contraction, decreasing the size of the cavity.

Ortiz-Monasterio and associates (1972) reported good results in 17 out of 21 reconstructions with the split technique. Of 32 patients who underwent the McIndoe operation (Thompson, Wharton, and Te Linde, 1951) satisfactory results were noted in 81 per cent; there were three rectovaginal fistulas, two urethral sloughs, and one postoperative hemorrhage. Garcia and Jones (1977) reported satisfactory results in 41 out of 43 patients treated with the split technique. Cali and Pratt (1968) noted seven complications and ten patients who required reoperations out of 123 patients; of 93 individuals who responded to questions about sexual function, 84 (90 per cent) said that function was satisfactory.

Complications of the split-thickness technique include stenosis, loss of the graft, rectovaginal fistula, and ureterovaginal fistula.

Squamous carcinoma has been reported in vaginas reconstructed from skin grafts. Careful yearly follow-up examination is recommended to monitor the graft for any signs of malignant degeneration.

The advantage of using a portion of the intestine to line the vaginal canal is that there is no need for frequent dilatation or stent wearing. The disadvantages of intestinal transfers include excessive mucus formation, especially with grafts from the small intestine, and a mortality rate between 1 and 2 per cent.

The disadvantages of the Frank technique of intermittent perineal pressure include the need for prolonged, periodic dilatation, and often inadequate results (the vagina being too short in depth).

The full-thickness graft technique is an advance beyond the split-thickness procedure. The latter technique requires stenting for periods of up to one year, and has a tendency for contracture when the stent is removed or when the patient does not have vaginal intercourse.

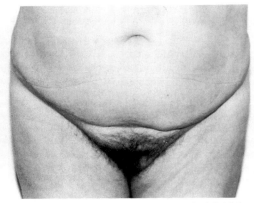

Figure 87–5. Appearance of donor sites for full-thickness skin grafts in the inguinal crease. (From Sadove, R. C., and Horton, C. E.: Utilizing full-thickness skin grafts for vaginal reconstruction. Clin. Plast. Surg., *15*:443, 1988.)

The favorable qualities of full-thickness skin grafts, well known in eyelid, hand, and hypospadias surgery, are the abilities to grow with the patient and to resist contracture. The same principle applies in the vaginal area. Once the vaginal tract is established with a full-thickness graft, the vagina does not contract; it grows at the rate of the remainder of the body and does not require prolonged stenting or care. Significantly, the small linear scars from the bilateral inguinal donor sites are much more esthetically acceptable than the scars in the split-thickness donor sites in the thigh or buttocks (Fig. 87–5). The size of donor sites required and their exposed locations create significant problems for the patient. Also, split-thickness donor sites have pigmentation irregularities in exposed areas (Fig. 87–6). There is an additional

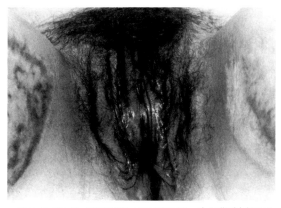

Figure 87–6. Unsightly appearance of split-thickness donor sites in the thighs, demonstrating pigment and contour irregularities. (From Sadove, R. C., and Horton, C. E.: Utilizing full-thickness skin grafts for vaginal reconstruction. Clin. Plast. Surg., *15*:443, 1988.)

risk of hypertrophic scar formation when split-thickness grafts are used.

Full-thickness skin grafts are superior for certain types of vaginal reconstruction. Their advantages include decreased contraction, a shorter period of postoperative stenting, correction at an earlier age, a lower risk of vaginal stenosis, and a cosmetically more acceptable donor site. In addition, the patient has the psychologic reassurance that she is normal as she develops through puberty and adulthood.

VAGINAL RECONSTRUCTION AFTER ABLATIVE SURGERY

History

Early Greek and Roman references to attempts at formation of the vagina relate largely to congenital absence. Although congenital agenesis of the vagina is rare, recurrent carcinoma of the cervix and pelvis after radiation therapy, radical surgery, or a combination of these remains a significant problem. Up to one-third of all patients treated for cervical cancer develop a recurrence, and in most the process is totally confined to the pelvis. Exenterative surgery for pelvic malignancy has been more useful in modern medicine, and in spite of the radical surgery necessary, the operative mortality rate remains low. The recent success of radiation therapy has decreased the need for exenteration. The plastic surgeon is invaluable in helping to repair the defects created by this extirpation. Radiation therapy, with resultant fibrosis and decrease in blood supply, further complicates reconstructive efforts in this area. Bulky, highly vascular flaps transferred to this area fill the pelvis and offer the greatest chance of successful primary healing.

Surgical Techniques

In 1953 Conway and Stark reported on the use of random gluteal and thigh pedicle flaps after radical pelvic surgery for carcinoma and irradiation. Pratt and Smith (1966) described the use of sigmoid loop for vaginal reconstruction following ablative gynecologic surgery. The large gluteal flap that had previously been delayed was rotated into the perineal defect. This procedure was not used primarily at the time of resection. The donor site of the gluteal flap was closed with a split-thickness skin graft.

Many methods have been proposed to repair these large, resulting defects. The authors consider it necessary to bring in a blood supply through a myocutaneous flap and reconstruct the vagina at the same time as the pelvic defect is covered. The use of immediate vaginal reconstruction fills the pelvic floor, and decreases the incidence of postoperative infection and small bowel obstruction. Delayed techniques for vaginal reconstruction can result in extreme difficulty in trying to dissect the space and plane without injuring the bowel that has become adhered to the adjacent pelvic walls and structures. The use of myocutaneous flaps decreases the morbidity and mortality rates of the original procedure and ensures a much smoother postoperative course.

Patients with a vulvar defect from extensive leukoplakia or carcinoma also are candidates for the use of myocutaneous flaps. To pull the tissue lateral to the defect into the vagina, where hair becomes an irritant and the introitus is destroyed, is no longer adequate for reconstruction. The use of a gracilis myocutaneous flap or an inferiorly based rectus abdominis myocutaneous flap has become routine in repairing large labial defects.

The gracilis myocutaneous flap is commonly employed for lower pelvic defects seen after total pelvic exenteration and abdominal perineal surgery. The low axis of this flap does not always allow transfer into the upper pelvis. It does, however, extend with confidence to the prominence of Si. The transverse and vertical rectus abdominis myocutaneous flaps add a high arch of rotation and allow them to obliterate massive dead space in high pelvic reconstruction. The rectus abdominis myocutaneous flap is supplied by the deep inferior epigastric vessels. The axis of this flap is determined by the location of these vessels and is usually transferred as a pure island flap through the posterior rectus sheath, rather than through the midline. The flap can be tubed to make a vagina, or the rectus abdominis muscle alone can be used as a muscle flap when the cutaneous segment is not needed. This flap can be used to reinforce suture lines in bladder sphincter repair, fill dead space to aid the surgical correction of incontinence, and produce an elevation of the mons in females with exstrophy. The gracilis myocutaneous flap has a high survival rate in the authors' experience. The rectus abdominis flap is even more reliable; it is larger and reaches higher positions in the pelvis, but it does require a laparotomy to insert into the pelvic defect. The gracilis flap can be used to correct a vesicovaginal fistula or to correct labial and lower vaginal deformities without the need for a laparotomy. Closure of both donor areas is not difficult, unless it is necessary to carry a large amount of rectus fascia with the muscle. The use of gracilis flaps or inferiorly based rectus abdominis myocutaneous flaps has been a significant advance in the treatment of pelvic and vaginal malignancy. To obliterate pelvic dead space and to repair massive defects of the perineum, groin, and pelvis, the plastic surgeon should be familiar with the advantages and disadvantages of these flaps in order to work as a team with the extirpative surgeon (see also Chap. 84).

GRACILIS FLAPS

McCraw and associates first reported the use of the gracilis myocutaneous flap for vaginal reconstruction in 1976. The patient is placed in a modified lithotomy position. The flap is outlined while the patient is awake; the anterior border of the flap lies on a line between the proximal adductor longus tendon and the distal semitendinosus tendon. The cutaneous portion of the flap extends 6 to 9 cm posterior to this line and is centered over the gracilis muscle. The flap is usually 20 to 25 cm in length and does not extend into the distal third of the thigh.

Elevation of the flap is begun proximally, first identifying the adductor longus tendon and its fascia. The adductor longus and adductor magnus muscles are then dissected, exposing the proximal neurovascular pedicle of the gracilis muscle. The neurovascular pedicle is surrounded by a layer of fascia that separates the adductor brevis and longus muscles. After identification of these structures, palpation is used to finally confirm the position of the gracilis muscle. The deep fascia that covers the adductor longus distally is incised to further outline the gracilis muscle. Together with the adjacent adductor longus and adductor magnus deep muscle fascia, the anterior border of the gracilis muscle is elevated. As the dissection continues inferi-

orly, the posterior margin of the sartorius muscle crosses the field obliquely. During elevation of the lower part of the flap, care must be taken to avoid injuring the saphenous nerve and vein. These structures should not be elevated with the flap.

Posteriorly, the semimembranous fascia is elevated with the flap. The dissection continues cephalad to the proximal gracilis neurovascular pedicle. The gracilis motor nerve, two muscular arteries, and four veins are identified. The vascular pedicles are then separated from the surrounding layer of areolar fascia. These vessels make up the rotational point or axis of the flap, which is located about 7 cm below the pubic tubercle. The deep fascia covering the proximal gracilis muscle is divided to complete the flap elevation. Division of the muscular origin is unnecessary. A subcutaneous tunnel is made under the skin bridge between the leg incision and the pelvic cavity. The flap is rotated posteriorly and passed beneath the skin bridge. The same procedure is performed on the other thigh.

The excess skin and fat is removed from the margin of the flaps, which are sutured into a pouchlike configuration, with the skin side facing internally. The new vaginal pouch is rotated caudally into the pelvic defect (Fig. 87–7). The tendinous ends are then anchored to the presacral fascia. The distal ends of the flaps become the apex of the vagina, and the proximal ends become the vaginal introitus. The new vaginal cavity is usually 13 to 15 cm in depth and 12 to 14 cm in circumference. The donor sites are closed primarily.

Occasionally, it may be difficult to center

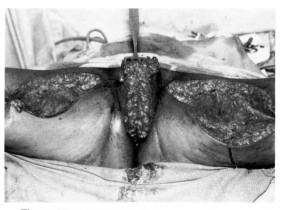

Figure 87–7. Paired gracilis flaps sutured together, skin surfaces opposed, before being rotated posteriorly into the pelvis.

the skin when outlining the flap because of thigh obesity, poor muscle tone, or inadequate hip abduction. An intraoperative solution for this problem was reported by Freshwater (1988). In McCraw's technique, a subcutaneous tunnel is made to pass the flap from the thigh to the perineal wound. To help identify the gracilis muscle, finger dissection from the perineal wound to the origin of the gracilis along the inferior pelvic ramus is performed. Because of the long and straplike configuration of the gracilis, its superior and inferior edges can be easily palpated through the tunnel. Accurate flap design can then be achieved from direct muscle belly palpation, bypassing the problems of obesity, poor muscle tone, or inadequate hip abduction.

Two other methods of intraoperative identification of the gracilis muscle have been reported. The first is to make a 5 cm transverse incision in the upper thigh at the proximal margin of the flap so that the progression of muscles from the abductor longus to the gracilis and to the semimembranosus can be seen. The second method is to identify the muscle at the distal margin of the flap through a second transverse incision to establish the position of the sartorius, gracilis, and semitendinosus and semimembranosus muscles from above, down. When both methods are used, the gracilis tendon can be elevated out of the distal portion of the wound. This causes the muscle to "bowstring" and outline the area of skin lying over the muscle. This also has the benefit of allowing further confirmation of the location of the gracilis muscle origin in the proximal transverse incision.

Vasconez, Bostwick, and McCraw (1974) also reported the use of rectus abdominis myocutaneous flaps to reconstruct the vagina after extirpative surgery. This technique has proved reliable and is the method of choice for reconstruction in many high pelvic defects.

STENOSIS

When radiation has caused such extensive scarring that the vaginal cavity is obliterated, it is possible to create a new vagina if the desired tract can be safely constructed. Unfortunately, adhesions in the pelvis make surgery for a new channel dangerous. Suturing the labia together to produce an external vaginal pouch has been recommended in these extreme cases.

If the patient is uncooperative or the stent is removed prematurely for any reason, stenosis, either complete or partial, may result. An attempt should be made to dilate whatever channel is present, but if this is unsuccessful, further surgery with reopening of the vagina is indicated. Full-thickness grafts should be used to resurface the cavity. Stent retention is mandatory for success.

VAGINAL FISTULAS

Trauma is the most common cause of vaginal fistulas. They may be due to unrecognized or unrepaired injury at the time of the surgical or gynecologic procedures. A high index of suspicion is recommended at the time of surgery to prevent fistula formation.

When located in the middle or distal third of the urethra, urethrovaginal fistulas may not be associated with incontinence, but the patient is likely to complain of vaginal discharge at the time of urination and of postmicturition dribbling.

The Symmonds and Hill (1978) technique remains popular. Rather than simply separating the urethra from the vagina and closing the two structures, a large U-shaped flap of vaginal mucosa containing the fistula is elevated. The fistula is closed, reinforced with pubococcygeus muscle or bulbocavernosus fat pad, and the flap is sutured to its original location.

When local tissues are compromised by radiation or scar, the interposition of a robust flap such as the gracilis or gluteal thigh flap between uroepithelium and the vagina helps to ensure primary healing. A well-vascularized flap reinforces the two separate suture lines, thereby preventing recurrent fistula formation.

Vesicovaginal fistulas are common subsequent to injury from cesarean section, hysterectomy, or unrecognized trauma at the time of previous surgery. Postoperative necrosis of small areas of bladder may occur secondary to the trauma or devascularization as a result of suturing. The possibility of multiple fistulas must always be considered.

Several excellent types of repair are popular. However, interposition of robust flaps as in the urethrovaginal repair is of particular benefit in cases of recurrence. The inferiorly based rectus abdominis muscle flap is ideally suited for reinforcing both bladder and vaginal walls after their repair.

LYMPHEDEMA OF THE VULVA

Just as there is lymphedema of the penis and scrotum in males (see Chap. 86), there can be lymphedema of the vulva in females. These patients have extremely large lateral protuberances of the vulva, the clitoral hood, and the vaginal tissues that cause excoriation, odor, and extreme physical displacement of the vaginal introitus. The cause of this condition usually is not similar to that of male lymphedema in the genital area, but rather relates to obstruction of the lymphatics in the labia due to chronic infection. Filariasis or leprosy are not found commonly in this area. Radiation and tumors are occasionally implicated, but the most common cause of lymphedema is idiopathic. The treatment for lymphedema of the labia is simple vulvectomy. If the vulva is so involved that the excision involves vaginal tissue, it is not desirable to pull the hair-bearing skin of the perineum into the vagina, because irritation will occur, and a chronic cyclic sequence of events will result in further lymphedema. Instead, reconstruction of the labia should be completed with either rectus abdominis or gracilis flaps so that circulation and lymphatic flow from a base outside the involved area can be secured. These myocutaneous flaps allow lymphatic distribution from the labial area to be taken into the circulation of the flap to bypass the obstructed labial area.

EXSTROPHY

There are peculiar problems with the escutcheon in females born with exstrophy of the bladder. Patients with exstrophy have displaced hair, a bifid clitoris, and an abnormally wide introitus with the labia minora and majora displaced; they frequently desire esthetic improvement in the contour of the area (Fig. 87–8). The umbilicus must be reconstructed. The wide-splayed pubic bones cause a depression in the mons area that may be visible through clothing. This is particularly true in dancers and individuals who must wear clothes that adhere to the pelvis.

W-flaps can be created to bring the laterally displaced hair over the superior portion of the pubic midline, but these are not always necessary in females. Wide excision of the midline scarring to join the bifid clitoris and labia in the midline is more desirable; the

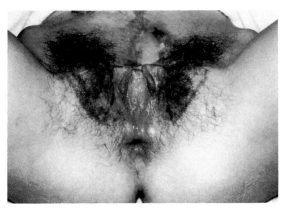

Figure 87–8. An exstrophy patient with displaced hair, midline scar, and bifid clitoris and labia minora.

wide introitus is thus reduced. As the scar progresses over the pubic area onto the abdominal wall, a large Z-plasty can be performed in the pubic hair-bearing area to break up the scar and produce a better mons prominence. Occasionally the patient desires more elevation of the mons; in this case a rectus abdominis flap can be used based on the inferior epigastric artery, and the muscle, without skin, can be transferred to the mons area to produce an elevation. If appropriate, a large bone graft can be taken from the iliac crest and secured to the pubic area bilaterally, to give contour to the pubic symphysis. The patient should be instructed about the possibility of vaginal delivery in case of pregnancy, because the bone graft may not expand like a normal pelvis. The authors are not familiar with cases of vaginal delivery in patients with epispadias or exstrophy who have had bone grafts to the pelvis. Cesarean section is probably indicated for these patients (see also Chap. 85).

REFERENCES

Abbé, R.: New method of creating a vagina in case of congenital absence. Med. Rec., *54*:836, 1898.

Baldwin, J. F.: The formation of an artificial vagina by intestinal transplantation. Ann. Surg. *40*:398, 1904.

Burian, F.: Autoplastie du Vagin au Moyen du Skin Inlay. Paris, l'Activité Scientifique et Medicale, 1935.

Cali, R. W., and Pratt, J. H.: Congenital absence of the vagina: long-term results of vaginal reconstruction in 175 cases. Am. J. Obstet. Gynecol., *100*:752, 1968.

Conway, H., and Stark, R. B.: Construction and reconstruction of the vagina. Surg. Gynecol. Obstet., *97*:573, 1953.

Fara, M., Vesely, K., and Kafka, V.: The reconstruction of vagina by thick graft. Acta Chir. Plast., *14*:17, 1972.

Frank, R. T.: The formation of an artificial vagina without operation. Am. J. Obstet. Gynecol. *35*:1053, 1938.

Freshwater, F.: Personal communication, 1988.

Garcia, J., and Jones, H. W.: The split-thickness graft technic for vaginal agenesis. Obstet. Gynecol., *49*:328, 1977.

Graves, W. P.: Operative treatment of atresia of the vagina. Boston Med. Surg. J., *163*:753, 1908.

Kanter, A. E.: Congenital absence of the vagina; a simplified operation with the report of one case. Am. J. Surg., *30*:314, 1935.

McCraw, J., Massey, F., Shanklin, K., and Horton, C.: Vaginal reconstruction using gracilis myocutaneous flaps. Plast. Reconstr. Surg., *58*:176, 1976.

McIndoe, A. H.: An operation for the cure of congenital absence of the vagina. Br. J. Obstet. Gynaecol., *45*:490, 1938.

Ortiz-Monasterio, F., Serrano, A., Barerra, G., and Ar-

aico, J.: Congenital absence of the vagina. Plast. Reconstr. Surg., *49*:165, 1972.

Pratt, J., and Smith, G.: Vaginal reconstruction with a sigmoid loop. Am. J. Obstet. Gynecol., *96*:40, 1966.

Sneguireff, W. F.: Zwei new Fälle von Restitutio vaginiae per Transplantationen Ani et Recti. Zentralbl. Gynäkol., *28*:772, 1904.

Symmonds, R. E., and Hill, L. M.: Loss of the urethra: a report of 50 patients. Am. J. Obstet. Gynecol., *130*:130, 1978.

Thompson, J. D., Wharton, L. R., and Te Linde, R. W.: Congenital absence of the vagina: An analysis of 32 cases corrected by the McIndoe operation. Am. J. Obstet. Gynecol. *74*:397, 1951.

Vasconez, L. O., Bostwick, J., and McCraw, J.: Coverage of exposed bone by muscle transposition and skin grafting. Plast. Reconstr. Surg., *53*:526, 1974.

Wells, W. F.: A plastic operation for congenital absence of the vagina. Am. J. Surg. 29:253, 1935.

88

Charles E. Horton
John F. Stecker
Gerald H. Jordan

Management of Erectile Dysfunction, Genital Reconstruction Following Trauma, and Transsexualism

MANAGEMENT OF ERECTILE DYSFUNCTION

Pathophysiology

The normal human penile erection requires the integration of neural, hormonal, vascular, and psychologic circuits. In order to understand the pathophysiology of erectile dysfunction as well as the diagnostic methods and surgical options for cure, it is necessary to examine the normal functioning of these circuits.

NERVOUS SYSTEM

The spinal nuclei responsible for erections are located in the intermediolateral gray matter at levels T10–L2 and S2–S4. Dorsal visceral efferent fibers from the S2–S4 nuclei emerge from the anterior root of S2–S4 and join sympathetic fibers to form the pelvic plexus, which branches to innervate the bladder, rectum, and penis. The autonomic cavernosal nerves (nervi erigentes) to the penis pass along the posterolateral aspect of the seminal vesicle and prostate and accompany the membranous urethra through the urogenital diaphragm. In the region of the bulbous urethra some fibers penetrate the tunica albuginea of the corpus spongiosum, while others enter the corpora cavernosa along the deep penile artery and cavernous vein. The terminal branches innervate the helicine arterioles and the erectile tissue within the corporal bodies. The dorsal nerve of the penis carries afferent sensory stimuli to the internal pudendal nerve, which runs with the pudendal vessels through Alcock's canal and the sciatic foramen, eventually terminating in the sacral cord segments S2–S4.

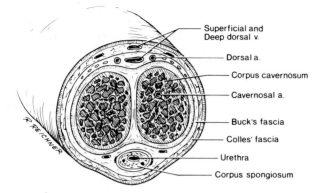

Superficial and
Deep dorsal v.

Dorsal a.

Corpus cavernosum

Cavernosal a.

Buck's fascia

Colles' fascia

Urethra

Corpus spongiosum

Figure 88–1. A cross sectional view of the penile shaft demonstrating the arterial supply and venous drainage of the penis.

VENOUS SYSTEM

A large network of subcutaneous veins runs on the dorsolateral surface between Colles' and Buck's fascia, and merges proximally to form the superficial dorsal vein. This vessel, usually single, drains most often into the left saphenous vein and less often into the right saphenous vein or both veins. The deep dorsal vein can be either single or multiple. Running beneath Buck's fascia and superficial to the tunica albuginea, this vein is formed from smaller branches from the glans penis (Fig. 88–1). The circumflex veins arise from the corpus spongiosum and empty into the deep dorsal vein. In addition, small emissary veins runs obliquely through the tunica albuginea of the corpora cavernosa and enter into the circumflex vein. Multiple communications do exist between the deep and superficial dorsal veins. One or two cavernosal veins run with the cavernosal artery within the corpora cavernosa and are formed by emissary veins from the proximal one-third of the penis. The cavernosal veins pass between the urethral bulb and crus of the penis, draining into the internal pudendal veins.

ARTERIAL SYSTEM

The internal pudendal artery, after giving off a perineal branch, enters the urogenital diaphragm as the penile artery. It branches near the urethral bulb into the bulbourethral artery, dorsal artery, and cavernous (deep) artery (Fig. 88–2). The bulbourethral artery enters the corpus spongiosum and passes along the urethra to the glans penis, giving off multiple branches. The dorsal artery courses between the deep dorsal vein and dorsal nerve, giving off three to ten circumflex branches that accompany the circumflex veins around the lateral surface of the corpora

cavernosa. The cavernous (deep) arteries arise from the internal pudendal or accessory pudendal artery. They enter the corpora cavernosa at the penile hilum and continue distally to the tip, giving off multiple branches (helicine arteries) supplying the cavernous spaces.

PHYSIOLOGY OF ERECTION

The lacunar spaces within the spongy erectile tissue of the corpora cavernosa are surrounded by smooth muscle. Stimulation of the cavernous nerve, either by erotic stimuli via the brain's limbic system or by tactile stimulation of the genitalia, results in active relaxation of the cavernosal smooth muscle. The neurotransmitters involved include acetylcholine released by cholinergic autonomic nerves and probably vasoactive intestinal polypeptide (VIP). In addition, the endothelial cells of the lacunar spaces may release prostaglandins and endothelial derived relaxation factor (EDRF), which further provide muscle relaxation. During erection, relaxation of the smooth muscle causes expansion of the lacunar spaces with a decrease in helicine artery resistance, thus increasing cavernosal blood flow. With filling of the spaces, the small venules within the erectile tissue become compressed, reducing venous outflow. With full erection, the subtunic venous plexus and emissary veins are compressed against the relatively noncompliant tunica albuginea, further restricting outflow to a minimum. Therefore, the increased penile blood flow and reduced venous outflow with erection is a passive phenomenon resulting only because of active smooth muscle relaxation produced by neural stimulation. In the flaccid state, the smooth muscle is contracted with loss of lacunar spaces. This muscle tone is maintained by the neurotransmitter norepinephrine. It thus can be seen that any pathologic condition involving arterial flow, lacunar endothelial cell smooth muscle function, or venous outflow could adversely affect erectile dynamics.

Evaluation of Erectile Dysfunction

Erectile dysfunction can be defined as the inability to obtain or maintain an erection suitable for the completion of the sex act to the satisfaction of both partners. Erectile impotence may be organic, psychogenic, or mixed. Obvious this distinction needs to be made in order to determine which patients may benefit from sex therapy and which may be candidates for a surgical or medical therapeutic approach.

A pragmatic systematic approach to the etiology of erectile impotence is required. Much information can be obtained from a detailed history and physical examination. Analysis of answers to a sexual function questionnaire (Table 88–1) is useful. Generally with organic impotence the patient describes an insidious onset that develops in association with the underlying causative systemic disease. A sequence of gradual deterioration of sexual function occurs, with an initial decrease in hardness and frequency of erections. Erections may be achieved but not maintained, and there is a progressive disappearance of nocturnal erections. Finally, a complete loss of erections occurs, even with masturbation. Generally, there is no loss of libido. In contradistinction, psychogenic impotence usually has an acute onset temporarily related to the particular emotional stress and generally intermittent in nature. There may be only limited or no impairment of erectile capacity with masturbation, and nocturnal penile tumescence is not affected.

The history should also include a complete review of systems with particular emphasis on the neurologic, genitourinary, endocrine,

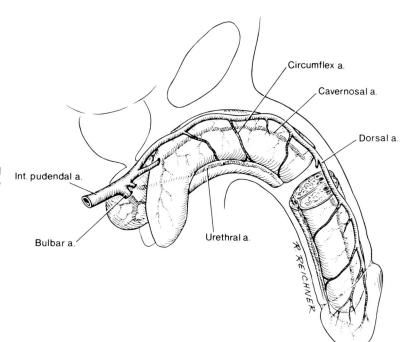

Figure 88–2. A longitudinal view of the penis showing the arterial blood supply.

Circumflex a.

Cavernosal a.

Dorsal a.

Int. pudendal a.

Urethral a.

Bulbar a.

R. REICHNER

The Trunk

Table 88–1. Sexual Function Questionnaire

1. Please describe in your own words your past sexual history and include in this description your current problem. How does this affect your life?
2. Describe your social and educational background (parents, marriage, children, social environment)
3. Do you have any erections at all?
   (a) Can you make a vaginal penetration?
       Yes ___ No ___ Rarely ___ Occasionally ___
   (b) Do you awaken with A.M. erection?
       If so, describe:
       Full ___ Partial ___ Poor ___
   (c) Does the quality of erection improve occasionally?
       Yes ___ No ___
   (d) Can you develop an erection with masturbation?
       Yes ___ No ___
4. Do you have orgasms?
   (a) If so, how are they achieved?
       Intercourse ___ Masturbation ___ Oral sex ___
       Others ___
   (b) Can you masturbate to orgasm but not achieve it with intercourse?
5. Are you concerned with the size of your penis? If so, what is the problem?
6. How strong is your desire for sexual intercourse?
   Slight ___ Poor ___ Fair ___ Strong ___
   Very strong ___
7. How strong is the desire of your wife or sexual partner for sexual intercourse?
   Slight ___ Poor ___ Fair ___ Strong ___
   Very strong ___
8. What is your partner's attitude about surgery to correct impotence?
9. Have you seen other physicians for this condition? If so, when and what therapy was given?
10. Have you consulted a psychiatrist for this problem? If so, please describe the results and give the name of the doctor.
11. Are you on any medications?
12. Have you had any major surgery? If so, what surgery? Describe the results.
13. Have you had a serious major illness or accident?
14. Is there any further information you feel is important to your problem?

From Stecker, J. F., Jr.: Surgical management of erectile impotence. In Paulson, D. F. (Ed.): Genitourinary Surgery. Vol. 2. New York, Churchill Livingstone, 1984, p. 590. By permission.

and cardiovascular systems. Special emphasis should be placed on any history of diabetes mellitus, lower extremity claudication, use of medications, and previous abdominal or pelvic surgery. Excessive alcohol intake may result in decreased libido, and chronic cigarette smoking can directly affect the cavernosal erectile tissue and result in organic impotence. Psychologic screening may be useful in eliciting underlying personality disorders or depression, or in helping to differentiate organic from psychogenic impotence. Beutler, Scott, and Karacan (1976) found the Minnesota Multiphasic Personality Inventory (MMPI) beneficial. Comparing patients' responses with those of patients with a defined psychopathologic pattern, the personality profile could be developed. In most of these patients, differentiation between psychogenic and organic impotence could be defined.

Physical examination should include examination of the penis for Peyronie's disease or hypospadias with chordee, which, because of resultant pain and angulation, may make intercourse impossible. Signs of reduced testosterone or elevated estrogen (e.g., gynecomastia, testicular atrophy) may explain reduced libido. Palpation of femoral pulses and examination of the lower extremities for ischemic disease are important. Neurologic examination should be undertaken if disease is suspected. Examination of the prostate may lead to a diagnosis of carcinoma.

Laboratory evaluation should include a complete blood count with differential and SMA-18 to rule out renal failure or systemic disease (e.g., cirrhosis, pernicious anemia). A glucose tolerance test is absolutely essential, since 50 per cent of patients with diabetes mellitus have a problem with erectile potency regardless of the duration or severity of the diabetes. In addition, about 5 per cent of patients with undiagnosed diabetes mellitus present with impotence as the primary complaint.

Endocrine problems are occasionally associated with impotence. Hyper- and hypothyroidism may be associated with loss of libido and decreased potency. Serum testosterone levels reflect the status of the hypothalamic-pituitary-testicular axis. Episodic daily fluctuations of serum testosterone within the normal range (300 to 1000 mg/dl) are common, and unless the testosterone value is below normal (300 mg/dl) no endocrine pathology should be suspected. However, if the serum testosterone level is below normal, the serum follicle stimulating hormone (FSH), luteinizing hormone (LH), and prolactin levels should be assayed.

Urinalysis and urine culture may identify those cases of urethritis, prostatitis, or cystitis that result in painful ejaculation and decreased sexual desire.

The most objective test of erectile potency, and one that usually allows differentiation of organic from psychogenic impotence, involves the measurement of noctural penile tumescence (NPT). Silicone mercury transducers are placed around the base and distal shaft of the penis so that changes in penile circumference with erection can be graphically recorded. As shown by Karacan, Scott, and Solis (1977), the normal adult male has three to five erections per night that occur with the stage of rapid eye movement (REM) sleep. Electroencephalographic (EEG) monitoring illustrates the periods of REM sleep and can usually be correlated with the appearance of erections. Changes in penile circumference, as well as the frequency and duration of erections, can be calculated. Generally, a deflection of greater than 15 mm in both the base and tip probes that is sustained for 10 to 15 minutes is considered a normal nocturnal erection. Fisher, Shiari, and Edwards (1977) quantitated results in two groups of patients with either organic or psychogenic impotence and found that T_{max} (maximal erection in millimeters) was four times greater in psychogenic impotence, and the frequency of occurrence of T_{max} was three times greater in these same patients. When T_{max} occurs, it is important to awaken the patient so that both the investigator and the patient can assess the turgidity of the erection. Measurement of nocturnal penile tumescence is accurate in about 80 to 90 per cent of patients in differentiating organic from psychogenic impotence.

The causes of organic impotence are myriad. They basically may be divided into systemic, endocrine, vascular, genital, neurologic, postsurgical injury, and drug-related causes (Table 88–2).

Erectile impotence occurs in 40 to 50 per cent of adult male diabetics and is apparently unrelated to the duration or severity of the diabetes. The pathology may involve corporeal smooth muscle myopathy or impairment in the release of EDRF.

Renal failure may result in reduced libido and impotence. Testosterone levels are low in patients on dialysis, but replacement of testosterone in these patients is of little value and actually may have an adverse effect on sexual potency. Recently it has been shown that prolactin levels are increased in renal failure, and this may explain the impotence and its lack of response to testosterone. Renal transplantation, if successful, restores potency as well as normalizing serum prolactin and testosterone levels.

Chronic ethanol injestion resulting in cirrhosis causes a decrease in circulating free testosterone, possibly secondary to a reduced level of gonadotropin hormone–releasing hormone. Gynecomastia, testicular atrophy, and reduced libido occur.

Endocrine disorders affecting the hypothalamus, pituitary, thyroid, adrenal, and testes can be associated with erectile impotence. Spark, White, and Connolly (1980) showed

Table 88–2. Causes of Organic Impotence

Systemic	**Neurologic**
Diabetes mellitus	Spina bifida
Renal failure	Spinal cord compression
Cirrhosis	Tabes dorsalis
Scleroderma	Multiple sclerosis
	Parkinson's disease
Vascular Disease	Pernicious anemia
Leriche's syndrome	
Bilateral renal transplantation	**Postsurgical or Postirradiation**
	Sympathectomy (bilateral lumbar)
	Retroperitoneal node dissection
Genital Disorders	Repair aortic aneurysm
Priapism	Radical prostatectomy or prostatocystectomy
Chordee	Abdominoperineal resection
Peyronie's disease	Radiation for pelvic carcinomas (prostate, bladder, etc.)
Epispadias-exstrophy	
Balanitis-urethritis	**Injuries**
	Penile
Drugs	Membranous urethral disruption
Ethanol	Spinal cord trauma
Sedatives	
Tranquilizers	**Endocrine**
Antihypertensives	Pituitary tumors
Parasympatholytics	Adrenal hyper- or hypofunction
Antiandrogens	Hyper- and hypothyroidism
Psychotropic agents	Hypogonadism (first or second degree)
Nicotine	

From Stecker, J. F., Jr.: Surgical management of erectile impotence. *In* Paulson, D. F. (Ed.): Genitourinary Surgery. Vol. 2. New York, Churchill Livingstone, 1984, p. 592. By permission.

that 37 of 105 patients with impotence (35 per cent) had abnormalities of the hypothalamic-pituitary-testicular axis. However, most of these patients had been diagnosed previously as having pituitary tumors (19 of 37) and had been initially referred to an endocrine clinic rather than presenting with the primary complaint of impotence. Generally, endocrine causes of organic impotence in most series are low. Vascular insufficiency of the pelvic vessels may result in impotence, as emphasized by Canning and associates (1963). Lower extremity claudication may also be present if the common or external iliacs are partially occluded (Leriche's syndrome). Ligation of both internal iliac arteries after renal transplantation usually also results in impotence. Genital disorders may contribute to sexual problems and are usually obvious on physical examination. Peyronie's disease, hypospadias with chordee, or chordee alone may cause painful angulation and distortion of the penile shaft with erection. The authors do not believe that the Peyronie's disease plaque interferes with the normal vascular engorgement of the corporeal bodies, or that it invades the dorsal neurovascular bundle. Nocturnal penile tumescence studies in most of our patients with Peyronie's disease did not demonstrate organic impotence. Any neurologic condition affecting the cerebral erection centers, the descending cord pathways, the sacral cord center, or the autonomic pelvic nerves can result in erectile dysfunction, as seen in multiple sclerosis, spina bifida, and cord compression.

Pelvic surgical procedures may produce impotence as a result of interference with the autonomic nerves. Radical prostatectomy or cystectomy, abdominoperineal resection, aortic aneurysm repair, and retroperitoneal node dissection may result in impotence. Injuries to the penis, disruption of the membranous urethra, or spinal cord trauma can be associated with erectile impotence. Drugs that may interfere with normal sexual activity are listed in Table 88–2. Ethanol is probably the most common offender, acting as a central nervous system (CNS) depressant as well as decreasing serum testosterone levels. Sedatives and tranquilizers also suppress the CNS and reduce libido. Antihypertensive agents may affect erectile ability by their sympatholytic action or effect on receptor sites. Propranolol hydrochloride (Inderal), a beta blocker, may also cause impotence. Antiandrogenic agents can block the action of testosterone on androgen receptor sites in the hypothalamus as well as peripherally. Psychotropic agents, including antidepressants, phenothiazine derivatives, and monoamine oxidase inhibitors, may depress potency, libido, and ejaculation. Nicotine from cigarette smoking can cause peripheral vasoconstriction as well as damage to the endothelial cells within the erectile tissue, thus contributing to erectile dysfunction.

If the NPT study suggest an organic pattern, more exhaustive testing can be carried out to determine the exact etiology by isolating a problem with arterial inflow, venous outflow, or the erectile tissue smooth muscle. Vasoactive drugs (phentolamine, papaverine) injected directly into the corpora cavernosa produce sustained erections in most patients with organic impotence, and can also be employed with dynamic measurements of arterial inflow, venous outflow and penile pressure changes occurring with erection. Lue and associates (1985) used a duplex ultrasound scanner with pulsed Doppler to measure changes in the diameter of the cavernosal artery that occur with papaverine-induced erection. Penile blood flow could be assessed, and in patients with a poor erection and minimal changes in penile diameter, blood flow found to be low could indicate large or small vessel arterial occlusive disease. Direct measurement of intracavernosal pressure changes after papaverine injection can also demonstrate poor arterial inflow. If saline is then infused into the corporeal bodies to maintain a pressure flow equilibrium, measurement of pressure and the rate of pressure fall after the infusion is discontinued can be used to determine whether there are venous leaks. Further information can be gained by infusing contrast material into the corporeal bodies and observing the venous drainage with fluoroscopy. The authors employ these diagnostic parameters, but consider them indicated in only those patients who fail to demonstrate an erection with the injection of vasoactive drugs.

Treatment of Impotence

With recent advances in the ability to diagnose the pathophysiology of erectile dysfunction, the treatment options have expanded, but still can be classified as nonsurgical or surgical.

NONSURGICAL

Patients with depressed libido and evidence of reduced serum testosterone respond favorably to androgen replacement therapy, usually intramuscular injection of testosterone enanthate (Delatestryl). This assumes that other endocrinopathies associated with a reduced testosterone level have been excluded.

The pharmacologic erection program (PEP) has had widespread acceptance by patients with erectile dysfunction. A combination of papaverine and phentolamine is injected by the patient into the corpus cavernosum. Papaverine probably releases VIP, which in turn causes relaxation of the smooth muscle of the erectile bodies. Phentolamine (Regitine) causes an alpha-adrenergic blockade, further increasing penile blood flow. Approximately 75 per cent of the authors' patients experienced erections with sufficient rigidity to complete coitus successfully, and this parallels most investigators' experience. Patients who fail to achieve adequate erections with the PEP should be further evaluated to determine whether poor arterial perfusion or venous leaks are present that may require alternative surgical therapy (discussed later). Patients on the PEP need to be monitored for the development of subcutaneous fibrous nodules or plaques similar to Peyronie's disease, which may require cessation of the test. An additional complication is the development of priapism, which can be managed by perinephrine irrigations of the corpora cavernosa to produce detumescence.

Vacuum-assisted devices have achieved some success in producing erections. These are plastic cylinders fitted over the penis and connected to a pump that produces a vacuum in the cylinder, thus increasing blood flow into the penis. A rubber band is then placed at the base of the penis to maintain an erection.

SURGICAL

Newer diagnostic parameters have illustrated that patients with organic impotence may require one of three different surgical approaches, depending on the cause of the impotence. Although the mainstay of surgical therapy for impotence remains the implantation of a penile prosthesis, patients with venous leaks or poor penile blood flow may need a different approach.

Arterial Revascularization. Many different surgical approaches have been used in an attempt to increase penile perfusion, including ligation of the penile veins, anastomosis of the inferior epigastric artery to the dorsal vein (venous arterialization) with or without a fistula to the corpus cavernosum, or direct anastomosis of the epigastric artery to a corpus cavernosum. Generally the success rate has not exceeded 50 per cent, with even fewer long-term (more than one year) successes. The advent of dynamic infusion cavernosometry, cavernosography, and selected internal pudendal angiography helps to select patients who may benefit from penile arterial revascularization. As Goldstein (1986) has shown, candidates are usually below the age of 40 years without vascular risk factors (e.g., diabetes mellitus, cigarette smoking, hyperlipidemia, hypertension, a history of myocardial infarction) whose impotence may be related to previous pelvic trauma. In patients over the age of 50 with significant vascular risk factors, the occlusive disease can be diffuse, and revascularization procedures usually yield poor results. Goldstein (1986) used a microsurgical technique, anastomosing the inferior epigastric artery to the dorsal penile artery in an end to end fashion. Of over 200 patients, 80 per cent were able to resume normal coitus.

Surgery for Venous Leaks. One of the first surgical methods to correct impotence involved ligation of the deep dorsal vein of the penis. Wooten (1903) and Lydstrom (1980) reported cure rates of around 50 per cent. The success rate can be enhanced with the use of dynamic cavernosometry and cavernosography to identify patients with either the congenital presence of excessively large veins draining the corpora cavernosa (primary impotence), or abnormal communications between the corpora cavernosa and the glans penis or corpus spongiosum. However, venous incompetence may be a secondary manifestation or symptom of underlying primary disease. Patients with endothelial cell damage within the erectile tissue, as seen in diabetes mellitus, atherosclerosis, cigarette smoking, elevated cholesterol levels, and hypertension demonstrate venous incompetence and yet do not respond well to venous ligation. Therefore, patient selection for ligation or removal of the deep dorsal vein should be limited to those with primary impotence, or those who have secondary impotence with large venous leaks without the underlying diseases listed above. Success rates following surgery are reported to be 75 to 80 per cent. An infrapubic (midline or lateral) approach allows exposure of the deep dorsal vein from just proximal to the glans to just under the pubic bone. If cavernosal or crural veins are found to leak, the suspensory ligament is detached from the pubic bone, thus allowing better exposure of these veins.

Penile Prostheses

Regardless of the type of prosthesis used (semirigid or inflatable) the goal of penile implantation surgery is to provide a penis rigid enough for vaginal penetration, and to ensure coitus that is satisfactory to both patient and partner. One of the earliest surgical attempts was undertaken by Bergman, Howard, and Barnes (1948), who implanted a rib graft. However, success was short-lived because the rib was reabsorbed. Goodwin and Scott (1952) were the first to report the use of synthetic (acrylic) implants placed in a pocket between the corporeal bodies. Later, Beheri (1966) pioneered the technique of placing the implants into each corpus. The use of Silastic in construction of the penile prosthesis was proposed by Pearman (1967). Small and Carrion (1975) reported a new prosthesis different from its predecessors in that it was formed of a silicone exterior with a silicone sponge interior, allowing it to be pliable and molded with a curved base. A similar prosthesis but with a hinged proximal portion was developed by Finney (1977). Semirigid malleable prostheses have also been developed by American Medical Systems (AMS) and the Mentor Corporation. The most recent modification, the Omniphase by Dacomed Corporation, is a nonhydraulic prosthesis that can be converted from the flaccid to the erect state by activating an internal cable system. This pulls a series of polysulfane segments together, with resulant rigidity. Lengthening the cable separates the segments, with consequent flaccidity. Activation and deactivation result by having the patient bend his penis down 120 degrees. This prosthesis must be placed through a subcoronal route since it cannot be bent for insertion.

Scott, Bradley, and Timm (1973) developed an inflatable prosthesis in an attempt to mimic tumescence and detumescence more closely. Many modifications have been made; the current product consists of triple-ply cylinders with a silicone inner and outer layer and a Dacron polyester woven fabric in the middle. The cylinders are connected to an inflate-deflate pump placed in the scrotum. A reservoir containing water and contrast material is placed in the retropubic space and connected with nonkink tubing to the pump. The advantage of this type of prosthesis is that it allows a fairly natural erection when inflated and a normal-appearing flaccid penis when deflated. Mentor Corporation has also developed an inflatable device, a recent advance being the elimination of the reservoir so that the fluid is now contained within the inflate-deflate pump within the scrotum. Also, Bioflex is used in producing the prosthesis rather than silicone; this material is apparently resistant to rupture or the formation of aneurysms. Finally, self-contained inflatable cylinders without a separate reservoir or pump have been developed by both Surgitex (Flexiflate) and AMS (Hydroflex). Both prostheses incorporate a prefilled cylinder with a nondistensible inner chamber. Compressing a distal tip pump within the cylinder transfers fluid from the outer to the inner chambers, resulting in rigidity of the cylinder. Deflation of the Flexiflate involves bending the prosthesis; increased pressure causes fluid to leave the inner chamber. With the Hydroflex, a deflate ring must be depressed while bending the cylinder.

SURGICAL TECHNIQUE

Selection of the prosthesis should involve a detailed discussion of the advantages and disadvantages of the various prostheses with the patient. The following guidelines are useful in allaying apprehension and patient misconceptions:

1. The prosthesis will not make the penis larger.
2. The prosthesis will not in itself produce glans rigidity.
3. No expansion of penile girth can be expected with the malleable, semirigid, and self-contained inflatable prostheses.
4. Orgasm and ejaculation will not be affected by the surgery.
5. Patients may continue to develop some natural erection around the prosthesis.
6. Mechanical failures can occur with the inflatable prosthesis.

The usual operative approaches for placement of the penile prosthesis are infrapubic, penile, penoscrotal, or perineal. These are selected on the basis of the type of prosthesis used, the familiarity of the surgeon with the approach, and the patient's circumstances. Regardless of the prosthesis and approach selected, certain preoperative and operative features remain the same:

1. Patients should be started on a broad-spectrum antibiotic (e.g., cephalosporin) one to two hours preoperatively, which is continued for eight to 12 hours postoperatively.

2. Patients should be shaved in the operating room and a povidone-iodine (Betadine) preparation used.

3. An antibiotic solution should be used for soaking the prosthesis and irrigating the wound.

4. Overdilatation of the corporeal bodies must be avoided.

5. A diagnosis of lower urinary tract outlet obstructive disease (benign prostatic hypertrophy, stricture) should be eliminated before implantation.

6. A 24-hour indwelling Foley catheter should be inserted.

7. There should be no activation of the prosthesis and no intercourse for four to six weeks.

Whether implanting a semirigid or an inflatable prosthesis, the authors routinely use an infrapubic approach extending from the base of the penis to or above the pubis (Fig. 88–3). However, if the patient has undergone

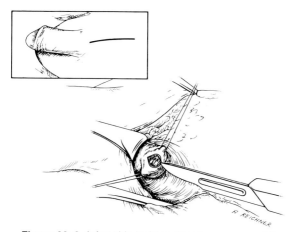

Figure 88–3. Infrapubic incision *(inset),* exposure of the corpus cavernosum, and placement of a 1.5 to 2.0 cm. incision through the tunica to expose the underlying erectile tissue. (From Stecker, J. F., Jr.: Surgical management of erectile impotence. *In* Paulson, D. F. (Ed.): Genitourinary Surgery. Vol. 2. New York, Churchill Livingstone, 1984, p. 594. By permission.)

previous surgery in the suprapubic or infrapubic area, a perineal or penile approach may be preferred; postoperative problems are reported to be minimal. Small (1978) uses a vertical perineal incision, the advantage being that the urethra is visualized, thus avoiding injury to this structure. Barry and Seifert (1979) advocated a vertical midline incision on the ventral shaft of the penis ending at the scrotum, but it is better to avoid incisions on the penile shaft, if possible. With an infrapubic approach, the corporeal bodies are isolated with blunt and sharp dissection so that the tunica albuginea of each corpus is exposed for 2 to 3 cm. A dorsolateral exposure of the tunica avoids injury to the dorsal midline neurovascular structures. A longitudinal incision is made through the tunica in each corpus between two previously placed stay sutures, thus exposing the underlying spongy tissue (Fig. 88–3). A plane is developed just beneath the tunica albuginea proximally and distally, using the tips of the Metzenbaum scissors, which facilitate developing the future pocket for the prosthesis. Dilatation is then carried out with progressively larger Hegar dilators up to a size 10. Care should be taken that the pocket is developed completely to the tip of the corpora under the glans distally and to the crural attachment proximally, with only gentle pressure usually required. Since the various semirigid prostheses are narrow at the base, dilatation of the proximal corpora can usually be stopped at a size 7 to 8 Hegar dilator. Care must be taken not to perforate the crus. Selection of the appropriate prosthesis size is important. Small-Carrion prostheses are available in three diameters (0.9, 1.1, and 1.3 cm) and 13 standard lengths (13 to 21 cm). Selection of a satisfactory length is aided by measuring the length of the Hegar dilator needed to reach the glans tip plus the length to the crural attachment. If the Flexi-rod hinge silicone prosthesis is used, the rigid shaft length can be determined by subtracting 20 mm from the measurement from the symphysis to the midglans of the maximally stretched penis. The total length can be adjusted by trimming the flexible base of the prosthesis with scissors. Flexirod prostheses are available in 9 and 12 mm diameters with lengths of 70 to 130 mm. If the Omniphase prosthesis is used, a subcoronal (circumcising) incision must be made because the prosthesis cannot be bent. This device consists of an activator body, with a distal tip and a rear tip, and is supplied in diameters of 10 and 12 mm. Length adjustment is made by using appropriate proximal and distal tips determined by the measurement of the corporeal length. Regardless of the prosthetic selection, a proper fit is most important; the prosthesis should be snug and smooth and should not buckle or twist. Longitudinal incisions in the tunica albuginea of the corpora are closed with interrupted 3-0 Vicryl. Irrigation of the corporeal bodies with a genitourinary irrigant is accomplished before wound closure. Subcutaneous sutures are placed and potential dead space is obliterated. No drains are used, and the skin is closed, as desired, with staples. A urethral catheter is left indwelling for 24 hours and antibiotic coverage is maintained for 12 hours. Patients are usually discharged on the first or second postoperative day. Intercourse should be avoided for four to six weeks or until all edema and pain have subsided.

The hydraulically inflatable penile prosthesis was devised by Scott, Bradley, and Timm (1973). Modifications have since been introduced in refining the pump mechanism, reservoir, and paired inflatable cylinders. Because of problems with nonuniform erections and cylinder aneurysms, a Dacron fabric middle layer was added to the cylinders, thus limiting cylinder expansion to 18 mm in diameter. As previously mentioned, Mentor Corporation and Surgitek produce an inflatable prosthesis combining the reservoir and pump into one unit that is placed in the scrotum. These devices most closely approximate the normal physiologic erection in that the cylinders expand longitudinally as well as circumferentially, and the penis is completely flaccid in the noninflated state. The prosthesis can be implanted by either a midline or transverse infrapubic approach or via a scrotal incision. The authors prefer a vertical incision just above the penis (Fig. 88–3). The rectus fascia is divided longitudinally and the rectus muscle bluntly separated in the midline, allowing entrance into the prevesical space. A compartment is developed by blunt finger dissection, usually on the same side as the future pump placement. A Kelly clamp is placed through the fascia in Hesselbach's triangle to exit in the previously dissected compartment, and the reservoir tubing is grasped and brought out near the external inguinal ring. The reservoir, previ-

ously evacuated of air and empty, is introduced into the compartment and filled with 65 ml of Conray 200 and water solution, and the rectus fascia is then closed. The preceding steps are not required with the Mentor or Surgitek inflatable prosthesis because these do not include a separate reservoir. The dorsolateral aspect of each erectile body is exposed as described for the semirigid prosthesis. Tunnels are created through a 1.5 to 3 cm incision placed longitudinally in the tunica. Dilatation with Hegar sounds through size 10 is used to expand the tunnels. With the Mentor, Flexiflate, and Hydroflex, dilatation through size 13 is usually required because the cylinders are larger in diameter. The Furlow inserter is introduced into the tunnels proximally and distally to determine the exact length of the corpus, thus allowing the selection of the appropriate cylinder size (Figs. 88–4, 88–5). Measurements are made from the distal edge of the incision proximally to the corpus attachment to the ischium. If the proximal measurement is greater than 4 cm, rear tip extenders must be used to allow the cylinder collar to lie just at the tunica albuginea incision, thus preventing the cylinder tubing from coming into contact with the cylinder wall. Furlow (1979) and others have found that continuous contact with the cylinder tubing against the silicone cylinder wall eventually causes cylinder leaks in 15 to 20 per cent of patients. For example, if the proximal measurement is 8 cm and the total corporeal length is 18 cm, 4 cm of rear tip extender is needed, since the distance from the cylinder collar to the proximal cylinder tip is 4 cm. However, the total cylinder length

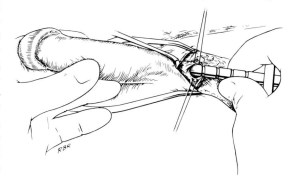

Figure 88–4. Use of the Furlow inserter to measure the distal corpus length from the distal edge of the incision to the glans tip. Stay sutures have been placed in the tunica. (From Stecker, J. F., Jr.: Surgical management of erectile impotence. *In* Paulson, D. F. (Ed.): Genitourinary Surgery. Vol. 2. New York, Churchill Livingstone, 1984, p. 596. By permission.)

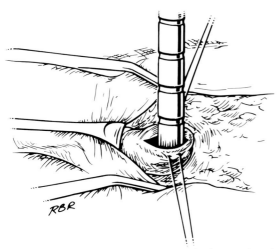

Figure 88–5. Measurement of the proximal corpus length with the Furlow inserter from the proximal incision edge to the ischial attachment. (From Stecker, J. F., Jr.: Surgical management of erectile impotence. *In* Paulson, D. F. (Ed.): Genitourinary Surgery. Vol. 2. New York, Churchill Livingstone, 1984, p. 596. By permission.)

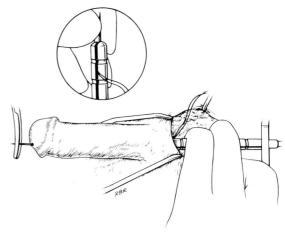

Figure 88–6. Placement of the Keith needle with cylinder strings into the tip of the Furlow inserter *(inset).* The Keith needle has now been passed through the dorsal glans by the Furlow inserter. (From Stecker, J. F., Jr.: Surgical management of erectile impotence. *In* Paulson, D. F. (Ed.): Genitourinary Surgery. Vol. 2. New York, Churchill Livingstone, 1984, p. 597. By permission.)

would then be increased by 4 cm, so 4 cm must be subtracted from the total length of 18 cm, thus providing for the use of a cylinder 14 cm in length with the 4 cm rear tip extenders added. Rear tip extenders are available in 1, 2, and 3 cm lengths; in this case two extenders (a 3 cm and 1 cm) are placed on each cylinder.

Insertion of the paired cylinder is easily accomplished using the Furlow inserter with a 2 inch Keith needle through which the cylinder strings have been passed (Fig. 88–6). Downward pressure on the glans ensures that the needle will not exit through the urethra or meatus. Gentle traction on the strings allows the cylinders to be inserted easily to the tip of the corpora under the glans (Fig. 88–7). The proximal nonexpanding portion of the prosthesis is inserted into each crus with the rear tip extenders, if needed (Fig. 88–8). Palpation of the proximal corporal crus ensures that the cylinder tip is not kinked or doubled on itself and extends to the end of the crus. The tunic incisions are closed with interrupted 2-0 Vicryl. A subcutaneous dartos pouch is developed low in the scrotum for the inflated-deflate mechanism (Fig. 88–9). An Allis clamp is placed just above the pump to hold it in place in the scrotum so that all tubing connections can be made. Right-angled connectors are used to attach the pump and cylinder tubing near the base of the penis subcutaneously (Fig.

88–10). The reservoir tubing is connected to the pump with a straight connector, avoiding kinks and excessive tubing length. The quick connect connectors are used if the patient is undergoing his first implantation. For a revision, plastic connectors doubly tied with 2-0 prolene are employed. The prosthesis is then activated three to four times to ensure proper function, and the wound is treated with a genitourinary irrigant. The wound is closed with 2-0 chromic, 2-0 plain catgut, and skin sutures. The prosthesis is left completely deflated. Drains are not placed unless the patient is markedly obese or moderate oozing is noted. In these instances, a subcutaneous Jackson-Pratt drain can be used to advantage for three to five days. Irrigation of the Jackson-Pratt drain twice daily with a genitourinary irrigant until the drain is removed reduces possible infection. A Foley catheter is

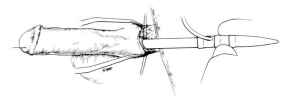

Figure 88–7. The cylinder is guided into the corpus pocket by gentle traction on the cylinder strings. Two rear tip extenders are shown. (From Stecker, J. F., Jr.: Surgical management of erectile impotence. *In* Paulson, D. F. (Ed.): Genitourinary Surgery. Vol. 2. New York, Churchill Livingstone, 1984, p. 597. By permission.)

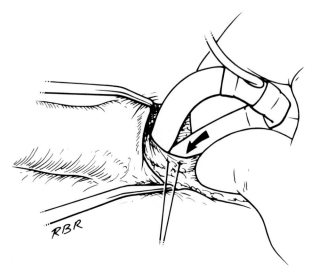

Figure 88–8. The proximal portion of the cylinder with rear tip extender is inserted into the proximal corpus pocket. (From Stecker, J. F., Jr.: Surgical management of erectile impotence. *In* Paulson, D. F. (Ed.): Genitourinary Surgery. Vol. 2. New York, Churchill Livingstone, 1984, p. 598. By permission.)

inserted and left for 24 hours. Antibiotic coverage is maintained for 12 to 24 hours postoperatively. No attempt is made to activate the prosthesis in the immediate postoperative period. Proper positioning is maintained by daily downward pulling of the pump so that it will not migrate upward in the scrotum. Patients usually return in four to six weeks for instruction in inflation and deflation of the prosthesis. They are told to inflate the prosthesis once or twice daily and leave it inflated for 10 to 15 minutes. Close observation of the following recommendations will help prevent complications:

1. Use pre- and postoperative prophylactic antibiotics.

2. Soak the prosthesis in a solution of genitourinary irrigant.

3. Avoid the introduction of air or blood into the prosthesis.

4. Clamp the tubing with silicone-shod instruments only.

5. Do not overdistend cylinders or reservoirs during filling.

6. Place the pump low in the scrotum.

7. Avoid sharp angles and kinks in the tubing and connectors.

RESULTS AND COMPLICATIONS

In order to assess the rate of success and possible complications, it is necessary to categorize penile prostheses into three groups: semirigid, inflatable, and self-contained inflatable.

Wound infections, prolonged pain, and hematoma may be seen with all three types of

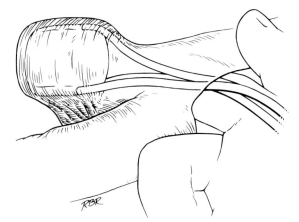

Figure 88–9. The pump is placed in a subcutaneous Dartos pouch in the lowermost portion of the scrotum. (From Stecker, J. F., Jr.: Surgical management of erectile impotence. *In* Paulson, D. F. (Ed.): Genitourinary Surgery. Vol. 2. New York, Churchill Livingstone, 1984, p. 598. By permission.)

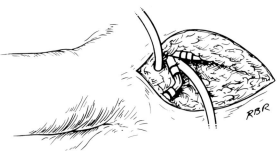

Figure 88–10. A straight metal connector has been used to connect the pump and reservoir tubing. A right-angled connector is shown connected to one cylinder tube and the pump tubing. The two free tubes (the remaining pump and cylinder) will also be connected with a right-angled connector. (From Stecker, J. F., Jr.: Surgical management of erectile impotence. *In* Paulson, D. F. (Ed.): Genitourinary Surgery. Vol. 2. New York, Churchill Livingstone, 1984, p. 599. By permission.)

Table 88–3. Complications with Semirigid Prostheses

Wound infection
Erosion into urethra or glans
Prolonged pain
Hematoma
Penile edema
"SST" deformity
Paraphimosis
Difficult concealment

From Stecker, J. F., Jr.: Surgical management of erectile impotence. *In* Paulson, D. F. (Ed.): Genitourinary Surgery. Vol. 2. New York, Churchill Livingstone, 1984, p. 599. By permission.

penile implants, whereas other complications are seen only with semirigid prostheses (Table 88–3). Wound infections occur in 0.5 to 1 per cent of patients; they can be prevented by the use of pre- and postoperative prophylactic antibiotics and the genitourinary irrigant intraoperatively. If an infection develops that involves the prosthesis, it must be removed. Superficial wound inflection not communicating with the prosthesis can be managed in a routine fashion.

Urethral erosion or glans penetration is usually due to improper length or width of the prosthesis, with resultant pressure necrosis of the tunica albuginea or adjacent urethra. In addition, unsuspected perforation of the tunica albuginea can occur during vigorous dilatation of the corpora.

Prolonged pain, usually in the glans, may result from an incorrect prosthetic size, but usually resolves with time. Rarely, intercourse is too painful to pursue and the prosthesis must be removed. Choosing a size that is excessively long may result in a flexion deformity of the penis (intraoperative sizing of the prosthesis avoids this). Insertion of the prosthesis may sometimes be extremely difficult, particularly in patients with extensive erectile tissue scarring due to priapism, inflammation, or penile trauma. In this case the smallest diameter of prosthesis should be selected. It may be necessary to completely excise the scarred erectile tissue and create a new corpus, utilizing Gore-Tex graft material. Penile edema or hematoma usually resolve with only conservative therapy.

Inadequate concealment is less of a problem with the hinged Flexi-rod and Omniphase prostheses than with the Small-Carrion, but in most cases this can usually be managed with tight-fitting jockey shorts. Urinary retention may develop in patients with unsuspected outlet obstruction (benign prostatic hypertrophy, neurogenic bladder, stricture). An outlet problem should be eliminated before surgery. Transurethral surgery, if necessary (after prosthesis insertion), is usually impossible without the use of a perineal urethrostomy, and open prostatectomy may be the procedure of choice. The overall results from implantation of the Small-Carrion prosthesis are reported as either excellent or poor. An excellent result means that patients have satisfactory sexual intercourse without pain or flexion deformity. If, for reasons of infection, erosion, or pain, the prosthesis had to be removed, the result would be considered poor. Small (1978) reported 260 patients in 251 of whom there was an excellent result. Four required removal of the prosthesis, and the status of five patients is unknown. Kramer and associates (1979) reported a similar series of 76 patients in which an excellent result was noted in 69. Removal of the Small-Carrion prosthesis was necessary in seven patients.

The immediate postoperative problems after implantation of the inflatable penile prosthesis, either AMS or Mentor, are similar to those with the semirigid type. Scrotal hematomas need to be drained immediately, otherwise a thick capsule develops around the pump and makes inflation and deflation difficult. Generally, penile pain and scrotal tenderness gradually resolve, as does subcutaneous fluid accumulation. The prosthesis should not be inflated or deflated until pain and edema have cleared, usually after about four weeks.

Complications related to mechanical problems with the AMS prosthesis are gradually being eliminated as improvements are incorporated into the basic inflatable prosthetic design. Fluid leaks are usually the result of cylinder wear with thinning of the silicone and eventual rupture. The use of rear tip extenders and new cylinder modifications (a CX cylinder with a middle layer of Dacron fabric) reduces weakening of the cylinder wall by limiting expansion and preventing cylinder buckling, ballooning, or rupture.

Aneurysmal dilatation (ballooning) of the old non-CX cylinder is usually the result of a weak area in the tunica albuginea of the corpora. Once ballooning occurs, it continues, as silicone has a "memory." Correction requires replacing the defective cylinder, with excision of the thinned, weakened area of the tunica albuginea, and replacement with a dermal graft or Gore-Tex patch. Inflation of the cylinder should then be completely avoided for at least four weeks after surgery.

In an American Medical Systems (AMS) survey (1979) of 21 implanting surgeons involved in 1243 procedures, the success rate was reported to be 92 per cent; 7 per cent were failures and 1 per cent were of unknown status. Sixty per cent of the patients with failures were pending prosthesis repair for mechanical problems. Scott and associates (1979) reported that of 245 patients with implants between 1972 and 1977, 234 were able to use the device to their satisfaction. Furlow (1979) reported a similar experience in the Mayo Clinic's first 175 patients; 168 had normally functioning prostheses. The initial high mechanical failure rate (20 to 30 per cent) was reduced to 10 per cent in 72 patients in 1978, and recent patient analysis found mechanical problems in only 1 to 2 per cent. Patient partner satisfaction with the AMS prosthesis approached 89 per cent. Reasons for dissatisfaction included inadequate firmness, cylinder ballooning, spontaneous device reinflation, and pain, most of which were corrected by additional surgery.

No results have been noted for the Mentor inflatable prosthesis, because not enough time has elapsed for long-term follow-up. However, there are no reports of cylinder rupture or ballooning with the Bioflex cylinders. If strict attention is not paid to proper fluid adjustment at the time of surgery, the patient may complain of inadequate rigidity with inflation, or inadequate flaccidity with deflation.

Self-contained inflatable prostheses, both the Flexiflate (Surgitek) and Hydroflex (AMS) types were first introduced in 1985. Fishman (1986) reported results in 50 patients implanted with the Hydroflex, 35 having been followed for a mean period of 11 months. Thirty of 35 were satisfied with the appearance and function of the prosthesis. Some patients complained of difficulty inflating and deflating the device or of spontaneous reinflation. In patients who had had a previous IPP, most felt that the length and girth of the Hydroflex were inferior to the IPP. Similar complaints have been voiced concerning the Flexiflate. Also, with vigorous coitus, the Flexiflate may suddenly deflate. Both prostheses require more than one instructional session with the patient, since it can be difficult mastering the inflate-deflate mechanism.

GENITAL RECONSTRUCTION FOLLOWING TRAUMA

The necessity to manage genital trauma in the male predates man's earliest recorded history. The stigmata of these injuries, with the accompanying fears of pain, loss of function, or loss of life, represent a major threat. The subject of genital trauma in the male includes the obvious injuries to the penis, scrotum, and scrotal contents. The less obvious trauma to the urethra must also be considered.

The incidence of trauma to the genitalia in the civilian population has increased. The age of mechanization and its accompanying accidents for the most part account for the increased incidence. In the past, large numbers of patients sustained their injuries in combat. In ancient civilizations, genital trauma was part of combat, but amputation of the penis in vanquished foes was part of the ritualistic plundering process rather than the result of the battle itself. Genital injuries still constitute a major portion of the injuries seen in current combat. However, these injuries are the result of weapons designed to cripple and maim the enemy. The axiom that it takes five men to manage a crippled soldier as opposed to one to manage a dead soldier has unfortunately influenced the design of modern weapons.

Civilian genital injuries are usually the result of motor vehicle accidents or accidents sustained while working around heavy machinery. Farm machinery seems to pose a particular risk. Currently, a few other cases occur as a result of felonious assault. In certain populations and ethnic groups around the world, these injuries abound. Athletic injuries or attempts at self-emasculation make up the remaining causes of genital trauma.

Anatomy

The anatomy of the male genitalia is complex, especially in the scrotum where there are multiple fascial layers. However, the fascial layers of importance in external genital trauma are the dartos-Colles' fascia of the penis and scrotum, Buck's fascia of the penis, and Colles' fascia as it reflects over the deep urethral structures and genitourinary diaphragm. The "butterfly" hematoma, frequently seen as a late sign in trauma to the perineum and genitalia, vividly demonstrates the posterior reflection of Colles' fascia. The dartos fascia of the penis becomes contiguous with Colles' fascia in the scrotum and perineum and continues over the lower abdomen as Scarpa's fascia. This fascial structure anatomically determines the patterns of spread or containment of urinary extravasation, periurethral phlegmon, hematoma, or purulent material. The external spermatic fascia assumes particular import when there is infection in the subdartos space. Because this fascia closely envelops the testicles and cord structures, even with fulminant abscess formation in the subdartos space, the testicle and spermatic cord usually are viable and uninvolved.

The male urethra begins at the bladder trigone and terminates on the glans penis as the urethral meatus. The urethra is divided into four anatomic areas: the posterior urethra, consisting of the prostatic urethra and the membranous urethra; and the anterior urethra, consisting of the bulbous urethra and the penile or pendulous urethra. The prostate is fixed to the pubic symphysis by the puboprostatic ligaments. The trigone is in continuity with the prostatic urethra, which then becomes the membranous urethra as it penetrates the pelvic diaphragm immediately beneath the triangular ligament. Realistically, the pelvic diaphragm does not exist as an anatomic entity, but rather is the plane between the decussation of the corpora cavernosa posterior to the ligament and anterior to the transverse perinei muscles. As the urethra emerges from the diaphragm it becomes enveloped by the spongy erectile tissue of the corpus spongiosum. The entire anterior urethra is enveloped by either the erectile tissue of the corpus spongiosum or the erectile tissue of the glans penis. The fossa navicularis is that portion of the anterior urethra that is enveloped by the glans penis, and consists of a slight fusiform dilation of the distal urethra. The precise function of this dilated portion of the anterior urethra remains to be defined. It can be theorized that the similarity in configuration of the shape of the fossa with a jug choke of a shotgun suggests that the fossa serves to condense and shape the urinary stream as it departs the "bone" of the urethral meatus.

The association of urethral trauma with pelvic fracture is well described. In posterior urethral injuries, the prostatic urethra is classically described as being "plucked" off the membranous urethra like an apple off the stem. Usually, however, the injury occurs at the interface of the membranous urethra and the envelopment of the urethra by the corpus spongiosum. In prepubertal males, injury to the prostatic urethra is not uncommon. The protection of the pubertal prostate, however, makes injury to the adult prostatic urethra a rarity.

Culp (1977) classified injuries to the external genitalia into five categories: (1) nonpenetrating (blunt trauma, contusions, fractures of the corpora/urethra/testicle); (2) penetrating (incisions, punctures, lacerations, amputations—self-inflicted or traumatic); (3) avulsions (degloving injuries of the penis, traumatic, emasculations); (4) burns (thermal/chemical/electrical); and (5) radiation injuries (direct, lymphedema). Isolated injuries to the urethra must be treated as a separate category of genital trauma, although they frequently accompany other injuries to the genitalia; as such they are covered separately in this chapter. The occurrence of urethral trauma in association with other genital trauma must always be considered, however.

The general principles of management of genital trauma are identical to the principles of trauma management that apply elsewhere in the body. The genitalia contain structures that are richly vascular, and special attention must be given to the acute blood loss associated with these injuries. Likewise, the high incidence of the injury to the urethra in association with other injuries to the genitalia often compounds the acute care that is required. The unusual nature of the highly compliant fascial structures likewise makes the management of scrotal infections unique. In the scrotum and penis, infections tend not to remain localized as in other superficial tissues of the body but rather to "run" along the fascial layers. Thus, the necrotizing inflammations of the fascia literally spread before one's eyes.

The injured patient must be stabilized. Associated cardiopulmonary, perineal, and intra-abdominal injuries must be identified or ruled out. The patient with genital injuries associated with other injuries may present in shock. If there is a urethral injury, the monitoring of the resuscitative phase is somewhat complicated by the inability to place a urethral catheter for close measurement of urinary output.

Once the acute respiratory and hemodynamic factors have been stabilized, a detailed examination of the penis, scrotum, and scrotal contents must be accomplished. The urethral meatus must be examined for the presence of bleeding or bloody discharge. A rectal examination must be made with special attention to rectal tone, rectal and anal competence, and the location of the prostate gland.

After physical examination, further investigation includes contrast studies to accurately define the suspected injury, along with intravenous pyelography and cystography as appropriate to rule out associated urologic injury. Two basic tenets apply: (1) to find genitourinary trauma, one must suspect it and search for it; and (2) the aggressive diagnosis of such trauma is often far more important than its aggressive treatment.

The management of acute posterior urethral trauma is controversial and is influenced by the expertise of the physician who first encounters the traumatized patient. In most surgeons' hands, the safest form of acute management of posterior urethral trauma consists of the placement of a suprapubic catheter only. The others advocate a urethral catheter to serve as a guide if possible. Attempts at urethral stenting, however, should be made only by a skilled urologist in a stable patient. Several methods for accomplishing the placement of a stenting catheter are advocated by various urologists. With posterior urethral trauma, the prostate often is displaced well into the pelvis. As the pelvic hematoma resolves and the pubic fragments stabilize, the bladder and prostate descend back to their near-normal positions. With a urethral catheter in place, the descensus occurs; the catheter serves as a guide to alignment of the prostatic urethra with the anterior urethra. It is emphasized that neither a suprapubic catheter nor a urethral guiding catheter will serve to prevent stricture formation. To all intents and purposes, the formation of stricture is determined at the time of impact. Placement of urethral and suprapubic catheters serves only to limit further complications of the initial trauma. The urethral catheter must never be placed to traction. Traction serves no beneficial purpose and has the potential for damaging the bladder neck. Definitive reconstruction of the posterior urethra can then be accomplished four to six months after the initial injury. Reconstruction of the posterior urethra is covered later in this chapter.

Injuries to the anterior urethra are likewise managed with diversion to prevent further sequelae of the initial injury. Often a urethral catheter serves as an adequate diversion. The anterior urethra is very seldom completely disrupted. The attempt at placement of a urethral catheter should be made only after the extent of injury has been carefully documented with contract studies. Again, the expertise of the surgeon encountering the traumatized patient must be taken into account. Diversion via a suprapubic catheter is always appropriate for the acute management of anterior urethral injuries. A period of four to six months must then be allowed before definitive urethral reconstruction can be attempted. The anterior urethra, unlike the posterior urethra, can often be definitively managed with internal urethrotomy. The definitive management of anterior urethral strictures is discussed later in this chapter.

Nonpenetrating Injuries

Nonpenetrating injuries to the genitalia result from crushing or sudden deforming forces applied to the penis or scrotum. These forces can be associated with severe damage to internal structures without disruption of the epithelium of the skin. When the penis is injured, an injury to the urethra must be assumed to be present until evaluation rules out such an injury. Fortunately, injury to the urethra with simple contusion is unusual. Hematomas resulting from such injuries are usually confined by the dartos fascia.

Not uncommonly, Buck's fascia is disrupted along with the immediate underlying structures. Simple contusions of the penis are relatively easily managed with analgesia, ice packs, bed rest, elevation of the area, and oral enzymes to add hematoma reabsorption.

A fracture of the penis implies a disruption of the tunica albuginea of the corpora cavernosa; this often occurs during vigorous intercourse. Not uncommonly, however, a patient will offer a history of rolling over on his erect penis. When the injury is associated with intercourse, the patient often reports noticing a distinct snapping feeling and sound. He then notes the immediate onset of pain and swelling of the penis. Buck's fascia is commonly disrupted. It is not unusual for the fracture also to involve the corpus spongiosum or the urethra, and retrograde urethrography is part of the routine evaluation of suspected penile fractures. These injuries are infrequent, making up only one in 175,000 hospital admissions.

When there is only disruption of the corpus spongiosum, the literature has reported good results from either conservative observation or immediate exploration and repair. However, the authors have seen a number of patients whose history is compatible with a fracture of the corpus cavernosum, who were treated conservatively, and who subsequently developed severe chordee. Likewise, the literature reports a significant incidence of penile deformity after fracture of the penis. This deformity can be severe enough to cause disability with intercourse (Fig. 88–11). This chordee seems to result from the fibrosis of the spongy erectile tissue as well as the tunica and immediately adjacent structures. Immediate exploration is favored, with evacuation of the hematoma, debridement, and anatomic repair of the disrupted tunica albuginea. This immediate exploration seems to limit subsequent scar formation and attendant chordee. If the urethra is involved, management is clear, the best results being obtained from immediate exploration and repair of the urethra and corpora cavernosa. A urethral or suprapubic catheter serves as adequate diversion and must be kept in place for seven to ten days; suprapubic diversion is preferred. Antibiotics are used liberally in all patients with genital trauma.

After exploration, a small suction drain is placed for 24 to 48 hours in the space superficial to Buck's fascia but deep to the dartos fascia. After repair of the deep structures, a meticulous anatomic closure of all the superficial layers of the penis is necessary to prevent troublesome adhesions between the tunica albuginea and the skin. In addition, manipulation of the skin of the penis during the healing phase helps to limit these adhesions between the elastic, compliant penile layers.

Contusions of the scrotum are easily treated with bed rest, ice packs, analgesia, scrotal elevation, and oral enzyme preparations. Scrotal elevation can be accomplished with a Bellevue-type bridge or a scrotal support. The differentiation between a scrotal contusion and a fracture of the testicle can be difficult, since both injuries present in an identical fashion. Scrotal ultrasonography is helpful. With a scrotal wall hematoma (contusion), the testicular anatomy is preserved while the scrotal layers demonstrate a mixed echogenic pattern compatible with the hematoma. With a fracture of the testicle, there is virtually always an associated hematocele. The hematocele serves as a sonographic window, and not uncommonly the extravasated seminiferous tubules are clearly demonstrated. As a general rule, a subdartos hematoma presents posteriorly to the testicle with the testicle pushed anteriorly against the skin. With a fracture of the testicle, the hematocele fills the space anterior to the testicle. Immediate surgical exploration of a fracture of the testicle with evacuation of hematocele, debridement of the damaged tubules, and repair of the tunica albuginea of the testis greatly reduces the morbidity of these injuries. If the scrotum does not demonstrate preservation of the testicular anatomy, testicular fracture must be presumed and exploration should proceed.

Patients not uncommonly present in a delayed fashion after a fracture of the testicle. The old literature suggested that delayed exploration inevitably led to orchiectomy. The author's experience does not support this concept; patients have been explored as long as 21 days after injury with repair accomplished easily and long-term follow-up demonstrating satisfactory salvage of the testicle.

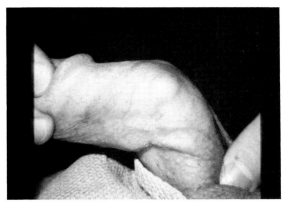

Figure 88–11. So-called "fracture" of the penis. The tunica is torn during trauma while erect. An unstable scar can result.

Penetrating Injuries

Penetrating injuries to the penis often involve the urethra, and all require exploration with irrigation of the area of penetration, removal of any foreign bodies or material, and an anatomic repair of the penile structures if possible. If the penis is amputated, replantation is favored. The ability to accomplish this is dependent on the time elapsed since amputation, the severity of injury to the amputated and nonamputated parts, and the care that has been given to the the amputated portion of the penis. If the amputating laceration is clean, if the remaining penis is relatively intact, and if the amputated portion is intact and has been cooled properly, replantation can be accomplished up to 16 to 18 hours after the trauma. The sooner replantation can be accomplished, however, the better.

With simple lacerations, primary closure is desirable, but (as with all wounds) if there is contamination, open dressing of the wound, drainage, and packing must be accomplished. Delayed primary closure should be performed when the wound is clean.

With replantation, meticulous anatomic closure of all layers of the penis must be accomplished. Reapproximation of the two dorsal arteries and the deep dorsal vein is a necessity; reapproximation of superficial veins is likewise desirable. The dorsal nerves of the penis begin as relatively substantial trunks in the area of the suspensory ligament. By the time these nerves reach the pendulous portion of the penis, they are arborized, and reapproximation of as many of these nerve branches as can be found gives the best functional result. Chronic preputial edema can occur after replantation. It is desirable, however, at the time of replantation to close the preputial or penile skin; if chronic edema results, excision at a later date is easily accomplished. Excision of the edematous tissue and coverage of the penis with a full- or split-thickness skin graft provides excellent functional and cosmetic results.

Purposeful emasculation in our culture fortunately is unusual. These patients often present in extremis owing to blood loss. Many times the amputated parts will have been disposed of. If the penis and testicles arrive with the patient and presentation has been prompt, microvascular replantation of all these structures should be undertaken. If the testicles are replanted, coverage by a primary closure of the remaining scrotum is optimal. If primary closure is not possible, the testicles should be placed in thigh pouches rather than being immediately covered with a split-thickness skin graft.

The penile and preputial skin derives its blood supply from the underlying deep structures. With replantation, revascularization of the penile and preputial skin is accomplished via the anastomosis of the dorsal penile arteries. On the other hand, the scrotum receives little blood supply from the deep structures. Dependable revascularization of the scrotal skin cannot be obtained by merely suturing it into place as a composite graft over the replanted spermatic cord structures.

In many cases, more skin than corporeal structures has been amputated. These cases are better managed by covering the exposed remaining corpora with a split-thickness skin graft. Primary closure in this situation often buries the remaining penis and it becomes nonfunctional. If the patient arrives without the amputated organs, primary closure or coverage must be accomplished. After hemostasis the penis can be closed in the same way as after an elective partial penectomy. Great care must be taken to create a widely spatulated neomeatus to prevent subsequent meatal stenosis.

Patients who have attempted self-mutilation are emotionally disturbed, but immediate surgery should not be delayed. Psychiatric care after surgery is essential, because many of these patients attempt to repeat or finish the job at the earliest opportunity. The patient with a known history of chronic psychotic disease may not be a candidate for replantation. An individual with an acute emotional decompensation, on the other hand, is a candidate, since the psychiatric disease is often short-lived and successfully treated. If in doubt, one should err by proceeding with replantation in as timely a fashion as possible.

The genitalia can also be harmed by human and animal bites. Because serious infections can occur from human bites, these wounds should not be closed. If necessary, the patient should be admitted to the hospital and appropriate antibiotic therapy instituted. The same principles should be followed with the occasional animal bite. Some animal bites can be serious, resulting in subtotal or total loss of the penis, scrotum, and testicles. Fournier in 1884 described a serious synergistic gangrene of the genitalia, an infection that spreads along superficial fascia and causes loss of the scrotal and penile skin. Often the testicles are not involved since they are protected by Colles' fascia. On bacteriologic study, cultures are positive for hemolytic streptococci and other bacteria such as *Staphylococcus aureus* and anaerobic streptococci. This syndrome is often associated with high morbidity and mortality rates. The infection should be controlled and a split thickness graft used to resurface the granulating area.

In larger trauma centers, penetrating injuries to the genitalia resulting from gunshot wounds are not unusual. Fortunately, these injuries generally occur as a result of small caliber, low velocity projectiles. Often, the patient is the victim of a jealous lover or girlfriend. In some cultures the genitalia seem to be the preferred target of felonious assaults of all kinds involving firearms. The testicles are often fractured beyond repair. Many of these patients are in extremis and have associated other pelvic and intestinal injuries; hence, repair of the testicles assumes a low priority.

In other cases, however, the testicles are reparable and reconstruction as for testicular fracture yields good results. As with all gunshot wounds, entry and exit wounds must be debrided. Copious irrigation of all bullet tracks must be accomplished. The repaired testicles must be drained and the bullet tracks packed. Broad-spectrum antibiotics are employed. A testicular nuclear scan is obtained on the fifth to seventh postoperative days to verify the viability of the repaired testicles. When there is infection or impaired viability, a sperm fistula almost always results. High velocity projections inevitably devastate the genital structures in their path. Realistically, management of the associated injuries to other pelvic structures will dominate the therapeutic procedures, and debridement of the genital structures is performed after the patient is stabilized.

Avulsion Injuries

Avulsion injuries of the genital skin frequently occur as the clothing becomes entangled in rotating machinery. The clothing twists and is stripped off, carrying the loose elastic skin of the genitalia with it. These injuries have also resulted from the use of suction devices for sexual arousal. Avulsion wounds can vary from a minimal laceration to injuries that are virtually emasculating. Because of the native elasticity of the genital skin, usually only the skin and dartos layers are avulsed, leaving the exposed corpora, urethra, and testicles. The competence of the urethra must be demonstrated, and a rectal examination performed to assess the anal sphincter. The avulsion usually occurs in an avascular plane, and profuse bleeding is seldom a problem.

Small avulsions can be managed as one simple laceration. Large injuries are treated by application of saline packs to the exposed areas. If there is clear demarcation between viable and nonviable skin, debridement with closure or coverage can be accomplished quickly. Ideally, closure should be accomplished within the first 12 hours. Usually, however, a clear demarcation is not obvious, and reevaluation after 48 hours will disclose the nonviable areas. Debridement can then be accomplished with skin coverage.

If the avulsion involves the penile shaft skin, debridement of the distal remaining penile or preputial skin to the area of a normal circumcision should be performed. This distal shaft skin is viable, but is prone to the development of chronic lymphedema in most cases. If the remaining skin is insufficient to close the wound, coverage can be accomplished with a split-thickness graft. Such grafts applied to the penis do not seem to contract and usually provide good functional coverage and cosmetic results.

If the avulsion is extensive and includes the scrotal skin, it has been recommended that the testicles be put into thigh pouches and the penis buried in a subcutaneous tunnel on the abdomen. The authors' experience shows, however, that neither the penis nor the testicles need be displaced from their normal anatomic position, since a split-thickness skin graft can be applied over all of these structures with good results. Some surgeons prefer a meshed graft over the scrotum with a nonmeshed graft on the penis. The meshing scars mimic the normal rugations of the scrotal skin. Before grafting, the testicles must be sutured together in the midline to prevent their migrating beneath the graft (Fig. 88–12).

Because with split-thickness grafts the numerous small vessels of the intradermal

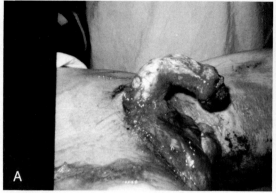

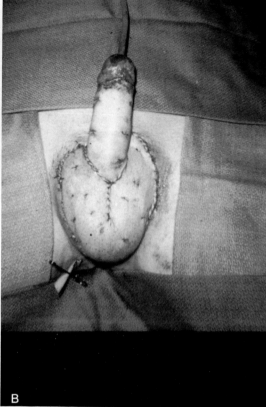

Figure 88–12. *A*, Penile and scrotal skin avulsion. *B*, Split-thickness grafts applied. *C*, After healing. Normal intercourse is possible.

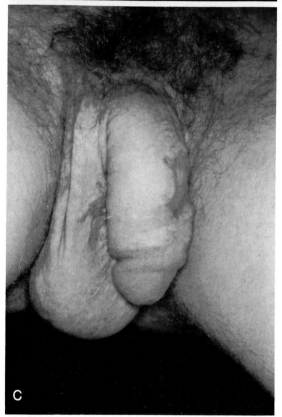

plexus are exposed to the graft bed, these grafts "take" in less than optimal situations. With full-thickness grafts, however, the less numerous vessels of the subdermal plexus are exposed to the graft bed, and hence the grafts often "take" only in optimal conditions. In the case of degloving injuries, the spermatic cords and testes are usually reliably healthy. Local skin flaps are not recommended for closure in these cases, because split-thickness grafts provide far better results. Diversion via a suprapubic catheter for approximately two weeks limits soiling of the bulky bolster dressings. In patients whose avulsions extend to near the anus, a diverting colostomy may also be required.

Because graft "take" generally requires 96 hours, patients are placed on strict bed rest for five days to diminish the chance of graft motion on the recipient bed. The bolster dressings are left in place for five to seven days. The patient's activities are severely limited for four to six weeks after grafting, by which time the graft is well established and can withstand the trauma of normal sedate activities. Patients are advised to refrain from intercourse for eight to ten weeks.

If the avulsion also involves the deep structures, i.e., the corpora or testicles, replantation is not an option. The injury damages the blood vessels and adjacent structures because of the "stretch before the snap" phenomenon that occurs. These patients require temporizing procedures with skin coverage and later penile and scrotal reconstruction.

The authors have treated a number of patients who have traumatic loss of the penis with free microvascular transfer flaps. At the time of flap transfer, microneural anastomosis to the remnant dorsal penile nerves creates an intact phallus with erogenous sensibility that is adequate for coitus. Currently in use is a radial forearm free flap for most cases of phallic reconstruction. The flap provides for a competent neourethra with the meatus located at the tip of the phallus. The patient can then void while standing. Care is taken during the dissection of the flap to preserve the lateral antebrachial cutaneous nerve. This nerve is anastomosed to branches of the dorsal penile nerves, thus allowing for subsequent erogenous sensibility. The radial artery is anastomosed to the deep inferior epigastric artery, and the accompanying vena comitans anastomosed to the saphenous vein or the deep inferior epigastric vena comitans.

The upper lateral arm flap has also been used for penile reconstruction. This flap has only a single vena comitans, which theoretically can be a problem for subsequent flap viability. In either flap, the urethra is formed on a lateral aspect of the flap. In the case of the radial forearm flap, the urethra is usually designed on the ulnar aspect, because this portion of the flap is usually less hirsute. The urethra is then tubularized with the epithelium toward the lumen. A strip about 1.5 to 2 cm is then deepithelized, which allows the remaining flap to be tubularized over the urethra with the epithelium outward. The "glans" is then formed by placing a small graft to create a coronal margin with the epithelium rolled to elevate the margin. Suprapubic diversion is employed with a small catheter per urethra to serve as a stent.

Avulsions can also accompany severe injuries that are tantamount to hemipelvectomy. The survival of these patients is critical and of first importance. Urinary and fecal diversions usually are always necessary in the initial treatment of these patients. If possible, one should allow the genital injuries to demarcate and then provide skin coverage. The degree to which erectile and urethral structures can be preserved significantly influences the patient's future.

Another injury that appears to have a classic presentation occurs when a person is run over by the wheels of a heavy vehicle. These injuries inevitably involve fractures of the pelvis and femur, and often a degloving injury of the lateral pelvis and upper thighs. The urethra may or may not be disrupted in association with the pelvic fracture. There inevitably is also a perineal laceration, which classically extends from the lateral anal verge anteriorly adjacent to the scrotum. The integrity of the anal sphincter is usually preserved, and the anus and rectal walls proper are seldom injured. The laceration extends into the ischial rectal fossa, and not uncommonly the surgeon can place the examining finger on the ischial tuberosity at the apex of the laceration.

Colostomy is always required. If the urethra is involved, suprapubic cystostomy is necessary. Care must be taken to examine the bladder closely at exploration, since intraperitoneal bladder rupture is not uncommon. This injury cannot be demonstrated before exploration without a good trainer cystogram. If the urethra is uninvolved as proved by retrograde urethrography, a Foley urethral catheter can be gently placed. Urethral catheterization need be continued for only a couple of days in the absence of a urethral disruption.

The perineal laceration should be packed gently. On about the tenth to 14th posttrauma days, the laceration is often cleanly granulated, and delayed primary approximation can be performed. The avulsion of skin from the lateral pelvis and thighs is often the tip of the iceberg, and severe underlying muscle damage becomes apparent two to three days after the injury. Complete debridement must be accomplished before any graft coverage is contemplated.

Burns

Emergency therapy for genital burns is similar to that for any burn. The genitalia can be dressed open with topical antibiotic creams or dressed by the closed method. A Foley catheter is required for monitoring during fluid resuscitation. The integrity of the urethra must be determined before placement of the catheter. If there is a urethral injury, no attempt at primary reconstruction should be made. Diversion can be accomplished via Foley catheterization through the area of injury or via a suprapubic tube, and maintained until the patient is allowed to void. If the urethra has been involved, voiding will occur through a urethrocutaneous fistula. Extensive debridement should be approached with caution as the erectile tissue usually is not reconstructable. When the burn surrounds the urethral meatus, meatal dilata-

tions instituted after discontinuation of the urethral catheter may help to prevent meatal stenosis.

Skin grafts to the penile shaft should be applied with the seam line placed on the ventral surface of the penis. In the past it was decreed that the seam line should be dorsal; however, it is cosmetically undesirable and is less easily visible if placed on the ventral aspect of the penis. If scars are associated with the suture line of the skin graft, they can be revised at a later date.

Chemical burns rarely involve structures deep to the skin. For the most part chemical burns, after copious irrigation with sterile water or saline, are managed in the same fashion as a thermal burn.

Electrical burns can create devastating tissue destruction. The electrical current is dissipated via the vessels, and extensive destruction of deep structures can occur despite the appearance of minimal skin loss and only superficial injury. In all cases an initial observation time of 12 to 24 hours is recommended. These patients all require suprapubic urinary diversion if the penis or the whole genitalia are involved. After the initial period of observation, the proximal limits of the deep tissue destruction can usually be determined and amputation and debridement to that point then accomplished. A nerve stimulator can be helpful in determining the viability of muscle. Later reconstruction can then be offered as the eventual situation becomes clear (Fig. 88–13).

Some authors recommend adding a weak acid to the irrigant in the case of a caustic burn. An acid burn typically looks worse in the initial period. A caustic burn, on the other

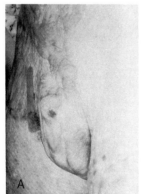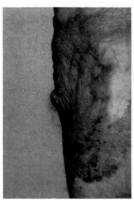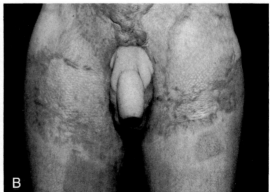

Figure 88–13. *A,* Electrical burn with loss of the penis. *B,* Microneurovascular reconstruction with a free flap. The patient has normal penile sensation.

hand, looks better early, but often converts to full thickness. Two particular chemical agents have specific antidotes. Hydrofluoric acid (HF) burns occur from industrial accidents, and are best treated with irrigation and subcutaneous injections of calcium gluconate into the wound areas. There is also a calcium gluconate paste that is produced for topical administration. Phosphorus burns are treated with calcium sulfite applied topically to the area of burning; this compound is nephrotoxic in large doses, and the patient must be watched closely.

Radiation Injuries

The genitalia can suffer radiation injury either from direct irradiation of the genitals or scatter radiation from treatment of structures in close proximity. Modern techniques of therapy have virtually eliminated scatter to the genitalia both by shielding and by the accuracy of delivery of the radiation.

At present the most frequent indication for direct irradiation of the genitalia is seen in young individuals with small (2 to 3 cm), superficial, noninvasive malignant lesions on the glans penis or coronal sulcus. Some patients refuse partial penectomy for larger or already metastatic lesions. Radiotherapy for this last group of patients can result in the significant complication of penile necrosis. Partial penectomy then becomes the procedure of choice.

Using small-field electron beam radiotherapy, the treatment of 2 to 3 cm superficial lesions is very successful and produces limited morbidity. Circumcision is mandatory before radiotherapy for the penis. An occasional patient who has undergone small-field electron beam radiotherapy to the penis combined with inguinal node dissection may have resultant chronic lymphedema.

Chronic lymphedema may follow radiotherapy to the genitalia and is seen after pelvic irradiation combined with lymph node dissection. The lymphatic channels themselves have remarkable tolerance to radiation, but perilymphatic fibrosis may obstruct the channels. Veins are easily injured by radiation. The combination of lymphatic obstruction and venous insufficiency causes chronic lymphedema.

The patient who presents after direct irradiation of the genitals with thickening and weeping of the skin is best treated conservatively. Therapy to improve the cosmetic appearance is not advised. Complications such as necrosis or gangrene require excision or, more frequently, partial penectomy.

However, the patient who presents with chronic lymphedema from pelvic lymphatic obstruction represents an entirely different situation. The use of full-thickness skin grafts or flap procedures is not recommended because of the frequent recurrence of edema. These patients can be managed successfully with excision of the edematous tissue to the level of Buck's fascia on the penis and the external spermatic fascia of the scrotum. The excision of the preputial skin must be carried distally to the coronal sulcus, obviating the development of a collar of edematous skin. The resultant defect then readily accepts a split-thickness graft (Fig. 88–14). The lack of the dermis layer prevents the recurrence of edema, and the split-thickness graft provides an excellent cosmetic result.

Other Injuries

Zipper injuries occur when the glans or prepuce becomes caught in the zipper teeth. The injuries are usually superficial and many require no therapy at all. The skin can be released by pulling the zipper apart. Several patients have presented late after a zipper injury with ulcerating lesions that are extremely painful. These ulcers culture *Staphylococcus aureus* and, if left untreated, can spread to the surrounding tissues. Treatment with sitz baths and antibiotics quickly halts the process and limits the eventual morbidity.

Foreign bodies in the genital area present

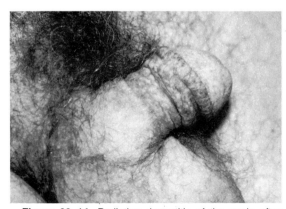

Figure 88–14. Radiation dermatitis of the penis after treatment for Peyronie's disease.

an interesting group of clinical problems. Pencils and other foreign bodies may be placed in the urethra, and other foreign bodies may be introduced through the skin (fragments of foreign materials and bullets). Occasionally, foreign bodies are placed circumferentially around the base of the penis and then cannot be removed because of distal edema. It may be necessary to give a general anesthetic before removal. Adequate evaluation after removal is important, and if necessary should include cystoscopy and proctoscopy. When rings have been placed around the penis, a general anesthetic is usually necessary, and manipulation of the ring with adequate soaping and oiling of the skin, or cutting of the ring, may be required. If industrial grade steel has been used in the ring, an industrial clamp may be used to crush the ring, which frequently shatters when adequate pressure is applied.

Rarely, a hair is concealed in an infant's diaper and wraps around the penis, causing constriction. Careful inspection should be made to diagnose and remove the hair. Partial amputation of the penis can result from such an incident.

In most cases, patients present with relatively minimal trauma. However, because of the complexity of the structures involved, minimal trauma can lead to significant disability later on. The process of erection requires correct functioning of the arterial, neurologic, and venous systems coupled with intact erectile bodies. The penis is composed of structures that are compliant and distensible to the limits of that compliance. These structures therefore tumesce in equal proportion to each other, allowing for straight erection. Relatively minimal trauma can upset this balance of elasticity and lead to disabling chordee. Likewise, relatively minimal injuries to the vascular erectile structures can cause significantly disabling spongiofibrosis.

The urethra is a conduit of paramount importance. The development of stricture is generally related to the nature of the trauma, but the extent of stricture and attendant complications are clearly functions of the immediate management. Overzealous debridement can greatly complicate subsequent reconstruction. A delicate balance must be struck between aggressive initial management and maximal preservation of viable structures.

Circumcision is one of the most commonly performed surgical operations. Approximately 55 per cent of American males were circumcised before 1985, although the incidence of circumcision is decreasing now. Many complications result from this operation. In the United States, circumcision is performed either with a mechanical device or by direct surgical excision.

The true incidence of complications from circumcisions is uncertain. They range from hemorrhage to catastrophic cases of total penile loss. These complications can be grouped into seven major categories: shortening of the shaft skin, meatal stenosis, urethral fistulas, partial or total loss of the phallus, psychologic grief caused by loss of the prepuce, and loss of preputial skin needed later to repair a congenital deformity such as hypospadias.

What appears to be inconsequential skin loss in the infant may become significant with growth. This loss may create a skin deficit and a contracting pull in one particular area, or may be associated with circumferential shortness of the entire shaft skin.

Therapy depends on the extent of the pathologic condition. If a simple tight band is present, a Z-plasty or scrotal or pubic flap can be used to correct linear noncircumferential tissue loss at the base of the penis.

Local flaps cannot correct extensive skin deficiency. When circumferential loss is severe, a graft is required (Fig. 88–15). Any circumferential flap or skin graft used for repair on the penis should be placed as distally as possible to facilitate drainage of underlying lymphatic tissue and prevent potential distal edema. When the scrotum is advanced abnormally distally onto the penile shaft with deficiency of penile skin, patients frequently complain of ventral tightness upon erection. In these cases, the scrotal skin can be retropositioned by the use of a Z-plasty or wedge excisions of the scrotum. In the usual short circumferential skin loss, a circumcising incision is made at the coronal sulcus and the unaffected skin retracted. The distal circumferential deficit is covered with a full-thickness skin graft. A donor site with the best color match and the least hair should be selected: the first choice is usually flank skin. All graft to graft suture lines should be on the ventral surface for the best esthetic result. A bolus dressing is used for five days and thereafter until the graft has "taken." A catheter for urinary drainage prevents the dressing from becoming soiled.

Scarring of the glans with adherence of the glans to the skin of the shaft is another

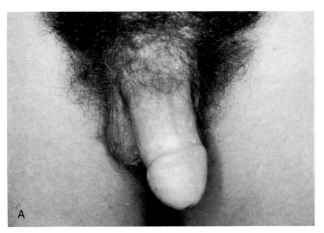

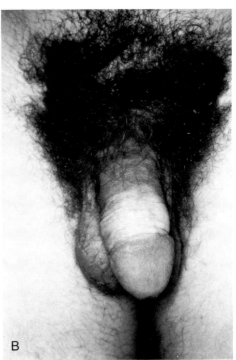

Figure 88–15. *A,* Tight penile skin after circumcision. *B,* Full-thickness skin graft applied to the distal penile shaft.

common complication, which may be associated with sensory loss. If the scar damage is localized, a full-thickness graft of "red" skin may be required. Full thickness grafts of scrotal skin are preferable because of its color. Excessive hair growth can be controlled with electrolysis. Postauricular skin occasionally possesses the necessary red color and may also be used. Small linear scar contractures between the glans and the shaft can be corrected with Z-plasties or local flaps. If the coronal sulcus is obliterated, a small full-thickness graft may be used to restore the sulcus.

Urethral fistula is a common complication of circumcision that usually results from the use of one of the mechanical devices. The ventral foreskin containing the anterior wall of the urethra is pulled beneath the crushing clamp, resulting in full-thickness loss of the urethra. These urethral fistulas are closed as previously recommended for hypospadias repair.

Partial or total loss of the phallus is the most tragic of all complications and also the most difficult to reconstruct. Even with only partial skin loss, the penis frequently heals with skin contracture, retractions, and scarring. If the existing corpora cavernosa can be advanced by freeing them proximally from the suspensory ligament and skin added,

greater length can be obtained. The amount of useable corpora cavernosa is difficult to determine, even with careful physical examination, and surgical exploration is frequently required. In infants, if the stretched length of the remaining penis is greater than 2 cm, the authors consider reconstruction with the remaining corpora rather than reconstruct a new phallus. Urethral repair is difficult, but is usually done by patch or tube grafting, if a graft can be covered with vascularized tissue. Occasionally, a microvascular free flap urethra may be required in reconstruction.

If erectile tissue of the corpora cavernosa is not present in newborns, consideration can be given to reassignment to the female gender. Immediate decisions are necessary, because later sex change is not desirable. In the past there was little option for such patients, since phallic construction was neither reliable nor desirable. With new operations for phallic construction, however, a sensate phallus with a fairly normal appearance can be reconstructed, and the conversion of these patients to the female gender is not now routinely recommended. These patients require psychologic counseling and may need early phallic construction at 6 to 10 years of age to allow them to meet their peers at school without psychologic damage. Later phallic construction may be required at a second stage after pubertal growth. However, the authors have seen these reconstructions in small children enlarge satisfactorily, and our present feeling is that it probably will not be necessary to perform a second total phallic reconstruction in these patients.

Many patients consult the plastic surgeon because they feel mutilated by circumcision and grieve at the loss of their prepuce. They consider that their body has been assaulted without their permission and they frequently voice anger at their parents and doctors. Sex therapy, not surgery, is the preferred treatment. Many patients accept the loss of their prepuce if the inability of reconstruction to return them to "normal" is adequately explained. Occasionally, a patient insists on reconstruction, which in rare circumstances can be attempted. Scrotal skin, using a bipedicle flap, has been recommended. Stretching by a ring on the skin of the penis, with a weight attached to the ring, has been utilized. More recently, the authors have used tissue expansion on the penis to produce excessive penile skin, which can later be fashioned into a prepuce. A V-Y advancement of the dorsal penile skin can be made, using the ventral skin to resurface the dorsal penis. A full-thickness graft can resurface the ventral denuded area, which is not easily visible to the patient (Fig. 88–16).

There have been reports of the circumcision of patients who had underlying congenital pathologic conditions, e.g., hypospadias. Tissue required for later reconstruction was removed. This frequency may reflect the use of inexperienced personnel, the intern or medical student, to perform this minor operation. It underscores the need for complete education of all personnel involved with neonates, both in recognizing congenital pathology and in understanding the requirements for correct repair. Many patients with congenital defects have been referred after circumcision with the usual notation: "We have cleaned up the area with a circumcision so that you can do the repair better." It is catastrophic that the well-meaning physicians did not realize they were discarding the tissue essential for later repair.

Reconstruction of the injured and multilated phallus requires not only knowledge of good surgical technique, but also an understanding of penile anatomy and physiology and patient psychology. Basic techniques of plastic surgery can be applied to solve each unique clinical problem of this area.

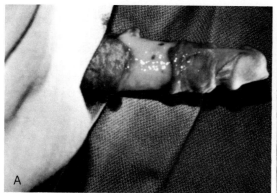

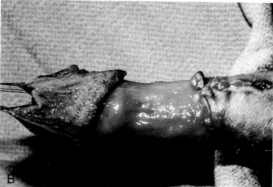

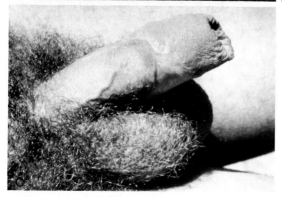

Figure 88–16. *A,* This patient was circumcised at birth. He desired foreskin reconstruction. *B,* Foreskin reconstruction using flaps and grafting. *C,* Final result.

Artificial erections are now commonly used to produce pathology noted by the patient upon normal erection. If a solution that is not easily tolerated by the body is accidentally injected (hypertonic saline), penile necrosis can result. Fibrosis of the vascular tissue inside the tunica may also be produced if irritating solutions are used in this space. Multiple artificial erections at surgery are recommended, but the nurse must be careful to inject only an isotonic solution (0.9 per cent saline) suitable for intravenous use into the penis.

Occasionally, patients wish to have their normal penis enlarged. Many substances have been used to inject into the soft tissue of the skin of the penis, paraffin and silicone being the two most common. Patients present with impotence, hypoesthesia, inflammation, and lymphedema. Ordinarily the penis is so disfigured from the injection, and the results of the weight of the injection causing distortion of the skin, that they are impotent and cannot insert the penis into the vagina.

Treatment of these patients is best carried out by total excision of the pathologic area. Ordinarily the entire skin of the penis has to be excised and the shaft resurfaced with either a split- or full-thickness graft. The silicone may be difficult to remove in its entirety, but most granulomas can be identified and reduced in size. Total excision is of course much better for the patient than leaving a foreign body in the wound and covering it with a skin graft.

TRANSSEXUALISM

Etiology

Transsexualism has been defined by Money and Gaskin (1970) as "a disturbance of gender identity in which the person manifests, with constant and persistent conviction, desire to live as a member of the opposite sex and progressively take steps to live in the opposite sex role full-time." The cause of this condition is unknown. Most authorities agree that there is such a condition and that no medication or psychiatric therapy is permanently helpful. For patients who are true transsexuals, sexual reassignment surgery is the best way to treat their problem at this time. The incidence of transsexualism has been reported as approximately one in 50,000. Male

to female transsexualism has been considered much more prevalent than female to male. This may not be accurate, since therapy was so much easier for the male to female patient, and the female to male patient was told of the difficulty of the surgery, which may have discouraged their conversion. More recent statistics show that the ratio of male to female and female to male transsexuals is approximately one to one. Now that newer techniques for phallus construction are available, the female to male transsexual desires the surgery to the same degree and in the same numbers as the opposite sex.

Transsexuals are normal people with normal chromosomes, with an unswerving conviction that they are members of the opposite sex. Homosexual individuals prefer sexual activity with the same sex. Psychopathic individuals exhibit bizarre, unnatural, abnormal behavior that is unacceptable to society. Transvestites wish to dress in the clothes of the opposite sex, but do not desire to convert to the opposite sex. Surgery for these individuals is contraindicated and should only be used in true cases of transsexualism. Cauldwell (1949) was the first in the United States to use the term "transsexualism." Harry Benjamin, an American endocrinologist, gave support to the theory of transsexualism and authored the first book describing this condition (Benjamin, 1966). He proposed that endocrine therapy be used for these individuals. The Harry Benjamin International Gender Dysphoria Association has been named for him and meets in various centers of the world to bring together psychologists, psychiatrists, urologists, plastic surgeons, general surgeons, gynecologists, and others interested in this disorder.

For centuries, an operation to correct vaginal agenesis has been known (see Chap. 87). McIndoe (1949) used split-thickness skin grafts for vaginal lining, and it was only necessary for Fogh-Anderson (1956) of Copenhagen to apply these principles to perform successfully one of the first documented sex reassignment procedures in 1952. Several types of vaginoplasty have been recommended by various authors. Bowel, dilators, split-thickness grafts, and full-thickness grafts all have champions. The authors have preferred full-thickness skin grafts.

The reconstruction of the penis is a much more difficult problem, however. To develop a technique by means of which an erection or a stiffness of the reconstructive phallus is possible, sensation is present, the urethra extends to the tip, and a normal shape and size of the penis and scrotum appear is much more difficult than to construct a vagina. Bogoras (1936) first used a tubed abdominal flap for phallus reconstruction. Until recently, there were abortive efforts to produce a sensate phallus by using scrotal skin flaps, by using vaginal lining to cover tubes, and by use of myocutaneous flaps. In the authors' center, we first started using microvascular free flaps with sensory innervation connecting the genital femoral and ileoinguinal nerves to the flaps, until the pudendal nerve was finally identified as the nerve of sexual stimulation for the patient. Since that time, we have been pleased with the innervated free flap and the pudendal nerve anastomosis with the nerve of the flap.

The first gender identity clinic was formed at Johns Hopkins University in 1963. Patient satisfaction was noted in such a high incidence of cases that this concept of forming a multifaceted health team to care for these individuals has been successful in many centers throughout the world.

It has been postulated that transsexualism may arise from a genetic or endocrine problem during prenatal or fetal development. This has not been proved. Other experts believe that the environment of child raising has more influence than genetic or endocrine problems. If a child notes aberrant family dynamics, a transsexual problem may exist. It is possible that both factors may influence the development of transsexualism. Because the diagnosis may be confusing, the etiology is unknown, and surgical treatment for this condition is irreversible, the physicians caring for this type of patient should be conservative in selecting patients for definitive sexual reassignment.

The Harry Benjamin Association has standardized guidelines for patients who may be surgical candidates and can be accepted into a program. There are no guidelines concerning cosmetic surgery in these patients. Augmentation mammoplasty, hysterectomy, oophorectomy, otoplasty, laryngeal sculpturing, body sculpturing, rhinoplasty, orchiectomy, mastectomy, may all be required by transsexual patients. These operations are not ordinarily regarded as being as complex as the irreversible sex change operation, and can be considered by the individual surgeon and the patient before the patient fulfills all the guidelines of the Association.

The Association recommends that six objectives must be met before a sex change operation is undertaken: (1) the patient must demonstrate a desire for sexual reassignment for at least two years; (2) a clinical behavioral scientist trained to deal specifically with transsexualism must make the diagnosis of gender dysphoria; (3) the patient must live and work exclusively in his or her chosen gender for not less than 12 months; (4) the patient must be under psychologic or psychiatric care for not less than six months before the surgery; (5) the patient must have hormonal sex reassignment and treatment for not less than six months before the surgery; and (6) throughout the evaluation process, peer review should be evaluated and the patient discussed by the appropriate clinicians. In the authors' clinic, preoperative consultation with a gynecologist, urologist, endocrinologist, psychologist, and psychiatrist is carried out.

With estrogen therapy, feminization of the body contours and breasts may occur. If desired, augmentation mammoplasty may be carried out using submuscular or subglandular positioning of implants. Surgical incisions may be inframammary, periareolar, or transaxillary. Reduction or osteoplastic rhinoplasty and otoplasty procedures are common in transsexuals. Patients with heavy hair growth often require electrolysis to remove body hair, particularly on the face. Sculpturing of the male thyroid cartilages may be necessary to form more female proportions. Mastectomy may be required in females. Some females who hate their breasts may have used binders so that the chest is scarred with repeated ulcerations and trauma due to the tightness of the binding. Hysterectomy and oophorectomy are frequently requested by the patient so that they will not have their menstrual periods and discharge from the vaginal area. These procedures allow the gender clinic to observe patients' reaction to surgery and to determine whether they are suitable candidates for the final sex change operation.

Hormonal therapy is usually given with slow release preparations of estrogens or endrogens. Medroxyprogesterone acetate (Depo-Provera) is administered every other week orally or perianally to male transsexuals; Depo-Testosterone is given to female transsexuals. This medication must be continued postoperatively. A complete endocrinologic study must be performed before placing these patients on the medication. They should be instructed about the potential hazards of long-term hormonal use. Many males develop enough breast tissue so that augmentation is not needed. Females on chronic androgen stimulation may have an enlargement of the clitoris to such a degree that they do not desire phalloplasty. The most common operation for female transsexuals is hysterectomy prior to phalloplasty. The inferior epigastric artery and veins and the rectus abdominis muscle must be preserved for subsequent phalloplasty surgery if the vascular anastomoses are to be used with these structures. A midline incision is the safest route to the uterus and ovaries. If a lower transverse incision is desired, this can subsequently be changed into a midline approach through the muscle fascia, and the epigastric artery and veins are protected.

Vaginoplasty

A one- or two-stage technique is usually advocated by most gender reassignment surgeons. Split-thickness skin grafts have been used for reconstruction of the vagina, but the disadvantages include marked contracture of the graft over long periods and a requirement that, to keep the vagina open, a stent be worn for several years after the surgery. The split-thickness skin graft donor site is also objectionable, although this technique has worked in hundreds of cases. The use of bowel for vaginal reconstruction has been advocated by many surgeons, particularly in Europe. There is a mucous discharge from a vaginoplasty with bowel, and the complication rate of this operation is, of course, much higher since invasion of the abdomen is necessary in order to obtain a bowel segment to be used for the vagina. Musculocutaneous flaps have been used for vaginal reconstruction after cancer surgery, but because the pelvic bone structures in transsexual patients leave little space for a vagina, the tissue required in a musculocutaneous flap is too abundant to make this technique worthwhile. Horton and associates (1977) described the use of full-thickness skin grafts to construct the vagina. These grafts can be taken from the groin area, which is relatively hairless, and the donor site can be closed in a transverse fashion, thereby producing a much more cosmetic defect for the patient than the split-thickness graft donor site. The full-thickness grafts are appropriately defatted and then formed around the vaginal stent, which consists of foam rubber covered with a condom. The penile urethra is preserved for approximately one-third of its length in the penis, and a penectomy is performed. The dorsal penile neurovascular bundle is identified and preserved. Orchiectomies are performed. All the penile skin is preserved and used to create the introitus. It is not adequate in length to create the vagina and the introitus, in the authors' opinion. The previously retained penile corporeal bodies or glands and urethra are brought through a hole in the flap and placed in a female position. In a plane between the prostate and the rectum, careful dissection is carried out to create a vaginal vault. A V-flap of posterior skin is inserted into the new vagina to avoid a circular contracting scar. Scrotal skin can be transposed posteriorly to construct normal-appearing labia (Fig. 88–17).

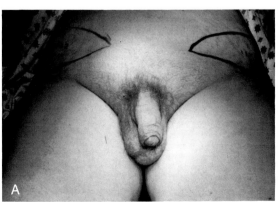 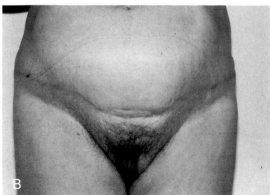

Figure 88–17. *A*, Preoperative male to female transsexual. *B*, Postoperative result.

The vaginal stent is left in position for five to seven days; under anesthesia, it is removed, the vaginal space is cleaned, and a new stent is placed in position. The incidence of vaginal stenosis following this technique has been low, and the advantage of the full-thickness graft is that a stent does not have to be worn for longer than six weeks postoperatively. Once the graft stabilizes, it does not contract like a split-thickness graft.

Phalloplasty

The construction of a penis has proved much more complex. As techniques develop to improve the cosmetic appearance and the function of the new phallus, the patient satisfaction rate has increased markedly. At the present time, the authors prefer a one-stage microsurgical procedure with the construc-

tion of a urethra. By using a neurotized flap to the pudendal nerve, erogenous sensation can be produced in the phallus. The newly created phallus can have enough bulk so that a stiffener can be used to allow insertion into the vagina. By means of a graft around the coronal sulcus area, an esthetically improved phallus can be constructed. Deficits still exist. The donor site flaps may be hairy and the penis may have abnormal-appearing hair; as a result, the construction of the urethra becomes more difficult. A full-thickness free graft for the urethra may be substituted. The ideal stiffener has not been found. Ordinary Silastic rods are probably best, but these may erode and cause difficulty in some patients. The donor site of the free flap is objectionable. In spite of these deficiencies, most female to male transsexuals are happy with a one-stage phallus microvascular construction. The best flap to date has been the radial forearm flap because it offers a reliable artery, vein, and

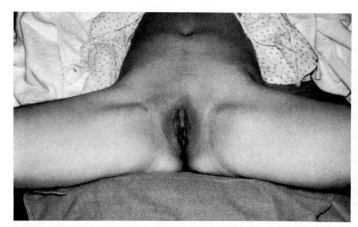

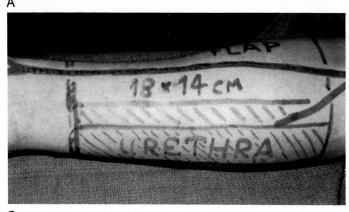

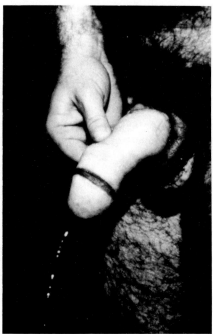

Figure 88–18. *A,* Preoperative female to male transsexual. *B,* Postoperative result. *C,* Outline of the flap on the radial aspect of the forearm.

nerve of adequate size. The lateral antebrachial cutaneous nerve is joined to one of the pudendal nerves. The clitoris, which is retained, remains innervated by the other pudendal nerve. If a new urethra can be constructed from the radial forearm flap, this repair is preferred (Fig. 88–18); however, if the arm is hairy, a free full-thickness skin graft must be used. The vaginal orifice is reduced in size, and occasionally excision of the vaginal mucous membrane is performed to remove all vestiges of this organ. Scrotal construction is achieved by using the labial tissue moved posteriorly or by use of a gracilis myocutaneous flap. Testicular prostheses can be utilized. Approximately 75 per cent of patients report erogenous sensibility in the new penis. They are able to achieve orgasms by manipulation of the neophallus. Fistula of the urethra continues to be a problem. Secondary procedures to correct a urethral fistula, to implant a prosthesis, and to improve the new phallus cosmetically are necessary in many patients.

A few patients do not want to go through the problem and expense of phallus construction. They prefer to have their somewhat enlarged clitoris exteriorized and covered with local flaps. This has never produced a phallus adequate in size, but some patients do not wish to use the new phallus for vaginal insertion.

The legal complications that may arise from transsexual surgery are numerous. It is possible for the independent operator to perform this surgery without adequate consultations and for many medical and legal complications to develop postoperatively. To protect the patient and the physicians who are caring for this complex kind of problem, the gender team is essential. More insurance companies are willing to compensate for associated surgical procedures and for the sex change operation. New and improved surgical techniques are leading to better phallus and vaginal reconstruction. It is the hope that in the future surgery will not be necessary for these individuals, and that medication can be found so that they will be happy with their sexual assignment by nature. Until that time, however, surgical reassignment appears to be the treatment of choice for these problems that cause severe and catastrophic psychologic and physical trauma.

REFERENCES

Abbé, R.: New method of creating a vagina in a case of congenital absence. Med. Res., *54*:836, 1989.

Alton, J. D.: Complete avulsion of the scrotum. *In* Broadbent, T. R. (Ed.): Transactions of the Third International Congress of Plastic Surgery. Amsterdam, Exerpta Media, 1963, p. 904.

Amercan Medical Systems: Inflatable penile prosthesis: clinical experience (1973–1979). Special report published at the Annual Meeting of the American Urological Association, May, 1979, by American Medical System, Inc. Copyright, American Medical Systems, Inc., Minneapolis, MN, 1979.

Barry, J., and Seifert, A.: Penoscrotal approach for placement of paired penile implants for impotence. J. Urol., *122*:325, 1979.

Beheri, G.: Surgical treatment of impotence. Plast. Reconstr. Surg., *38*:92, 1966.

Benjamin, H.: The Transsexual Phenomenon. New York, Julian Press, 1966.

Bergman, R., Howard, A., and Barnes, R.: Plastic reconstruction of the penis. J. Orol., *59*:1174, 1948.

Beutler, L., Scott, F., and Karacan, T.: Psychological screening of impotent men. J. Urol., *116*:193, 1976.

Bhanganada, K., Chayavatana, T., Pongnumkul, C., Tonmukayakul, A., Sakolsatayadorn, P., et al.: Surgical management of an epidemic of penile amputations in Siam. Am. J. Surg., *146*:376, 1983.

Bogoraz, N. A.: Über die volle plastische Wiederherstellung eines zum Koitus Fähigen Penis (Peniplastica totalis). Z. Chir., *63*:1271, 1936.

Canning, J., Bowers, L., Lloyd, F., and Cottrell, T.: Genital vascular insufficiency and impotence. Surg. Forum, *14*:298, 1963.

Cauldwell, D. O.: Psychopathia transsexualis. Sexology, *16*:276, 1949.

Chang, T. S., and Hwang, W. Y.: Forearm flap in one stage reconstruction of the penis. Plast. Reconstr. Surg., *74*:251, 1984.

Chopp, R., and Mendez, R.: Sexual function and hormonal abnormalities in uremic men on chronic dialysis and after renal transplantation. Fertil. Steril., *29*:661, 1978.

Cohen, B. E., May, J. W., Daly, J. S., and Young, H. H.: Successful clinical replantation of an amputated penis by microneurovascular repair. Plast. Reconstr. Surg., *59*:276, 1977.

Crown, S. (Ed.): Transsexuality (gender dysphoria) desire to "change sex" and psychosexual problems. New York, Academic Press, 1976.

Culp, D. A.: Genital injuries: etiology and initial management. Urol. Clin. North Am. *44*:143, 1977.

Culp, D. A., and Huffman, W. D.: Temperature determination in the thigh with regard to burying the traumatically exposed testis. J. Urol., *76*:436, 1956.

d'Allessio, E., Rossi, F., and d'Allesio, R.: Reconstruction in traumatic avulsion of penile and scrotal skin skin. Ann. Plast. Surg., *9*:120, 1982.

Devine, C. J., Jr.: Urethral strictures. *In* Guerriro, W. G., and Devine, C. J., Jr. (Eds.): Urologic Trauma. E. Norwalk, CT, Appleton-Century-Crofts, 1984, pp. 171–188.

Devine P. C., and Devine, C. J., Jr.: Posterior urethral injuries associated with pelvic fractures. Urology, *20*:467, 1982.

Devine, P. C., Winslow, B. H., Jordan, G. H., Horton, C. E., and Gilbert, D. A.: Reconstructive phallic surgery. John A. *In* Libertino, J. A. (Ed.): Pediatric and Adult Reconstructive Urologic Surgery. 2nd Ed. Baltimore, Williams & Wilkins Company, 1987, p. 553.

Eckhardt, C.: Untersuchungen über die Erection des Penis beim Hunde. Beitr. Anat. Physio., *3*:123, 1863.

Edgerton, M. T., Knorr, N. J., and Callison, J. R.: The surgical treatment of transsexual patients. Plast. Reconstr. Surg., *45*:38, 1970.

Farah, R. N., Stiles, R., Jr., and Cerny, J. C.: Surgical treatment of deformity and coital difficulty in healed traumatic rupture of the corpora cavernosa. J. Urol., *120*:198, 1978.

Finney, M.: Flexi-flate penile prosthesis. Semin. Urol., *4*:244, 1986.

Finney, R.: New hinged silicone penile implant. J. Urol., *118*:585, 1977.

Fisher, C., Shiari, R. and Edwards, A.: Quantitative differences in nocturnal penile tumescence (NPT) between impotence of psychogenic and organic origin. Sleep Res., *6*:49, 1977.

Fishman, I.: Experience with the Hydroflex penile prosthesis. Sem. Urol., *4*:239, 1986.

Fogh-Anderson, P.: Transvestism and transsexualism—surgical treatment in a case of autocastration. Acta Med. Leg. Social., *9*:1, 1956.

Forsberg, L., Gustarii, B., Hagerbock, T., and Olsson, A.: Impotence, smoking and beta-blocking drugs. Fertil. Steril., *31*:589, 1979.

Friedreich, J.: Versuch einer Literargeschichte der Pathologie and Therapie der Psychishen. Wurzburg, Krankheiten, 1830.

Furlow, W.: Inflatable penile prosthesis: Mayo Clinic experience with 175 patients. Urology, *13*:166, 1979.

Furlow, W., and Barrett, D.: Inflatable penile prosthesis: new device design and patient-partner satisfaction. Urology, *24*:559, 1984.

Geiderman, J. M., and Paris, P. M.: Fracture of the penis. Ann. Emerg. Med., *9*:8, 1980.

Gerstenberger, D., Osborne, D., and Furlow, W.: Inflatable penile prosthesis: followup study of patient-partner satisfaction. Urology, *14*:583, 1979.

Gibson, T.: Traumatic avulsion of the skin at the scrotum and penis: use of avulsed skin as a free graft. Br. J. Plast. Surg., *6*:283, 1954.

Gibson, T.: Avulsion of penile and scrotal skin. *In* Horton, C. E. (Ed.): Plastic and Reconstructive Surgery of the Genital Area. Boston, Little, Brown & Company, 1973, pp. 463–466.

Gilbert, D. A., Horton, C. E., Terzis, J. K., Devine, C. J., Jr., Winslow, B. H., and Devine, P. C.: New concepts in phallic reconstruction. Ann. Plast. Surg., *18*:128, 1987.

Gillies, H., and Harrison, R. J.: Congenital absence of the penis, with embryological considerations. Br. J. Plast. Surg. *1*:8, 1948.

Glass, R. E., Flynn, J. T., King, J. B., and Blandy, J. P.: Urethral injury and fractured pelvis. Br. J. Urol., *50*:578, 1978.

Goldstein, I.: Penile revascularization. *In* Mundy, A. (Ed.): Current Operative Surgery: Urology. Eastbourne, Bailliere Tindall, 1986.

Goldstein, I., Saenz De Tajeda, I., and Blanco, R.: Impotence in diabetes mellitus. *In* Larner, J., and Pohl, S. J. (Eds.): Methods in Diabetes Research. New York, John Wiley & Sons, 1985.

Goldwin, R.: History of attempts to form a vagina. Plast. Reconstr. Surg., *3*:59, 1977.

Goodwin, W., and Scott, W.: Phalloplasty. J. Urol., *68*:903,1952.

Gorden, G., Altman, K., and Southrun, L.: Effect of alcohol (ethanol) administration on sex-hormone metabolism in normal men. N. Engl. J. Med., *295*:793, 1976.

Gordon-Taylor, G.: Injuries of urinary tract in peace and war. *In* Riches, E. W. (Ed.): Modern Trends in Urology. London, Butterworth & Company, 1953, p. 431.

Green, R.: Mythological, historical and cross-cultural aspects of transsexualism. *In* Benjamin, H. (Ed.): The Transsexual Phenomenon. New York, Julian Press, 1966.

Gross, M.: Rupture of the testicle: the importance of early surgical treatment. J. Urol., *101*:196, 1969.

Horton, C. E., McCraw, J. B., Devine, C. J., Jr., et al.: Secondary reconstruction of the genital area. Urol. Clin. North. Am., *4*:133, 1977.

Jordan, G. H. and Devine, C. J., Jr.: Reconstructive surgery of the urethra. *In* Cass, A. S. (Ed.): Genitourinary Trauma. Boston, Blackwell Scientific Publications (in press).

Jordan, G. H., and Gilbert, D. A.: Male genital trauma. AUA Update Series, Lesson 20, Vol. IV, 1985.

Jordan, G. H., Gilbert, D. A., Winslow, B. H., and Devine, P. C.: Single-stage phallic reconstruction. World J. Surg., *5*:14, 1987

Karacan, I., Scott, B., and Solis, P.: Nocturnal penile tumescence (NPT) and diabetic impotence. Sleep Res., *6*:53, 1977.

Kolb, L. C., and Brodie, H. K.: Modern Clinical Psychiatry. 10th Ed. Philadelphia, W. B. Saunders Company, 1982.

Koranyi, E. K.: Transsexuality in the Male. Springfield, IL, Charles C Thomas, 1980.

Kramer, S., Anderson, E., Bredael, J. and Paulson, D.: Complications of Small-Carrion penile prosthesis. Urology, *13*:49, 1979.

Levine, J. I., and Crampton, R. S.: Major abdominal injuries associated with pelvic fractures. Surg. Gynecol. Obstet., *116*:223, 1963.

Lewis, R., and Puyua, F.: Procedures for decreasing venous drainage. Semin. Urol., *4*:263, 1986.

Lin, S. D., Lai, C. S., and Su, P. Y.: Replantation of the testis by microsurgical technique. Plast. Reconstr. Surg., *76*:620, 1985.

Lue, T. F., Hricak, H., Marich, K. W., and Tanagho, E. A.: Evaluation of arteriogenic impotence and intracorporal injection of papaverine with the duplex ultrasound scanner. Semin. Urol., *3*:43, 1985.

Lue, T. F., Hricak, H., Schmidt, R. A., and Tanagho, E. A.: Functional evaluation of penile veins by cavernosography in papaverine-induced erection. J. Urol., *135*:479, 1986.

Lue, T. F., Takamura, T., Umraiya, M., Schmidt, R. A., and Tanagho, E. A.: Hemodynamics of canine corpora cavernosa during erection. Urology, *24*:347, 1984a.

Lue, T. F., Zeineh, S. J., Schmidt, R. A., and Tanagho, E. A.: Neuroanatomy of penile erection: its relevance to iatrogenic impotence. J. Urol., *131*:273, 1984b.

Lydstrom, G.: The surgical treatment of impotency. Am. J. Clin. Med., *15*:1571, 1908.

Mancharda, R. L., Singh, R., Keswani, R. K., and Sharma, C. G.: Traumatic avulsion of scrotum and penile skin. Br. J. Plast. Surg., *20*:97, 1967.

Masters, F. W., and Robinson, D. W.: The treatment of avulsions of the male genitalia. J. Trauma, *8*:430, 1968.

McAninch, J. W.: Personal communication, 1985.

McConnell, J. D., Peters, P. G., and Lewis, S. E.: Testicular rupture in blunt scrotal trauma—review of 15 cases with recent application of testicular scanning. J. Urol., *128*:309, 1982.

McDougal, W. S., and Persky, L.: Traumatic injuries of the genitourinary system. *In* International Perspectives in Urology. Vol. I. Baltimore, William & Wilkins, Company, 1981.

McDougal, W. S., Peterson, H. D., Pruitt, B. A., and Persky, L.: The thermally injured perineum. J. Urol., *121*:320, 1979.

McIndoe, A.: The treatment of congenital absence and obliterative conditions of the vagina. Br. J. Plast. Surg., *2*:254, 1949.

Meares, E. M., Jr.: Traumatic rupture of the corpus cavernosum. J. Urol., *105*:407, 1971.

Money, J., and Gaskin, R.: Sex reassignment. Int. J. Psychiatry, *9*:249, 1970.

Montyel, M. de: De la maladie de scythes. Ann. Med. Psychol., *1*:161, 1877.

Morehouse, D. D.: Emergency management of urethral trauma. Urol. Clin. North Am., *9*:251, 1982a.

Morehouse, D. D.: Emergency management of urethral trauma. Urol. Clin. North Am., *9*:251, 1982b.

Morehouse, D. D., and MacKinnon, K. J.: Urological injuries associated with pelvic fractures. J. Trauma, *9*:479, 1969.

Muir, I. F., and Morgan, B. D.: Burns of the genitalia and perineum. *In* Horton, C. E. (Ed.): Plastic and Reconstructive Surgery of the Genital Area. Boston, Little, Brown & Company, 1973, pp. 443–449.

Padma-Nathan, H., Goldstein, I., Asadzoi, K., Blanco, R., Saenz de Tejada, I., and Krane, R. J.: In vivo and in vitro studies on the physiology of penile erection. Semin. Urol., *4*:209, 1986.

Padma-Nathan, H., Goldstein, I., and Krane, R.: Evaluation of the impotent patient. Semin. Urol., *4*:255, 1986.

Palomer, J. M., Halikiopoulos, H., and Polanco, E.: Primary surgical repair of the fractured penis. Ann. Emerg. Med., *9*:5, 1980.

Pearman, R.: Treatment of organic impotence by implantation of a penile prosthesis. J. Urol., *97*:716, 1967.

Peltier, L. F.: Complications associated with fractures of the pelvis. J. Bone Surg., *47A*:1060, 1965.

Pennal, G. F.: Fracture dislocation of the pelvis. Report presented at the 31st Annual Meeting of the Royal College of Physicians and Surgeons of Canada, Toronto, January, 1962.

Quinby, W. C., Jr.: Fractures of the pelvis and associated injuries in children. J. Pediatr. Surg., *1*:353, 1966.

Rodgers, B. O.: History of external genital surgery. *In* Horton, C. E. (Ed.): Plastic and Reconstructive Surgery of the Genital Area. Boston, Little, Brown & Company, 1973, pp. 3–47.

Ross, M. W., Walinder, J., Lundstrom, B., and Thuwe, I.: Cross-cultural approaches to transsexualism: a comparison between Sweden and Australia. Psychiatr. Scand., *63*:75–82, 1981.

Saario, I., Vsenious, R., and Vusi-Penttila, S.: Rupture of the penis. Ann. Chir. Gynaecol., *68*:67, 1979.

Saenz de Tejada, I., Goldstein, I., Blanco, R., Cohen, R., and Krane, R.: Smooth muscle of the corpora cavernosa: role in penile erection. Surg. Forum, *36*:623, 1985.

Schuster, G.: Traumatic rupture of the testicle and a review of the literature. J. Urol., *127*:1194, 1982.

Scott, F. B., Bradley, W. E., and Timm, G. W.: Management of erectile impotence. Use of implantable inflatable prosthesis. Urology, *2*:80, 1973.

Scott, F. B., Byrd, G. J., Karacan, I., Olsson, P., Beutler, L. E., and Altia, S. L.: Erectile impotence treated with an implantable, inflatable prosthesis. J.A.M.A., *241*:2609, 1979.

Semans, J. and Langworthy, O.: Observations on neurophysiology of sexual function in the male cat. J. Urol., *40*:836, 1938.

Shrom, S., Lief, H., and Wein, A.: Clinical profile on experience with 130 consecutive cases of impotent men. Urology, *13*:511, 1979.

Small, M. P.: The Small-Carrion prosthesis. Urol. Clin. North Am., *5*:549, 1978.

Small, M. P., and Carrion, H. M.: A new penile prosthesis for treating impotence. Cont. Surg., *7*:29, 1975.

Socarides, C.: The desire for sexual transformation: a psychiatric evaluation of transsexualism. Am. J. Psychiatry, *125*:1419, 1969.

Spark, R., White, R., and Connolly, M.: Impotence is not always psychogenic: newer insights into hypothalamic-pituitary-gonadal dysfunction. J.A.M.A., *243*:750, 1980.

Sperber, M. A., and Jarvik, L. F.: Psychosocial, ethical and legal considerations. *In* Transsexual: Mind Versus Body. Psychiatry and Genetics. New York, Basic Books, 1976.

Stecker, J., Jr., and Devine, C., Jr.: Evaluation of erectile dysfunction in patients with Peyronie's disease. J. Urol., *132*:680, 1984.

Sullivan, L.: Information for the Female-to-Male Cross-Dresser and Transsexual. 2nd ed. 1985.

Tuerk, M., and Weir, W. H.: Successful replantation of a traumatically amputated glans penis. Plast. Reconstr. Surg., *48*:499, 1971.

Turner-Warwick, R.: A personal view of the management of traumatic posterior urethral strictures. Urol. Clin. North Am., *4*:111, 1977.

Velvant, J.: Arterial perfusion of hydrofluoric acid burns. Hum. Toxicol., *2*:233, 1983.

Vincent, M. P., Horton, C. E., and Devine, C. J.: An evaluation of skin grafts for reconstruction of the penis and scrotum. Southeastern Society Meeting, 1984.

Wasserman, M., Pollak, L., and Spielman, A.: Differential diagnosis of impotence: the measurement of nocturnal penile tumescence. J.A.M.A., *243*:2038, 1980.

Wespes, E., and Schulman, C.: Venous leakage: surgical treatment of a curable cause of impotence. J. Urol., *133*:796, 1985.

Westpahl, C.: Die contrare Sexualempfindung. Arch. Psychiat. Nerv., *2*:73, 1879.

Wooten, J.: Ligation of the dorsal vein of the penis as a cure for atonic impotence. Texas Med. J., *18*:325, 1903.

Zenteno, S.: Fracture of the penis. Plast. Reconstr. Surg., *52*:669, 1973.

Zorgniotti, A. W., and Lefleur, R. S.: Auto-injection of the corpus cavernosum with a vasoactive drug combination for vasculogenic impotence. J. Urol., *133*:39, 1985.

Index

Index

Anesthesia *(Continued)*
  for upper extremity
    for replantation or revascularization, 4362
    patient evaluation for, 4302–4305
    regional, 4302
  for upper lip reconstruction, 2027, *2027*
  general, 153–155
    for cleft palate repair, 2739
    for soft tissue wounds in face, 902
    techniques for, 155
    vs. local, for suction-assisted lipectomy, 3967–3968
  ketamine, 157–158
  legal aspects of, 139–140
  local
    allergic reactions to, 144
    chemistry of, 143
    for soft tissue wounds in face, 902
    mechanism of action of, 143
    toxicity of, 144, 144*t*
    vs. general, for suction-assisted lipectomy, 3967–3968
  neural complications of, 4304–4305
  pediatric, 155–157, 156*t*
Aneuploidy, midline posterior cervical lymphatic cysts and, 3243–3245, *3245*
Aneurysms, arterial
  local, abnormal blood flow and, 452
  true, 5007
Angiofibromas, 3184
Angiogenesis
  dependency, hemangiomas and, 3199
  stages of, 281
Angiography
  for arteriovenous malformations, 3256
  for venous malformations, 3252
  of orbit, 1586, *1587*, 1588
Angiokeratoma circumscriptum, *3234*, 3235–3236
Angiokeratoma corporis diffusum universale, 3236, *3236*
Angiokeratomas
  fucosidosis, 3236
  histopathologic criteria for, 3234
  of Fordyce, 3235, *3236*
  of Mibelli, 3235
Angioma cavernosum, 3192
Angioma simplex, 3192
Angiosarcoma
  of head and neck, 3371
  of jaw, 3359
Angiosomes
  concept of, *343–350*, 347, 349, 351–352
  definition of, 334–335, *341*
Angle-rotation flap, for removal of cheek scars, 2167, 2169, *2168, 2170–2171*
Animal bites
  delayed primary wound closure and, 900–901
  hand infections from, 5534–5535, *5534*, 5535*t*
Ankle
  cutaneous arteries of, *371*, 373–374
  suction-assisted lipectomy of, 4019, *4020, 4021, 4023*
Ankles, suction-assisted lipectomy of, complications of, 3978
Ankylosis, of temporomandibular joint, 1494–1496, *1495*
Anomalies, minor, 78–81, *79*, 80*t*
  frequency of, *80*

Anomalies *(Continued)*
  significance of, 81*t*
Anophthalmos
  primary congenital, 1639–1640, *1641, 1642*, 1644–1646, *1644–1646*
  secondary, 1640
Anoxia, skeletal muscle and, 550
Antacids, for prevention of ulceration, 809
Anterior interosseous nerve syndrome
  characteristics of, 4831
  etiology of, 4832
  management summary for, 4832–4833
  surgical indications for, 4832, *4832, 4833*
Anterior neural plate, embryological development of, 2517, *2517*
Anthelical fold, restoration of, 2116–2117, *2117*
Anthrax, 5550
Antibiotics, for suction-assisted lipectomy, 4026
Antibodies, production of, 190–191
Anticoagulants, 458
Anticoagulation, 458–459
Anticonvulsants, craniofacial cleft formation and, 2928–2929
Anti-inflammatory agents, for reflex sympathetic dystrophy, 4910–4911
Antilymphocyte globulin, immunosuppression by, 194–195
Antimetabolic agents, craniofacial cleft formation and, 2929
AO fracture healing, *591*, 591–592
Aortic bodies and sinuses, embryological development of, 2478, *2479*
Apertognathism. *See* Open bite deformity.
Apert's syndrome
  clinical presentation of, 3021, *3022*, 5293, 5296, *5296*
    hand configuration in, 5296, *5297, 5298*
  craniofacial manifestations of, 2488
  face proportions in, 30–32, *30, 32*
  hydrocephalus in, 3025
  inheritance of
    dominant type of, *91*
    sporadic occurrence of, 89, *90*, 104
  maxillary deformities in, 1360
  pathogenesis of, 97–98
  radiologic findings in, 3021, *3022*
  treatment of, 5298–5300, *5299*
  visual abnormalities in, 3025–3026
Apical ectodermal ridge (AER), 2482, 5217, 5219, *5218*
Aplasia cutis congenita, 1540–1542, *1541–1544*
Aponeurosis, 630
Aponeurosis surgery, for ptosis, *1758*, 1759, 1765–1766
Apron flaps, for intraoral reconstruction, 3438, *3441*
Arch and band appliances, for mandibular fixation, 3500, *3500–3506*
Arch bars, 1035, *1037*, 1216, *1217*
  for intermaxillary fixation, 922, *923–926*, 925–926
  prefabricated, for intermaxillary fixation, 944, *945, 946*
Arch wires, cable, 944
Areola, reconstruction of, *3907, 3908*
Argon laser
  characteristics of, 3666
  lesions amenable to, 3667–3669, *3667–3669*
Arhinencephaly, orbital hypotelorism and, 3005, *3005*
Arion prosthesis, for eyelid paralysis, 2310

Metacarpal hand, *4338*, 4338–4339

Metacarpals

distraction lengthening of, for congenital hand deformities, 5252, *5253, 5254,* 5255

extension of, tendon tranfer for, in radial palsy, *4944,* 4944–4945

fractures of, without joint injury, 4598–4601, *4598–4601*

lengthening of, for thumb reconstruction. *See* Thumb reconstruction, by bone lengthening.

malunion or non-union of, 4601

transposition of, 5248

transverse absence of, 5246, 5248, *5249–5251, 5252, 5253–5254,* 5255

Metacarpophalangeal block, in flexor tendon repair, 4543, *4543*

Metacarpophalangeal joint

anatomy of, 4254–4255, *4254,* 4257–4258, *4258, 4259,* 4655–4656, *4656, 4657*

arthrodesis of, small joints, 4671. *See also* Arthrodesis.

indications for, small joints, 4671

deformities of, after burn injury, 5467

dislocations of, 4612–4616, *4613–4615*

fracture-dislocations of, 4616–4617, *4617*

locking of, 4728–4729

pathophysiology of, 4655–4656, *4656, 4657*

stiffness of

age and, 4661

from edema, 4657–4658

from immobility, 4656–4657

from mechanical obstruction, 4661, *4661*

from scar contracture, 4658–4661, *4659–4661*

hand therapy for, 4665–4666, *4666, 4667*

mobilization vs. immobilization for, 4663–4665, *4664, 4665*

subluxations of, 4612–4616, *4613–4616,* 4616–4617

Metacarpotrapezial joint

first, *4256,* 4256–4257

ligaments of, 4257, *4257*

Metal tray with bone chips, for mandibular defects, 1413–1414

Metals, in alloplastic implants, 703–706, 704*t,* 705*t*

Metatarsal artery, variability of course of, *1444*

Metatarsus, vascularized grafts of, 625

Methotrexate, 195

Methylmethacrylate implants, for craniofacial surgery, 1561–1562, *1563*

Metopic synostosis, 3032, 3035, *3034*

Meyer-Abul-Failat technique, for lower lip reconstruction, 2020, *2021*

MHC (major histocompatibility complex), 187

Mibelli lesions, 3235

Microcirculation, 449, *450, 451*

Microfilaments, 636

Microgenia

chin augmentation for, *1307,* 1307–1308

clinical presentation of, 1260, 1305–1306

contour restoration for

by alloplastic implant, 1308–1309, 1312, *1307, 1309–1311*

by cartilage or bone grafts, 1323, 1329, *1330*

by horizontal advancement osteotomy, 1312, 1318, *1313–1321*

by skin graft inlay and dental prosthesis, 1329, *1331, 1332, 1332*

Microgenia *(Continued)*

diagnosis and preoperative planning for, 1306–1307

surgical correction of, in Down syndrome, 3170, *3170, 3171*

with mandibular prognathism, 1258, *1259*

Micrognathia

definition of, 3123

mandibular, *1261*

contour restoration in, 1289, *1290*

etiology of, 1260–1262

maxillary, 1360

Micrognathia-retrognathia, maxillary

onlay bone grafts for, 1367, *1367, 1368*

treatment for, 1366, *1366*

Microneurovascular muscle transfers

for facial paralysis, 2298–2300, *2300–2303*

of skeletal muscle, 555–556, *556*

Microphthalmos, 1640–1642, *1643*

orbital expansion for, 1644–1646, *1646*

Microscope, operating, 412–414, *413, 414*

maintenance of, 415

preoperative preparation of, 414–415

Microsomia, craniofacial. *See* Craniofacial microsomia.

Microsurgery

development of, 20

for auricular replantation, 2125

interfascicular and perineural nerve repair, for facial paralysis, 2258–2259

of hand, operating room organization for, 4290

Microtia

auricular reconstruction method, 2100–2101

bilateral, 2108, 2110

complete

clinical characteristics of, 2099–2100

correlation of surgery with facial deficiency surgeries, 2100

general treatment considerations for, 2100

deformities associated with, 2099, *2099*

etiology of

hereditary factors in, 2098

specific factors in, 2098–2099

incidence of, 2097–2098

indications for timing of middle ear surgery, 2146

middle ear problem in, embryology and, 2096–2097, *2097*

middle ear surgery for, timing of, 2149

repair of, historical perspective of, 2094–2095

Microtubules, 636

Microvascular composite tissue transplantation, for breast reconstruction, 393

Microvascular free flaps, 3448–3449, *3449*

for Romberg's disease treatment, 3140, *3141*

Microvascular surgery

artery to vein repair ratio in, 4369

blood flow in, abnormal, 449, 451–453

continuous suturing in, 434–435

definition of, 4356

end-to-end anastomosis in

exposure for, 421

for normal or near-normal vessel tension, 423

for repair of normal vessels, 421–422, *422*

for similar diameter vessels, 423

operative technique for resection to normal vessels of, 423–427, *423–434,* 429–434

position and preparation for, 420–421

technique for, 421

Velopharyngeal incompetence *(Continued)*
  management of, 2910–2914
    choice of surgery for, 2914–2915
    operative technique for, 2915, *2916*, 2917
  postoperative speech therapy, 2917–2918
  surgical correction of, historical aspects of, 2907–
    2908, 2910, *2907, 2909–2911*
Velopharyngeal sphincter
  in speech production, 2903–2904
  inability to close. See Velopharyngeal incompetence.
  lace of movement for speech, velopharyngeal incom-
    petence and, 2906
Veloplasty, intravelar, 2742
Venae comitantes, 353, *354, 355, 355*
Venae communicantes, 353
Venous anatomy, in great toe vs. thumb, 5165–5167,
  5166
Venous malformations
  clinical findings in, 3250, *3251*, 3252
  histology of, 3249–3250
  of hand, 5316, *5318, 5318–5319, 5320–5322*
    combined with lymphatic malformations of, 5324
  terminology for, 3249
  treatment of, 3252–3254, *3253*
Venules, microstructure of, 449, *451*
Venus, necklace of, 29, *29*
Veratrum californicum, craniofacial cleft formation
  and, 2930
Vermilion. *See also* Lip(s), upper.
  adjustments of, 2187
  anatomy of, 2184
  deficiency or deformity of, 2790–2791, *2791–2796*,
    2793, 2796
  of upper lip, reconstruction of, 2027–2028, *2028–
    2031*, 2030–2031
  reconstruction of, 2013–2105, *2014–2016*
  repair of, perimeter flaps from lingual tip for, 3490,
    3490–3492, 3492
  secondary deficiency of, from bilateral cleft lip repair,
    2853, *2854*
Vermilionectomy, 2014–2015, *2015*
Verruca vulgaris
  clinical description of, 3561–3562, *3562*
  epidemiology of, 3561
  etiology of, 3560
  incidence of, 3560–3561
  malignant transformation of, 3563
  of perionychium, 4509–4510
  pathology of, 3562–3563
  treatment of, 3563, 3565, *3564, 3565*
Vertebrobasilar insufficiency, transient, 5007
Vessel wall tension, microvascular surgery and, 444–
  445
Vestibule, nasal
  anatomy of, 1797–1798, *1797*, 1925
    ventilation and, *1807*, 1807–1808
  atresia of, 1882
Vestibules, nasal, 1804
V-excision, for lower lip reconstruction, 2015
Vibrio hand infections, 5551
Vincula, 4268, *4268*
Viral infections
  craniofacial cleft formation and, 2928
  of hand, 5553, *5554*
  squamous cell carcinoma and, 3630
Viral warts, of perionychium, 4509–4510

Visceral arches
  embryologic development of, 2468, *2468t, 2469*, 2470
  growth centers in, 2455, 2481–2483, *2484*
  in development of voluntary muscles, 2471, *2472*,
    2743
  of head and neck, 2519, *2520*
Vision
  abnormalities of, in craniosynostosis, 3025–3026
  decreased, after orbital or nasoethmoido-orbital frac-
    tures, 1105
  obstruction of, by hemangiomas, 3206–3207
Visual acuity, 1117, 1581, *1582*
Visual evoked response (VER), 1118
Visual examination techniques, for optic nerve injury,
  1117–1118
Visual field testing, 1118
Visual loss, with frontobasilar region fractures, 1115
Vital dye tests, for flap perfusion assessment, *319t,*
  321–322
Vitamin A, corticosteroids and, 179
Vitamin deficiencies, cleft palate and, 2546
Vitamin supplements, cleft lip/palate prevention and,
  2535–2537
Volar advancement flap, for soft tissue injuries of
  thumb, 5092–5093, *5092–5094*
Volkmann's canals, 583
Volkmann's ischemic contracture
  development of, 4286–4287
  differential diagnosis of, 4905–4906, *4906*
  historical aspects of, 5033
  management of
    in evolutionary stage, 5036
    in final stage
      with clawhand, *5037,* 5037–5038
      without clawhand, 5036, *5037*
    in initial stage, *5034,* 5034–5036
  pathophysiology of, 5033–5038
  surgical treatment of
    for correction of type I deformity, 5038–5039, *5039*
    for correction of type II deformity, 5039–5040, *5040*
    for correction of type III deformity, 5040
    to restore sensation, 5040
  treatment of, for initial stage, 5034–5036, *5035*
Volume loading, for abdominoplasty, 3935–3936
Vomer
  anatomic distortion of, in cleft palate, 2730
  deformities of, in unilateral cleft lip and palate,
    2590–2591, *2591*
  in cleft lip and palate, 2583–2584, *2584*
Von Langenbeck operation, for cleft palate repair,
  2742–2744, *2743*
Von Recklinghausen's disease. *See also* Neurofibromatosis.
  in children, 3181–3183, *3183*
V-Y advancement
  double, for vermilion deformities, 2793, *2795,* 2796
  flap design for, 289, *289*
  for soft tissue injuries of thumb, 5090–5092, *5090,
    5091*
  for vermilion border misalignment, 2791, *2791*
V-Y advancement flaps
  design of, 65–66
V-Y biceps femoris flap, for genital reconstructive surgery, 4147–4148
V-Y volar flaps, for coverage of digital tip amputation
  stumps, 4488, *4489*